Modern System of Ophthalmology (MSO) Series

Theory and Practice of
Squint and
Orthoptics

Third Edition

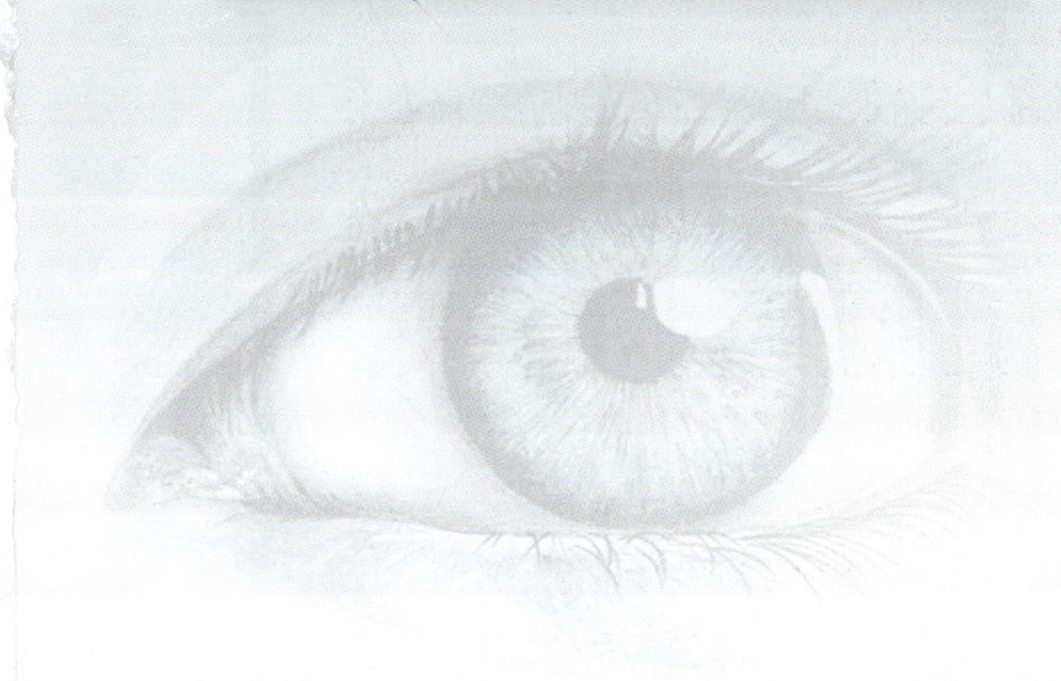

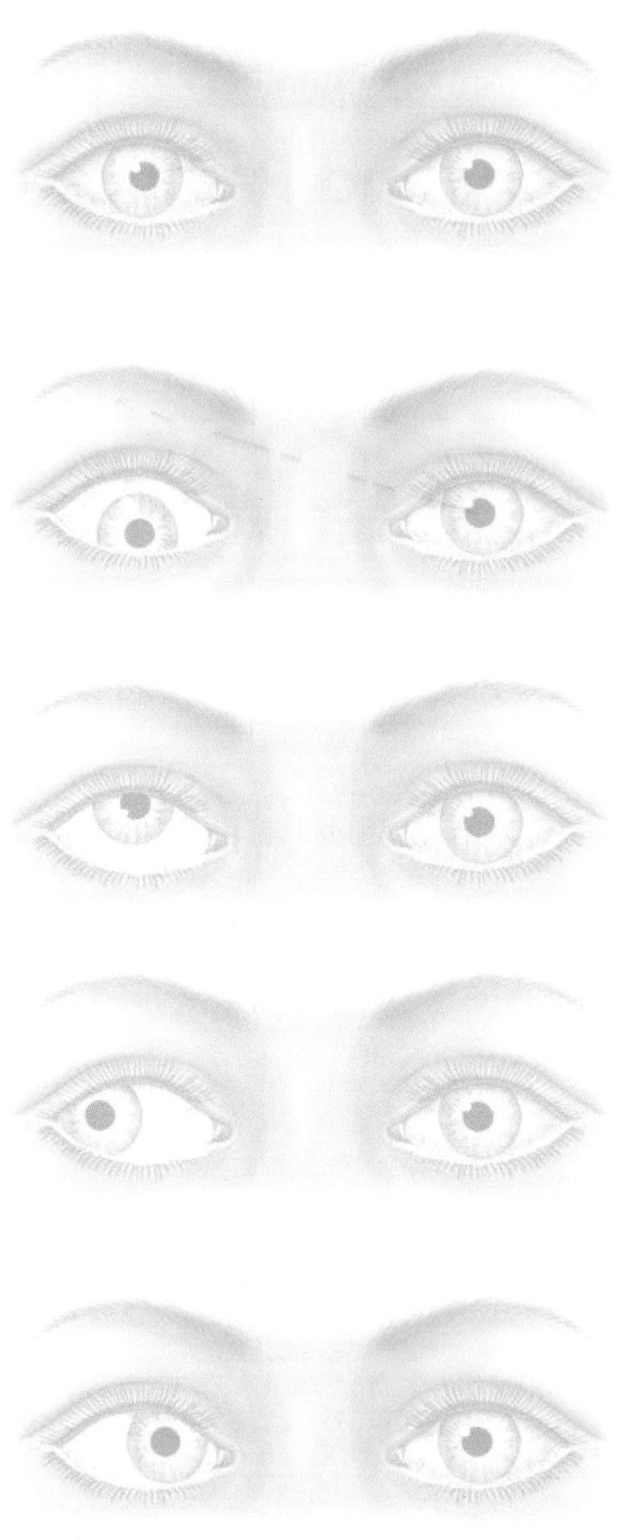

Modern System of Ophthalmology (MSO) Series

Theory and Practice of
Squint and
Orthoptics

Third Edition

AK Khurana MS, CTO (London), FAICO
Senior Professor and Head
Paediatric Ophthalmology, Squint and Oculoplasty Services
Regional Institute of Ophthalmology
Pt. BD Sharma Postgraduate Institute of Medical Sciences
Rohtak, Haryana

Assisted by

Aruj K Khurana DNB, FICO, FVR, FNN
Consultant Vitreo-Retina Services
Nirmal Eye Institute
Rishikesh, Uttarakhand

Bhawana Khurana MS, DNB, FICO, FNN
Consultant Orbit, Oculoplasty and Ocular Oncology,
Paediatric Ophthalmology and Squint
Nirmal Eye Institute
Rishikesh, Uttarakhand

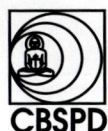

CBSPD

CBS Publishers & Distributors Pvt Ltd

New Delhi • Bengaluru • Chennai • Kochi • Kolkata • Lucknow • Mumbai
Hyderabad • Jharkhand • Nagpur • Patna • Pune • Uttarakhand

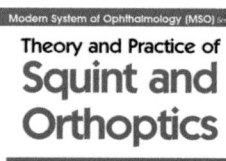

Modern System of Ophthalmology (MSO) Series

Theory and Practice of
Squint and Orthoptics
Third Edition

ISBN: 978-93-87085-81-7

Copyright © AK Khurana

Third Edition: 2018
Reprint: 2019, 2021, 2022
First Edition: 1999
Second Edition: 2013

Published by Satish Kumar Jain and produced by Varun Jain for
CBS Publishers & Distributors Pvt Ltd
4819/XI Prahlad Street, 24 Ansari Road, Daryaganj, New Delhi 110 002, India
Ph: 011-23289259, 23266861, 23266867   Website: www.cbspd.com
Fax: 011-23243014   e-mail: delhi@cbspd.com; cbspubs@airtelmail.in.

Corporate Office: 204 FIE, Industrial Area, Patparganj, Delhi 110 092, India
Ph: 011-4934 4934   Fax: 011-4934 4935   e-mail: publishing@cbspd.com;
publicity@cbspd.com

Branches

- **Bengaluru:** Seema House 2975, 17th Cross, KR Road, Banasankari 2nd Stage, Bengaluru 560 070, Karnataka, India
  Ph: +91-80-26771678/79   Fax: +91-80-26771680   e-mail: bangalore@cbspd.com
- **Chennai:** 7, Subbaraya Street, Shenoy Nagar, Chennai 600 030, Tamil Nadu, India
  Ph: +91-44-26680620, 26681266   Fax: +91-44-42032115   e-mail: chennai@cbspd.com
- **Kochi:** 42/1325, 1326, Power House Road, Opp KSEB, Power House, Ernakulam Kochi 682 018, Kerala, India
  Ph: +91-484-4059061-65,67   e-mail: kochi@cbspd.com
- **Kolkata:** 147, Hind Ceramics Compound, 1st Floor, Nilgunj Road, Belghoria, Kolkata-700056, West Bengal, India
  Ph: +033-25633055, 033-25633056   e-mail: kolkata@cbspd.com
- **Lucknow:** Basement, Khushnuma Complex, 7 Meerabai Marg (Behind Jawahar Bhawan),Lucknow-226001, UP, India
  Ph: +0522-4000032   e-mail: tiwari.lucknow@cbspd.com
- **Mumbai:** PWD Shed, Gala no 25/26, Ramchandra Bhatt Marg, Next to JJ Hospital Gate no. 2, Opp. Union Bank of India,
  Noorbaug, Mumbai-400009, Maharashtra, India
  Ph: 022-66661880/89   e-mail: mumbai@cbspd.com

Representatives

- Hyderabad   0-9885175004
- Patna   0-9334159340
- Jharkhand   0-9811541605
- Pune   0-9623451994
- Nagpur   0-9421945513
- Uttarakhand   0-9716462459

Printed at Nutech Print Services, Faridabad, Haryana, India

to
My parents
and
teachers for their blessings

My wife, Indu
for her understanding

My children Aruj, Bhawna, Arushi and Gurukripa for
their love and affection
&

My grandson Agastya for providing endless joy

Modern System of Ophthalmology (MSO) series comprises separate volumes on different subspecialties of ophthalmology. Each volume is planned with a very specific aim to cater to the needs of postgraduate students in ophthalmology.

Salient Features of MSO Series

- Each volume is edited by different editors, yet the layout and organization has been kept similar.
- Editors of different volumes are masters in their subspecialty with an uncanny knack of picking up the right perspectives.
- Text matter is designed to meet the needs of residents in ophthalmology with a comprehensive coverage in a concise manner. Text is complete and up-to-date with recent advances incorporated.
- Text is organized in such a way that the students can easily understand, retain and reproduce it. Various levels of headings, subheadings, bold face and italics given in the text will be helpful for a quick revision of the subject.

Theory and Practice of Squint and Orthoptics, a volume of *Modern System of Ophthalmology [MSO] Series,* in its third edition presents an updated and thoroughly revised text in a simplified from, so that the complex and intricated physiology of neuromuscular co-ordination of extraocular muscles can be easily understood. This flavour of the book makes the strabismus a fascinating interesting entity.

This book, in its third edition, continues its aim of providing information on basic principles of squint and orthoptics to the residents in ophthalmology as well as students of orthoptics and optometry. However, it is hoped that the book would be equally useful for the practising ophthalmologists, optometrists and orthopticians as well. To keep it a basic book, advanced theories and many diverse opinions have been excluded. I hope, the experienced strabismologists and researchers in this field will bear this with me.

The text has been organized into fifteen chapters. First four chapters have been devoted to the anatomical and physiological aspects of extraocular muscles, faculty of vision, and binocular vision. The remaining eleven chapters have been planned to provide a clear insight of the various disorders of ocular motility.

Salient Features of the Book

- The text has been organized in such a way that the students can easily understand, retain and reproduce the facts. Various levels of headings, subheadings, boldface and italics given in the text should be helpful for a quick revision of the text.
- A brief list of the contents given in the beginning of each chapter provides a clear layout of the text.
- The text has been illustrated with high quality clear line diagrams and photographs depicting vivid and lucid details in colour.
- The text matter in the chapters 'Evaluation of Strabismus and Orthoptic Instruments' and 'Principles of Non-surgical and Surgical Management of Strabismus' has been discussed in length.
- Operative steps of various surgical techniques have been elucidated in a self-explanatory manner.

Key Features of Third Edition

- Thorough revision of each chapter has been done to keep abreast with the newer concepts and principles of investigative modalities, treatment modalities and surgical procedures evolved over the period.
- The concept of 'muscle pulley' and 'active pulley hypothesis' has been explained in detail.
- Chapter on 'Visual Acuity' has been expanded and reorganised.
- Amblyopia Treatment Studies (ATS) have been summarized in tabulated form and the recomendations incorporated in the management of amblyopia.
- Chapter on Nystagmus and related Ocular Oscillations, written as per new system of classification and newer terminologies evolved by National Eye Institute's working group called the 'Classification of Eye Movement Abnormalities and Strabismus' (CEMAS), has been further simplified.
- Chapters on 'Vertical Strabismus' and 'Incomitant Strabismus' have been uniquely, classified and organised.

The thorough revision and updating of the third edition of the book has been possible as a result of active assitance from Dr Aruj K Khurana and Dr Bhawna Khurana and the active criticism, suggestions and generous help received from many teachers and students from all over India. Surely, I owe sincere thanks to them all. I must thank Dr Kanwar Mohan from Chandigarh, Dr Kalpana and Dr Sandra from Arvind Eye Hospital, Coimbatore, and Dr Shubhangi Bhave from Nagpur for providing valuable photographs of their patients. I acknowledge with gratitude the special help rendered by Dr Subhash Dadeya, Director Prof GNEC, MAMC and Chief Editor DOS Times and Dr Sonam Yangzes and Dr Savleen Kaur from AEC, PGIMER, Chandigarh, for allowing to reproduce the Ambyopia Treatment Study Reports. The help received from faculty memberms of RIO, PGIMS, Rohtak in general and Dr Reena Gupta Singh, Associate Professor from Paediatric Ophthalmology Unit in particular is highly appreciated. I also acknowledge the help rendered by Dr Amit Matrey from HIMS, Jolly Grant and the residents RIO, PGIMS, Rohtak, especially Dr Kamal Garg. I also appreciate Dr CS Dhull, Head RIO, Dr MC Gupta, Director, PGIMS and Dr OP Kalra, Vice-Chancellor, UHS, Rohtak for providing the conducive environment.

The enthusiastic co-operation received from Mr SK Jain, Managing Director, Mr YN Arjuna Senior Vice-President Publishing, Editorial and Publicity, and Ms Ritu Chawla, AGM Production, CBS Publishers and Distributors, New Delhi, need special acknowledgement. Ms Jyoti Kaur, DTP Operator and Mr Sanju graphic artist, need special mention because of their efforts to provide considerable beauty to this volume.

Finally, I feel proud in expressing my sincre gratitude to my son-in-law Dr Gurukripa and daughter Dr Arushi, Virginia Commonwealth University (VCU), Virginia, USA; and my wife Dr Indu Khurana, Professor of Physiology and Dean-cum-Principal, World College of Medical Sciences and Research, Gurawar, Jhajhar for their ever available love and encouragement.

Sincere efforts have been made to verify the correctness of the text. However, in spite of the best efforts, ventures of this kind are not likely to be free from human errors, some inaccuracies, ambiguities and typographic mistakes. Therefore, the users are requested to send their feedback and suggestions which will be highly appreciated and duly acknowledged. The importance of such views in improving the future editions of the book cannot be overemphasized.

AK Khurana

Preface to the First Edition

Strabismus, being an interesting subject, has always fascinated most of the ophthalmologists. However, the extremely complex physiology and pathology of binocular vision and an intricated neuromuscular co-ordination of the extrinsic ocular muscles have made strabismus an untouchable entity for majority of the residents in ophthalmology as well as the practising general ophthalmologists. Therefore, an attempt has been made in this book to present the subject in a more easily understood form. In a bid to simplify the text, at places the description looks more dogmatic than is warranted by the facts.

This book is intended to provide information on basic principles of squint and orthoptics to the residents in ophthalmology and, students of orthoptics and optometry. It is hoped, the book would be equally useful for the practising ophthalmologists and orthopticians as well. To keep the book a basic text, advanced theories and many diverse opinions have not been included. I hope, the experienced strabismologists and researchers in this field will bear this with me.

First four chapters of this book have been picked up as such from the book, 'Anatomy and Physiology of Eye'—a joint venture of mine with my wife. This would definitely extend some relief to the students as this new text, comprising of fifteen chapters would practically get down to eleven chapters. This becomes particularly relevant when the uncopable advances in the field of ophthalmic technology has beset the present day residents in ophthalmology with the voluminous texts on different aspects of the discipline. Some of the salient features of this book are as follows:

- The text has been organised in such a way that the students can easily understand, retain and reproduce it. Various levels of headings, subheadings, boldface and italics given in the text should be helpful for a quick revision of the text.

- A brief list of the contents given in the beginning of each chapter provides a clear layout of the text.

- The text has been well illustrated with high quality clear line diagrams depicting vivid and lucid details.

- The text matter in chapters on 'Evaluation of Strabismus and Orthoptic Instruments' and 'Treatment Modalities and Outlines of Strabismus Management' has been discussed in length. Operative steps of various surgical techniques have been illucidated in a self explanatory manner.

Volumes like this are impossible without the contribution of several people. The significant efforts put in by Dr. Vinod Kumar Sharma are loudly acknowledged. He has rendered an unprecedented help in completion of this book. I am thankful to Dr. R. C. Nagpal, Prof. and Head, Deptt. of Ophthalmology and Prof. D. S. Dubey, Director, Pt. B.D. Sharma PGIMS, Rohtak for affording me a working atmosphere.

I am deeply indebted to my dear friend and old batchmate and a well known strabismologist, Dr. Kanwar Mohan, Assoc. Prof., Deptt. of Ophthalmology, PGI Chandigarh, for providing the valuable photographs of patients with palsy of third and fourth cranial nerves (Figs 12.42 and 12.19) and Duane's retraction syndrome (Figs 12.43 to 12.45).

It is a special pleasure to acknowledge the most assured co-operation and skill of Mr. Mahesh, Mr.Updesh and M/s CBS Publishers & Distributors in general, and Mr. S. K. Jain, Managing Director and Mr. V. K. Jain, Production Director, in particular. Mr. Dharamvir deserves a special appreciation for his sincere efforts in streamlining the text. Lastly, I feel proud in admitting that the main force behind all the little I am able to do, is my wife Dr. (Mrs.) Indu Khurana, Assoc. Prof. in the Deptt. of Physiology, PGIMS, Rohtak. I must also register my thanks to her for allowing me to lift the first four chapters from the book 'Anatomy and Physiology of Eye' of which she is a co-author.

It is unequivocal that in spite of the best efforts,ventures of this kind are not likely to be free from human errors, some inaccuracies, ambiguities and typographic mistakes. However, a feedback and active criticism from the users is always of invaluable help in rectifying such pitfalls. I shall eagerly await the response from all the learned readers.

AK Khurana

Contents

Chapter

1

Anatomy of Extraocular Muscles and Related Structures

Chapter Outline

EXTRAOCULAR MUSCLES AND ORBITAL FASCIA

Extraocular muscles

- Rectus muscles
- Oblique muscles
- Nerve supply
- Blood supply
- Actions
- Structural characteristics

Orbital Fascia

- Fascia bulbi
- Sleeves (fascial sheaths) of extraocular muscles
- Intermuscular septa (anterior pulley slings)
- System of muscle pulleys and related facial expansions

Applied Anatomical Aspects

ANATOMY OF THIRD, FOURTH AND SIXTH CRANIAL NERVES

- Oculomotor nerve
- Trochlear nerve
- Abducent nerve

EXTRAOCULAR MUSCLES AND ORBITAL FASCIA

A set of six extraocular muscles (4 recti and 2 obliques) controls the movements of each eye (Fig. 1.1). Rectus muscles are superior rectus (SR), inferior rectus (IR), medial rectus (MR) and lateral rectus (LR). The oblique muscles include superior oblique (SO) and inferior oblique (IO).

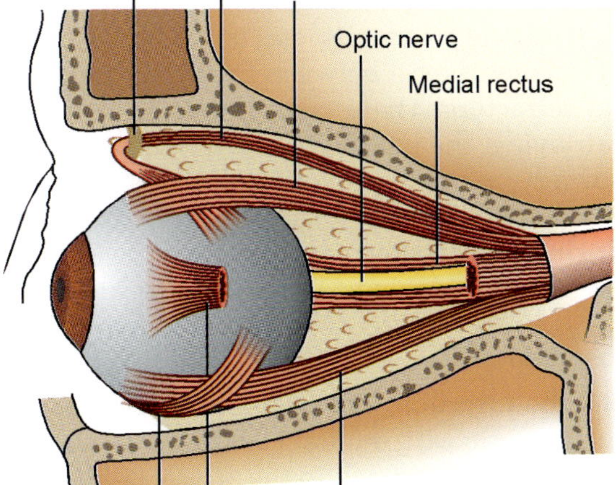

Fig. 1.1 *Extraocular muscles.*

EXTRAOCULAR MUSCLES

RECTUS MUSCLES

Origin

The four rectus muscles originate from a common tendinous ring (the annulus of Zinn), which is attached at the apex of the orbit encircling the optic foramina and medial part of the superior orbital fissure (Fig. 1.2). The *annulus of Zinn* appears oval on cross-section. Medial rectus arises from the medial part of the ring, superior rectus from the superior part, inferior rectus from the inferior part and lateral rectus from the lateral part by two heads which join in a 'V' form. Due to slope of the orbital roof, the origin of the superior rectus and medial rectus is slightly at the anterior plane to others. The superior rectus and medial rectus are closely attached to the dural sheath of the optic nerve at their origin. This attachment accounts for the characteristic pain in a case of retrobulbar neuritis, felt during upward and inward movements of the globe.

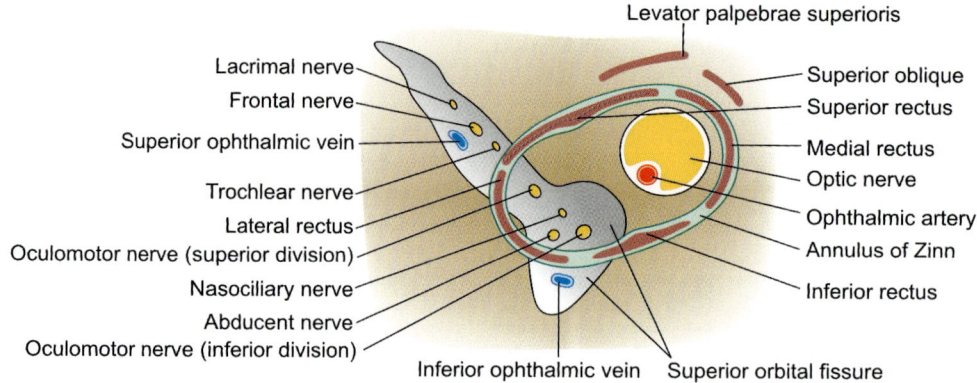

Fig. 1.2 *Origin of the rectus and superior oblique muscles.*

Course

All the four recti from their origin run forward around the eyeball. The medial and lateral recti follow the corresponding walls of the orbit in most of the part of their course, and the inferior rectus remains in contact with the orbital floor for only about half its length. The superior rectus muscle is separated from the orbital roof by the levator palpebrae superioris muscle. The course of the four recti, starting from the apex of the orbit, is diverging, however, somewhat in front of the equator they turn towards the eyeball in a gentle curve to get inserted on the sclera.

Medial rectus (MR) muscle follows the medial wall of the orbit in most part of its course. This proximity to the medial orbital wall accounts for its inadvertent damage during standard or endoscopic ethmoid sinus surgery. Medial rectus muscle is the only rectus muscle that does not have a facial attachment to an oblique muscle; and because of this fact, it is at the greatest risk of slippage or loss during surgery.

Lateral rectus (LR) muscle, after arising from the lateral part of annulus of Zinn, follows the lateral orbital wall in most of the part of its course. Its inferior border passes just superior to the insertion of inferior oblique (IO) muscle (Fig. 1.1). The facial connections between LR and IO muscles at this point, which is 8–9 mm posterior from the insertion of LR, allow the surgeon to retrieve the, inadvertently lost LR muscle during surgery, at this point.

Suprior rectus (SR) muscle after origin from the superior part of annulus of Zinn runs anteriorly,

slightly laterally and superiorly in the superior orbit. In most of its course, it is separated from the orbital roof by the levator palpebrae superioris (LPS) muscle. In primary position, SR muscle forms an angle of 23° with the visual axis. This angle determines the secondary and tertiary actions of the SR muscle in primary position. Anteriorly, prior to insertion, the SR muscle courses between the tendon of superior oblique and LPS muscles. Fascial attachments from the SR muscle extend to SO and LPS muscles.

Inferior rectus (IR) muscle, after arising from the inferior part of the annulus of Zinn, runs anteriorly, slightly inferiorly and laterally making an angle of 23° with the visual axis in its primary position. In posterior half of its course, the IR muscle remains in contact with the orbital floor. Anteriorly, the IR muscle courses between the globe and inferior oblique (IO) muscle prior to its insertion (Fig. 1.1). Facial attachments exist between the IR, IO and lower lid retractors. These connections are useful in retrieving, the inadvertently slipped IR during surgery, in the region of Lockwood's ligament. Further, failure to dissect these connections during IR recession or resection may lead to eyelid fissure widening or narrowing, respectively.

Insertion

At the insertion, the striated muscle fibres of recti muscle with minimal tendinous connective tissue, directly attach to the sclera. All the four rectus muscles are inserted into the sclera just anterior to the equator of globe at different distances from the limbus as under (Fig. 1.3A):

	(Fuchs, 1884)	(Apt, 1980)
Medial rectus :	5.5 mm	5.3 mm
Inferior rectus :	6.5 mm	6.8 mm
Lateral rectus :	6.9 mm	6.9 mm
Superior rectus :	7.7 mm	7.9 mm

Thus the insertions of the recti, being not equidistant from the limbus, do not form a circle concentric with the limbus; rather form a spiral (*the spiral of Tillaux*).

The *insertion lines* (Fig. 1.3A) of medial and lateral rectus muscles show slight convexity facing the limbus. The lines of insertion of superior and inferior rectus muscles show marked convexity towards the limbus and are obliquely placed in such a way that the lateral end of their insertion line is posteriorly placed as compared to the medial end.

▉ OBLIQUE MUSCLES

Superior Oblique Muscle

Origin

The superior oblique muscle arises from the bone (body of sphenoid) above and medial to the optic foramen (Fig. 1.2) by a narrow tendon, partially overlapping the origin of levator palpebrae superioris.

Course

The muscle moves forward between the roof and medial wall of the orbit to reach the *trochlea* of the superior oblique muscle. The trochlea is a thick fibrous cartilagenous pulley attached to spina trochlearis on the under aspect of the frontal bone, at the superomedial angle, between the anterior most parts of the superior and medial walls of the orbit. After passing the trochlea, the superior oblique muscle turns posterolaterally. At about distal third of the direct portion (about 10 mm behind the trochlea), the muscle becomes tendinous and remains so in its post-trochlear or reflected part also.

The reflected tendon of the superior oblique (so) passes under the superior rectus muscle and fans out to get inserted on to the sclera. The fibres of this fan-shaped tendinous part of SO muscle make an angle of 51° with the visual axis in primary position. Functionally, these fibres can be separated into two parts:

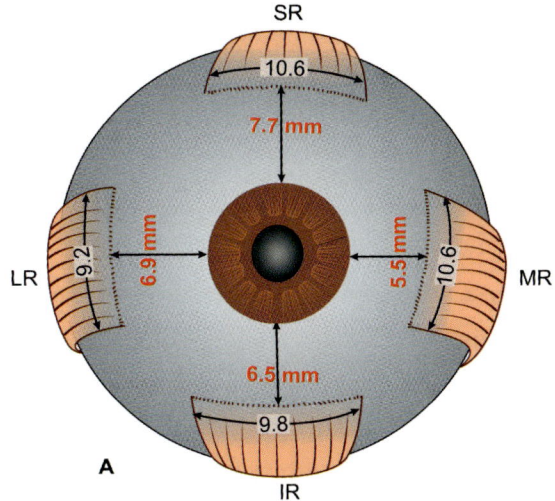

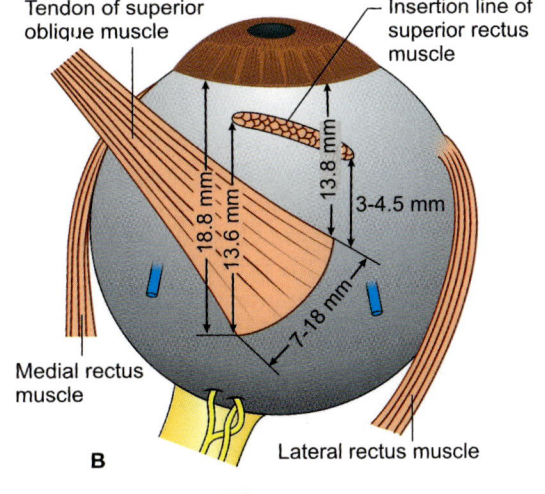

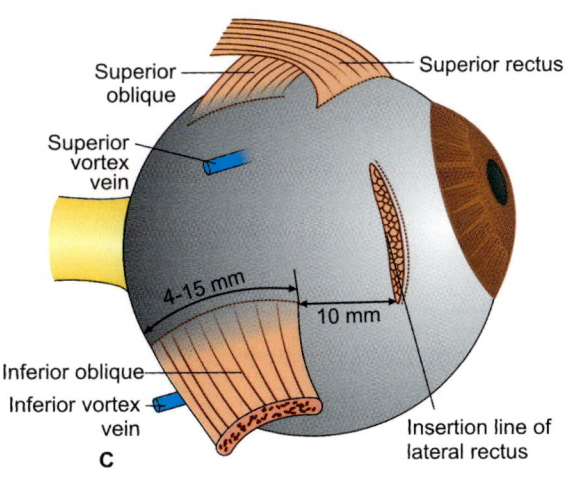

Fig. 1.3 *Insertion lines of the extraocular muscles on the sclera as seen from (A) front; (B) above; and (C) lateral side. (SR, superior rectus; MR, medial rectus; IR, inferior rectus; LR, lateral rectus).*

- *Anterior one-third* fibres of the tendon are exclusively responsible for the incyclotorsion of the globe. Therefore, only these fibres of SO muscle are manipulated to enhance incyclotorsion action in Harada-Ito procedure.
- *Posterior two-third* fibres of the fan-shaped tendon of SO function to depress and abduct the globe.

Insertion

The fanned out reflected tendon of the superior oblique is inserted onto the upper and outer part of the sclera behind the equator (Fig. 1.3B).

The insertion line is curved with its concavity facing the trochlea with following landmarks:

- *Anterior end* of insertion lies some 13.8 mm behind the limbus and about 3 to 4.5 mm behind the lateral end of the insertion line of the superior rectus muscle.
- *Posterior end* of the insertion line lies about 18.8 mm behind the limbus and some 13.6 mm behind the medial end of the insertion line of superior rectus muscle.
- *Medial or posterior end of the insertion line* lies about 8 mm from the posterior pole.
- *Width of the insertion* line is about 11 mm, but it varies greatly from 7 to 18 mm.

The superior oblique is the *longest and thinnest* of all the extraocular muscles. The length of its direct part is about 40 mm and that of the reflected tendon is about 19.5 mm (total being 59.5 mm). From a physiologic and kinematic standpoint, the trochlea is the origin of the muscle.

Inferior Oblique Muscle

Origin

The inferior oblique muscle arises by a rounded tendon from a shallow depression on the orbital plate of maxilla just lateral to the orifice of the nasolacrimal duct (Fig. 1.4). Some fibres arise from the lacrimal fascia. It is the only muscle which takes origin from front of the orbit.

Course

From its origin, the muscle passes laterally and backward, between the inferior rectus muscle and floor of the orbit (Fig. 1.1). It is almost wholly muscular with a short tendon at origin and insertion. It is the *shortest* of the eye muscles, being only 37 mm long. The anterior fibres of the muscle are primarily responsible for extorsion and posterior fibres for the elevation.

Insertion

It is inserted by a short tendon (1 to 2 mm long) in the lower and outer part of the sclera behind the equator (Fig. 1.3C). The insertion line is

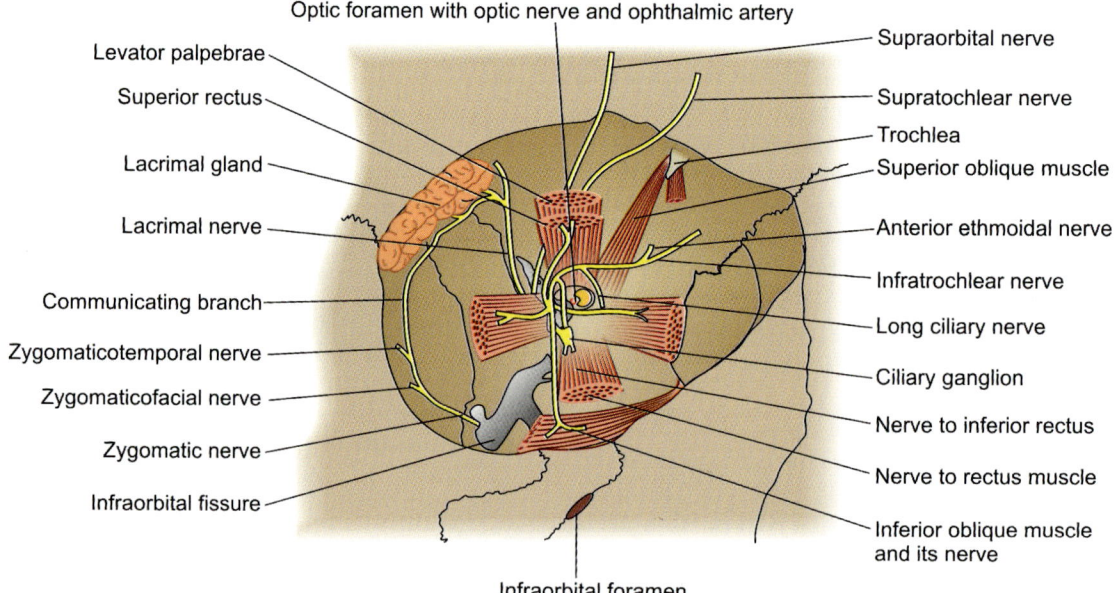

Levator palpebrae
Superior rectus
Lacrimal gland
Lacrimal nerve
Communicating branch
Zygomaticotemporal nerve
Zygomaticofacial nerve
Zygomatic nerve
Infraorbital fissure

Optic foramen with optic nerve and ophthalmic artery
Supraorbital nerve
Supratrochlear nerve
Trochlea
Superior oblique muscle
Anterior ethmoidal nerve
Infratrochlear nerve
Long ciliary nerve
Ciliary ganglion
Nerve to inferior rectus
Nerve to rectus muscle
Inferior oblique muscle and its nerve

Infraorbital foramen

Fig. 1.4 *Origin of inferior oblique muscle and innervation of extraocular muscles.*

curved with a concavity facing the origin, with following landmarks:

- Its average width is around 9 mm. However, it varies widely from 5 to 14 mm.
- Its anterior end is about 10 mm behind the lower edge of the insertion of the lateral rectus muscle.
- Its posterior end is about 1 mm below and 1 to 2 mm in front of a point corresponding with the foveal region.
- Near the insertion, the inferior vortex vein is in relation to its posterior border.

Comparative Dimensions

The comparative dimensions of the extraocular muscles are shown in Table 1.1. The table depicts the following:

- Superior oblique is the longest and thinnest muscle.
- Inferior oblique is the shortest muscle.

NERVE SUPPLY OF EXTRAOCULAR MUSCLES

The extraocular muscles are supplied by third, fourth and sixth cranial nerves (Fig. 1.4).

Third cranial nerve (oculomotor) supplies the medial, superior and inferior recti and inferior oblique muscles. The branches enter their respective muscles from their bulbar surfaces. The branches from the inferior division of third nerve supply the medial rectus (enters its belly 15 mm from origin), inferior rectus (enters at the junction of the posterior and middle thirds of the belly) and inferior oblique (enters just after the muscle passes lateral to the inferior rectus muscle) muscles. The branches for the superior rectus muscle originate from the upper division of the oculomotor nerve and enter the muscle at the junction of the posterior and middle thirds.

Fourth cranial nerve (trochlear) innervates the superior oblique muscle. Unlike other muscles, the nerve to this muscle enters from its outer (orbital) surface near the lateral border. The nerve divides into three or four branches. The most anterior branch enters the belly at the junction of posterior and middle thirds of the muscle and the most posterior at about 8 mm from its origin.

Sixth cranial nerve (abducent) innervates the lateral rectus muscle by entering the muscle on the bulbar side 15 mm from its origin.

BLOOD SUPPLY OF EXTRAOCULAR MUSCLES

Muscular arteries, usually two—medial and lateral (with a few fine twigs), are branches of the ophthalmic artery. The *medial muscular* branch, larger of the two, supplies the medial rectus, inferior rectus and inferior oblique muscles. The medial rectus also receives a branch from the lacrimal artery and the inferior rectus and inferior oblique muscles receive branch from the infraorbital artery. The *lateral muscular branch* supplies the lateral rectus, the superior rectus, the levator muscle and the superior oblique muscle.

Table 1.1 *Comparative dimensions of various extraocular muscles in mm*						
Dimension	*Superior rectus*	*Inferior rectus*	*Lateral rectus*	*Medial rectus*	*Superior oblique*	*Inferior oblique*
• Total length	42	40	48	40	60	37
• Tendon length	5.8	5.5	8.8	3.7	20	1 to 2
• Muscle breadth	9	9	9	9	9	9
• Tendon breadth at insertion (insertion line)	10.8	9.8	9.2	10.3	11	9.4
• Distance of mid-point of insertion line from the limbus	7.7	6.5	6.9	5.5	16.3	18.4
• Arc of contact	6.5	6.5	12	7	7–8	15
• Cross-sectional area in mm						
– Volkmann	11.3	14.8	16.7	17.4	8.4	6.7
– Nakagama	11.4	15.0	17.5	16	7.9	9.5

Note: These are average figures and may vary greatly among individuals.

Anterior ciliary arteries arise from the muscular branches. These are usually seven—two each from the superior, inferior and medial recti and one from the lateral rectus muscle.

Veins from the extraocular muscles correspond to the arteries and empty into the superior and inferior ophthalmic veins.

ACTIONS OF THE EXTRAOCULAR MUSCLES

Detailed actions of each extraocular muscle, along with the mechanics of the ocular movements, are described in the section on physiology of ocular movements (page 22–30). However, a summary of actions of each extraocular muscle in primary position of gaze (Fig. 1.5) is depicted in Table 1.2.

STRUCTURAL CHARACTERISTICS OF EXTRAOCULAR MUSCLES

Muscle capsule, a thin connective tissue covering of the belly of each extraocular muscle (EOM), extends from its origin to insertion. The

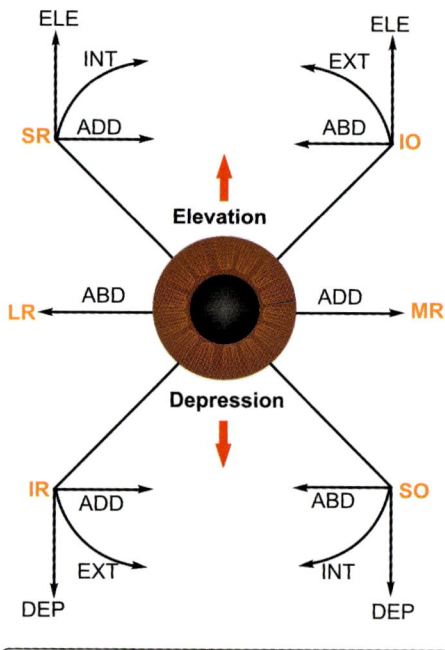

MR = Medial rectus	INT = Intorsion
LR = Lateral rectus	EXT = Extorsion
SR = Superior rectus	ADD = Adduction
IR = Inferior rectus	ABD = Abduction
SO = Superior oblique	ELE = Elevation
IO = Inferior oblique	DEP = Depression

Fig. 1.5 *Actions of extraocular muscles.*

Table 1.2 *Actions of extraocular muscles in primary position of gaze*

Muscle	Primary action	Secondary action	Tertiary action
Medial rectus	Adduction	—	—
Lateral rectus	Abduction	—	—
Superior rectus	Elevation in abduction	Intorsion	Adduction
Inferior rectus	Depression in abduction	Extorsion	Adduction
Superior oblique	Intorsion	Depression	Abduction
Inferior oblique	Extorsion	Elevation	Abduction

smooth avascular surface of the muscle capsule allows the muscle to slide easily over the globe.

Extraocular muscles are voluntary striated muscles. However, the EOMs differ from the *typical skeletal muscle* with the following characteristics:

- Diameter of these fibres is small.
- Contain an enormous amount of fibroelastic tissue
- Contain both slow and fast fibres
- Richly supplied by vessels
- Richly innervated at a ratio of nerve fibre to muscle fibre up to 10 times that of skeletal muscle.

Note: The above characteristics of the EOMs allow quick as well as smooth eye movements. Further the EOMs have high contraction speed and participate in motor acts that are among the fastest (saccadic eye movements) in human body and among the most sustained gaze fixation and vergence movements.

Structural characteristics of EOM, which need to be elaborated are:

- Global and orbital layers of EOMs
- Transverse compartmentalization of EOMs

GLOBAL AND ORBITAL LAYERS OF EOMs

The muscle belly of each EOM can be divided into two distinct portions: the superficial part or the orbital layer (OL) and the deep part or the global layer (GL). Both zones are distinctly separated from each other.

- *In rectus muscles,* the GL is located adjacent to globe (eyeball) and OL on the orbital surface of muscles.
- *In oblique muscles,* the GL is located in the central core and OL forms the concentric outer layer.

Global layer

Global layer of each rectus EOMs passes through its muscle pulley (described on page 10–11) becomes contigenuous with its small terminal tendon and is inserted onto the sclera (Fig. 1.6A). This global layer (GL) is responsible for eye movements. It is mainly (90%) composed of singly innervated fibres (SIFs) with only 10% multiply innervated fibres (MIFs)

- *Singly Innervated fibres (SIFs)* are fast twitch generating and fatigue resistant fibres, and thus allow for large, rapid and precise eye movements. SIFs can be subdivided into three groups (red, intermediate and white), based on the mitochondrial content, with the red fibres being the most fatigue resistant and the white fibres, the least.
- *Multiple innervated fibres (MIFs),* which constitute only 10% of the GL, are thought to be involved in fine control of fixation and in smooth and fine graded eye movements, particularly the vergence control movements.

Orbital layer

- *In rectus muscles,* the orbital layer (OL) is inserted into their respective muscle pulleys and not the sclera (Fig. 1.6A).
- *Orbital layer (OL) of IO muscle* inserts on the IR and LR pulleys.
- *Orbital layer (OL) of SO muscle* inserts via the SO sheath on the medial aspect of SR pulley.

Types of muscle fibres

OL for each EOM contains 80% SIFs and 20% MIFs.

- *SIFs of OL* are specialized for an intense oxidative metabolism, have a large blood supply and are fatigue resistant. They are considered the major contributor to sustained EOM force in primary and deviated position, by allowing most sustained pulley tension. Of all muscle fibre types, this type is most affected by dennervation from damage to the motor nerves or the end plates, as occurs after botulinum toxin injection.
- *MIFs of OL* are thought to play the same role as that of GL.

TRANSVERSE COMPARTMENTALIZATION OF EXTRAOCULAR MUSCLES

Concept of transverse compartmentalization of EOM fibres and their innervation has been suggested in many studies to explain the different functions being performed by a group of fibres from each EOM.

Anatomical compartmentalization of EOMs and their innervation is reported as below:

- *Lateral rectus (LR) muscle:* The abducent nerve, supplying LR muscle, often divides into two or more trunks. Further, longitudinal LR splitting is evident in several congenital cranial deinnervation disorders (CCDDs).
- *Medial rectus (MR) muscle:* Motor nerve to MR also bifurcates into superior and inferior divisions.
- *Inferior rectus (IR) muscle* has a selective lateral trunk overlapping arborization of another trunk throughout the entire muscle length.
- *Superior rectus (SR) muscle* is, however, reported to lack selective compartmental innervation.
- *Superior oblique (SO) muscle* is reported to be innervated by two (medial and lateral) divisions of trochlear nerve in non-overlapping medial and lateral compartments. The medial compartment of SO muscle is contiguous with tendon fibres which are inserted on the equatorial sclera, and produce incycloduction. While the lateral compartment of SO muscle is contiguous with tendon fibres which are predominantly inserted posterior to equator and produce infracycloduction.
- *Inferior oblique (IO) muscle* is also reported to be innervated in compartmental fashion by separate motor nerve trunks.

Functional anatomical compartmentalization of EOMs has also been demonstrated on MRI studies. A few observations are as below:

Change in posterior partial volume (PPV) is the best contractility index, observed on MRI studies. It robustly correlates with the ductions for horizontal rectus EOMs.

Horizontal rectus EOMs (MR as well as LR) have been divided into superior and inferior halves (compartments) on MRI studies. Inferior compartments are slightly larger than the superior compartments of both MR as well as LR muscles.

In lateral rectus (LR) muscle, MRI studies, the contractility for convergence as well as adduction is reported to be similar in both superior as well as inferior compartments.

In medial rectus (MR) muscle, however, the superior compartment exhibited much greater contractility in adduction than in convergence.

During vertical duction on MRI studies, no differential compartmental changes were noted in vertical recti (SR and IR). However, superior compartments of MR muscles showed changes in maximum cross-section and PPV. But no change was noted in inferior MR compartments and in LR muscle compartments.

During vertical fusional vergence (VFV), induced by a 2 PD base up prism, the LR and SO muscles are reported to exhibit differential compartmental contraction. These observations suggest that the EOM mechanisms that normally compensate for the vertical heterophoria are highly complex.

Compartmental brainstem control for the differential compartmental behaviour of the EOMs has also been reported in the neuroanatomic studies.

Compartmental involvement of extraocular muscles has also been reported in nerve palsies as below:
- *Greater atrophy of superior than inferior compartment of LR muscle* is reported in about 30% cases of abducens palsy. An ipsilesional hypotropia, suggesting preserved inferior compartment function, is also reported in some cases.
- *Hypertropia, that increases in abduction,* reported in many cases of isolated LR palsy, suggests relationship to the residual LR contraction.

ORBITAL FASCIA

The orbital fascia is a thin connective tissue membrane lining the various intraorbital structures. Recent studies have shown that this is a complex interwoven connective tissue joining the various intraorbital contents. Though the orbital fascia is one tissue, for descriptive convenience, it can be described under the heads of (Fig. 1.6):
- Fascia bulbi,
- Sleeves (fascial sheaths) of extraocular muscles,
- Extraocular muscle pulleys,
- Anterior pulley slings (intermuscular septa), and
- Fascial expansions of extraocular muscles.

FASCIA BULBI

Fascia bulbi, or Tenon's capsule, envelops the globe from the limbus to the optic disc. Its inner surface is well defined and lies in close contact with sclera to which it is connected by fine trabeculae. The outer surface of the fascia bulbi lies in contact with orbital fat posteriorly and with subconjunctival tissue anteriorly with which it merges near the limbus. Tenon's capsule is separated from the sclera by episcleral space (Tenon's space), which can be readily injected. Tenon's capsule can be divided into anterior and posterior portions:
- *Anterior Tenon's capsule* is the subconjunctival membrane that extends from the limbus to the level of penetration of the rectus muscles (About 10 mm posterior to the insertion of rectus muscles, i.e. just posterior to the equator).
- Anteriorly, it fuses with the conjunctiva 2 to 3 mm posterior to the limbus. When suturing a muscle during strabismus surgery, it is important to clear anterior Tenon's capsule off the tendon insertion to avoid complication of a slipped muscle.
- *Posterior Tenon's capsule* extends from the penetration of the recti muscles to the optic nerve and thus separates the orbital fat from the sclera.

Around the distal end of optic nerve, the posterior Tenon's capsule is fused with the dural sheath of the optic nerve. Schwalbe, however, considered it to be continuous as a membrane surrounding the dural sheath to form a

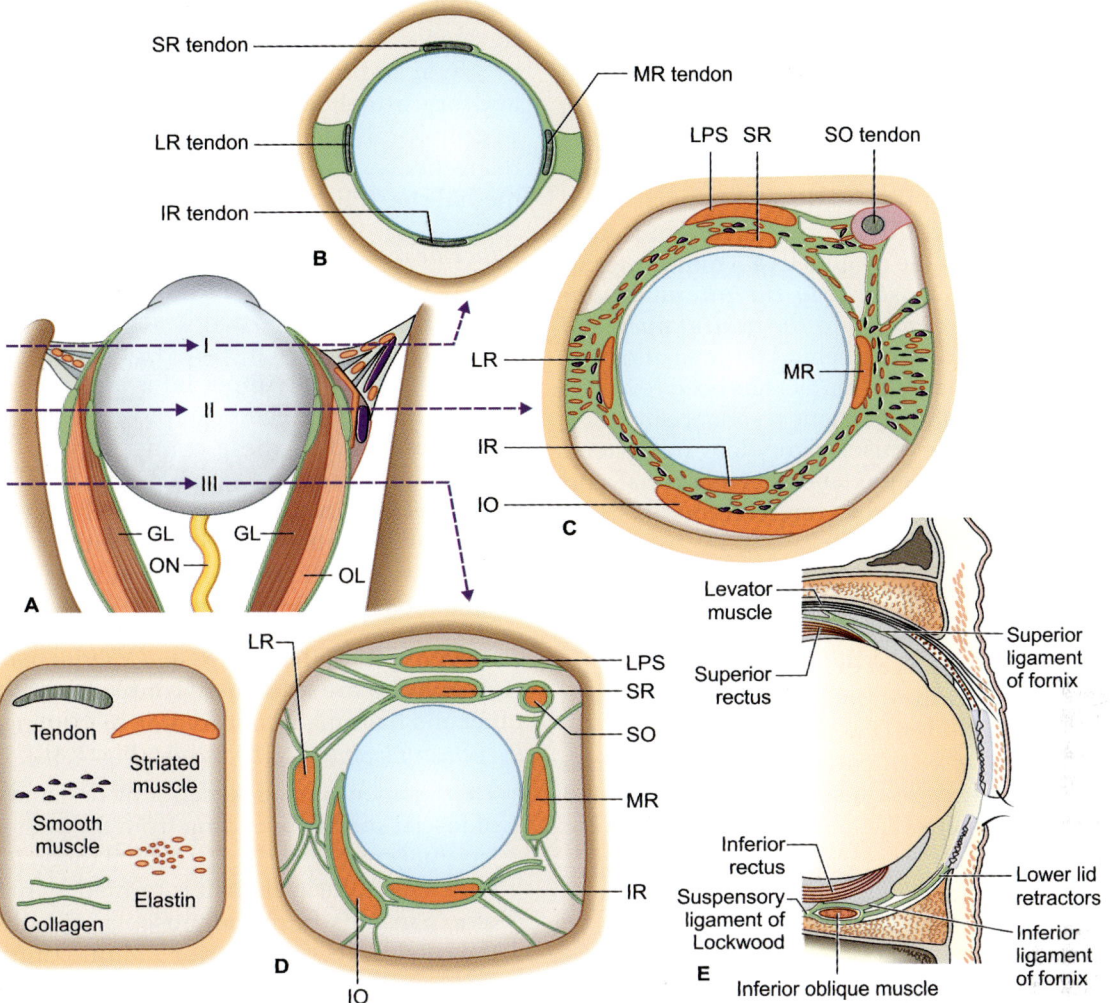

Fig. 1.6 *Schematic depiction of orbital connective tissues: A, Axial view; B, C and D are coronal sections at levels I, II and III, respectively; E, schematic section of lower eyelid showing suspensory ligament of Lockwood and inferior suspensory ligament of the fornix and upper lid showing superior suspensory ligament of fornix. GL, global layer; OL, orbital layer; ON, optic nerve; SR, superior rectus; MR, medial rectus; LR, lateral rectus; SO, superior oblique; IR, inferior rectus; LPS, levator palpebrae superioris; IO, inferior oblique.*

supravaginal lymph space, a view which is now considered doubtful.

Fascia bulbi is pierced posteriorly by the optic nerve, ciliary nerves and vessels, just behind the equator by venae vorticosae, and near the equator by six extraocular muscles; where it becomes continuous with the fascial sheaths of these muscles.

SLEEVES (FASCIAL SHEATHS) OF EXTRAOCULAR MUSCLES

At the points near the equator, where the fascia bulbi is pierced by an extraocular muscle, it sends a tubular reflection, which clothes the muscles like a glove and are called sleeves or sheaths of extraocular muscles.

Note. The anterior Tenon's capsule, posterior Tenon's capsule, and the muscle sleeves are very important structures, since they form the barriers between the orbital fat and globe and extraocular muscles. When posterior capsule or muscle sleeve is traumatically violated, fat adherence can occur. The fat adherence can occur as a complication of almost any extraocular surgery, e.g. strabismus surgery, buckling procedure for retinal detachment or periocular trauma.

INTERMUSCULAR SEPTA (ANTERIOR PULLEY SLINGS)

The sleeves and pulleys of the four rectus muscles are joined to each other by a fascial membrane called the intermuscular septum *(anterior pulley sling)* (Fig. 1.6A to D). This membrane divides the orbital cavity and orbital fat into a central (canal) and a peripheral (extraconal) part. Anteriorly the intermuscular septa fuse with the conjunctiva 3 mm posterior to the limbus. *Posteriorly the intermuscular septa do not extend up to the orbital apex* and vanish a short distance behind the area of globe–optic nerve junction. This fact has been revealed on high-resolution magnetic resonance imaging (MRI). Thus, the muscle cone does not extend up to the orbital apex and that the conal and extraconal spaces become one continuous space near the apex of the orbit.

SYSTEM OF MUSCLE PULLEYS AND RELATED FACIAL EXPANSIONS

Fascial expansions of extraocular muscles. The muscular sheath of each extraocular muscle sends expansions to the surrounding structures which along with muscle pulleys form a complex system of muscle pulley and related facial expansions (Fig. 1.6).

Muscle pulleys refer to stiff concentric ring-like structures present around the belly of EOMs. These consist of collagen, elastin and smooth muscle fibres.

Pulleys of rectus EOMs, about 2–3 mm in length, are present close to the equator of globe, i.e. beginning at the points where the rectus muscles penetrate the Tenon's capsule. Thus, the rectus muscle pulleys are co-axial with the underlying collagenous sleeves around the EOMs.

- The rectus muscle pulleys are stiff and are *stabilised by* septa which are attached around the facial bulbi, intramuscular septa and periorbita.
- Dynamic MRI studies have shown that the pulleys act mechanically as the *functional origins* of the muscles and thus effectively modify the direction of pull of the rectus muscles.
- *Pulleys also serve to stabilise the muscle path,* preventing the sides slipping or movement perpendicular to the muscle axis.
- Anteriorly, the pulleys merge with muscle sleeves.

Pulleys of MR and LR muscles are well developed. Fascial expansions from the pulleys of lateral and medial rectus muscles are strong and are attached to orbital tubercle on the zygomatic bone and to the lacrimal bone, respectively. These are also called lateral and medial **check ligaments**.

Superior rectus muscle pulley is attached to the pulley of levator palpebrae superioris. This attachment ensures synergic action of the two muscles. Thus, when the superior rectus makes the eye look up, the upper lid is also raised. In maximal levator resection for ptosis, hypotropia can be induced, if these connections are not severed. A dense band extends from the lateral border of conjoint SR-LPS pulley to the superior border of LR pulley. This band contains dense collagen and elastin throughout and divides the orbital lobe of lacrimal gland.

Pulleys of inferior rectus (IR) and inferior oblique (IO) muscles are intimately coupled with each other and have main contribution in forming the *suspensory ligament of Lockwood* (Fig. 1.6E).

- This ligament is a thickened sling or hammock of fascial sheath extending from the posterior lacrimal crest to the lateral orbital tubercle, on which rests the eyeball. It is formed by fusion of expansions from the muscular sheaths of the medial rectus, inferior oblique, inferior rectus and lateral rectus muscles joined with the thickened inferior part of Tenon's capsule.
- *Expansion from the inferior rectus muscle* is attached to the capsulopalpebral fascia, a tissue analogous to levator aponeurosis in the lower lid and the sheath of inferior oblique muscle. This relationship is important because an inferior rectus muscle recession can result in lower lid retraction with lid fissure widening while resection results in lid advancement with lid fissure narrowing. Another importance of this relationship is that when the inferior rectus is inadvertently disinserted or lost during surgery, these connections will hold the inferior rectus to the inferior oblique and keep it from retracting posteriorly. Therefore, the lost inferior rectus can usually be found lying between the inferior oblique muscle and the sclera.

Superior oblique (SO) pulley, also known as trochlea, is a thick fibrocartilaginous pulley present at the superomedial angle of the orbital wall. Around it turns the SO tendon. Orbital layer (OL) of the SO muscle is inserted, via the SO sheath, on the medial aspect of SR pulley.

- *Superior transverse ligament of the Whitnall.* It is a thickened band of orbital fascia which extends from the trochlear pulley to the lacrimal gland and its fossa. It is formed by a condensation of the superior sheaths of the levator muscle joined medially by the sheath of the reflected tendon of superior oblique muscle. It forms a true check ligament of the levator muscle.

- *Suspensory ligaments of the fornices* are also well recognized. Superior suspensory ligament of the fornix is formed by the continuation forward of the fibrous tissue between the superior rectus and levator muscles to the upper fornix. During ptosis surgery, if this ligament is cut, fornix conjunctiva can prolapse. Similarly, the *inferior suspensory ligament of the fornix* is formed by the continuation forward up to the inferior fornix of the fibrous tissue of lower lid retractors (Fig. 1.6E).

- *Orbital septa* of elastic and collagenous tissue are well developed in the adults. These septa pass inward from the periorbita to the intermuscular septa (membrane pulleys and muscle sleevs) (Fig. 1.6B). Such septa also pass to and between the extraocular muscles and provide specific supportive channels for the ophthalmic veins.

◼ APPLIED ANATOMICAL ASPECTS

1. *Nerves to the rectus muscles and the superior oblique muscle* enter the muscles about one-third of the distance from the origin to the insertion (or trochlea, in the case of the superior oblique muscle). It is difficult, but possible, to damage these nerves during anterior surgery. However, if an instrument is thrust more than 26 mm posterior to the rectus muscle's insertion, injury to the nerve may occur.

2. *Nerve supplying the inferior oblique muscle* enters the lateral portion of the muscle where the muscle crosses the inferior rectus muscle; it can be damaged by surgery in this area. Since the parasympathetic innervation to the sphincter pupillae and ciliary muscle accompanies the nerve to the inferior oblique muscle, pupillary abnormalities may also result from surgery in this area.

3. *Inferior rectus muscle is distinctly bound to the lower eyelid* by the fascial extension from its sheath. Recession of the inferior rectus muscle tends to widen the palpebral fissure, and resection of the inferior rectus muscle tends to narrow the fissure. Therefore, any alteration of the inferior rectus muscle may be associated with palpebral fissure change.

4. *Superior rectus muscle is loosely bound to the levator palpebrae superioris muscle.* The eyelid may be pulled forward following resection of the superior rectus muscle, thus narrowing the palpebral fissure; also, in hypotropia, a pseudoptosis may be present.

5. *Blood supply to the extraocular muscles* provides almost all of the temporal half of the anterior segment circulation; it provides the majority of the nasal half of the anterior segment circulation, of which some blood is supplied by the long posterior ciliary artery. Therefore, simultaneous surgery on three rectus muscles may induce anterior segment ischaemia, particularly in older patients.

6. *Whenever muscle surgery is performed*, special care must be taken to avoid penetration of Tenon's capsule; if the integrity of Tenon's capsule 10 mm posterior to the limbus is violated, fatty tissue may prolapse through Tenon's capsule and may form a restrictive adhesion and limit ocular motility.

7. *During resection or transposition of extraocular muscles*, the intramuscular septal connections and check ligaments attached to the Tenon's capsule should be carefully severed. This prevents the relocation of adjacent muscles and fat compartments. For example, if the attachments between LR on IO are not severed, the IO is moved anteriorly during resection of the LR.

8. *During rectus muscle recessions*, the severing of the intramuscular septal connections is not necessary.

9. *Posterior dissection* during the rectus muscles surgery may result in pulley damage, so special care is required.

10. *When surgery is performed in the domain of the vortex veins,* accidental severing of a vortex vein is possible. The procedures that present the greatest risk for damaging a vortex vein are inferior rectus and superior rectus muscle recession or resection, inferior oblique muscle weakening and exposure of the superior oblique muscle tendon.

11. *The sclera is thinnest just posterior to the four rectus muscle insertions.* This is the site for most muscle surgery, especially for recession procedures. Therefore, the risk of scleral perforation is always present during eye muscle surgery. This risk can be best minimized by using spatulated needles with swedged sutures; working with a clean, dry, and blood-free surgical field; using loupe magnification; and employing a head mounted fibreoptic light source in addition to the overhead operating lights.

ANATOMY OF THIRD, FOURTH AND SIXTH CRANIAL NERVES

OCULOMOTOR NERVE

The oculomotor (third cranial) nerve is entirely motor in function. It supplies all the extraocular muscles except lateral rectus and superior oblique.

Oculomotor nuclear complex

The oculomotor nucleus complex has two motor nuclei: (a) *the main motor nucleus* of large multipolar neurons, and (b) *the accessory parasympathetic nucleus* (Edinger-Westphal nucleus) of small multipolar neurons.

a. *The main motor nucleus* is composed of the subnuclei (Fig. 1.7A and B) supplying individual extraocular muscles as follows:

1. *Dorsolateral nucleus*: Ipsilateral inferior rectus.
2. *Intermedial nucleus*: Ipsilateral inferior oblique.
3. *Ventromedial nucleus*: Ipsilateral medial rectus.
4. *Paramedial (scattered) nucleus*: Contralateral superior rectus.
5. *Caudal central nucleus*: Bilateral levator palpebrae superioris.

b. *The accessory motor nucleus* (Edinger-Westphal nucleus). It is situated posterior to the main oculomotor nucleus mass. It sends preganglionic parasympathetic fibres along the other oculomotor fibres.

Course and distribution

For the purpose of description, the course of the oculomotor nerve can be divided into: Fascicular, basilar, intracavernous and intraorbital parts.

Fascicular part

The fasciculus consists of efferent fibres which pass from the third nerve nucleus through the red nucleus and the medial aspect of the cerebral peduncle. They then emerge from the midbrain and pass into the interpeduncular space (Fig. 1.8).

Basilar part

The basilar part starts as a series of 15 to 20 rootlets in the interpeduncular fossa. These coalesce to form a large medial root and a small lateral root, which unite to form a flattened nerve, which get twisted bringing the inferior fibres superiorly and superior fibres inferiorly; and thus the nerve becomes a rounded cord. The nerve then runs forwards to reach the cavernous sinus (Fig. 1.9).

Intracavernous part

After entering the cavernous sinus, the nerve descends to the lateral wall of the sinus, where it lies above the trochlear nerve (Fig. 1.10). In the anterior part of the cavernous sinus, the nerve divides into superior and inferior divisions which enter the orbit through the middle part of the superior orbital fissure within the annulus of Zinn (Fig. 1.11). In the fissure, the nasociliary nerve lies in between the two divisions, while the abducent nerve lies inferolateral to them.

Intraorbital part

In the orbit (Fig. 1.9), the smaller *superior division* ascends on the lateral side of optic nerve and supplies the superior rectus and the levator palpebrae superioris. The larger, *inferior division* divides into three branches: (1) *nerve to the medial rectus* passes inferior to the optic nerve, (2) *nerve to inferior* rectus passes downward and enters the muscle on its upper aspect and (3) *nerve to inferior oblique* (longest of the three branches)

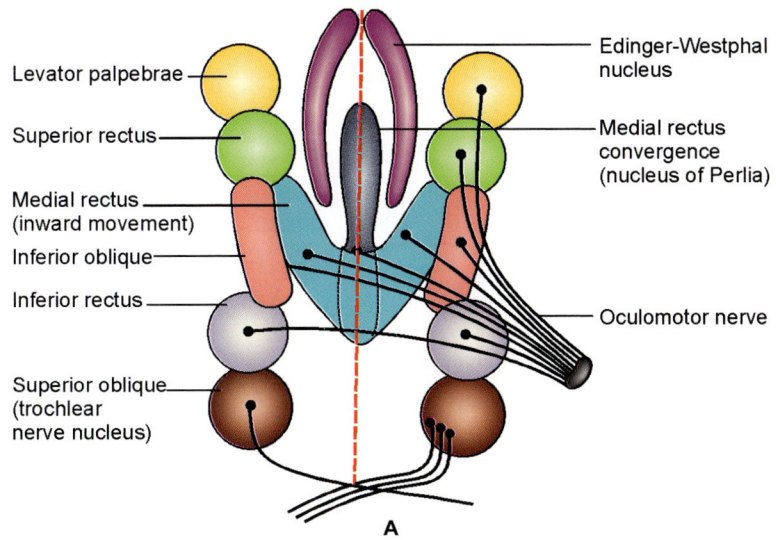

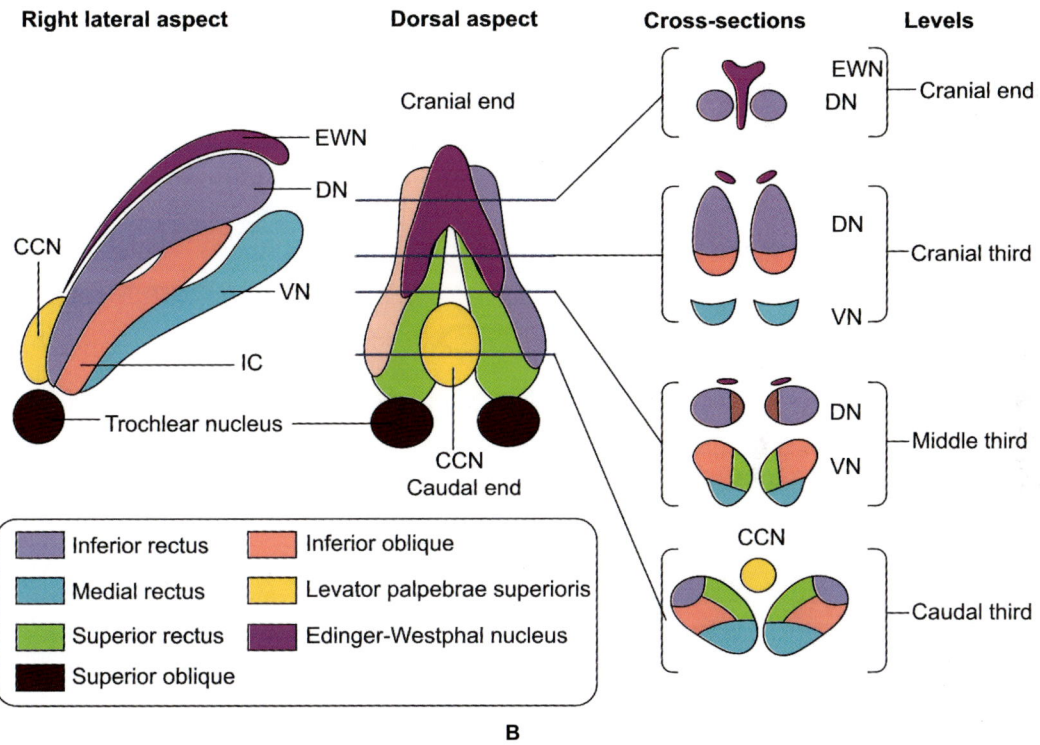

Fig. 1.7 *Scheme to show components of oculomotor nucleus complex. A: old outdated concept, B: modern concept (Warwick, 1953) (EWN, Edinger-Westphal nucleus; DN, Dorsal nucleus VN, Ventral nucleus, IC, intermediate column; CCN, caudal central nucleus).*

passes in between the inferior rectus and lateral rectus and supplies the inferior oblique from its posterior border. It gives off the motor root to the ciliary ganglion.

TROCHLEAR NERVE

The trochlear (fourth cranial) nerve is entirely motor in function and supplies only the superior oblique muscle of the eyeball.

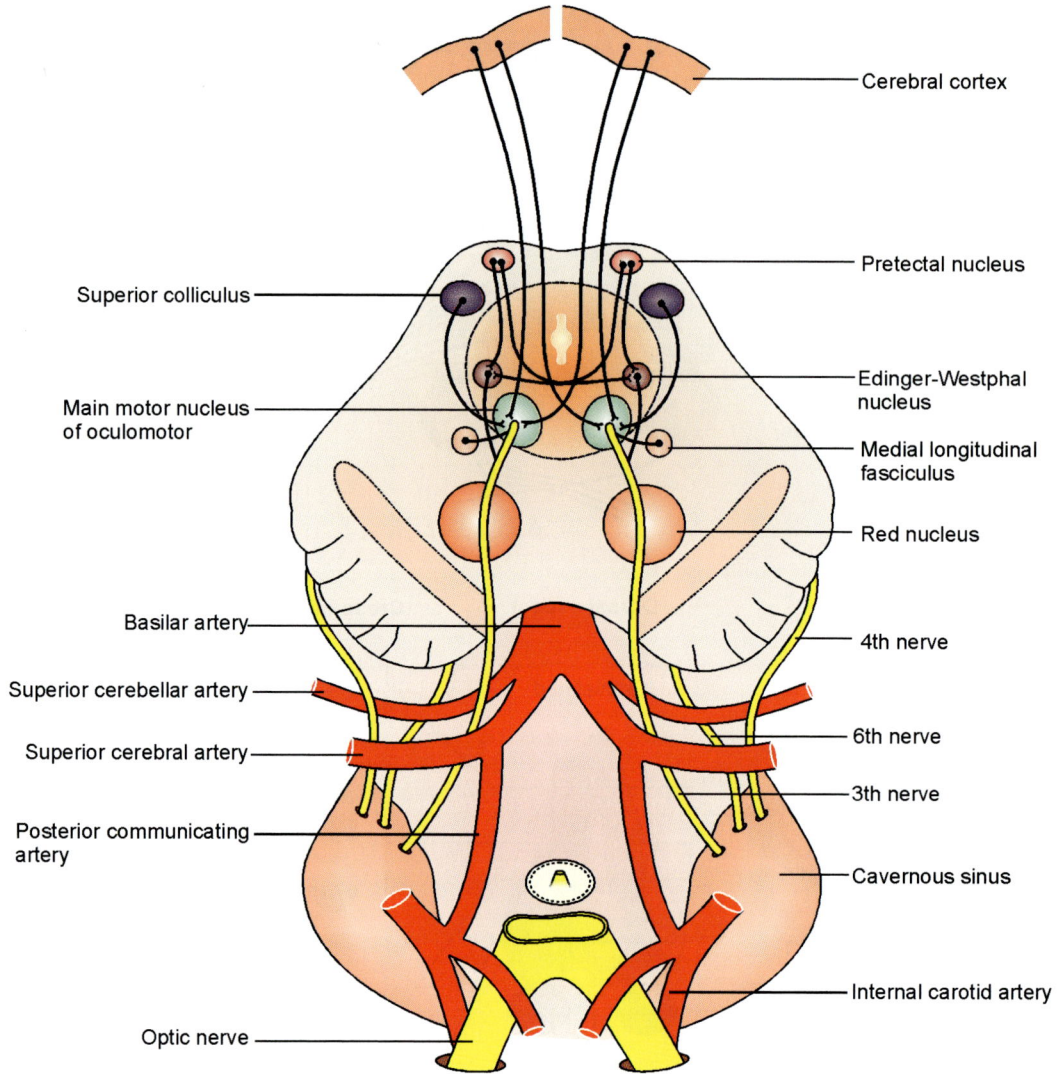

Superior colliculus

Main motor nucleus
of oculomotor

Basilar artery

Superior cerebellar artery

Superior cerebral artery

Posterior communicating
artery

Optic nerve

Cerebral cortex

Pretectal nucleus

Edinger-Westphal
nucleus

Medial longitudinal
fasciculus

Red nucleus

4th nerve

6th nerve

3th nerve

Cavernous sinus

Internal carotid artery

Fig. 1.8 *Oculomotor nerve nuclei, their central connections and course of fascicular and basilar parts of the nerve.*

Nucleus

The trochlear nucleus is situated in the ventromedial part of the central grey matter of the midbrain at the level of inferior colliculus (Figs 1.12 and 1.13). It is caudal to and continuous with the third nerve nucleus complex.

Course and distribution

For the purpose of description, the course of the trochlear nerve can be divided into fascicular, precavernous, intracavernous and intraorbital parts.

Fascicular part

The fasciculus consists of efferent fibres which after leaving the nucleus, pass posteriorly around the aqueduct in the central grey matter and decussate completely in the anterior medullary velum (Fig. 1.13).

Precavernous part

The trochlear nerve trunk after emerging from the dorsal aspect of midbrain winds round the superior cerebellar peduncle and the cerebral peduncle just above the pons. It then runs forwards and enters into the cavernous sinus.

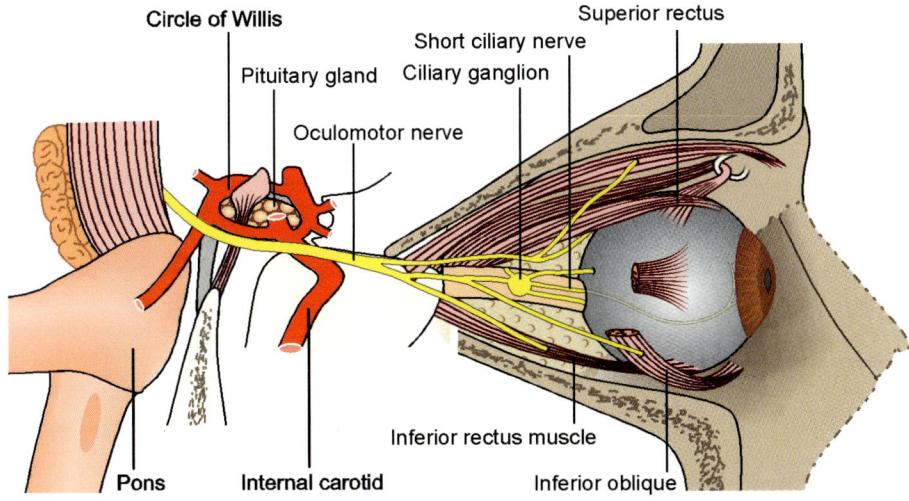

Fig. 1.9 *Showing the course of oculomotor nerve.*

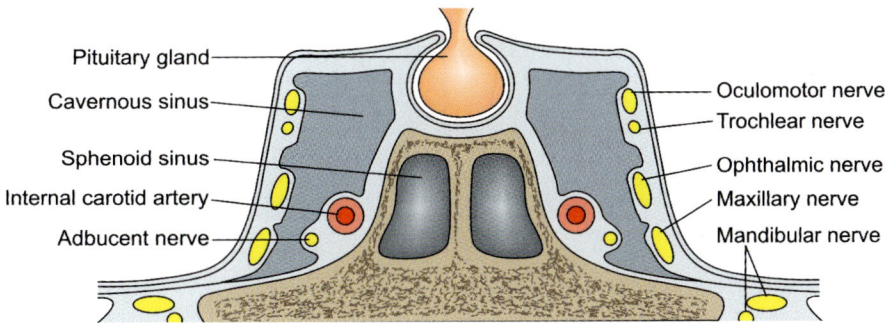

Fig. 1.10 *Coronal section through the middle cranial fossa showing the relations of cranial nerves (3rd, 4th, three divisions of 5th and 6th) with each other in the lateral wall of the cavernous sinus.*

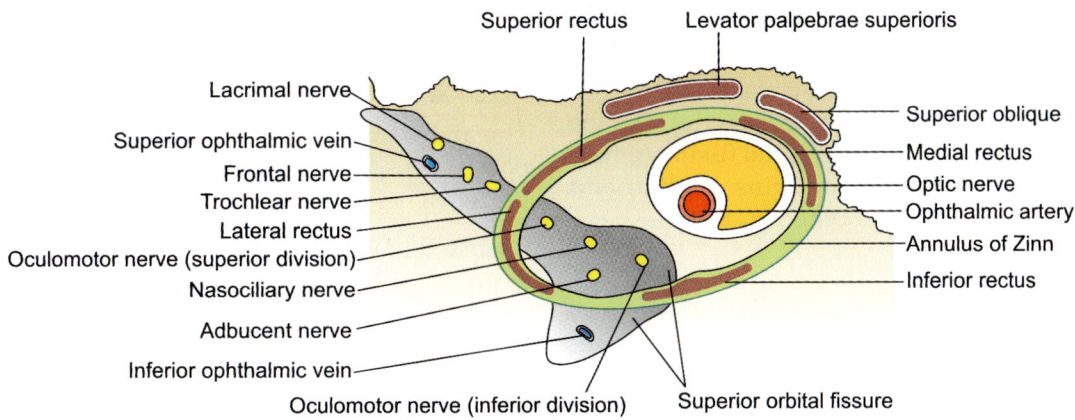

Fig. 1.11 *Apical part of the orbit showing the origin of extraocular muscles, the common tendinous ring and the structures passing through the superior orbital fissure.*

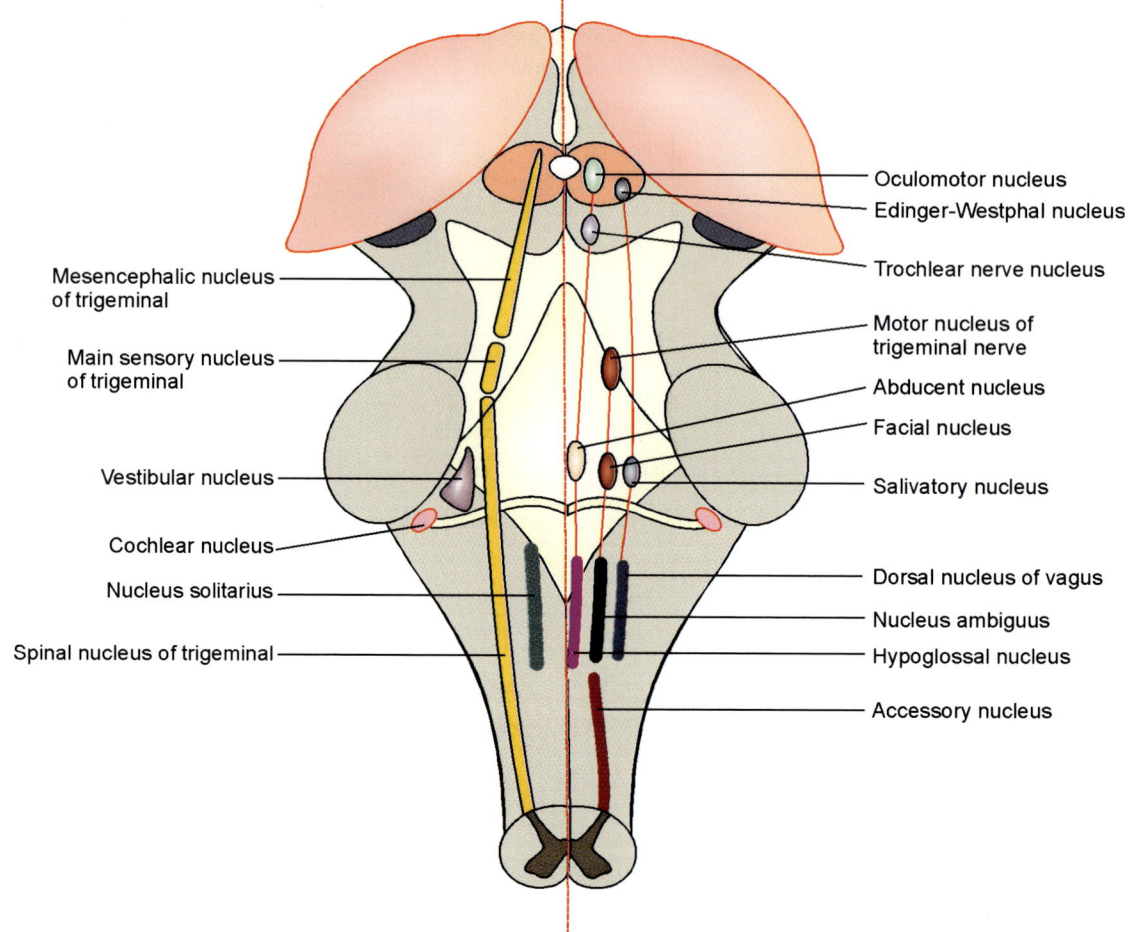

Fig. 1.12 *Scheme to show the cranial nerve nuclei as projected onto the posterior surface of the brainstem.*

Intracavernous part

In the cavernous sinus, the nerve runs forwards in its lateral wall lying below the oculomotor nerve and above the first division of the fifth cranial nerve (Fig. 1.10). In the anterior part of the cavernous sinus, it rises, crosses over the 3rd nerve and leaves the sinus to pass through the lateral part of the superior orbital fissure (where it lies superolateral to annulus of Zinn and medial to the frontal nerve) (Fig. 1.11).

Intraorbital part

After entering the orbit through the lateral part of the superior orbital fissure, the nerve passes medially above the origin of levator palpebrae superioris (Fig. 1.14) and ends by supplying the superior oblique muscle through its orbital surface.

■ ABDUCENT NERVE

The abducent (sixth cranial) nerve is a small, entirely motor nerve that supplies the lateral rectus muscle of the eyeball.

Nucleus

The abducent nucleus is situated in the lower part of pons, closely related to the fasciculus of the facial nerve (Fig. 1.15).

Course and distribution

For the purpose of description, the course of the abducent nerve can be divided into: Fascicular, basilar, intracavernous and intraorbital parts.

Fascicular part

The fasciculus consists of efferent fibres which start from the nucleus, pass forward and emerge

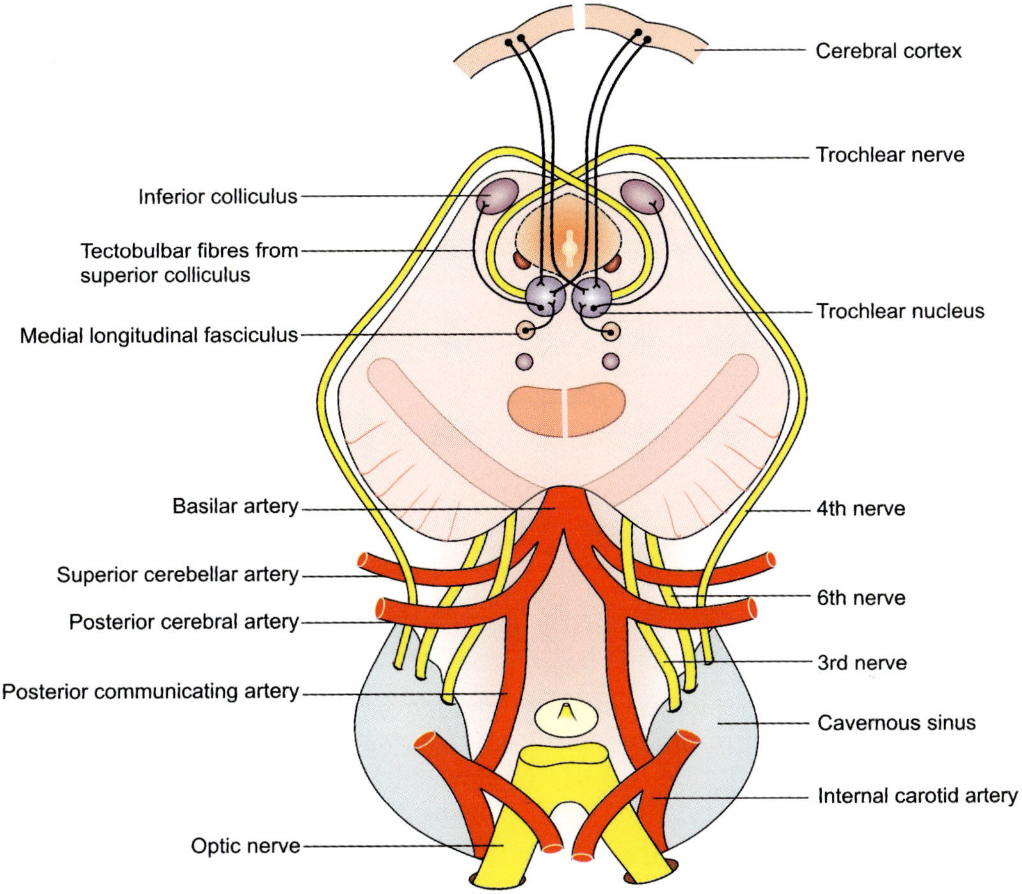

Cerebral cortex

Trochlear nerve

Inferior colliculus

Tectobulbar fibres from superior colliculus

Trochlear nucleus

Medial longitudinal fasciculus

Basilar artery

4th nerve

Superior cerebellar artery

6th nerve

Posterior cerebral artery

Posterior communicating artery

3rd nerve

Cavernous sinus

Internal carotid artery

Optic nerve

Fig. 1.13 *Trochlear nerve nucleus, its central connections and course of fascicular and basilar parts of the nerve.*

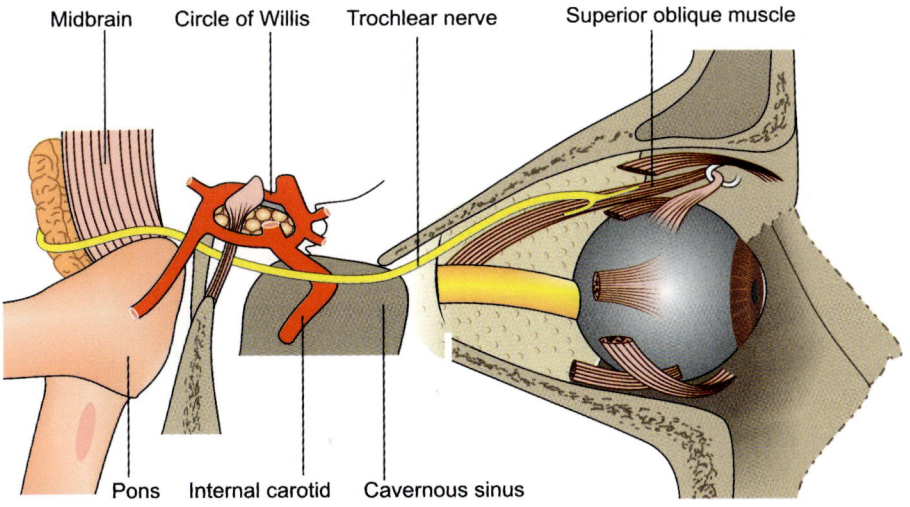

Midbrain   Circle of Willis   Trochlear nerve   Superior oblique muscle

Pons   Internal carotid   Cavernous sinus

Fig. 1.14 *Showing the course of trochlear nerve.*

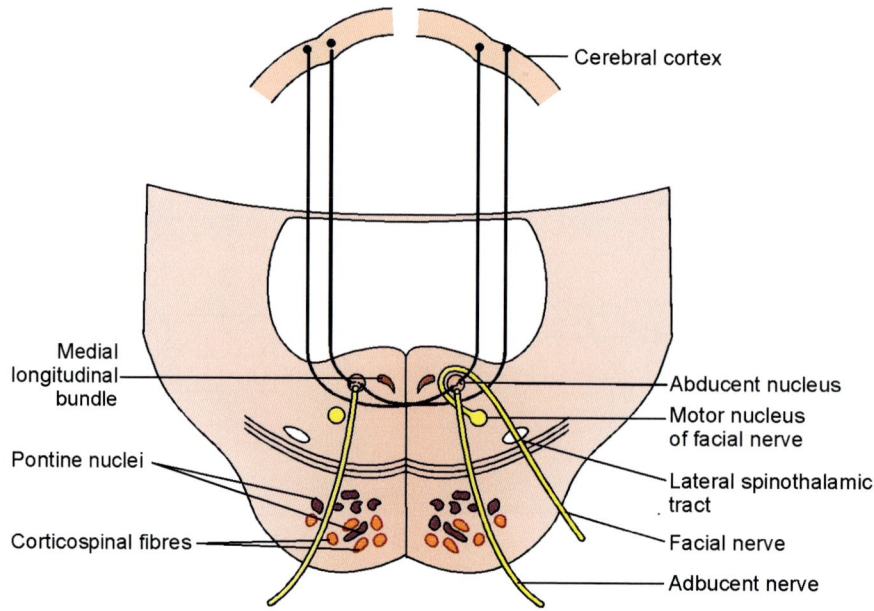

Fig. 1.15 *Abducent nerve nucleus and its central connections.*

by some 7 to 8 rootlets from the junction of pons and medulla which join to form one nerve (Fig. 1.15).

Basilar part

The nerve then runs forwards, upwards on the back of the petrous temporal bone near its apex. At the sharp upper border of the petrous bone, the nerve bends forward at right angle and enters the cavernous sinus.

Intracavernous part

In the cavernous sinus, the nerve runs almost horizontally forward, occupying a position below and lateral to the internal carotid artery (Fig. 1.10). The nerve then leaves the cavernous sinus to enter the orbit through the middle part of the superior orbital fissure within the annulus of Zinn (Fig. 1.11). In the superior orbital fissure, the abducent nerve lies inferolateral to the oculomotor and nasociliary nerves.

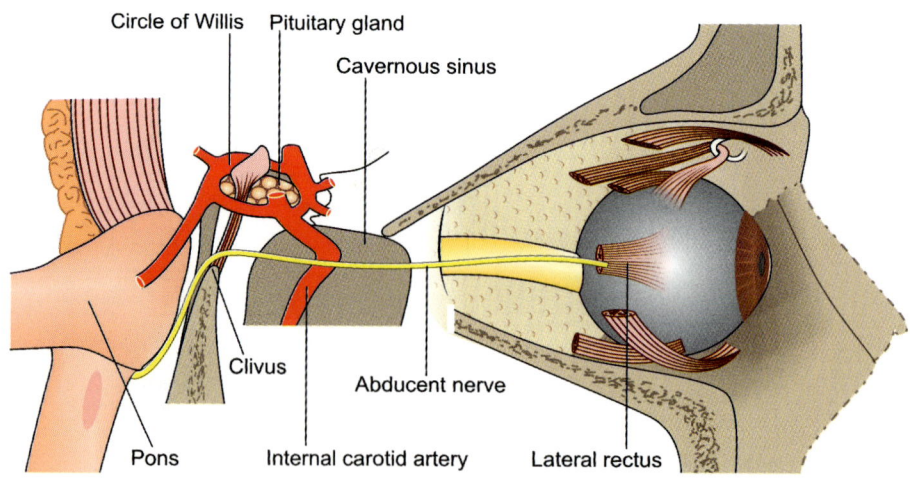

Fig. 1.16 *Course of sixth cranial nerve.*

Intraorbital part

In the orbit, the nerve runs forwards and enters the ocular surface of the lateral rectus muscle just behind its middle portion after dividing into three or four branches (Fig. 1.16).

BIBLIOGRAPHY

1. Bisaria KK. Cavernous portion of the trochlear nerve with special reference to its site of entrance. J. Anat. 159:29–35, 1988.
2. Duane's Ophthalmology, Chapter 32 Embryology and Anatomy of the Orbit and Lacrimal System. (eds Tasman W, Jaeger EA) Lippincott/Williams & Wilkins, 2007.
3. Hoya K, Kirino T. Traumatic Trochlear Nerve Palsy Following Minor Occipital Impact. Neurol Med Chir 40:358–360, 2000.
4. Joseph L. Demer (April 2002). "The Orbital Pulley System: A Revolution in Concepts of Orbital Anatomy". Annals of the New York Academy of Sciences. Neurobiology of eye movements: from molecules to behavior. 956: 17–32. doi:10.1111/j.1749-6632.2002.tb02805.x.
5. Mehta MP; Perry JD (2015). "Medial orbital wall landmarks in three different North American populations". Orbit. 34 (2): 72–8. PMID 25804299. doi:10.3109/01676830.2014. 997394.
6. Orbit at the US National Library of Medicine Medical Subject Headings (MeSH).
7. Tenon JR, Naus J, Blanken R (March 2003). "Anatomical observations on some parts of the eye and eyelids. 1805". Strabismus. 11 (1): 63–8. PMID 12789585. doi:10.1076/stra.11.1.63. 14089.
8. Vilensky, Joel; Robertson, Wendy; Suarez-Quian, Carlos (2015). The Clinical Anatomy of the Cranial Nerves: The Nerves of "On Olympus Towering Top". Ames, Iowa: Wiley-Blackwell. ISBN 978-1-118-49201-7.

Chapter

2

Physiology of Ocular Motility

BASIC KINEMATICS

POSITIONS OF GAZE

To understand the ocular movements and their mechanics, a frame of reference against which the movements may be quantitated is necessary. The primary position of the eye is that position from which all other ocular movements are initiated, changing the position of eyeball from primary to secondary or tertiary. All the extraocular muscles have a given tone for every position of gaze. A total of 9 positions of gaze have been described. These include one primary, 4 secondary and 4 tertiary positions (Fig. 2.1).

Primary position of gaze

The primary position has been defined by Scobee as that position of the eyes in binocular vision when, with the head erect, the object of regard is at infinity and lies at the intersection of the sagittal plane of the head and a horizontal plane passing through the centres of rotation of the two eyeballs (Fig. 2.1E).

Secondary positions of gaze

These are the positions assumed by the eyes while looking straight up (supraversion), straight down (infraversion), to the right (dextroversion) and to the left (levoversion) (Fig. 2.1B, D, F, H).

Tertiary positions of gaze

These describe the positions assumed by the eyes, when combination of vertical and horizontal movements occurs. These include position of eyes in dextroelevation, dextro-depression, levoelevation and levodepression (Fig. 2.1A, C, G, I).

Cardinal positions of gaze

These are the positions which allow examination of each of the 12 extraocular muscles, of the two eyes, in their main field of action. There are six cardinal positions of gaze, viz., dextroversion, levoversion, dextroelevation, levoelevation, dextrodepression and levodepression (Fig. 2.1A, C, D, F, G, I).

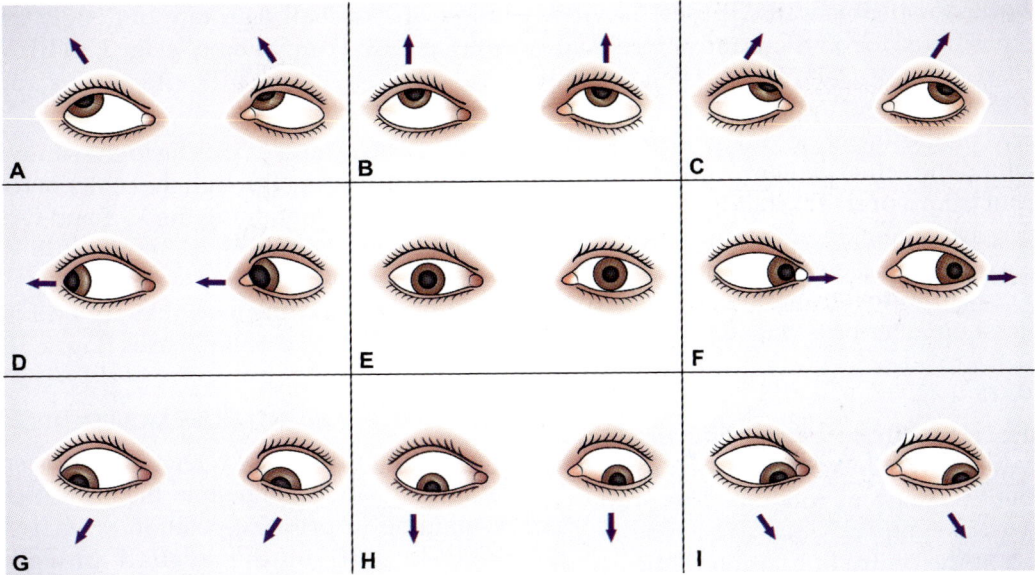

Fig. 2.1 *Diagnostic positions of gaze. Primary position (E); secondary positions (B, D, F, H); tertiary positions (A, C, G, I); cardinal positions (A, C, D, F, G, I).*

CENTRE OF ROTATION

It refers to a hypothetical point around which the eyeball performs rotatory movements. Earlier this has been assumed that the centre of rotation is a fixed point. However, newer experiments indicate that translatory movements do take place to some extent (i.e. laterally, vertically, or in or out), and that the centre of rotation of the eye does not have zero velocity. It has been reported that the centre of rotation moves in a semicircle in the plane of rotation.[1] This locus has been called the *space centroid* (Fig. 2.2).

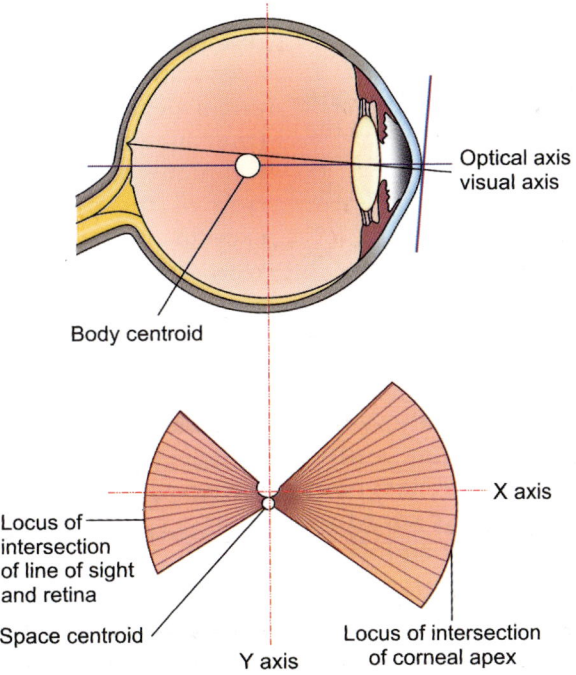

Fig. 2.2 *Position of space centroid as computed by Park and Park.[1]*

However, for all practical purposes, the globe can be considered to rotate around a fixed point. In primary position, the centre of rotation lies some 13.5 mm behind the apex of cornea, when measured on the line of sight. This is in reality a little behind the actual geometrical centre of the globe; but from a practical standpoint, it will be considered to coincide with the centre of the globe. In big myopic eyes, the centre of rotation is a bit farther posterior and in small hyperopic eyes, it is a bit anterior to this ideal position.[2]

FICK'S AXES

Fick described three axes (co-ordinates) to analyse all movements of the globe around the hypothetical centre of rotation. The proposed three axes are perpendicular to each other and intersect at the centre of rotation of the eye. In Fick's system, these coordinates (Fig. 2.3A) are as described below.[3] Recently, oblique axis has also been described.

X (horizontal) axis

It lies horizontally, when the head is in an upright position. Rotation around the horizontal (X) axis results in *elevation* (sursumduction) or *depression* (deosursumduction) (Fig. 2.3B II and VIII).

Y (anteroposterior) axis

The anteroposterior axes of the two eyes are parallel to each other and perpendicular to the horizontal axis. Rotation of the globe around the anteroposterior (Y) axis (Fig. 2.3A) produces the torsional movements named according to the movement of the 12 o'clock meridian of the cornea as *extorsion* (excycloduction) and *intorsion* (incycloduction).

Z (vertical) axis

It extends vertically (direction of gravity), when the head is in an upright position, and is perpendicular to the X and Y axes. Rotations of the globe around vertical (Z) axis are known as *adduction* and *abduction* (Fig. 2.3B IV and VI).

Oblique axis

The Listing's plane also contains two oblique axes 0–0 and 0'–0' (Fig. 2.3B I and III) which allow the eyeball to rotate obliquely up and in (Fig. 2.3B I), up and out (Fig. 2.3B III), down and in (Fig. 2.3 B VII) and down and out (Fig. 2.3B IX).

Note. The X, Z and O axes lie in the same plane. This plane passing through the centre of rotation of the eye and containing the X, Z and O axes is called *Listing's plane* (Fig. 2.3A and 2.3B V). The eyeball can reach all positions of gaze by rotations around the axes that are on Listing's plane, i.e. Z, X and oblique axes (Fig. 2.3B).

TRANSLATORY AND ROTATORY MOVEMENTS

Translatory movements refer to the movements of the eyeball as a whole in the orbit, with eye remaining in primary position of gaze. These include shift of the eyeball upwards or downwards, anteriorly or posteriorly and sideways. *Rotatory movements* occur along the three axes of rotation around a fixed centre of rotation as discussed above.

POSITION OF REST

Position of rest, i.e. a position without actions of extraocular muscles is very hard to document. Even in death, rigor mortis may make the extraocular muscles pull the eye away from the true rest position. It has been reported that the eye positions of orthophoric normal individuals under deep anaesthesia with curare paralysis (measured by an accurate photographic technique) are probably the closest approximation of the position of rest. Under such experiments, an exotropia of 2.25° in each eye which increases with age has been observed in young adult eyes.[4]

MECHANICS OF ACTIONS OF EXTRAOCULAR MUSCLES

FACTORS INVOLVED IN MECHANICS OF EXTRAOCULAR MUSCLE ACTIONS

1. Cross-sectional area of the muscle. Cross-sectional areas of the extraocular muscles as described by Volkmann[5] and Nakagama[6] are shown in Table 2.1. On the basis of the cross-sectional area of the muscles, following comments have been made:

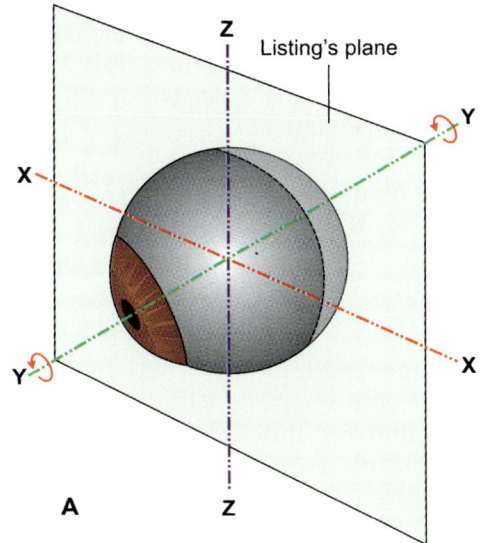

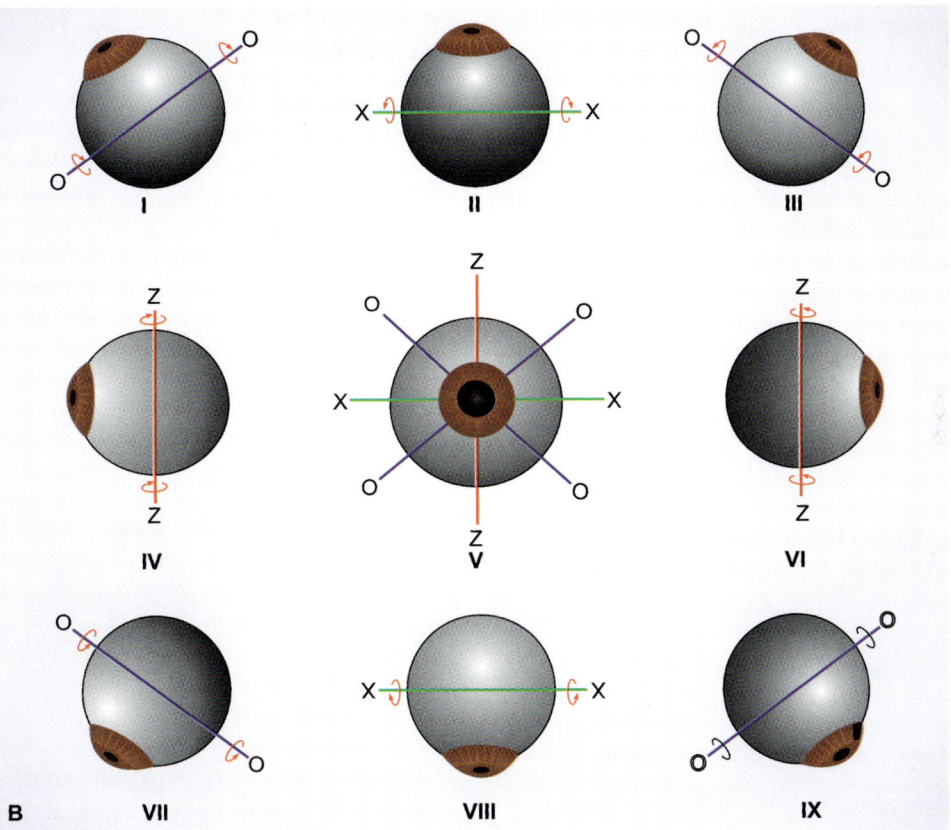

Fig. 2.3 A. *Fick's axes and Listing's plane*, B. *Note that eyeball can reach all positions of gaze by rotations around axes that are on Listing's plane, i.e. Z, X and O (oblique) axes.*

- Cross-sectional area of the horizontal recti is maximum. This is sensible, since they alone are horizontal movers.
- The vertical recti average about 75% and the obliques about 50% the size of the horizontal muscles.
- In general, antagonists such as medial and lateral recti are similar in size, thereby balancing opposing forces.
- Muscles exert force in proportion to their cross-sectional area.

2. Length of the muscle. The average length of various extraocular muscles is shown in Table 2.1. It has been reported that for the normal amplitude of rotation (45°–50° each way from the primary position), approximately 10 mm (about 25% of the normal resting length) change in muscle length is required in each direction. Therefore, a sacrifice of muscle length during resection of the muscles usually reduces the amplitude of eye rotation.

3. Arc of contact. The distal portion of each extraocular muscle or muscle tendon lies flush against the globe for a variable distance before it blends into the sclera (*anatomic insertion*). The point at which the centre of the muscle or its tendon first touches the globe is the *tangential point*. It is also referred to as the *physiologic or effective insertion* of the muscle, since from a mechanical point of view, a tangent to the globe at this point indicates the direction of pull of that muscle. The position of this point changes, when the muscle contracts or relaxes and the globe rotates (Fig. 2.4).

The arc of contact is the distance on the scleral circumference between the tangential point (T) and the centre of anatomic insertion of the muscle (A) on the sclera. The lengths of the contact area for various extraocular muscles in primary position of the gaze are given in Table 2.1.

The arc of contact represents the lever arm in the mechanical system. The arc of contact varies with the position at tangential point, e.g. as the eye is abducted, the arc of contact of lateral rectus is reduced (Fig. 2.4B), while in adduction, it is increased (Fig. 2.4C). However, the location of the tangential point with respect to the centre of rotation of the eye (C) and the point of origin of the muscle (O) remains unchanged (Fig. 2.4A, B and C); so that the *torque* (i.e. the force of rotation) also remains constant. This holds true

Table 2.1 *Lengths of the contact arc for various extraocular muscles in primary position of the gaze*

Muscles	Lengths of contact arc
Lateral rectus	15 mm
Medial rectus	6 mm
Superior rectus	8.4 mm
Inferior rectus	9 mm
Superior oblique	5 mm
Inferior oblique	17 mm

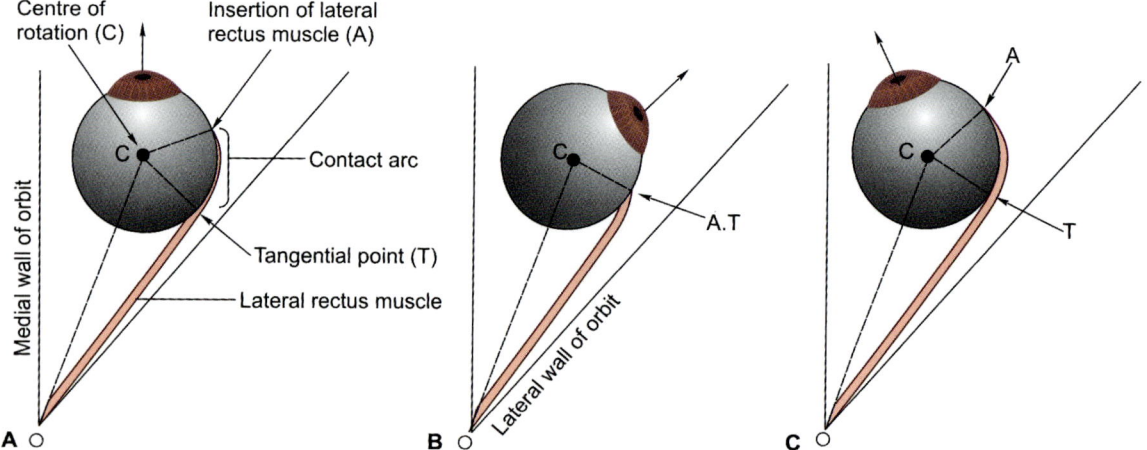

Fig. 2.4 *The arc of contact of the lateral rectus muscle.*

till arc of contact is practically zero that is, the tangential point coincides with the anatomical insertion.

Since the power of a muscle is proportionate to its length and arc of contact, retroplacement of the insertion of muscle (recession) weakens the action of the muscle by shortening its effective length and by reducing its arc of contact in the various positions of gaze. Advancement of an extraocular muscle has a strengthening effect because of the increase in the effective length as well as its arc of contact.

4. *Muscle plane.* It is an imaginary plane which passes through the midpoints of origin of the muscle (O), anatomical insertion (A), functional insertion, i.e. tangential point (T) and the centre of rotation of the globe (C) (Fig. 2.5). Thus each muscle plane runs through the long axis of the muscle. The angle formed by a muscle plane with the visual direction or line of fixation depends on the position of the globe. When the line of fixation lies in or parallel to the muscle plane, the angle is zero.

The ocular muscles are paired, each pair having a common muscle plane. These pairs are the medial and lateral recti [their muscle plane coincides with the horizontal plane of the globe], superior and inferior recti [their muscle plane makes an angle of 23° with the visual line in primary position (Fig. 2.6)] and superior oblique tendon from the trochlea to globe and the inferior oblique [their muscle plane makes an angle of about 51° with the visual line when the eye is in the primary position (Fig. 2.7)].

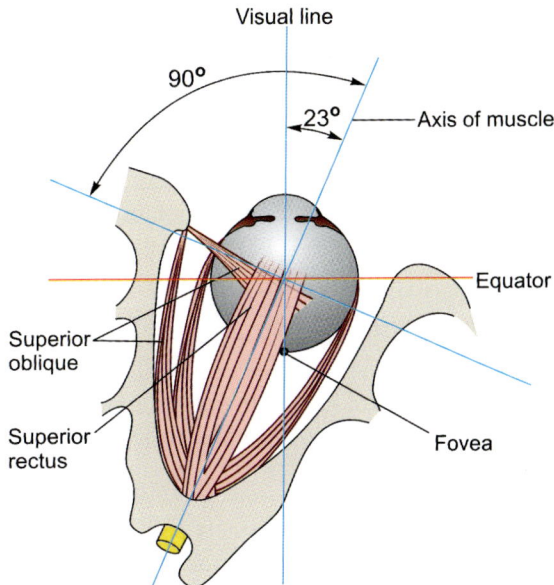

Fig. 2.6 *Relation of muscle plane of superior and inferior recti with the visual line in primary position.*

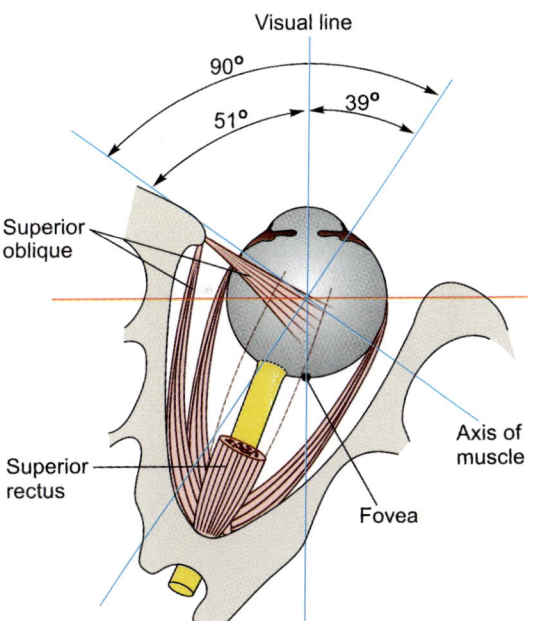

Fig. 2.7 *Relation of muscle plane of superior and inferior obliques with the visual line in primary position.*

5. *Muscle axis of rotation.* It is perpendicular to the muscle plane erected in the centre of rotation. The individual muscle pulling on the eye will rotate the globe around this axis through the centre of rotation.

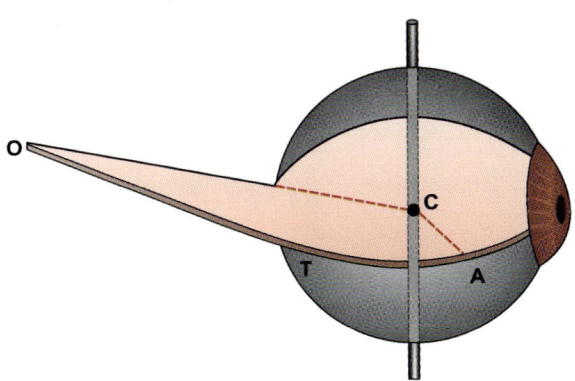

Fig . 2.5 *Schematic presentation of muscle plane (TACO).*

6. *Role of muscle pulleys.* Muscle pulleys, formed by stiff connective tissue have been described to exist for rectus muscles as part of their sleeves at or just posterior to the equator of globe. The muscle pulleys redirect the extraocular muscles and act as their functional origins; and thus affect the ocular movements in different positions of gaze.

CLASSICAL CONCEPT OF ACTIONS OF THE EXTRAOCULAR MUSCLES

The basic and classical concept implies that the actions of the extraocular muscles depend upon the position of the globe at the time of muscle contraction. The *primary action* of a muscle is its major effect, when the eye is in the primary position. The additional effects (other than the primary action) in the primary position are called subsidiary (secondary and tertiary) actions. Duane[7-9] proposed that opposed vertical muscles act as synergists in certain gaze positions and that their functions vary with change in direction of gaze.

Based on the old classical concept by Duane,[7-9] the muscle actions may be summarized as below.

Horizontal rectus muscles

The horizontal recti have a common muscle plane which is horizontal in primary position and their axis of rotation coincides with the 'Z' axis of the globe.

When the eye is in primary position, the horizontal recti are purely horizontal movers around the vertical 'Z' axis and have only a primary action. Thus lateral rectus causes *abduction* and medial rectus causes *adduction*.

Vertical rectus muscles

The superior and inferior rectus muscles have a common muscle plane which is in the same line as the orbital axis and thus form an angle of 23° with the optical axis (Fig. 2.6).

Actions of superior rectus

- In the *primary position,* the *primary* action of the superior rectus is elevation (Fig. 2.8A). This movement occurs about the horizontal 'X' axis. The *secondary* action is *intorsion* (around 'Y' axis) and tertiary action is adduction (around 'Z' axis).
- *When the globe is abducted 23°,* the axis of rotation of superior rectus muscle and optical axis coincide so that the muscle has no subsidiary actions and can only act as *elevator* (Fig. 2.8B). This is, therefore, the best position of the globe for testing the function of the superior rectus muscle.
- *If the globe could be adducted 67°,* the superior rectus would produce pure incycloduction (Fig. 2.8C). Since the globe cannot adduct, therefore, there is some elevating component to the action of superior rectus even in adduction.

Actions of inferior rectus

Actions of inferior rectus are analogous to the superior rectus, i.e.:

- In *primary position,* its primary action is depression, secondary action is extorsion and tertiary action is adduction.

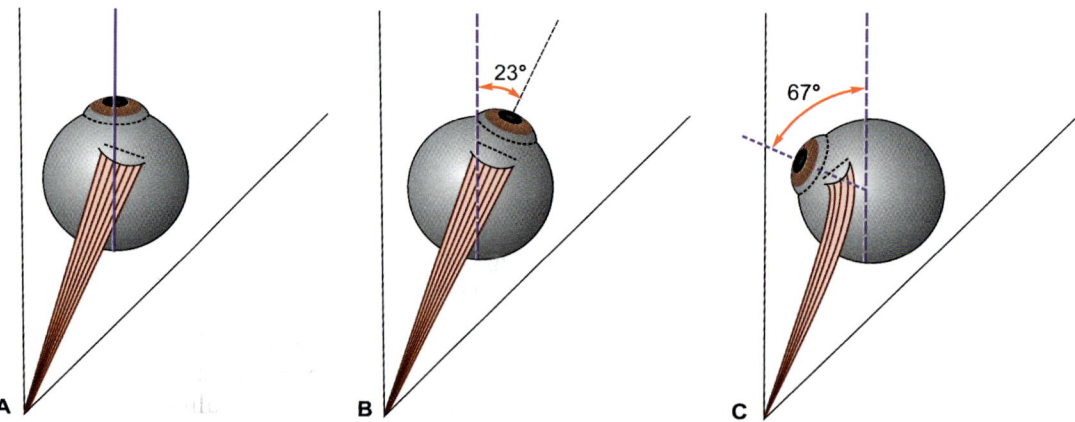

Fig. 2.8 *Actions of superior rectus muscle. A, in primary position; B, when the globe is abducted 23°; and C, when the globe could be adducted 67°.*

- When the globe is abducted 23°, its only action is *depression*.
- If the globe could be adducted 67°, inferior rectus will produce only *extorsion*.

Oblique muscles

The oblique muscles are inserted behind the equator and form an angle of 51° with the optical axis (Fig. 2.7) and thus have following actions.

Actions of superior oblique

- *In primary position*, the primary action of superior oblique is *intorsion* (Fig. 2.9A), which occurs about anteroposterior (Y) axis; the secondary action is depression and the tertiary action is abduction.
- *When the globe is adducted 51°*, the axis of muscle rotation coincides with the optical axis so that it can only act as a depressor (Fig. 2.9B). This is the best position of the globe for clinically testing the action of superior oblique muscle.
- *When the eyeball is abducted by 39°*, the optical axis and line of pull of the superior oblique make on angle of 90° with each other. In this position, the superior oblique can only cause intorsion (Fig. 2.9C).

Actions of inferior oblique

These are analogous to the superior oblique as follows:

- *In primary position*, main action is extorsion, secondary action is elevation and tertiary action is abduction.

- *When the globe is adducted 51°*, its only action is *elevation*.
- *When the globe is abducted 39°*, its only action is *extorsion*.

Contribution of different extraocular muscles in vertical eye movements

The vertical recti are primary elevators and depressors, while the obliques are the primary torsional muscles.

Elevation in primary position and in abduction is contributed by superior rectus—60%, inferior oblique—30% and the rest 10% by the medial and lateral recti. While in adduction between 10° and 30°, the contribution of superior rectus, inferior oblique and horizontal recti is about 40%, 30% and 30%, respectively.

Depression in primary position, in abduction and up to 10° adduction is contributed by inferior rectus—80%, superior oblique—10% and horizontal recti—10%. The corresponding figures in a position of adduction between 10° and 30° are inferior rectus—50%, superior oblique—20% and horizontal recti—30%.

KINEMATICS OF MUSCLE PULLEYS

Rectus muscle pulleys are fundamental to ocular kinematics. Mechanics of action of extraocular muscles is presently being considered on the basis of kinematics of muscle pulleys.[9a]

Anatomical aspects of system of muscle pulleys and their connections are described on page 10–11.

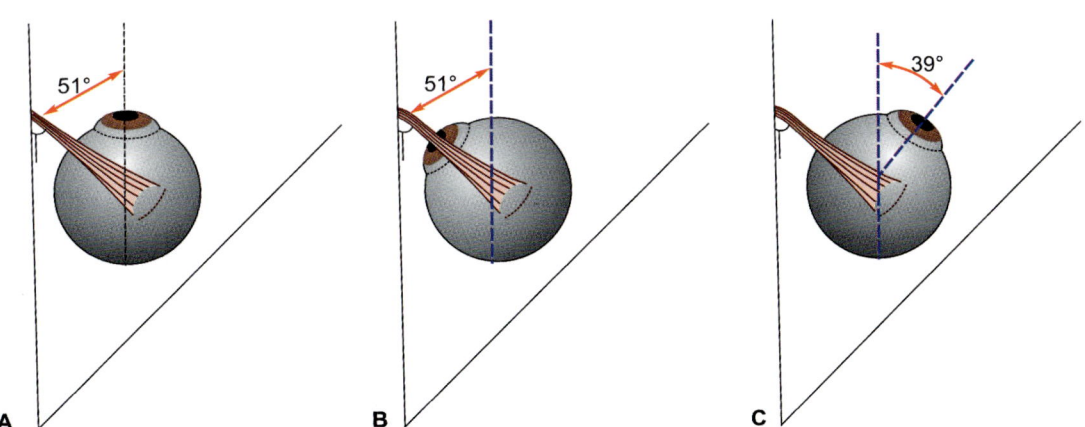

Fig. 2.9 *Actions of superior oblique muscle.* A, *in primary position;* B, *when the globe is adducted 51°;* and C, *when the globe is abducted 39°.*

Physiological aspects, i.e. kinematics of pulleys need delibrations on the following:
- Relationship of the pulley to rotational axis of EOMs.
- Half-angle-rule
- Pulley suspension forces
- Kinematics of individual EOM pulley

Relationship of pulley to rotational axis of EOMs

- *Pulleys of rectus EOM* located just behind the equator, serve as functional origin of the muscles (Fig. 2.10).
- *Rotational axis of all rectus EOMs* is perpendicular to the segment between the

pulley and scleral insertion and thus vertical in central gaze (Fig. 2.10A).
- *Muscle pulley is pulled posteriorly during EOM contraction by the orbital layer (OL) of the muscle inserted over it. These muscle pulleys move in coordination with the insertion and the sclera.*

Half-angle-rule

- *Rotation axis of the eyeball shifts equivalent to half of the angle* by which eyeball moves during duction movement from the primary position. This has been depicted on dynamic MRI studies. For example, if in supraduction the eyeball moves up by angle β, the horizontal

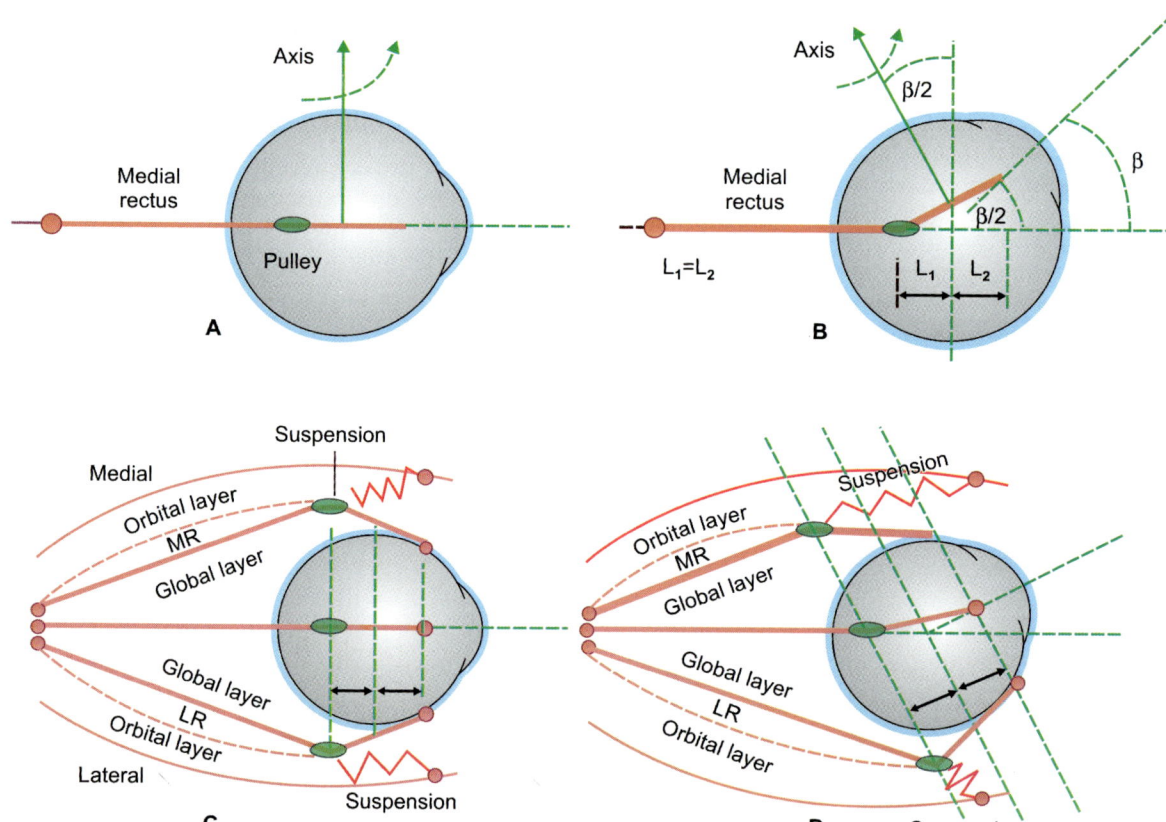

Fig. 2.10 *Schematic depiction of relationship of pulleys to the rotational axis of horizontal rectus muscles: A, Rotational axis of medial rectus (MR) muscle is perpendicular to the segment between the pulley and scleral insertion, and is thus vertical in central gaze; B, In supraduction by angle β, the distance L_1 from the pulley (ring) to globe center is equal to distance L_2 from globe center to the insertion, this causes the rotational axis of MR to tilt posteriorly by approximately angle β/2, the half-angle rule to implement Listing's law; C, Axial view showing pulleys (depicted as spindles) of the horizontal rectus muscles in central gaze; D, In adduction, the orbital layer of contracting MR shifts its pulley posteriorly, while the relaxing lateral rectus (LR) orbital layer allows its pulleys to move anteriorly (modified from Demer II, Invest Ophthalmol Visc Sci 2004).*

axis, around which supraduction occurs, moves posteriorly by half the angle (i.e. β/2) (Fig. 2.10B).

- *Half-angle-rule is maintained due to appropriate location of the rectus muscle pulleys* in such a way that the distance from pulley ring to centre of globe rotation (L_1) is equal to the distance from center of rotation to the muscle insertion on the sclera (L_2) (Fig. 2.10B).
- *Half-angle-rule allows the prerequist for the Listing's law*, which states that the eyeball can reach all positions of gaze by rotations around the axis that lie on the Listing's plane (vertical plane passing through the centre of rotation of eyeball).

Pulley suspension forces

As mentioned above, the muscle pulleys move along the length of the EOMs by the action of orbital layer of the muscles. However, the pulleys are located quite stably and stereo-typically in the transverse direction. Stability is provided by the suspensory forces due to interconnections of the pulleys to muscle sleeves, intermuscular septa, pulleys of other muscles and the periorbita (*see* Fig. 1.6)

Pulley kinematics of individual EOMs

Active pulley hypothesis (APH) states that the pulley shifts during the eye movements are generated by the contractile activity of the orbital layer of EOMs.

- Figure 2.10C is the diagrammatic depiction of the muscle pulleys, horizontal recti and the suspension forces in the central gaze (axial view)
- During adduction, the contracting orbital layer of the MR muscle pulls its pully posteriorly, while the relaxing lateral rectus orbital layer allows its pulley to move anteriorly (Fig. 2.10D).

Rectus EOMs activity during eye movements is as below:

- *Global layer* (GL) contraction leads to movement of eyeball. The mechanical load of GL is predominately the viscosity of relaxing antagonist EOMs and a load proportional to the speed of rotation.
- *Orbital layer* (OL) contraction moves the pulley posteriorly by the same distance as the scleral

insertion. The mechanical load of OL is due to the elasticity of the pulley suspension. This load is independent of speed of eyeball movement but proportional to the gaze angle.

- *Neural command needed by OL and GL of EOMs during contraction* is different. The ratio of motor nerve fibre to muscle fibre in GL is low (about 1:1) for rectus EOMs, reflecting high precision for ocular rotation.

However, for OL this ratio is higher (1:5 in horizontal recti and 1:2.5 in vertical recti); reflecting less percision for pulley control.

Inferior oblique (IO) muscle kinematics are as below:

- *Half-angle-kinematics* is also observed by IO muscle.
- *Orbital layer* (OL) of IO muscle is inserted on the pulley of IR and LR, and so the pulley of IO moves by half of the vertical ocular duction.
- *During oblique gaze shift* from supraducted adduction to infraducted abduction, the IO pulley moves anteroposteriorly by half the movement of IR pulley.

Superior oblique pulley and its kinematics is as below:

- *Superior oblique pulley is fixed* and so does not move during ocular movements.
- *Half-angle-kinematics* is also exhibited by SO, since the distance from trochlea to centre of globe is approximately equal to the distance from its insertion to centre of globe; so the rotational axis of SO muscle shifts by half the horizontal duction.

FIELD OF ACTION

This term is used in two ways to describe entirely separate and distinct concepts. Field of action may be used: (1) to indicate the direction of rotation of the eye, when a muscle contracts, and (2) to refer to the gaze position in which the effect of the muscle is most readily observed. The field of action for lateral rectus muscle and medial rectus muscle is same by both the concepts, i.e. abduction and adduction, respectively. However, they are not the same for other muscles, for example, the inferior oblique muscle creates some vertical, torsional, and horizontal movements whenever it contracts. Furthermore, the amount of vertical, horizontal, and torsional changes depends on the position of the eye. Thus, a field of action is not a single unvarying movement for the inferior oblique muscle. Also, only attempted elevation of the eye increases inferior oblique muscle activity; it does not increase with attempted abduction. (The vertical rectus muscles also tend to remain at similar levels of innervation across the horizaontal plane.) "*Field of activation*" would perhaps be a better term for this innervation sense of what a muscle does. The inferior oblique muscle is usually tested by its contribution to vertical eye movement in the adducted position; however, this is only because this is its field of greatest vertical action.

Thus, one must keep in mind three separate things: (1) the plane of the muscle action, (2) the gaze direction, which increases or decreases the innervation to the muscle, and (3) the vector distribution of the muscle's force (vertical, horizontal, torsional) in various gaze positions.

The importance of fields of action is that a deviation (strabismus) that increases with gaze in some directions is possibly due to weakness of the muscle normally pulling the eye in that direction. For example, esotropia increasing with gaze to the right may be due to right lateral rectus weakness.

inferior oblique from one eye act as *synergistic elevators*; however, in respect to torsion movement, they act as antagonists, as the superior rectus produces intorsion while the inferior oblique produces extorsion.

Each extraocular muscle has two synergists and two antagonists with exception of medial and lateral recti which have two synergists and three antagonists (Table 2.2).

Yoke muscles (contralateral synergists)

It refers to a pair of muscles (one from each eye) which contract simultaneously during version movements, e.g. right lateral rectus and left medial rectus muscles act as yoke muscles for dextroversion movement. The yoke muscle pairs for six cardinal positions of gaze are listed in Table 2.3.

According to recent theories, a pair of muscles in one eye can be yoked with a pair in the other eye.[10] For example, the elevators of one eye (superior rectus and inferior oblique muscles), are yoked as a unit to the elevators of the fellow eye. Similarly, a pair of depressors of one eye are yoked with a pair of depressor from the fellow eye. Further, yoking may change according to the different types of eye movement; e.g. left medial rectus is yoked with right lateral

AGONIST, SYNERGISTS, ANTAGONISTS AND YOKE MUSCLES

Agonist

It refers to any particular extraocular muscle producing a specific ocular movement; e.g. for producing abduction in right eye, the right lateral rectus muscle is agonist.

Synergists

Two muscles moving an eye in the same direction are called *synergists*. For example, superior rectus and inferior oblique muscles of the same eye act as *synergists* for elevation movement.

Antagonists

These are the muscles having opposite action in the same eye, e.g. medial and lateral recti. Further, as we know the superior rectus and

Table 2.2 Agonist, synergist and antagonist extraocular muscles

Agonist	Synergists	Antagonists
Medial rectus	Superior rectus	Lateral rectus
	Inferior rectus	Superior oblique
		Inferior oblique
Lateral rectus	Superior oblique	Medial rectus
	Inferior oblique	Superior rectus
		Inferior rectus
Superior rectus	Inferior oblique	Inferior rectus
	Medial rectus	Superior oblique
Inferior rectus	Superior oblique	Superior rectus
	Medial rectus	Inferior oblique
Superior oblique	Inferior rectus	Inferior oblique
	Lateral rectus	Superior rectus
Inferior oblique	Superior rectus	Superior oblique
	Lateral rectus	Inferior rectus

which is moving right and left, up and down. Thus, the pursuits help to keep the image of a moving object on the fovea constantly.

Characteristic features of pursuits are as follows:

- Images moving away from the fovea constitute the strongest stimuli for pursuit movements.
- Pursuit movements are elicited after a latency of 125 msec.
- Smooth following movements can keep up with targets moving up to 30° to 40°/sec. Beyond that point, the eyes tend to fall behind and saccades have to be made to catch up.
- The system has a very limited ability to follow targets moving back and forth; beyond 2 Hz, it breaks down.
- Only one image can be tracked normally.
- Usually, pursuits are performed to track an image of some real object in space. But it can also be an after image placed on the retina of some real object in space or a bright light. Also, a few people are able to track hallucinated targets, suppressing the saccadic system.
- The effectiveness of pursuit system is dependent on the degree of alertness.

3. *Position maintenance movements.* These help to maintain a specific gaze position by means of rapid micromovements called '*flicks*' and slow micromovements called '*drifts*'.

4. *Stabilization movements.* These include dynamic and tonic movements:

- *Dynamic movements.* Suppose one is sitting in a bus watching a bird out of the window. As the bus bounces, the eyes of the observer do not go off the target; since there is an immediate correction from the *vestibular system* to the eye muscles to correct for rotation of the head. Thus if the head is turned to the right, the eyes turn to the left.
- *Tonic movements.* Gravity and other linear accelerations also influence eye position by *labyrinthine reflexes* from the otoliths. These influences persist with head position and are not transient inputs just during the head movements. Examples of tonic movements: (1) when one is lying supine and the head is rotated to the right, the eyes will rotate to the left (and vice versa); (2) if while standing erect,

the head is tipped backward, the eyes will rotate downward (and vice versa). This phenomenon of tonic eye movements is also called as '*doll's eye*' mechanism.

Note: In monocular vision, the saccades, pursuits, position maintenance movements and the stabilization movements are a form of ductions.

VERGENCES

Vergences are disjugate, synchronous and symmetric movements of the two eyes in opposite direction. Vergences are tonic movements and are much slower than the versions (with a velocity of 80 to 250 times per second). A vergence may be a voluntary movement or an optomotor reflex. The same muscle in one eye may be involved in both versions and vergences. However, the underlying neuro-muscular mechanism may be quite different. For example, in the pathologic condition of a lesion interrupting the medial longitudinal fasciculus in the midbrain between the left sixth nerve nucleus on one side and the opposite right third nerve nucleus, the right medial rectus may show impairment of adduction on a movement of *levoversion.* However, it may demonstrate good adduction on convergence. This condition is known as internuclear ophthalmoplegia.

Types of vergences

Depending on the direction of movement, vergences are of following types:

1. *Convergence.* It is simultaneous and synchronous inward rotation of both eyes which results from co-contraction of the two medial rectus muscles. For details, see page 152.

2. *Divergence.* It is simultaneous and asynchronous outward rotation of both eyes which results from co-contraction of the two lateral rectus muscles. For details, see page 161.

3. *Vertical vergence.* By definition, vertical vergence refers to disjugate vertical movements of the two eyes in opposite direction, i.e. one eye should rotate upward and the other downward. However, in practice, the vertical vergence movements are classified as *positive* *vertical divergence* (in which, the right eye rotates upward in relation to the left one and so also called as right supravergence or right sursumvergence) and *negative vertical divergence* (in which, the left eye rotates upward in relation to the right one and so also called as left supravergence or left sursumvergence).

In practice, the vertical vergence movements are said to occur in a bid to correct the vertical heterophoria. Hence, these are also reflexly controlled and stimulated by retinal image disparity. The amplitude of vertical fusional vergences is much smaller than the amplitude of horizontal fusional vergences. The average amount of vertical fusional vergence is reported to be 3D to 8D.

4. Cyclovergence. Cyclovergence is the disjugate torsional movement in which the vertical meridians of the two eyes move in opposite directions to each other. *Incyclovergence* is a torsional disjugate movement in which the upper end of the vertical meridian (superior pole or 12 o'clock position) in each eye tilts towards the nose. *Excyclovergence* is opposite to incyclovergence, i.e. in it the upper end of the vertical meridian in each eye tilts away from the nose. Cyclovergences are also involuntary movements stimulated by retinal image disparity due to cyclophoria and thus occur in the interest of fusion to compensate for the cyclophoria. Their amplitude is expressed in degrees with average values being 6° to 10° for incyclovergence and 4° to 8° for excyclovergence. Thus, these movements are slow, of low amplitude, and their significance in compensating for a manifest cyclodeviation is not clear. These findings do not invalidate the concept that cyclofusion occurs predominantly on a sensory basis.[16]

BIBLIOGRAPHY

1. Park GS, Park GE: The center of ocular rotation in a horizontal plane. Am J Physiol 104:542, 1933.
2. Donders FC: On the Anomalies of Accommodation and Refraction of the Eye. R/London, Hatton, 1952, p 404.
3. Howard IP, Templeton WB: Human Spatial Orientation, London, John Wiley, 1966.
4. De Groot JA, Scott AB, Sindon A, Authier L: The human ocular anatomic position of rest: a quantitative study. In Fells P (ed): Second Congress International Strabismological Association, 1974, Marseilles, Marseilles, Diffusion Generale de Librairie, 1976, pp 408–414.
5. Volkmann AW: On the mechanics of the eye muscles. In Berichte der K sachs Ges d Wissensch math-phys K1 21:28, 1869. Summarized by H von Helmholtz in: Physiological Optics, 3rd ed, Leipzig, 1910. Translated and edited by JPC Southall. R/New York, Dover, 1962, III, p 128.
6. Nakagama T: Topographic anatomic studies on the orbit and its contents. Acta Soc Ophthalmol Jap 69: 2155, 1965.
7. Duane, A: A new classification of the motor anomalies of the eye, Ann. Ophthalmol. Otolaryngol. 5:969, 1896.
8. Duane, A: The basic principles of the diagnosis in motor anomalies of the eye, Arch. Ophthalmol, 48:2, 1919.
9. Duane, A: Anomalies of ocular muscles, Arch. Ophthalmol, 11:394, 1934.
9a. Demer II. Pivotal role of orbital connective tissues in binocular alignment and strabismus. The fundamental lecture. Invest Ophthalmol Vise Sci 2004, 45;72–38.
10. Boeder, P: Cooperative action of extraocular muscle, Br J Ophthalmol. 46:397, 1962.
11. Donders, FC Beitrag zur Lehre von den Bewegungen des menschlichen Auges, Holiand Beitr. Anat. Physiol. Wiss. 1:104, 384, 1848.
12. Listing, JB: Reported from Listing's original work. In Ruete, C.g.Th., Lehrbuch der Ophthalmologie fur Aerzte und Studirende, ed. 2, vol 1, Braunschweig, 1855. Friedr Vieweg and Sohn GHBH. 37ff.
13. Hering, E: die Lehre vom Binocularen Sehen, Leipzig, 1868, Wilhelm Engelmann.
14. Sherrington, CS: Experimental note on two movements of the eyes, J Physiol (Lond.) 17:27, 1894.
15. Daroff, RB: Physiologic, anatomic and pathophysiologic considerations of eye movements, Trans. Ophthalmol. Soc. U.K. 90:409, 1970.
16. Noorden, GK von: Clinical and theoretical aspects of cyclotropia, J Pediatr Ophthalmol Strabismus 21:126 1984.

Chapter

3

Visual Acuity and Contrast Sensitivity

VISUAL ACUITY

GENERAL CONSIDERATIONS

The vision or visual perception is a complex integration of light sense, form sense, contrast sense and colour sense. *Visual acuity* is considered a measure of form sense, so it refers to the spatial limit of visual discrimination. Technically speaking, visual acuity measurement involves the determination of a threshold. In terms of visual angle, the visual acuity is defined as the reciprocal of the minimum resolvable visual angle measured in minutes of arc for a standard test pattern. Therefore, to understand visual acuity, the knowledge about visual angle is essential.

VISUAL ANGLE

Visual angle is the angle subtended at the nodal point of the eye by the physical dimensions of an object in the visual field (Fig. 3.1). Visual angle is a useful and convenient mode of specifying the spatial extent of objects or elements in the visual field.

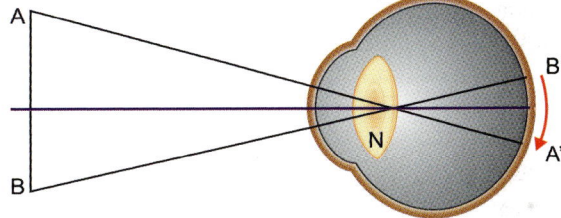

Fig. 3.1 *Visual angle (ANB) subtended at the nodal point by the physical dimensions (AB) of the object.*

It has been observed that the two adjacent points can be seen clearly and discretely only when these two points (say A and B in Fig. 3.1) produce a visual angle not less than 1 minute. The dimensions of the visual angle depend upon the size of the object as well as its distance from the eye. Therefore, to be seen clearly either the object should be large enough or it should be placed near the eye (at an appropriate distance). In terms of the length of the retinal image, it has been seen that the two points (A and B) will be seen clearly when their image size (A9B9) is more than 4.5 m. This is so, because the diameter of individual cone stimulated by the image points A9 and B9 is 1.5 m each and at least one

37

cone in between (of 1.5 m diameter) must be unstimulated. The retinal image size for a given visual angle may vary slightly with changes in viewing distance and associated changes in accommodation of the lens, but this effect is relatively small.

COMPONENTS OF VISUAL ACUITY

In clinical practice, measurement of the threshold of discrimination of two spatially separated targets (a function of the fovea centralis) is termed visual acuity. However, in theory, visual acuity is a highly complex function that consists of the following components:

- Minimum visible,
- Resolution,
- Recognition, and
- Minimum discriminable.

MINIMUM VISIBLE

The ability to determine whether or not an object is present in an otherwise empty visual field is termed *visibility* or *detection*. This kind of task is referred to as the *minimum visible* or *minimum detectable*.

RESOLUTION (ORDINARY VISUAL ACUITY)

Discrimination of two spatially separated targets is termed resolution. The minimum separation between the two points, which can be discriminated, is known as *minimum resolvable*. Measurement of the threshold of discrimination is essentially an assessment of the function of the fovea centralis and is termed *ordinary visual acuity*. The distance between the two targets is specified by the angle subtended at the nodal point of the eye. The normal angular threshold of discrimination for resolution measures approximately 30–60 seconds of an arc; it is usually called the minimum angle of resolution (MAR). The clinical tests determining visual acuity measure the form sense or reading ability of the eye. Thus, broadly, resolution refers to the ability to identify the spatial characteristics of a test figure. The test targets in these tests may either consist of letters (Snellen's chart) or broken circles (Landolt's ring). More complex targets include gratings and checkerboard patterns.

RECOGNITION

It is that faculty by virtue of which an individual not only discriminates the spatial characteristics of the test pattern but also identifies the patterns with which one has had some experience. Recognition is thus a task involving cognitive components in addition to spatial resolution. For recognition, the individual should be familiar with the set of test figures employed in addition to being able to resolve them. The most common example of recognition phenomenon is identification of faces. An average adult can recognize thousands of faces.

MINIMUM DISCRIMINABLE OR HYPERACUITY

Minimum discriminable refers to spatial distinction by an observer when the threshold is much lower than the ordinary acuity. The best example of minimum discriminable is *vernier acuity*, which refers to the ability to determine whether or not two parallel and straight lines are aligned in the frontal plane. The threshold values of vernier acuity (Fig. 3.2) are in the range of only a few seconds (2–10) of arc. Hyperacuity should not be confused with the threshold for the minimum visible, where merely the presence or absence of a target is being judged. The mechanism subserving hyperacuity is not clearly known, but so much is clear; no contradiction is involved with the optical and receptor mosaic factors that limit ordinary visual acuity.

MEASUREMENT OF VISUAL ACUITY

As discussed earlier, the visual acuity is a highly complex function that consists of:

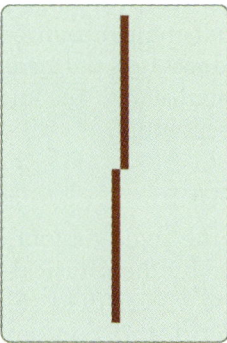

Fig. 3.2 *Typical target configuration for detecting vernier acuity.*

- *Minimum visible*, i.e. detection of presence or absence of stimulus,
- *Minimum separable*, i.e. judgement of location of a visual target relative to another element of the same target, and
- *Minimum resolvable* (ordinary visual acuity), i.e. the ability to distinguish between more than one identifying feature in a visible target.

In clinical practice, the measurement of visual acuity is considered synonymous with the measurement of 'minimum resolvable'. (However, in theory, it is not so, as is clear from the above.) The threshold of the minimum resolvable is between 30 seconds and 1 minute of arc. Therefore, all the clinical tests employed to measure the visual acuity are designed taking into consideration the threshold of the one minimum resolvable. Based on this basic principle, many visual acuity charts have been developed.

■ MILESTONES IN DEVELOPMENT OF VISION

Before discussing the various methods of visual assessment in infants, children, and adults, it will be worthwhile to have a quick look on the visual development. Important milestones in development of vision are summarized in Table 3.1.

Table 3.1 *Milestones in the development of vision*		
Age	*Visual milestone*	*Visual acuity*
Newborn	• Pupillary reaction to light • Blinking to light stimulus • Conjugate horizontal gaze developed	6/360 to 6/120 (by OKN)
1 week	• Vestibulo-ocular reflex	
2 weeks	• Small saccades develop • Follows horizontal moving objects	
1 month	• Fixation developing • Can watch mother's face for prolonged time	6/480–6/120 (by PL tests)
2 months	• Bifoveal fixation • Large saccades • Pursuits and convergence movements • Conjugate vertical gaze developed	6/120–6/60
3 months	• Watches movements of own hands and reaches out towards interesting objects • Prefers photographs to patterns	
4 months	• Foveal differentiation complete • Sensory fusion and accommodation begins to develops	6/120–6/30
5 months	• Blink response to visible threat (menace response) • Grasps and explores objects • Stereopsis begins to develop	6/90–6/24 6/12–6/6 (by VER)
6 months	• Accommodation well developed • Fusionalvergence well developed	6/90–6/24 6/12–6/6 (by VER)
9 months	• Visual differentiation of objects • Picks up small objects	6/48–6/12 6/6 (by VER) 18
18 months	• Visual acuity at adult levels on paediatric acuity card • Myelination of optic nerve completed	6/18–6/7.5
2–3 years	• Best visual acuity approaches near adult levels, but may not be 6/6 • Can play picture or letter recognition games • Can respond to some binocular vision tests • Contrast sensitivity well developed	6/12–6/6 (36 months)
5 years	• Stereopsis fully developed	6/6–6/5
8–10 years	• Critical period of monocular deprivation ends	6/6–6/5

TESTS FOR VISUAL ACUITY ASSESSMENT

Various visual acuity tests available can be grouped as follows:

I. *Detection acuity tests.* These assess the ability to *detect* the smallest stimulus without recognizing correctly. Common detection acuity tests are:
1. Dot visual acuity test
2. Catford drum test
3. Boek candy bead test
4. STYCAR graded ball's test
5. Schwarting metronome test

II. *Recognition acuity tests.* These are designed to assess the ability to recognize the stimulus or to distinguish it from other competing stimuli. These include:

A. *Direction identification tests*
1. Snellen's E-chart test
2. Landolt's C-chart test
3. Sjogren's hand test
4. Arrows test

B. *Letter-identification tests*
1. Snellen's letter chart test
2. Sheridan's letter test
3. Flook's symbol test
4. Lipman's HOTV test

C. *Picture identification charts (miniature toy test)*
1. Allen's picture cards test
2. Beale Collins picture charts test
3. Domino cards test
4. Lighthouse test
5. Miniature toy test of Sheridan

D. *Tests based on picture identification on behavioural pattern*
1. Cardiff acuity cards test
2. Bailey Hall cereal test

III. *Resolution acuity tests*
1. Optokinetic nystagmus (OKN) test
2. Preferential looking test (PLT)
    i. Two-alternative forced choice test
    ii. Operant variation looking test
    iii. Teller acuity cards test
3. Visually evoked response (VER)

Tests employed for visual acuity assessment at various age groups are summarized in Table 3.2.

MEASURMENT OF VISUAL ACUITY IN INFANTS

ASSESSMENT OF VISUAL ACUITY FROM BIRTH TO 3 MONTHS

At birth, visual acuity is 1/60 which improves very fast to 2/60 at 1 month and 6/60 at 4 months. With 1/60 vision, the child is able to fix a face moving within one metre. The fixation reflex and following reflexes take about 6–8 weeks to develop before which an infant may fix for a few seconds and give up. There are a few bizarre movements which appear till the development of definite fixation reflex. Neonates have sporadic jerky movements made up of saccadic eye movements without smooth pursuit. So, Visual acuity in a newborn and infant up to 3 months of age can be determined by the tests given below.

1. Blink reflex test. Blink reflex is present since birth (after 30 weeks of gestational age). It is occasionally present in decorticate infants as well. When bright light is shown, a normal infant should respond by blinking.

2. Pupillary light reflex test. Presence of pupillary light reflex indicates intact afferent visual neurologic pathways to the level of the brachium of the superior colliculus and efferent pathways to the iris sphincter. This reflex is present in premature babies over 29–31 weeks of gestational age. *This is most reliable test to determine presence of vision except in cortical blindness.* The test is best performed in a semi-darkned room because the infant's pupils are smaller than that of a normal adult and constrict in the presence of bright light in the room. In the semi-dark room, the pupil comes to a state of semi-dilatation that reacts briskly. The light used should be small, well focused and bright. Visualization in very young children sometimes requires a magnifying glass, as their pupils are smaller than those of the older children (because of decreased sympathetic tone) and the light responses are of small amplitude.

3. Vestibulo-ocular reflex. The vestibulo-ocular reflex (VOR) is generally tested by turning the newborn's head on his/her long axis and observing for the doll's eyes response (the eyes deviate opposite to the direction of head rotation).

Age	Tests for assessment of vision	Type of visual acuity
Birth–3 months	• Blink reflex • Pupillary light reflex • Vestibulo-ocular reflex test • Eye popping test • OKN • VER	Resolution acuity
3–6 months	• Fixation and following of objects or small toys • CSM (central, steady and maintained) fixation • Response to occlusion • OKN • VER	Resolution acuity
6–12 months	• Preferential looking tests (Teller acuity tests) • Catford drum test	Resolution acuity Detection acuity
1–3 years	• Cardiff acuity tests • Marble game test • TYCAR ball test • E game test • Boeck candy test	Resolution + Recognition acuity Detection acuity
3–5 years	• Broken wheel test • Landolt C test • Isolated hand figure test • Pictorial vision chart tests • Tumbling E test • HOTV test • Snellen's numbers • Snellen's letters	Recognition acuity
Above 5 years	• Snellen's numbers • Snellen's letters chart • LogMAR chart	Recognition acuity

Table 3.2 *Commonly used visual assessment tests at various age groups*

4. Eye popping test. Another behaviour that is unique to babies is *eye popping*. Sometimes, for a variety of reasons, very young infants don't show any distinguishable visual behaviour at all. In this case, the eye popping reflex indicates at least the baby's ability to detect changes in the room illumination. When the room lights are suddenly dimmed, the baby's upper eyelids should pop open wide for a moment. The baby will often close its eyes when the lights are brought up back, but will again pop its eyes open when the lights are dimmed. This behaviour is documented as "positive eye popping.

5. Optokinetic nystagmus (OKN) test. It is an objective method of visual assessment in infants and uncooperative children as well as adults. In this test, nystagmus is elicited by passing a succession of black and white stripes by means of OKN drum of the size 10 × 8 inches diameter, which is rotated at 8–10 rpm through the patient's field of vision (Fig. 3.3). Eyes respond with a slow movement in the direction of drum lasting about 0.2 sec and fast phase in the reverse direction of 0.1 sec. The visual angle subtended by the smallest strip width that still elicits an eye movement (minimum separable) is a measure of visual acuity. The only cooperation required in this test is that the infant be awake and should hold both eyes open. It is reported that OKN acuity is at least 6/120 in the newborns and improves fairly rapidly during the first few months of life, reaching to a level of 6/60 at 2 months, 6/30 at 6 months and 6/6 by 20–30 months. OKN is asymmetric in

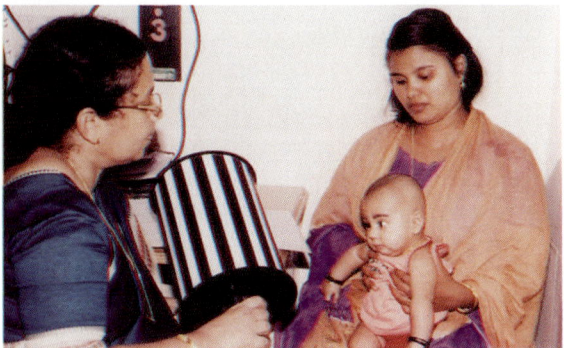

Fig. 3.3 *Optokinectic nystagmus test for visual acuity (Courtesy: Dr Elizabeth Joseph).*

newborns and becomes symmetric by 4–6 months of age.

6. Visual evoked response (VER). It refers to electroencephalographic (EEG) recording made from the occipital lobe in response to visual stimuli. VER is the only clinically objective technique available to assess the functional state of the visual system beyond the retinal ganglion cells. It is quite useful in assessing visual function in infants. It reflects acquity from the central retina and thus forms a good macular function test.

Flash VER is usually preformed in very young children or those incapable of fixing on a target. It just tells about the integrity of the macular and visual pathway.

Pattern reversal VER is recorded using some patterned stimulus, as in the checkerboard (Fig. 3.4). In it, the pattern of stimulus is changed (e.g. black squares go white and white become black), but the overall illumination remains the same. The pattern reversal VER depends on form sense and thus gives a rough estimate of the visual acuity. VER studies have shown visual acuity in infants to be 6/120 at the age of 1 month, which reaches to 6/60 at 2 months and 6/6–6/12 at the age of 6 months to 1 year.

Drawbacks of VER include:
- Expensive
- Time consuming
- Limited availability
- Not standardized
- Little clinical relevance

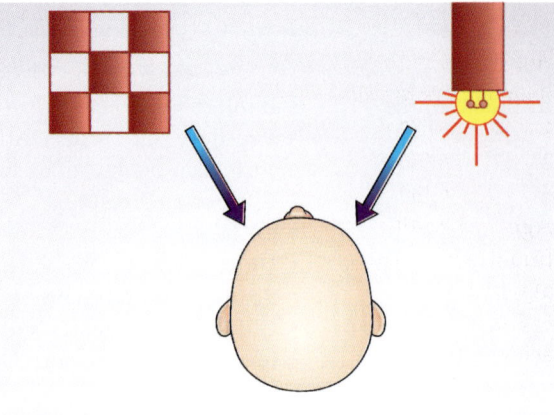

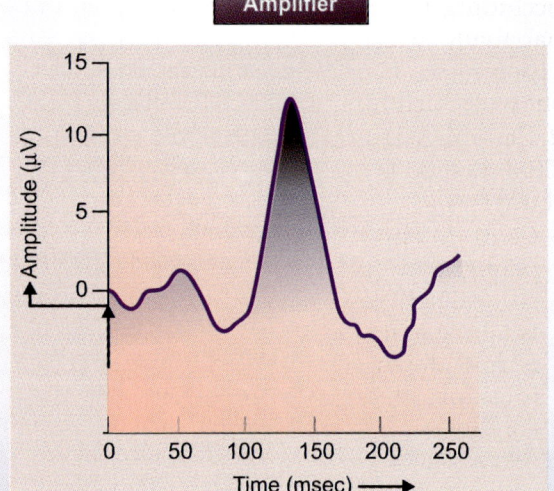

Fig. 3.4 *Technique of recording visually evoked response (VER) and record of normal VER pattern.*

Note: The discrepancy between estimated visual acuity values with optokinetic nystagmus, preferential looking test and visually evoked response at 6 months of age must be kept in mind while performing these tests (Table 3.3).

ASSESSMENT OF VISUAL ACUITY FROM 3 TO 6 MONTHS

Since the fixation develops to moving objects by 3-4 months of age, the visual acuity in this age group can be assessed, in addition to the above mentioned tests, the help of following tests based on fixation behaviour of the infant.

1. Fixation behaviour test. Ability of the child to fix and follow the face of the examiner, toys or

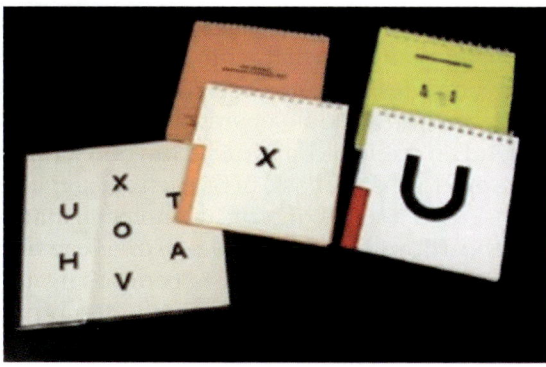

Fig. 3.10 *Sheridan–Gardiner single letter optotypes.*

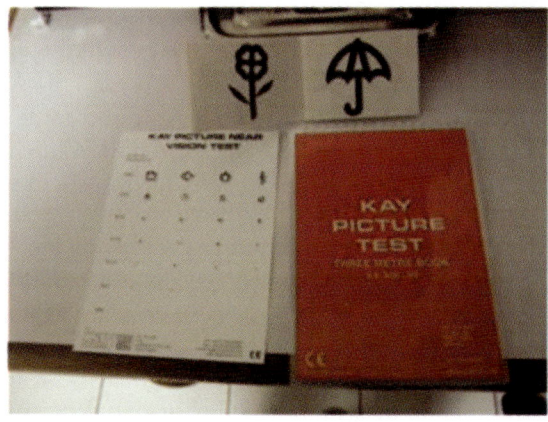

Fig. 3.12 *Kay picture test.*

7. *Pictorial vision charts*. When the child is able to verbalize, visual acuity chart showing pictures, rather than symbols, may be used. Many such charts have been devised, and one should be chosen that presents pictures of objects with which the child is likely to be familiar. Pictorial vision charts include Kay picture test, Allen cards test, Lae symbols test and BUST.

- *Allen cards test* (Fig. 3.11). In this test, seven optotypes are presented to the child for recognition at a test distance of 15 feet (20/40) at 3 years of age and 20 feet (20/30) at 4 years of age.
- *Kay pictures* (Fig. 3.12) is another picture optotype developed to assess visual acuity in young children at distance as well as at near. The figures are child friendly with matching cards for children who cannot speak. The individual elements subtend a visual angle of 1 min of arc and the total figure subtends 10 minutes of arc at the eye. The available test

booklets are for 6 m and 3 m distance. The 3 m booklet used for younger children who will not be attentive at 6 m. Near point cards are also available to assess near visual acuity.

- *Lae symbols test* (Fig. 3.13) was developed by Dr Lea Hyvärinen, a Finnish paediatric ophthalmologist, who developed a vast array of testing devices that have been standardized using four pictures—circle, square, house and apple. Lea numbers were developed in 1993 and calibrated in 1994. These optotypes can be presented as single characters, as a wall chart at a distance of 10 to 20 feet. They can be presented on a video display terminal screen or in the form of a flip book. With the Landolt C type being the reference optotype since 1988, earlier to which Snellen E chart was the reference optotype, the size of the 1.0 (20/20,6/6) optotypes was reduced from 7.5 to 6.84 minutes of arc.

Lea symbols now have two important basic features of good optotypes that they blur equally and are calibrated against the Landolt–C. This is a good way of testing

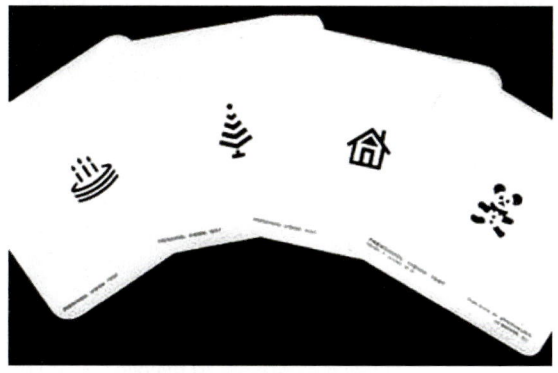

Fig. 3.11 *Allen cards test.*

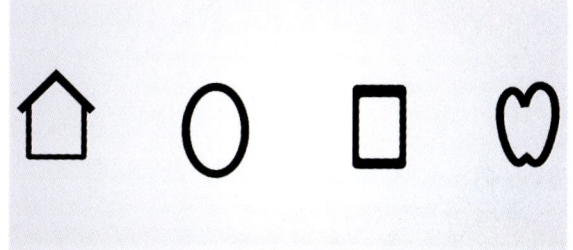

Fig. 3.13 *Lae symbols test.*

individuals who do not use the western alphabet. Hence it eliminates the problem with language barriers.

- *BUST is* another picture test designed to test visual acuity of children with vision impairment and developmental handicaps. BUST is an acronym for the Swedish words for "visual acuity and picture perception test". The range of visual acuity for distance acuity measurement values goes from 0.02 to 1.6 (20/1000to 20/10).

7. *Boek candy bead test.* The child is asked to match beads at 40 cm. Snellen's visual acuity equivalent of 20/200 is estimated by this method.

8. *Light home picture cards.* A chart containing an apple, a house and an umbrella (Fig. 3.14), arranged in Snellen's equivalents of 20/200–20/10 is used, and the child is asked to identify the pictures along the lines. The test is carried out at 10 ft.

MEASUREMENT OF VISUAL ACUITY IN SCHOOL CHILDREN (ABOVE 5 YEARS) AND ADULTS

- *Snellen's visual acuity charts* are most commonly employed in this age group. Illiterates E charts and Landolt's C charts are used as alternative to Snellen's test types.
- *LogMAR charts* enable a more accurate estimate of acuity as compared to other charts. Because of high accuracy, these are the most commonly used charts in research settings/clinical trials.

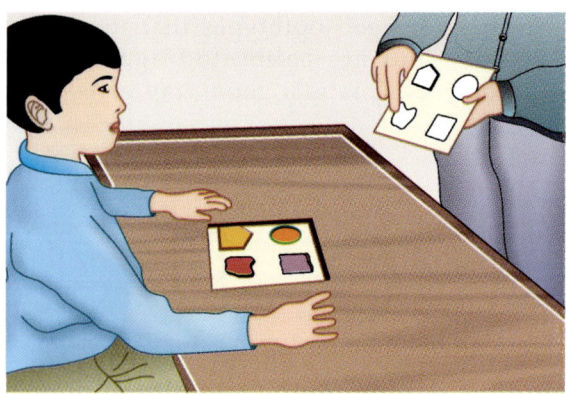

Fig. 3.14 *Light home picture cards.*

1. Snellen's test types

The distant central visual acuity is usually tested by Snellen's test types. The fact that two distant points can be visible as separate only when they subtend an angle of 1 minute at the nodal point of the eye forms the basis of Snellen's test types. It consists of a series of black capital letters on a white board, arranged in lines, each progressively diminishing in size. The lines comprising the letters have such a breadth that they will subtend an angle of 1 minute at the nodal point. Each letter of the chart is so designed that it fits in a square, the sides of which are five times the breadth of the constituent lines. Thus at the given distance, each letter subtends an angle of 5 minutes at the nodal point of the eye (Fig. 3.15). The letter of the top line of Snellen's chart (Fig. 3.16) should be read clearly at a distance of 60 m. Similarly, the letters in the subsequent lines should be read from a distance of 36, 24, 18, 12, 9, 6, 5 and 4 m.

Landolt's test types It is similar to Snellen's test types except that in it instead of the letter the broken circles are used. Each broken ring subtends an angle of 5 minutes at the nodal point and is constructed similar to letter of Snellen's test types (Fig. 3.17).

With Snellen's letters, the end point consists of letter recognition; with Landolt's rings, it consists of the detection of the orientation of the break in the circle. Each method has advantages and disadvantages. Letter targets represent a practical visual test. However, the ability to recognize the target is influenced by literacy and past experience, even if the targets are somewhat blurred. Landolt's rings were designed to eliminate these factors and present a more objective test. However, since the gap can be placed in only four positions (up, down, left and right), guessing becomes an important factor.

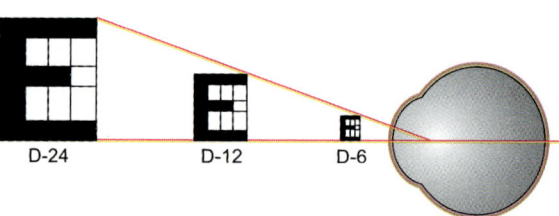

Fig. 3.15 *Principle of Snellen's test types.*

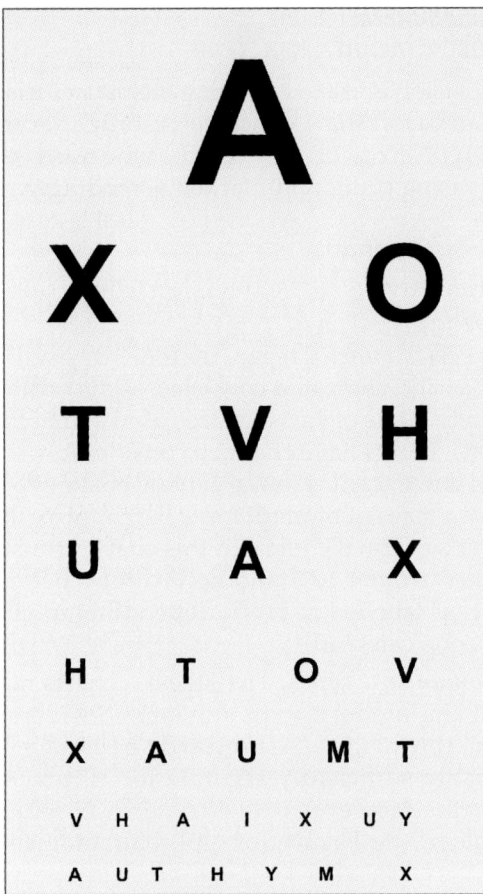

Fig. 3.16 *Snellen's test types.*

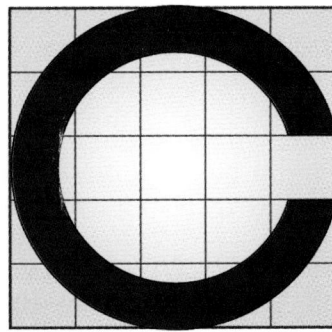

Fig. 3.17 *Construction of Landolt's visual acuity target.*

Also letter tests remain much less confusing for the patient and the examiner, since the identification of letters is both immediate and unequivocal.

Procedure of testing. For testing distant visual acuity, the patient is seated at a distance of 6 m from the Snellen's chart, so that the rays of light are practically parallel and the patient exerts minimal accommodation. The chart should be properly illuminated (not less than 20 footcandle). The patient is asked to read the chart with each eye separately and the visual acuity is recorded as a fraction, the numerator being the distance of the patient from the letters and the denominator being the smallest letters accurately read.

When the patient is able to read up to 6-m line, the visual acuity is recorded as 6/6, which is normal. Similarly, depending upon the smallest line that the patient can read from the distance of 6 m, his or her vision is recorded as 6/9, 6/12, 6/18, 6/24, 6/36 and 6/60. If one cannot see the top line from 6 m, he or she is asked to slowly walk towards the chart till one can read the top line. Depending upon the distance at which one can read the top line, the vision is recorded as 5/60, 4/60, 3/60, 2/60 and 1/60.

If the patient is unable to read the top line even from 1 m, he or she is asked to count fingers (CF) of the examiner. His or her vision is recorded as CF-39, CF-29, CF-19 or CF close to face, depending upon the distance at which the patient is able to count fingers. When the patient fails to count fingers, the examiner moves his or her hand close to the patient's face. If one can appreciate the hand movements (HM), visual acuity is recorded as HM positive. When the patient cannot distinguish the hand movements, the examiner notes whether the patient can perceive light (PL) or not. If yes, vision is recorded as PL positive and if not it is recorded as PL negative.

2. LogMAR visual acuity charts

LogMAR stands for **Log**arithm of the **M**inimum **A**ngle of **R**esolution. A LogMAR chart comprises rows of letters and has equal number of letters in each line (Fig 3.18). It is used at a distance of 4 meters. It is designed to enable a more accurate estimate of acuity as compared to other charts (e.g. the Snellen chart), for this reason, it is recommended in research settings.

An observer who can resolve details as small as 1 minute of visual angle scores LogMAR 0, since the base-10 logarithm of 1 is 0; an observer

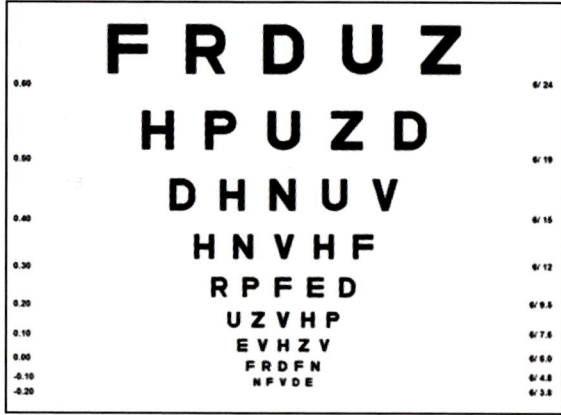

Fig. 3.18 *LogMAR visual acuity chart.*

who can resolve details as small as 2 minutes of visual angle (i.e. reduced acuity) scores LogMAR 0.3, since the base-10 logarithm of 2 is 0.3; and so on.

Visual acuity equivalents in different notations

Table 3.4 indicates different ways for specifying visual acuity levels, viz. Minimal angle of resolution (MAR), Snellen's acuity, efficiency rating, Snellen's fraction (that is the reciprocal of the MAR) and the logarithm of Snellen's fraction.

Near vision is tested by asking the patient to read a near-vision chart which consists of a series of different sizes of 'printer types' arranged in decreasing order and marked accordingly.

Near-vision charts

Commonly used near-vision charts are as follows.

1. *Jaeger's chart.* Jaeger, in 1867, devised the near-vision chart that consisted of the ordinary printers' fonts of varying sizes used at that time. Printers' fonts have changed considerably since then; however, it is now a general custom to use various sizes of modern fonts that approximate Jaeger's original choice. In this chart, prints are marked from 1 to 7 and accordingly patient's acuity is labelled as J1–J7, depending upon the print one can read.

2. *Roman test types.* The Jaeger's charts made from the modern fonts deviate considerably from the original standard, but they are probably sufficiently accurate for all practical purposes. However, to overcome this theoretical problem, the Faculty of Ophthalmologists of

Table 3.4 *Visual acuity equivalents in different notations*						
MAR or minimum angle of resolution (minutes of arc)	Snellen's visual acuity ft	m	Snell-Sterling visual efficiency (%)	Loss of central vision (%)	Snellen's fraction acuity relative 20/20	LogMAR acuity relative to
0.5	20/10	6/3	109	0	2.0	0.3
0.75	20/15	6/4.5	104	0	1.33	0.1
1.00	20/20	6/6	100	0	1.0	0
1.25	20/25	6/7.5	96	4	0.8	−0.1
1.5	20/30	6/9	91	9	0.67	−0.18
2.0	20/40	6/12	84	16	0.5	−0.3
2.5	20/50	6/15	76	24	0.4	−0.4
3.0	20/60	6/18	70	30	0.33	−0.5
4.0	20/80	6/24	58	40	0.25	−0.6
5.0	20/100	6/30	49	50	0.2	−0.7
6.0	20/120	6/36	41	60	0.17	−0.78
7.5	20/150	6/45	31	70	0.133	−0.88
10.0	20/200	6/60	20	80	0.10	−1.0
20.0	20/400	6/120	3	90	0.05	−1.3

Great Britain in 1952 devised another near-vision chart. It consists of 'Times Roman' type fonts with standard spacing (Fig. 3.19). According to this chart, the near vision is recorded as N5, N6, N8, N10, N12, N18, N36 and N48.

3. Snellen's near-vision test types. Snellen introduced the so-called 'Snellen's equivalent for near vision' on the same principles as his distant types. The graded thickness of the letters of different lines is about 1/17th of the distant-vision chart letters. In this event, the letters equivalent to 6/6 line subtend an angle of 5 minutes at an average reading distance (35 cm/ 14 in.).

The unusual configuration of letters of this chart, however, cannot be constructed from the available printers' fonts. It can only be reproduced by a photographic reduction of the standard Snellen's distant-vision test types to approximately 1/17th of their normal size. Further, such a test has never become popular.

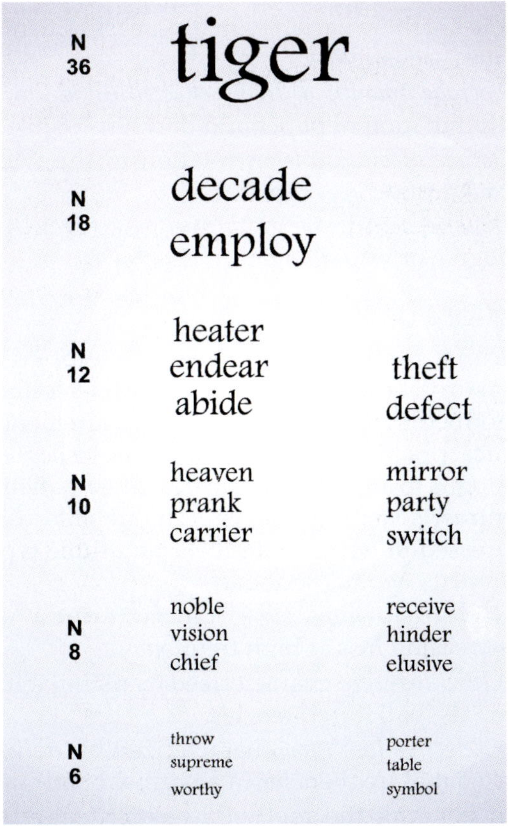

N 36	tiger	
N 18	decade employ	
N 12	heater endear abide	theft defect
N 10	heaven prank carrier	mirror party switch
N 8	noble vision chief	receive hinder elusive
N 6	throw supreme worthy	porter table symbol

Fig. 3.19 *Near-vision chart.*

The graded sizes of pleasing types of passages from literature, the reading of which helps in the interpretation, are habitually employed.

4. Lea near-vision cards. This test assesses a child's functional vision at near distances. It can also be used to familiarize child with testing procedure before introducing a distance test. It consists of cards measuring 8" × 10" (20.3 cm × 25.4 cm) which contain proportionally spaced (logMAR) lines on one side and more tightly-spaced symbols on the opposite side. Line sizes range from 20/400 to 20/10 (6/120 to 6/3) equivalent, 0.05 to 2.00. Response key is printed on test card. Testing distance is about 16 inches/ 40 cm.

Procedure of testing

For testing the near vision, the patient is seated in a chair and asked to read the near-vision chart kept at a distance of 25–35 cm, with a good illumination thrown over his or her left shoulder. Each eye should be tested separately. The near vision is recorded as the smallest type that can be read comfortably by the patient. A note of the approximate distance at which the near-vision chart is held should also be made. Thus near vision (NV) is recorded as:

- NV 5 J_1 at 30 cm (in Jaeger's notation)
- NV 5 N_5 at 30 cm (in Faculty's notation)

Near-vision equivalents in different notations

These are shown in Table 3.5.

CONTRAST SENSITIVITY

INTRODUCTION

Contrast sensitivity is the ability to perceive slight changes in luminance between regions that are not separated by definite borders and is just as important as the ability to perceive sharp outlines of relatively small objects. It is only the latter ability that is tested by means of the Snellen's test types. In many diseases, loss of contrast sensitivity is more important and disturbing for the patient than is the loss of visual acuity. Further, contrast sensitivity may be impaired even in the presence of normal visual acuity.

Visual angle (minutes)	Snellen equivalent	American Medical Association notation	Decimal notation	Jaeger notation	Faculty's Roman test types notation	Metre notation (m)	Central visual efficiency for near (%)	Vision loss (%)
5.00	20/20	14/14	1.00	J1	N5	0.37	100	0
6.25	20/25	14/17	0.80	J1	N6	0.43	100	0
7.50	20/30	14/21	0.66	J2	N8	0.50	95	5
10.00	20/40	14/28	0.50	J4	N10	0.75	90	10
12.50	20/50	14/35	0.40	J6	N12	0.87	50	50
15.00	20/60	14/42	0.33	J8	N14	1.00	40	60
20.00	20/80	14/56	0.25	J10	N18	1.50	20	80
25.00	20/100	14/70	0.20	J1	N24	1.75	15	85
50.00	20/200	14/140	0.10	J17	N36	3.50	2	98

Table 3.5 *Equivalent visual acuity notations for near*

TYPES OF CONTRAST SENSITIVITY

1. Spatial contrast sensitivity

Spatial contrast sensitivity refers to detection of striped patterns at various levels of contrast and spatial frequencies. In its measurement, patient is presented with sine wave gratings of parallel light and dark bands (Arden gratings) and is asked to tell the minimum contrast at which the bars can be seen at each frequency. The width of the bars is defined as spatial frequency which expresses the number of pairs of dark and light bars subtending an angle of 18 at the eye. A high spatial frequency implies narrow bars, whereas a low spatial frequency indicates wide bars.

2. Temporal contrast sensitivity

Here the contrast sensitivity function is generated for time-related (temporal) processing in the visual system by presenting a uniform target field modulated sinusoidal in time, rather than as a function of spatial position.

Both temporal and spatial contrast sensitivity testing yield significantly more complete and systematic data on the status of visual performance than the conventional tests.

MEASUREMENT OF CONTRAST SENSITIVITY

When a subject is presented with the grating frequencies and contrast below which resolution is impossible, it indicates the threshold level; and the reciprocal of this contrast threshold gives the contrast sensitivity.

Contrast sensitivity is measured as $(L_{max} 2 L_{min})/(L_{max} 1 L_{min})$, where L is the luminance recorded by photocells scanning across the gratings.

VARIABLES IN THE MEASUREMENT

There are three variables in the measurement of contrast sensitivity:
- *Average amount of light reflected* depends on illumination of paper and darkness of ink.
- *Degree of blackness* in relation to the white background, i.e. contrast.
- *Distance between the grating periods* or cycles per degree of visual angle.

METHODS OF MEASUREMENT

Various methods have been developed to measure contrast sensitivity. Bodis-Wollner, introducing contrast sensitivity measurement in clinical practice, suggested the name *visuogram*, analogue to an *audiogram*, to describe a patient's 'contrast sensitivity curve'. The deficits were expressed in terms of decibels, and three types of deficits were described:
- *High-frequency type* characterized by increasing loss at high frequency.
- *A level-loss type* characterized by a similar loss for all spatial frequencies.
- *A selective-loss type* characterized by deficits of spatial frequencies in a narrow band.

In general, the methods recommended to measure contrast sensitivity include: simple plates, cathode ray tube display on a screen, letter acuity charts, laser interferometer (LI) which produces grating on the retina, visual field testing using low contrast rings on stimuli, pattern discrimination test, prototype for forced choice printed test, visually evoked cortical potentials to checkerboard pattern reversal dependent contrast threshold measurement, two-alternative forced choice test and many more.

Some of the simple, inexpensive but reliable methods of measuring contrast sensitivity are described in brief in the following text.

1. Arden gratings. Arden, in 1978, introduced a booklet containing seven plates: one *screening plate* (No. 1) and six *diagnostic plates* (No. 2–7). The contrast changes from top to bottom and covers a range of approximately 1.76 log units. The plates are studied at 57 cm, with spatial frequency increasing from 0.2 cycles/degree to 6.4 cycles/degree, each being double the frequency of the previous one. A score of 1–20 is assigned to each plate, depending upon the amount of plate uncovered. Sum of six plates with an upper limit of 82 was established for normal subjects together with an interocular difference of less than 12.

2. Cambridge low-contrast gratings. Cambridge low-contrast gratings consist of a *set of ten plates* containing gratings in a spiral bound booklet. To perform the test, the booklet is hung on a wall at a distance of 6 m. The pages are presented in pairs, one above the other. One page in each pair contains gratings and the other is blank (Fig. 3.20), but the pages have the same mean reflectance. The subject is simply required to choose which page, top or bottom, contains the gratings. The pages are shown in order of descending contrast and are stopped when the first error is made. Four descending series are shown separately to each eye. When no error is made at plate 10, then a score of 11 is given. Depending upon the total score of the patient from four series, the contrast sensitivity is noted from the conversion table (Fig. 3.21).

3. Pelli-Robson contrast sensitivity chart. This chart consists of letters that subtend an angle of 38 at a distance of 1 m. The chart is printed on both the sides. The two sides have different letter

Fig. 3.20 *Cambridge low-contrast gratings.*

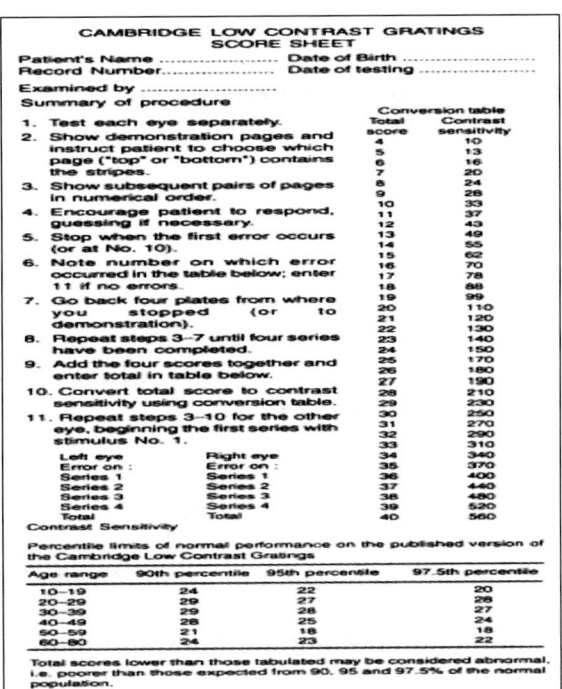

Fig. 3.21 *Cambridge low-contrast gratings score sheet and conversion table.*

sequence but are otherwise identical. The letters on chart are organized as triplets, there being two triplets in each line (Figs 3.22A and B). The contrast decreases from one triplet to the next. The log contrast sensitivity varies from 0.00 to 2.25.

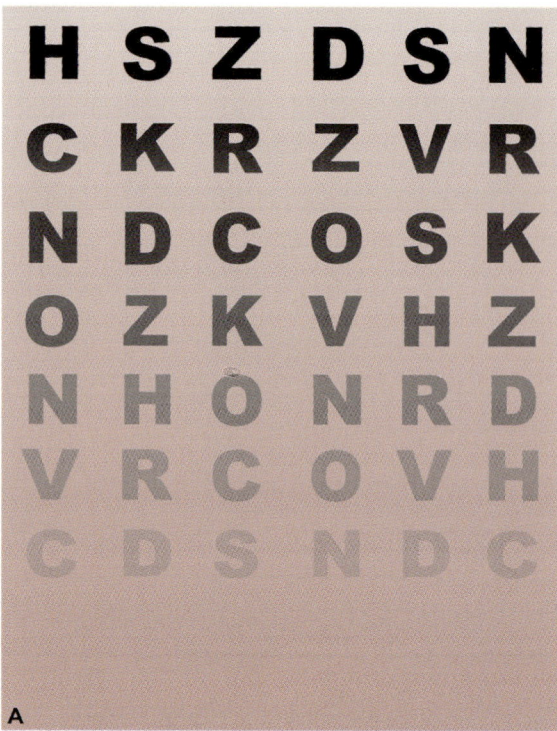

A

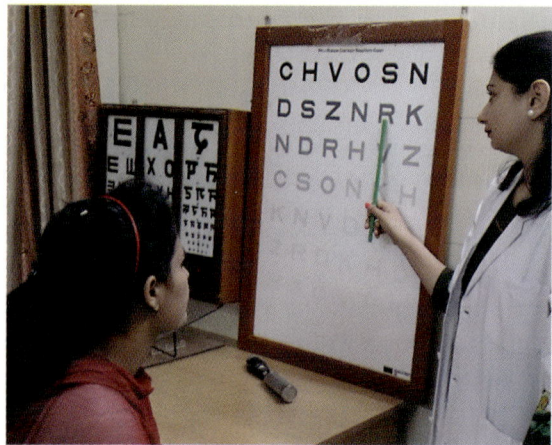

Fig. 3.23 *Measurement of contrast sensitivity with Pelli-Robson chart.*

0.00	H S Z	D S N	0.15
0.30	C K R	Z V R	0.45
0.60	N D C	O S K	0.75
0.90	O Z K	V H Z	1.05
1.20	N H O	N R D	1.35
1.50	V R C	O V H	1.65
1.80	C D S	N D C	1.95
B 2.10	K V Z	O H R	2.25

Fig. 3.22 *Pelli-Robson contrast sensitivity chart. A, Photograph; B, Log contrast sensitivity score of each triplet.*

To perform the test, the chart is hung on the wall, so that its centre is approximately at the level of the subject's eye. The chart is illuminated as uniformly as possible, so that the luminance of the white areas is between the acceptable range of 60 and 120 cd/m, which corresponds to a photographic exposure between 1/15 and 1/30 second at f/5.6 with an ASA of 100. The luminance is determined with the help of a light meter.

While recording, the subject sits directly in front of the chart at a distance of 1 m (with the best distance correction) (Fig. 3.23). The subject is made to name or outline each letter on the chart, starting from the upper left corner and reading horizontally across the line. Subject is made to guess, even when he or she believes that the letters are invisible. The test is concluded when the subject guesses two of the three letters of the triplet incorrectly. The subject's sensitivity is indicated by the finest triplet for which two of the three letters are named correctly.

4. The Vistech chart. This chart consists of sine wave gratings and is used at a distance of 3 m from the subject. In this test, contrast is assessed at several spatial frequencies (distance of the separation of the grating bars) and the subject has to identify the orientation of the grating, i.e. whether vertical or 158 clockwise, or anti-clockwise.

5. Vector vision chart. Vector vision CSV 1000 (USA) chart test frequency of 3,6,12 and 18 cpd.

6. Fact CS chart. The fact CS chart tests for 1.5, 3, 6, 12 and 18 cpd.

BIBLIOGRAPHY

1. Alpern M: Accommodation. In Davson H (ed): The Eye, Vol 3. Muscular Mechanisms. New York, Academic Press, 1962, pp 191–229.
2. Arden GB, Jacobson JJ. A simple grating test for contrast sensitivity. Preliminary results indicate

value in screening for glaucoma. Invest Ophthalmol Visual Sci 1978;17: 23–32.

3. Arden GB. Testing contrast sensitivity in clinical practice. Clin Vis Sci 1988; 2(3): 213–24.

4. Arden GB. Testing contrast sensitivity in clinical practice. Clin Vision Sci 1988; 2 (3); 213–24.

5. Arden GB. Visual loss in patients with normal visual acuity. Trans Ophthalmol Soc UK 1978; 98:219–23.

6. Arundale K. An investigation in to variation of contrast sensitivity with age and ocular pathology. Br J Ophthalmol 1978; 62:213–15.

7. Bahrick HP, Bahrick PO, Wittlinger RP. Fifty years of memory for names and faces: a cross-sectional approach. J Exp Psychol Gen 104:54–75, 1975.

8. Barlett NR. Thresholds as dependent on some energy relations and characteristics of the subject. In: Graham CH(ed). Vision and Visual Perception. New York, Wiley, 1965, pp 154–84.

9. Berlyne DE. The influence of the albedo and complexity of stimuli on visual functions in the human infant. Bt. J. Psychol 49–315, 1958.

10. Bodis Wollner L. Visual acuity and contrast sensitivity in ptients with cerebral lesions. Science 1972; 178: 769–771.

11. Brown JL, Black JE. Criticalduration for resolution of acuity targets. Vision Res 16:309–15, 1976.

12. Brown JL, Mueller CG. Brightness discrimina-tion and brightness contrast. In: Graham CH(ed). Vision and Visual Perception. Wiley, New York, 1965, pp 208–50.

13. Butler T and Westheimer G. Interference with stereoscopic acuity: spatial, temporal and disparity tuning, Vision Res. 18:1387, 1978.

14. Campbell FW, Green DG. Optical and retinal factors affecting visual acuity. J Physiol 1965; 181:576–93.

15. Campbell FW, Robson JG. Application of Fourier analysis to the visibility of gratings. J Physiol 1968; 197: 551–56.

16. Dala Sala S, Bertoni G, Somazzi L. Impaired contrast sensitivity in diabetic patients with and without retinopathy. A new technique for rapid assessment. Br J Ophthalmol 1985; 69: 136–42.

17. Ditchburn RW and Ginsborg BL (1952). Vision with a stabilised retinal image, Nature, 170, 36–37.

18. Dobson V and Teller D. Visual acuity in human infants: a review and comparison of behavioral and electro-physiological sutdies,, Vision Res. 18: 1469, 1978.

19. Dobson V, Teller D, Lee CP and Wade B. A behavioral method for efficient screening of visual acuity in young infants. I. Preliminary laboratory development. Invest. Ophthalmol. Vis Sci. 17:1142, 1978.

20. Drum B et al. Pattern discrimination perimetry. A new concept in visual field testing. Doc Ophthalmol Proc Ser 1987; 49:433.

21. Emsley HH. Irregular astigmatism of the eye. Effect of correcting lenses, Trans. Opt. Soc. Lond. 27:28, 1925.

22. Fantz R. Pattern vision in young infants, Psychol, Rec. 8:43, 1958.

23. Flom MC, Weymouth FW, Kahneman D. Visual resolution and contour interaction. J Opt Soc Am 53:1026, 1963.

24. Hartridge H. The visual perception of fine detail. Philos Trans R Soc Lond (Biol Sci) 232; 519–671, 1947.

25. Hecht S, Mintz EV. The visibility of single lines at various illuminations and the retinal basis of visual resolution. J Gen Physiol 22:593–612, 1939.

26. Hecht S, Ross S, Mueller CG. The visibility of lines and squares at high brightnesses. J Opt Soc Am 37: 500–07, 1947.

27. Hecht S. Vision. II. The nature of the photoreceptor process. In: Murchison C(ed). A Handbook of General Experimental Psychology, Worcester MA, Clark University Press, 1934, pp 704–828.

28. Howe JW, Mitchell KW, Mahabateswara M, Abdel-Katek MN. Visual evoked potential latency and contrast sensitivity in patients with posterior chamber intraocular lens implants, Br J Ophthalmol 1986; 70: 890–4.

29. Hoyt CS, Nickel BL and Billson FA. Ophthalmological examination of the infant: developmental aspect, Surv. Ophthalmol. 26:177, 1982.

30. L Schade O. Optical and photoelectric analogue of eye. J Opt Soc Am 1956; 46:721–39.

31. Leibowitz H: The effect of pupil size on visual acuity for photometrically equated test fields at various levels of luminance, J. Opt.Soc. Am. 42:416, 1952.

32. Lempert P, Hopcroft M, Lempert Y. Evaluation of posterior subcapsular cataracts with spatial contrast acuity. Ophthalmology 1987; 94(S): 14–18.

33. Lythgoe RJ. The measurement of visual acuity. Med Res Council Sp Rep Ser, No. 173, 1932.

34. Marg E, Freeman DN, Peltzman P, and Goldstein P. Visual acuity development in human infants:

evoked potential measurements. Invest. Ophthalmol. 15:150. 1976.

35. Mayer L, Fulton A, and Rodier D. Grating and recognition acuities of pediatric patients, Ophthalmology 91:947, 1984.

36. Pelli DG, Robson JG, Wilkin AJ. The design of a new letter chart for measuring contrast sensitivity. Clin Vis Sci 1988; 2(3): 187–99.

37. Pirenne MH, Marriott FHC, and O'Doherty EF. Individual differences in night-vision efficiency. Med Res Council Sp Rep Ser, No 294, 1957.

38. Regan D, Neima D. Low contrast letter charts as a test of visual function. Ophthalmology 1983; 90: 1192.

39. Riggs LA, Ratliff F, Cornsweet JC, and Cornsweet EF (1953). The disappearance of steadily fixated visual test objects. F. opt. Soc.Amer., 43,495–501.

40. Riggs LA. Visual acuity. In Graham CH (ed). Vision and Visual Perception. New York, Wiley, 1965, pp 321–49.

41. Rodieck RW. The Vertebrate Retina. San Francisco, WH Freeman and Co, 1973.

42. Shlaer S. The relation between visual acuity and illumination. J Gen Physiol 21:165–88, 1937.

43. Skalka WH. Effect of age on Arden grating acuity. Br J Ophthalmol 1980; 84:21–23.

44. Sokol S, Measurement of infant visual acuity from pattern reversal evoked potentials, Vision Res. 18:33, 1978.

45. Teller DY and Movshon JA. Visual development, Vision Res. 26:1483, 1986.

46. Teller DY, and Movhson JA: Visual develop-ment, Vision Res. 26:1483, 1986.

47. Teller DY. The forced choice preferential looking procedure. A psychophysical technique for use with human infants, infant Behav. Dev. 2:135, 1979.

48. Tomlinson E and Martinez D. The measurement of visual acuity: comparison of Teller acuity cards with Snellen and MBL results, Am. Orthopt. J. 38:130,1988.

49. Vaegan F, Halliday BL. A forced choice test improves clinical contrast sensitivity testing. Br J Ophthalmol 1982; 66: 477–91.

50. Weale RA. The Aging Eye. London, Leis, 1963.

51. Westheimer G and Hauske G. Temporal and spatial interference with vernier acuity, Vision Res. 15:1137, 1975.

52. Westheimer G and Hauske G: temporal and spatial interference with vernier acuity. Vision Res 15:1137, 1975.

53. Westheimer G and Mckee SP. Visual acuity in the presence of retinal-image motion, J. Opt. Soc. Am. Am 65:847, 1975.

54. Wilcox WW, Purdy DM. Visual acuity and its physiological basis. Br J Psychol 23:233–61, 1933.

55. Wilkins AJ, Delia SS, Somazzi L, Smith N. Age related norms for the Cambridge low contrast gratings, including details concerning their design and use. Clin Vision Sci 1988; 2(3): 201–12.

56. Wolf E, Gardiner JS. Studies on the scatter of light in the dioptic media of the eye as a basis of visual glare. Arch Ophthalmol 74:338–45, 1965.

57. Woodson WE: Human Engineering Guide for Equipment Designes. Los Angeles, University of California Press, 1954.

58. Wulfing EA: Uber den Kleinsten Gesichts-winkel. Z Biol 29:199, 1892.

59. Yamazaki H, Adachi-Usami E, Chiba J. Contrast thresholds of diabetic patients determined by VECP and psychophysical measurements. Acta Ophthalmol 1982; 60:386–92.

Chapter

4

Binocular Vision

BINOCULAR VISION: DEFINITION AND GRADES

DEFINITION

Romano and Romano[1] defined binocular vision as that state of simultaneous vision with two seeing eyes (neither of which needs necessarily be normal) that occurs when an individual fixes his visual attention on an object of regard. By and large binocular vision implies binocular single vision (fusion) and a high level stereoacuity.

Though, cursorily binocular vision may be defined as the coordinated use of the two eyes to produce a single mental impression, its full definition includes its full scope, i.e. grades of binocular vision.

GRADES OF BINOCULAR VISION

Thus, binocular vision may be defined to consist of following:

Simultaneous perception (first grade of binocular vision)

Simultaneous perception exists when signals transmitted from the two eyes to the visual cortex are perceived at the same time. The term simultaneous perception does not imply that both eyes see the same object and transmit identical information to the visual centre, nor does it imply that the two pictures can be seen superimposed. It consists of power to see two dissimilar objects simultaneously. It can be demonstrated by presenting separate stimuli to the two eyes, such as a picture of a cage to one eye and a picture of bird to the other eye. If both cage and the bird are seen at the same time, then simultaneous perception is present (Fig. 4.1A).

Further, there is a fundamental difference between seeing with two eyes alternately and simultaneous binocular perception. An animal whose eyes are situated laterally in the head so that the visual fields of the two eyes never overlap or overlap in only a very small portion and thus can use one eye at a time. This is alternate use of the two eyes, rather than simultaneous use of the two eyes. It can be further classified by the typical example that, when a bird sees a worm on the ground and tilts its head so that it obtains a clear image of the worm with the right eye, the left is directed upward. Since the simultaneous image of this eye would detract considerably from the perception of the worm, there is a reason to think that one image is suppressed mentally. The bird may direct its attention at will to the image of the left eye and ignore the image of right eye temporarily. This would surely happen, if under these circumstances a hawk were to fly overhead. Under certain conditions, human beings suppress the image from one eye with both eyes open. Simultaneous perception ceases to exist under these circumstances. For example, when using a monocular microscope, one suppresses the image of the other eye.

Fusion (second grade of binocular vision)

Fusion constitutes second grade of binocular vision. It implies the ability of the two eyes to produce a composite picture from two similar pictures, each of which is incomplete in one small detail. For example, there are two rabbits each lacking either a tail or a bunch of flowers. If fusion is present, one rabbit complete with tail

and holding a bunch of flowers will be seen (Fig. 4.1B). It should not be confused with the superimposition of two dissimilar (but not mutually antagonistic) pictures, such as a cage and a bird. So, when a person sees the bird inside the cage (Fig. 4.1A), it is not fusion, but simply a simultaneous perception in the same direction.

Stereopsis (third grade of binocular single vision)

Stereopsis implies the ability to obtain an impression of depth by the superimposition of two pictures of the same object which have been taken from slightly different angles, such as a bucket that is appreciated in three dimensions (Fig. 4.1C). Stereopsis should not be considered synonymous with the depth perception, since, depth perception is the perception of distances of objects from each other or from the observer. Even a monocular observer is quite capable of judging distances and of obtaining an impression of spatial order. Therefore, stereopsis refers to the visual appreciation of three dimensions during binocular vision.

PSYCHOPHYSICS AND SENSORY ASPECTS OF BINOCULAR VISION

The various facts about the psychophysics and sensory aspects of the binocular vision (revealed by psychophysical and experimental physio-

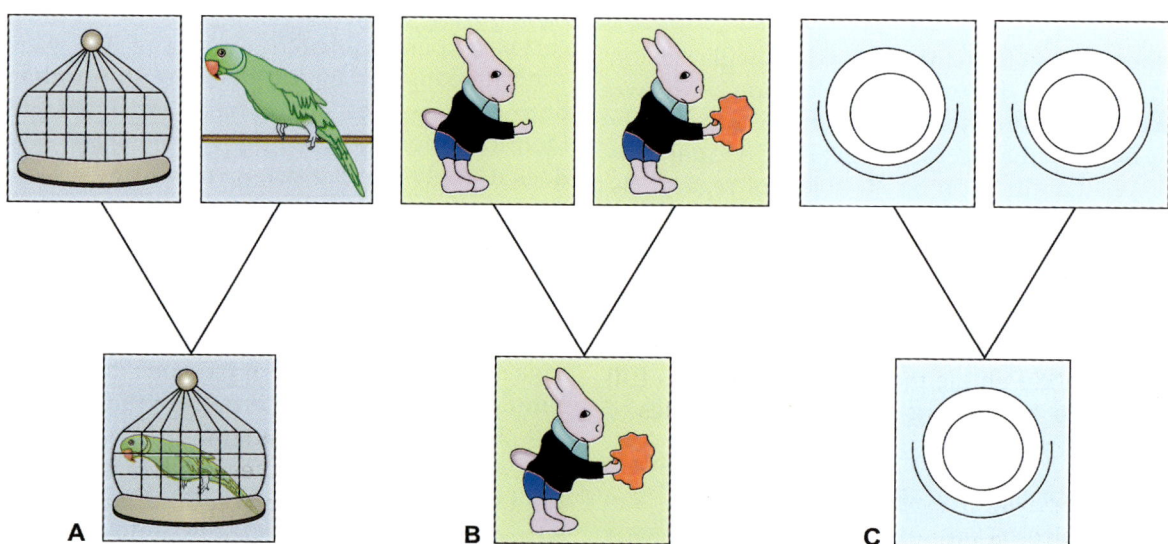

Fig. 4.1. *Grades of binocular single vision: A, simultaneous perception; B, Fusion; C, Stereopsis.*

logical studies), for the purpose of descriptive convenience, can be compiled as below:

1. *Visual direction and the horopter*
   - Visual space versus physical space
   - Visual directions
   - Corresponding points and normal retinal correspondence
   - Horopter
   - Physiological diplopia
2. *Binocular fusion*
   - Sensory fusion
   - Concept of Panum's area
   - Fixation disparity
   - Theories of binocular fusion
3. *Dichoptic stimulation*
   - Depth with fusion
   - Depth with diplopia
   - Diplopia without depth
   - Binocular rivalry and suppression
4. *Stereopsis*
   - Physiological basis of stereopsis
   - Stereopsis and fusion
   - Stereoscopic acuity
   - Neurophysiology of stereopsis
5. *Depth perception*
   - Stereopsis
   - Nonstereoptic binocular clues
   - Monocular clues
   - Influence of accommodation and convergence
6. *Integration of motor and sensory systems* into binocular vision.

VISUAL DIRECTION AND THE HOROPTER

VISUAL SPACE VERSUS PHYSICAL SPACE

Perception of space and spatial localization are extremely intricate functions that are not fully understood. The perception of spatial order is a mental phenomenon based on innate anatomic and physiologic systems, on visual clues, and on learning. The order in which objects are seen in visual space is a subjective perception. Therefore, visual space is referred to as subjective space. The subjective space is distinct from the physical space of real objects. Location of an object is its position in physical space, whereas localization is the position of an object in the subjective visual space. The experiments of Hering[7,8] demonstrate that objects, which may be widely separated in physical space, may have a common direction in subjective space. It is important to recognize that the anatomic distribution of retinal elements and the physiologic distribution of spatial values do not coincide. There are many examples that demonstrate the difference between physical space and its subjective interpretation. For example, if a vertical line is presented to a single eye in the absence of other visual clues, it appears to be slanted or tilted. Disclination (temporal shift) or conclination (nasal shift) of the vertical meridian in subjective space will occur. This demonstrated that the spatial values of the retinal receptors above and below the horizontal midline differ.

Another example of the difference between subjective space and physical space is the Kundt-Munsterberg illusion. In this illusion, the temporal half of a horizontal line, when viewed monocularly and kept at right angles to the line of sight at the point of bisection, will appear shorter than the nasal half of that bisected line. Because of this illusion, when an attempt is made with one eye to bisect the horizontal line, the temporal segment will be longer than the nasal. The distribution of subjective retinal spatial values differs between the nasal and temporal halves of the retina.

VISUAL DIRECTIONS

Oculocentric visual direction (monocular vision)

When an object is viewed, its image falls on the foveola. The visual direction of the object can be represented by a line joining the object to the centre of foveola—principal visual line or visual axis. The position of all other objects in the monocular field can be fixed by their oculocentric visual directions with respect to the visual axis. Thus each point on the retina can be thought of as having its own particular visual direction or visual line passing out through the nodal point of the eye. A visual line is, therefore, the locus of all points fixed relative to the eye whose images stimulated a given point on the retina.

For a given position of the eye, objects having superimposed retinal images will be seen as being in alignment in the visual field (law of oculocentric visual direction), although at different distance from the eye along the same visual line.[7, 8]

Egocentric visual direction (binocular vision)

Retinal points in the two eyes are said to be corresponding, if, when stimulated separately, they appear to have the same common visual direction.

Because each eye sees the world from different view point, the oculocentric frame of reference is necessarily different for the two eyes. However, in binocular vision, a single system of visual direction is needed whose frame of reference is related to the head (egocentric) rather than two eyes. When we use two eyes we seem to see the visual space through some imaginary single eye (cyclopean eye) situated in the head midway between the two eyes (Fig. 4.2).[9]

Foveae have a common subjective visual direction (Hering's law of identical visual direction). Hering[8] described it by the following classical experiment (Fig. 4.2): Let the observer stand 1/2 metre from a window which affords a view of outdoors, hold his head very steady, close the right eye and direct the left eye to an object located somewhat to the right, e.g. a triangle. While fixing the triangle with the left eye, a black mark (F) is made on the window pane at a spot in line with the triangle. Now left eye is closed and the right eye is opened and directed at the spot (F) on the window and beyond that to some object in line with it, e.g. a hut. Then with both eyes open and directed at the spot, the latter will appear to cover parts of the triangle and the hut both, which will be seen simultaneously.[8]

CORRESPONDING POINTS AND NORMAL RETINAL CORRESPONDENCE

Each retinal element has a directional or spatial value without which localization in space is impossible. These are intrinsic, not learned, values. The spatial value of retinal elements is

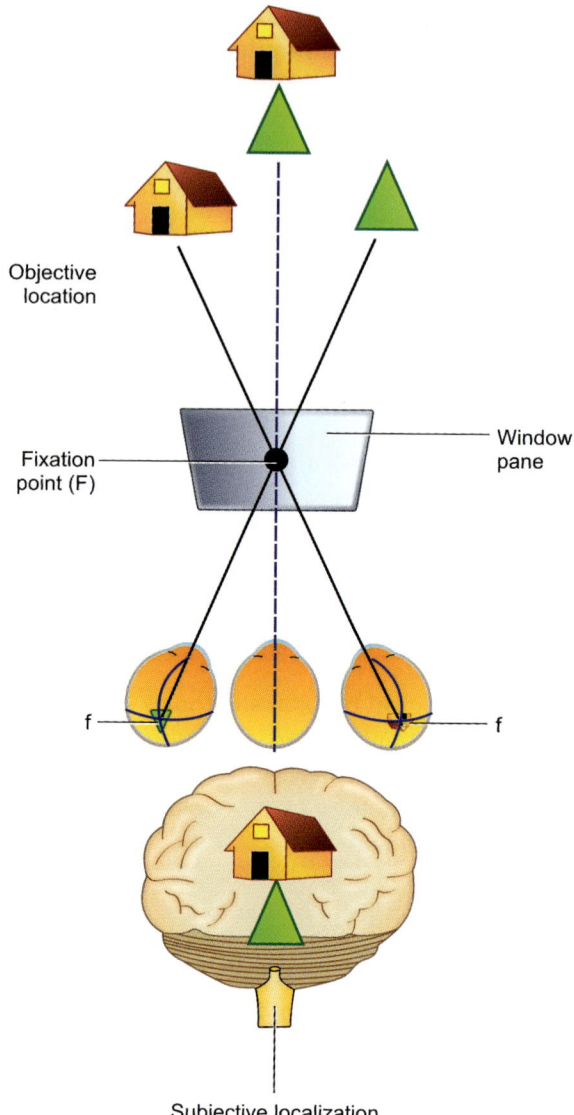

Fig. 4.2. *Concept of cyclopean eye. (diagrammatic representation of Hering's law of identical binocular direction) (Alter Howard and Templeton[9]).*

relative, not absolute. They are related to the spatial value of the fovea in each eye. The fovea, therefore, is the principal spatial value or principal directional value of each eye.

In order to understand normal retinal correspondence, it must be clearly understood that correspondence refers only to the relative localization of objects in space to each other under binocular conditions. The relationships of objects in space to ourselves—that is, to a coordinate system surrounding our person or our "ego centre"—is called absolute localization.

The information gained from relative localization is only one of many clues used in the process of absolute localization. Other information related to the vestibular mechanism, an ocular motor monitoring system, and possible proprioceptive feedback mechanisms is utilized by the brain to make the subjective interpretation of absolute localization.

Burian[10] states that corresponding retinal elements are those elements of the two retinae, the stimulation of which in binocular vision, gives rise to the localization in one and the same visual direction, no matter whether the stimulus reaches the retinal elements in one eye alone, or its corresponding partner in the other eye alone, or both simultaneously.

The fovea normally determines the principal visual direction. The correspondence mechanism is based on the assumption that each retinal receptor, when stimulated under monocular conditions, dictates a subjective visual direction determined by the relationship of that receptor to the fovea. The retinal receptors in both eyes that dictate a common visual direction under binocular conditions are called corresponding points or elements. Bagolini[11] has shown that this is an area-to-area relationship rather than a point-to-point relationship. Under binocular conditions, the correspondence process analyses the information relayed from each eye and may modify it in making the determination of absolute localization.

In normal retinal correspondence, both foveae have the same space value—zero—the value of the principal visual direction. The other receptor elements correspond to each other in fair approximation to their geometric locations so that a receptor 5° temporal to the fovea in one eye corresponds to a receptor 5° nasal to the fovea in the other eye.

Images falling on corresponding points give rise to a single mental impression to visual direction that we call sensory fusion. Corresponding retinal elements, therefore, have a common visual direction and permit a single visual impression. They do not permit double

vision. The mental image resulting from the fusion of the two retinal images can be conceived as the image or mental image received by a cyclopean eye. This is an eye, presumably located in the middle of the forehead, that sees in visual space the fused images of the two individual eyes (Fig. 4.3).[12] Normal retinal correspondence is thus the basis for normal binocular single vision. If, during fixation of an object, one eye of the observer would be passively turned with forceps, the object would no longer be imaged on corresponding retinal points. While the images would fall on the fovea in the one eye, it would be received somewhere on the peripheral retina in the deviated eye. Since these two areas are non-corresponding and have different spatial values, diplopia would be present (i.e. the object would be seen double).

HOROPTER

The term horopter, which literally means the horizon of vision, was introduced by Aguilonius.[13] As we know, when, in normal binocular vision, both eyes fixate the same object point, this point will be imaged on corresponding retinal elements of the two eyes—the foveae. At the same time, there will be other object points in space besides the fixation point that also will be imaged on corresponding retinal elements of the

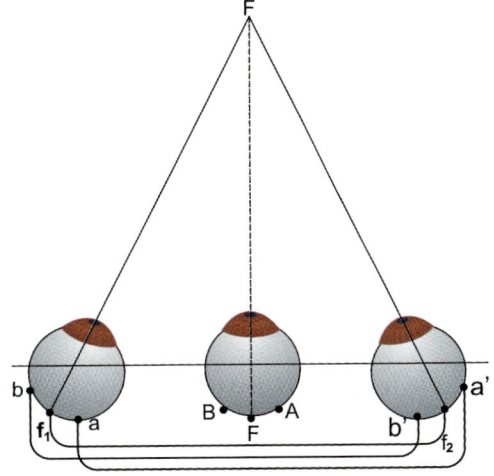

Fig. 4.3. *Normal retinal correspondence. The visual direction of f_1 and f_2 proceed from F the fovea of the imaginary cyclopean eye. A and B represent the points from which the visual direction belonging to a and a´, b and b´ would proceed (From Bielschowsky[12]).*

two eyes. If the position of these other points is determined theoretically, a circle will be found passing through the fixation point and the entrance pupils of the two eyes. This circle is known as the theoretical or geometric horopter (Vieth-Muller horopter).[14,15] Theoretically, any point on it will stimulate corresponding retinal elements in the two eyes, because every point on the horopter will form an angle with the two entrance pupils that is equal to the angle formed by the fixation point and the two entrance pupils (Fig. 4.4). It follows that there is a different horopter for each fixation distance.

In other words, the horopter can be defined as the sum total of points in physical space that stimulate corresponding retinal elements of the two eyes. It is a complex mathematical model having all three dimensions. The longitudinal horopter is that surface that determines horizontally distributed object points in space.[13] The longitudinal horopter curve is a line formed by the intersection of the visual plane and the longitudinal horopter plane. The visual plane is determined by the fixation point and the centres of the two pupils.[16, 17]

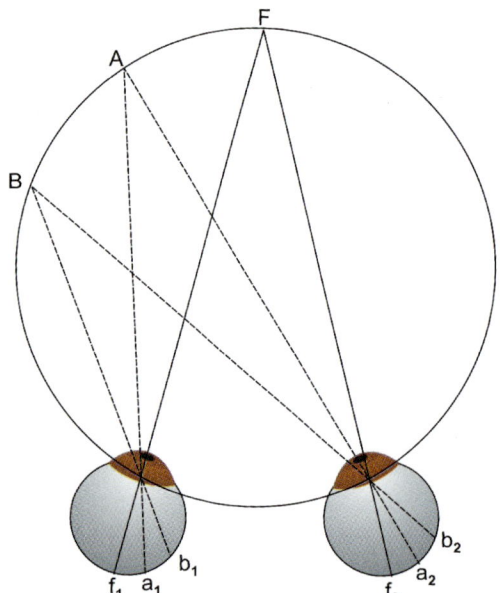

Fig. 4.4. *Diagrammatic representation of the theoretical horopter (Vieth-Muller horopter circle). Points F, A and B fall on geometrically corresponding retinal points f₁ and f₂, a₁ and a₂ and b₁ and b₂, respectively.*

The horopter can be determined with an instrument utilizing movable, vertically placed wires set at a certain distance. While fixation is maintained upon a central wire, those on either side in the periphery are adjusted forward or backward by the subject until they appear to lie in the same visual plane. In determining the horopter, the difference between subjective visual space and physical space is again demonstrated. Subjectively, the movable wires appear to lie in the same visual plane; however, they actually lie on a curved surface. Thus, the horopters found experimentally do not actually coincide with the theoretical horopters. They are called empirical horopters.

PHYSIOLOGIC DIPLOPIA

Since only object points which lie on the horopter will be imaged on corresponding retinal elements, all objects that are either nearer or farther away than the horopter will be imaged on disparate (i.e. non-corresponding) retinal elements and, consequently, will be seen double.

Point a in Fig. 4.5 A, located closer than the horopter (point b), is imaged temporal to the fovea in each eye. The right eye will see this point as being on the left side of the fixation point, while the left eye will see it to the right of the fixation point. In other words, point a will be seen double (a₁ and a₂). Since each eye perceives it as being on the opposite side, this is referred to as crossed diplopia. With respect to the retina, point a shows temporal disparity. Conversely point a, which is located beyond the horopter (point b) in Fig. 4.5B; will be imaged on the nasal retinae of both eyes and, therefore, will also appear double. However, this time the diplopia will be uncrossed—the right eye will localize the object to the right of the fixation point, while the left eye will place it to the left. The retinal images will have nasal disparity.

Physiologic diplopia can be demonstrated by holding two pencils vertically in front of the eyes with one pencil about twice as far away as the other. If either one of them is fixated, the other will be seen double. If the more distant one is fixated, crossed diplopia will be experienced. If the closer one is fixated, the diplopia will be uncrossed.

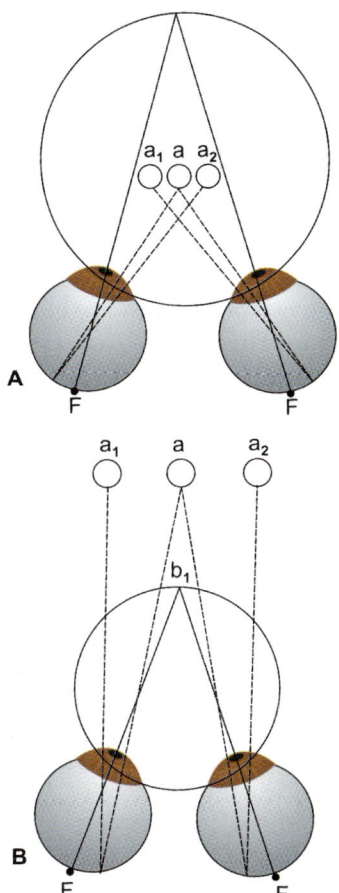

Another contributing factor is the low visual acuity of the peripheral retina, which frequently does not yield sufficient resolution of peripherally located objects for the recognition of diplopia.

BINOCULAR FUSION

When images of an object fall on corresponding retinal points, in the normal subject, they seem to be fused into a single mental impression. The sensory fusion should be distinguished from motor fusion, which refers to the ability to align the eyes in such a manner that sensory fusion can be maintained. The stimulus for these fusional eye movements is retinal disparity. Unlike sensory fusion, the motor fusion is exclusive function of the extra-foveal retinal periphery. Under normal conditions, sensory fusion occurs when corresponding retinal elements of the two eyes are stimulated by images from the same object. However, fusion will also take place when the stimuli in the two eyes are not identical but only similar. The dissimilarity may be one of form, size, colour, luminosity, distinctness or contrast. To a limited extent, it is also possible to fuse signals from non-corresponding points (see discussion on fixation disparity below).

Fig. 4.5. *Diagram illustrating physiological diplopia. Points a and b which are not located on the horopter, are imaged on non-corresponding retinal points and so physiological diplopia either crossed (A) or uncrossed (B) is produced.*

This demonstration will not be immediately successful in all subjects, since one of the images may be suppressed from conscious perception, a process which also is physiologic, as is explained later in this chapter.

In view of what has been said about the horopter and physiologic diplopia, it should be expected that one would have constant diplopia during casual daily vision, with the exception of the object of fixation and the few objects that happen to be on the horopter for the momentary fixation distance. Obviously, this is not the case; and it is not primarily suppression that prevents the occurrence of physiologic diplopia, but the exclusiveness with which our attention is usually directed to the fixated object. Although diplopia is present, this rarely enters consciousness.

The anatomic basis which allows sensory fusion to occur is the course of the visual nerve fibres. By crossing in the chiasma, nerve fibres from the nasal retina are brought to the same side as their counterparts from corresponding points of the temporal retina of the other eye. While ascending in the visual pathway, the fibres from corresponding retinal points converge until finally they are adjacent to each other. They terminate in the same cortical cell complexes.

But for our knowledge of the anatomic arrangement, little definite information exists on the physiology of sensory fusion. It is probable that fusion occurs in the cortex. It is not certain, however, whether the two signals transmitted separately from two corresponding points are synthesized so that they simultaneously contribute to the resulting single perception, or whether the two signals are mutually exclusive and are utilized alternately to be combine into the resulting single constant perception so that first one eye and then the other contributes its stimulus to a given point of the whole.

At birth, coordinated conjugate eye movements are absent, visual perception is poor, and fusion is not established as a stable binocular function. If development proceeds normally, fusion evolves later as a conditioned reflex. If there is a significant abnormality in the optical performance of the eyes, in the function of the nerve elements that are concerned with the transmission or perception of visual stimuli, or in the motor cooperation of the two eyes, fusion may never develop normally. It is conceivable that there may be individuals in whom a basic ability for fusion does not exist.

PANUM'S AREA

As stated previously that only object points which lie on the horopter and which stimulate corresponding retinal points in the two eyes are seen as single is not quite exact and must be qualified. When a horopter is determined experimentally, it is found that an object may be located a certain distance in front of or behind it without producing diplopia. The field in front of and behind the horopter, in which the expected diplopia does not occur is known as Panum's fusional space.

Panum's fusional space is smallest at the fixation point (Fig. 4.6). Toward the periphery,

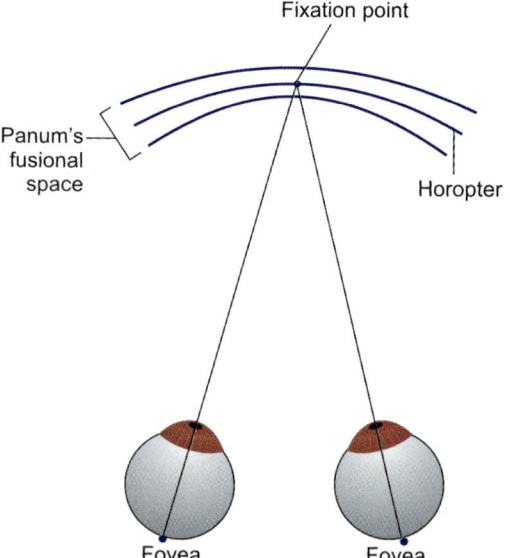

Fig. 4.6. *Diagram of Panum's fusional space.*

it gains increasingly in depth, so that objects located peripherally may be farther from the horopter without producing diplopia than objects located more centrally. Any point not on the horopter is not imaged on corresponding retinal areas but will stimulate disparate retinal areas. If, despite the disparity, no diplopia occurs, fusion of signals from non-corresponding points must have taken place. Thus, a signal from a given retinal point not only is fused with the signal from its corresponding point in the other eye, but also may be fused with signals from a limited area surrounding that corresponding point. Such a retinal Panum's area corresponds in size to the depth of Panum's fusional space. Since the latter is small in the vicinity of the fixation point, Panum's areas in the fovea are also small, actually in the order of 5' of arc. Away from the fixation point, Panum's fusional space enlarges (i.e. the size of Panum's areas in the peripheral retina increases). Since retinal disparity in the horizontal meridian can be overcome to a larger extent than disparity in the vertical meridian, Panum's areas have the shape of an oval with the longer axis horizontal. If the fixation distance is more than 20 m, objects lying behind the horopter will always be seen as single, since the disparity of their images is always smaller than Panum's areas.

FIXATION DISPARITY

Under laboratory conditions, it can be demonstrated that, during binocular fixation, the point of fixation is rarely ever imaged exactly on corresponding points of the two foveae but that the primary line of sight of one eye misses the fixation point very slightly, being either under-converged or over-converged (Fig. 4.7). This phenomenon is called fixation disparity. It does not give rise to diplopia, because the disparity with which the fixation point is imaged on the two retinae is less than the size of Panum's area.

Thus, in fixation disparity, one eye will fixate the object directly with the central fovea, while the other eye will fixate slightly eccentrically. However, the horopter simply passes through the actual point of fixation rather than through the fixation stimulus. Fixation disparity may

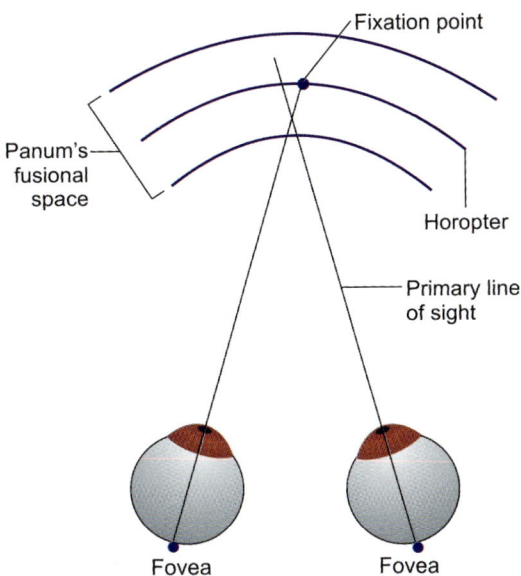

Fig. 4.7. *Diagram illustrating fixation disparity.*

arise from a small foveal scotoma or from an oculomotor imbalance which is tending to pull the eyes away from the appropriate angle of convergence. An example of a horopter showing fixation disparity was obtained by Olge[18] on his own eyes.

DICHOPTIC STIMULATION

Dichoptic stimulation simply refers to a different stimulation in the two eyes, which occurs when binocular stimuli fall on non-corresponding points on the two retinae. There are five classes of percepts which are obtained, depending upon the degree of non-correspondence between the stimuli:

1. Depth with fusion;
2. Depth with diplopia;
3. Diplopia without depth;
4. Binocular rivalry and suppression; and
5. Binocular lustre.

DEPTH WITH FUSION AND DEPTH WITH DIPLOPIA

Strictly speaking, these are not generally referred to as dichoptic stimuli, since the two retinal patterns are sufficiently similar to be combined into a unified impression (particularly for fused stereopsis). Therefore, these will be dealt in the section of stereopsis.

DIPLOPIA WITHOUT DEPTH

When the degree of non-correspondence is such that no fusion occurs and diplopia results without depth perception. Depending upon the location of non-corresponding points stimulated, the diplopia may be homonymous or uncrossed (Fig. 4.5B) and heteronymous or crossed (Fig. 4.5A). Sensory adaptations which may occur to compensate for the annoying diplopia include: suppression, amblyopia, and abnormal retinal correspondence. Motor mechanisms which compensate for diplopia are an abnormal head posture and certain permanent changes in the extraocular muscles such as inhibitional palsy, overaction and contractures.

RETINAL RIVALRY AND SUPPRESSION

When dissimilar contours are presented to corresponding retinal areas (having same visual direction), fusion becomes impossible, since two dissimilar objects localized in the same place give rise to a conflict and confusion. The conflict which results when contradictory and incompatible signals are transmitted from corresponding points to the visual cortex is termed retinal rivalry. The phenomenon of retinal rivalry, also termed as binocular rivalry, must be clearly distinguished from local adaptation, or Troxer's phenomenon.[24] Binocular rivalry may also be produced by uniform surfaces of different colour (colour rivalry) and unequal luminances of the two targets. Many combinations of contours, colours and luminances have been studied exhaustively since the days of Panum,[25] Fechner,[26] Helmholtz[27] and Hering.[28]

- *Retinal rivalry* is a very normal event, since corresponding areas are consistently exposed to dissimilar images from objects located outside Panum's fusional space.

The visual system responds to retinal rivalry by rejecting the signals transmitted from a given area of one retina in favour of those coming from the corresponding parts of the other retina. Thus, only information from one retina becomes a visual perception while the information simultaneously transmitted from corresponding parts of the other retina is not used, so that the involved area may be considered temporarily blind. This reaction to the influx of conflicting information is called suppression.

■ *Suppression* is an innate, involuntary process. Under certain conditions, all the signals from one retina may be suppressed so that no information from that eye reaches the threshold of conscious perception.[29-33] Usually, however, responding to the demand of the momentary conditions, suppression is restricted to limited areas in both retinae so that those portions of the subjective visual field in which fusion cannot occur may be composed, like a mosaic, of pieces of information from only one or the other retina in constant variation (Fig. 4.8).

Although an eye may be suppressed for long periods, suppression basically is a transient phenomenon, present only momentarily when needed. Because it is a physiologic function that does not have to be learned but is readily available, it frequently becomes the firstline of defence against pathologic interruption or embarrassment of bifoveal single vision. For example, a patient who has a marked refractive error in only one eye may show suppression of that eye to eliminate the disturbing effect of the blurred image. In patients with strabismus, a condition in which objects are not imaged on

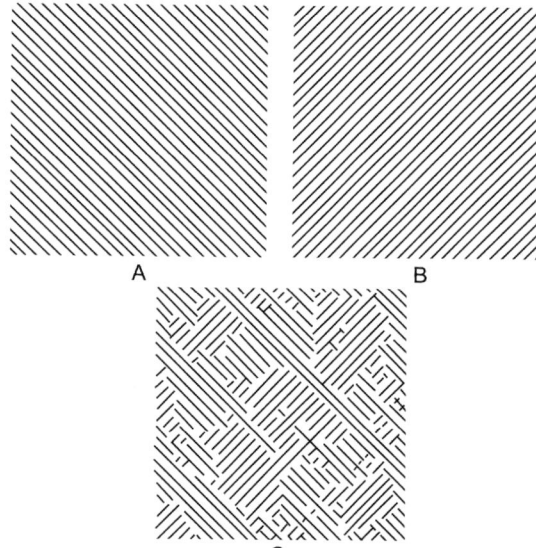

Fig. 4.8. *Retinal rivalry produced by dissimilar contours: A, pattern viewed by left eye; B, Pattern viewed by right eye; C, binocular impression (mosaic of pieces). After Panum.*[25]

normally corresponding retinal areas, suppression is a frequent response to solve the problem of incompatible information transmitted from corresponding areas of the two eyes. It has been shown experimentally that retinal rivalry and the suppression resulting from it are influenced by certain conditions. If non-fusable patterns are presented to the two eyes, it is found that perception from corresponding areas alternates equally between the two eyes, if the objects are of equal brightness, size and prominence. The rate of alternation under such test conditions is influenced by the brightness of the field, the size of the target area, the distinctness of the targets, and the location of the stimulated area in the retina. If any of these factors is impaired equally for both eyes, the rate of alternation will decrease. If the visual conditions are improved, it will increase. However, suppression will always alternate equally between the two eyes.

In contrast, by changing the stimulus conditions for only one eye, the rate of alternation can be changed markedly in its favour or disfavour.

Retinal or binocular rivalry fluctuations are similar in many respects to fluctuations of attention, and are widely supposed to be under voluntary control to some extent. Actually, a number of studies have found that there is very little voluntary control over which eye dominates at any given time.[34] The change of dominance is not affected by eye blinks[35] or by variations in accommodation or pupil size.[36] In fact, the fluctuations in rivalry are well described by a sequentially independent random variable with no periodicities, as though the arrival of each change in dominance had no effect on the occurrence of subsequent changes.[37]

The phenomenon of retinal rivalry has been explained in neurophysiologic terms by the presumption that separate channels are present for the right and left eyes which compete for access to the visual cortex. A third binocular channel is activated only by fusible input.[38,39] Because of this competition and inhibition elicited, only fragments of the image seen by each eye are transmitted to the visual cortex in the case of non-fusible binocular output. This hypothesis looks logical but needs experimental verification.

BINOCULAR LUSTRE

The lustrous appearance of surfaces like a waxed surface, tabletop or a car body is essentially due to binocular lustre. It results from the different position of partially reflected objects in the surface by virtue of the different position of the two eyes. The partial reflection provides a fixation place at which the partially reflected image usually has a large disparity and hence areas of binocular luminance difference. The lustrous region is not localizable in depth, but it seems unitary and does not fluctuate in the manner of binocular rivalry. Binocular lustre was described by early authors in visual science, such as Panum[19] and Helmholtz,[21] as a kind of lustrous or shimmering surface of indeterminate depth.

The detection of binocular lustre during static and dynamic random dot stereogram testing is even more rapid than the detection of depth changes.[40-42]

STEREOPSIS

Stereopsis is the visual appreciation of three dimensions during binocular vision. It occurs through fusion of signals from disparate retinal elements.

As shown in Fig. 4.9, if one views two posts, A and B, situated at slightly different distances, with both eyes open, their separation in depth is readily apparent to a normal person. This perception of depth is maintained as long as both eyes are used. If either eye is closed, the effect of depth then vanishes. If the right eye is closed, the appearance of the two posts is that shown on the left hand side of Fig. 4.9, and, if the left eye is closed, the appearance is that shown on the right side of the figure. The only difference between these two images is that the posts seem to be farther apart in the frontoparallel plane when seen with the left eye than when seen with the right. This difference in lateral separation is due to the fact that the receptors stimulated in the left eye are more widely separated from each other than those in the right retina (note distance between a and b of two eyes in Fig. 4.9).

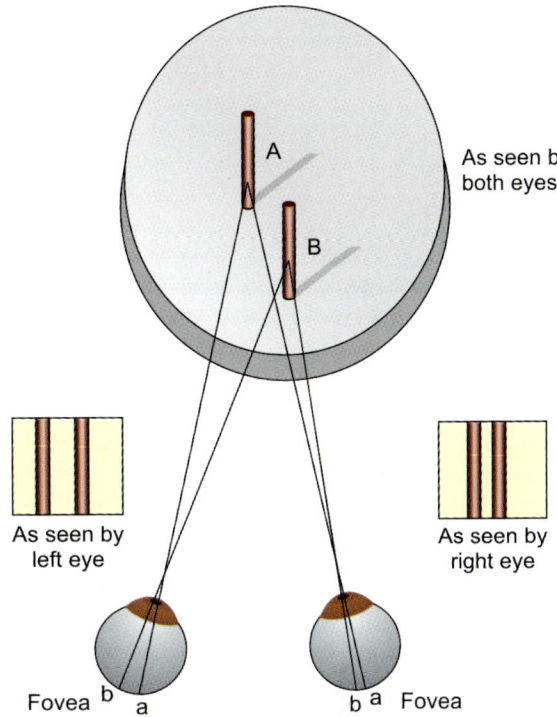

Fig. 4.9. *Disparateness of retinal images producing stereopsis.*

An object point which is located in front of the fixation point but is still within the limits of Panum's fusional space will stimulate disparate retinal elements. The disparity will be temporal, each image being temporal to the point that corresponds to the location of the image in the other eye. Although both images are fused since they are within the limits of Panum's area, the fact that they are temporarily desparate is not lost in the resulting single perception but gives the perception of its additional quality of nearness relative to the fixation point. Conversely, when an object is located behind the horopter but still within the Panum's fusional space, nasal disparity will exist, adding the quality of farness to the perception. Thus, it can be seen from Fig. 4.10 that, when the images do not fall on exactly corresponding retinal points, an impression that the image is in front or behind a given frontal plane is produced. In the figure 4.10, F and F' are the foveae fixating a point C, straight ahead. This point determines the frontal plane, XX'. An object A, whose image falls on a in the left eye produces an image at b' in the right eye. b' is not the corresponding point,

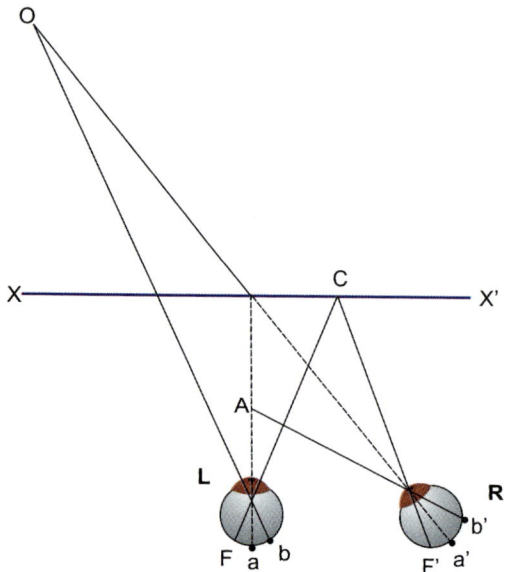

Fig. 4.10. *Scheme showing the effect produced by stimulation of slightly incongruous retinal points. a-a', corresponding points; b-b' corresponding points; F-F', the foveas*

which is a'. Because of this, the impression is that the point A lies nearer the eyes than the frontal plane, XX'. Similarly, an object O, whose image falls on b in the left eye produces its image at a' in the right eye. The corresponding retinal point of b is b'. The image of object O lies to the nasal side of this point at a' in the right eye. The impression is gained, therefore, that point O lies behind frontal plane XX'.

Thus, it proves that in general nasal disparity gives the impression of remoteness of an object, and temporal disparity gives the impression of nearness of an object.

Stereopsis is a unique cognition, a distinct perceptual quality of its own. If one does not have it, one cannot learn it even in the presence of all requirements such as bifoveal fixation, fusion, and good visual acuity. Although stereopsis is the most important factor in judging distances, especially at close range, additional information about the absolute and relative distances of objects is gained in several other ways. While in bifoveal vision these other means are only an addition to stereopsis, they are the only source of information on which a monocular observer can base his distance judgement.

Worth classified fusion in three degrees. *First-degree fusion* was the simultaneous macular perception of two different non-fusable objects. *Second-degree fusion* was characterized as the ability of the motor system to align the eyes in such a way that sensory fusion was possible. *Third-degree fusion* was stereopsis. Worth's classification of third-degree fusion, however, is not entirely correct since stereopsis is a separate quality of the visual system, a sensory responsiveness to disparate stimuli that can occur, under certain conditions, without second-degree fusion being present.

In a two-dimensional representation, certain colours seem to stick out and others do not. *Colour stereopsis* is related to the differential refraction for various wavelengths of light. The different blur circles can stimulate disparate retinal points within Panum's area and thus give true stereopsis to a flat picture in which there is no lateral or horizontal separation of the retinal images.

PHYSIOLOGICAL BASIS OF STEREOPSIS

Stereopsis a function of spatial disparity

Stereopsis arises when horizontally disparate retinal elements are stimulated simultaneously.[43] The fusion of such disparate images results in a single visual impression perceived in depth, provided the fused image lies within Panum's area of single bionocular vision. Vertical disparities produce no stereoscopic effect. A solid object placed in the median plane of the head produces unequal images in the two eyes due to horizontal separation of the two eyes (Fig. 4.11). The sensory fusion of the two unequal retinal images results in a three-dimensional percept.

A stereoscopic effect can also be produced by two-dimensional pictures, some elements of which are imaged on corresponding retinal points to give the frame of reference for the relative localization of other elements of figures constructed to provide horizontally disparate imagery. Such figures must be viewed separately but binocularly in a stereoscope or some haploscopic device.

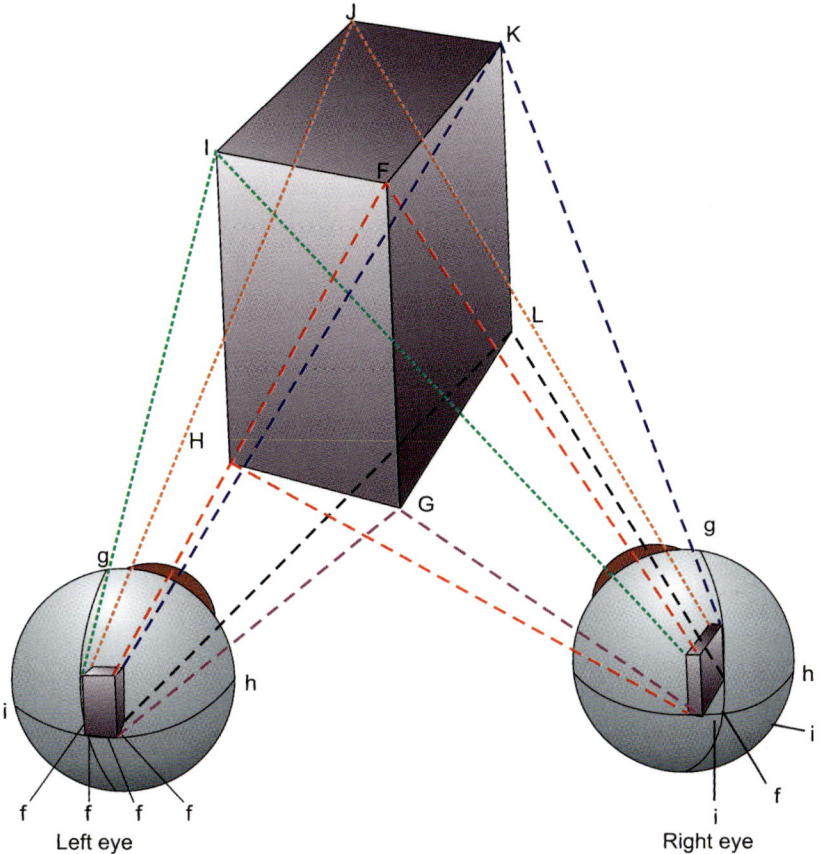

Fig. 4.11. *A solid object placed in the midline of the head creates slightly different or disparate retinal images, the fusion of which results in a three-dimensional sensation.*

Local and global stereopsis

Julesz[44,45] studied stereopsis perception utilizing random stereogram and put forward the concept of local and global stereopsis. The term local stereopsis is used to denote stereopsis elicited by the dot-by-dot or square-by-square matching process that occurs between the right and left stereogram.

When there is ambiguity as to which elements in the two retinal images correspond to each other, a global process is needed that evaluates different possible sets of corresponding pairs and selects one set of matched pairs that, by their depth values, can provide the data for recognition of a three-dimensional form. Julesz refers to this additional mechanism as global stereopsis, since the problem of ambiguities can only be resolved on a global basis. Therefore, a satisfactory theory for binocular depth perception must obviously take account of both local and global stereopsis.

Fine versus coarse stereopsis

Fine stereopsis is a highly specific pattern matching process involving very local features of the two retinal images and operating over a relatively narrow range of spatial disparities probably no more than about 0.5 degrees.

Dissimilar images cannot be simultaneously perceived. If binocular vision is to occur, the two retinal images must be closely similar, otherwise there is retinal rivalry and suppression of one or other of the antagonistic image features.

Coarse stereopsis is a much less specific process that can operate on visual images quite dissimilar in form, luminance and contrast and separated by several degrees in spatial position- up to as much as 7 to 10 degrees of retinal image disparity. Since coarse stereopsis acts beyond the range of retinal rivalry, dissimilar images can be simultaneously perceived. For coarse fusion (single vision), however, the images must again be similar, but the disparity limits over which fusion can take place (Panum's area of up to about 7 degrees) are much larger than they are for fine stereopsis. Coarse single vision may occur in the absence of fine fusion, but fine single vision is always accompanied by coarse fusion.

STEREOPSIS AND FUSION

Fusion is not absolutely required for stereopsis. Stereopsis is independent of fusion, but it is necessary that similar parts of stereograms be fused (stimuli reaching corresponding elements), since these form the place of reference.

The presence of sensory fusion, that is ability to unify images falling on corresponding retinal areas, in itself does not guarantee the presence of stereopsis. A patient may fuse similar targets but have no stereopsis. Such patients suppress selectively the disparately imaged elements of a stereogram seen by one eye.

A certain degree of stereopsis may occur in diplopia. Conversely, there may be fusion without stereopsis. Some people are capable of motor and sensory fusion but have no perceptual resonse to disparate stimuli and, therefore, have no stereopsis. Peripheral stereopsis may exist where central stereopsis does not. Our methods primarily test central retinal areas. There are persons who show regional suppression but who have peripheral stereopsis.

Experiments of Burian[10] and others have shown that a sense of depth still occurs under certain conditions even though the disparity of the receptors stimulated is such that they lie outside of Panum's area and, therefore, are not seen single, but double. Figure 4.12 shows the regions, as determined by Ogle,[46] in which there is single vision without depth (determined as the horopter), single vision with stereoscopic depth (determined as Panum's area), and finally, outside the Panum's area a crude sense of depth and diplopia. As Burian[10] points out, it is not strictly correct to call stereopsis third-degree fusion. It is more than that. It is a sense sui genesis.

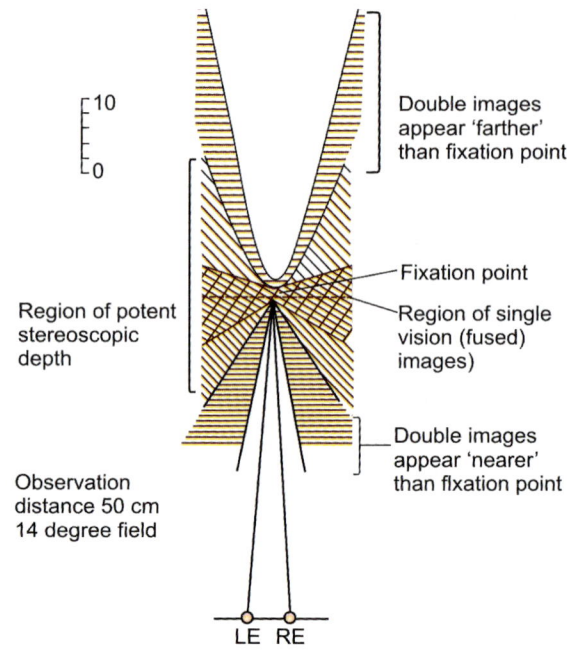

Fig. 4.12. *The regions of obligatory and qualitative stereoscopic perception of depth about the point of fixation. From Angle[46]*

The degree of responsiveness to disparate stimulation is also related to visual acuity. All other things being equal, the better the visual acuity, the better the stereoscopic acuity. Good visual acuity, however, does not guarantee stereoscopic acuity. Reduced visual acuity, such as that with monocular amblyopia, does not preclude stereopsis. While fusion and acuity are important factors in stereopsis, there is no linear relationship between them. It is important to realize that a shift of visual directions takes place in stereopsis. In other words, objects viewed by stereopsis produce a visual impression and a visual direction unlike the visual direction initiated by either eye alone.

STEREOSCOPIC ACUITY

Stereopsis is one of the finest spatial discriminations of which the human visual system is capable. There is minimal disparity beyond which no stereoscopic effect is produced. This limiting disparity characterizes a person's stereoscopic acuity.

Stereoacuity of as low as 2 to 7 sec of arc have been found. But a threshold of 15 to 30 sec obtained in clinical tests may be regarded as excellent. There are no standardized clinical stereoscopic acuity tests comparable to visual acuity tests.

Under normal conditions, most observers with no ocular abnormalities can discriminate a depth differ-ence between two images with a relative disparity of only about 10 arc sec (0.0028°). For the closest fixation of 10 inches away, the best stereoscopic threshold corresponds to the appreciation of a depth of one thousandth of an inch.[25]

Beyond 600 metres, there is no true stereopsis. At this distance, monocular clues take over for the perception of depth. This allows stereoscopic discrimination of depth in some types of clouds. These limits provide useful stereopsis over an extensive range of environmental conditions.

Stereoacuity is excellent at the fovea, but decreases from the centre to the periphery of retina. Stereopsis rapidly becomes very poor beyond about 20° eccentricity, or outside the circle passing through the two blind spots in the binocular visual fields.[47]

DEPTH PERCEPTION

Depth perception is the perception of distances of objects from each other or from the observer. It is somewhat ambiguous term since it is also used to imply the visual perception of three-dimensional space.

Using it in its first connotation, it is independent of the appreciation of three dimensions and does not require binocular vision. A monocular observer is quite capable of judging distances and of obtaining an impression of spatial order. Little is known about the quality and mechanism of absolute depth perception where a judgement cannot be based on any additional clues, as, for instance, when estimating the distance of a point light source in an absolutely dark room. In a normal visual environment, several factors contribute to the perception of depth: stereopsis, parallactic movements, interposition of objects, size in which an object is seen, distance of an object from the horizon, perspective, shadows, and aerial perspective.

I. STEREOPSIS

As discussed earlier, stereopsis is the relative localization of visual objects in depth which can occur only under conditions of binocular vision. As described in detail (page 67–71), stereopsis is based on a physiologic process derived from the organization of sensory visual system. Stereopsis is apparently innate, not acquired through experience and is unequivocal and inescapable.

II. NON-STEREOSCOPIC CLUES TO THE PERCEPTION OF DEPTH UNDER BINOCULAR CONDITIONS

Under binocular conditions, retinal disparity gives a clue to depth without stereopsis. When there is temporal retinal disparity, an awareness of nearness occurs. When there is nasal retinal disparity, an awareness of distance occurs.

III. MONOCULAR CLUES (NON-STEREOSCOPIC CLUES TO SPATIAL ORIENTATION)

Stereopsis is restricted to relatively short visual distances and is not the only means we have for spatial orientation. There is a set of monocular or experimental clues that play an important role in our estimation of the relative distance of visual objects. They are the result of experience and are equivocal. Monocular clues include the following:

1. Parallactic movements

Next to stereopsis, parallactic movements are most important in the perception of depth. They are the apparent movements made by objects when the observer moves his head. A slight shift of the head in any direction while fixation is maintained on the same point results in a change of the relative position of all objects in the direction of gaze. Objects beyond the fixation point appear to move in the same direction as the observer's head, whereas objects closer than the fixation point appear to move in the opposite direction. Greater the displacement of an object relative to the fixation point the more distant the object is from the fixation point.

2. Linear perspective

Object points having a constant size appear to subtend smaller and smaller angles as they recede from the subject, e.g. railroad tracks which are in fact parallel seem to approach each other in the distance. This is an example of the perspective in which the three-dimensional object space imaged geometrically in two dimensions on the retina creates an impression of depth. The geometric reproduction in two dimensions is not only of theoretical interest with respect to the translation of such two-dimensional retinal stimuli into a three-dimensional perception, but is also of great importance in creating the feeling of depth in drawings and paintings. Its most prominent feature is the fact that lines which are parallel in object space and at an angle with the picture plane seem to be directed to one point, the vanishing point (Fig. 4.13).

3. Overlay of contours

By superimposing or interposing the contour of configuration, one can find distance clues. Interposition of objects gives an absolute clue as to their relative position, since the outline of one object interrupts or hides the contour of another object behind it (Fig. 4.14).

4. Size

The size in which an object is seen is another important factor in the judgement of distances, provided the actual size is known to the observer. Objects encountered in daily life, such as people and cars, allow a definite judgement

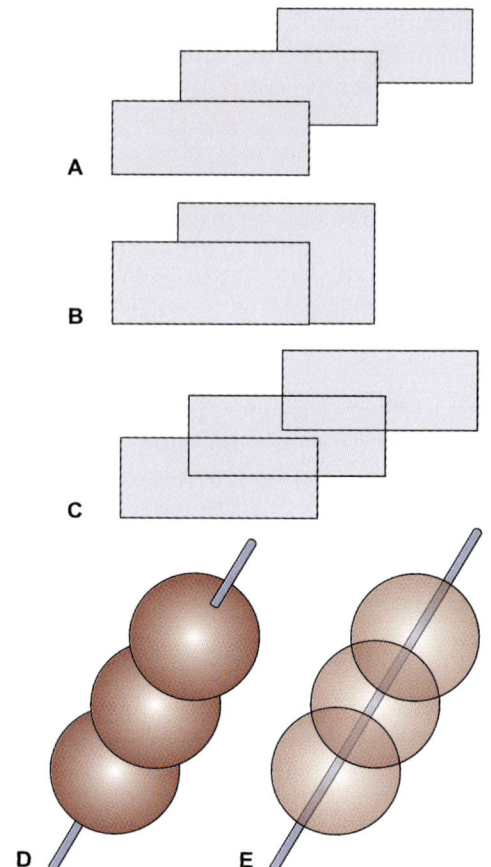

Fig. 4.14. *Effect of overlay of contours; A and D, depth is achieved by interposing one object in front of the other; B, C and E, the same forms are drawn to avoid a clue of depth.*

of their distance. If the actual size of an object is unknown, however, and a comparison with a known object is impossible, marked errors occur. This may be the case, for example, when looking at a bird against the sky. If its real size is unknown to the observer, then distance judgement is merely a guess. The difficulty is particularly obvious at night if an attempt is made to estimate the distance of a light source of unknown size.

5. Distance from horizon

The distance of an object from the horizon or its relative height in the visual field gives an important clue to distance. Since the eyes of an observer are at a certain height above the ground, it appears as if the ground is rising toward the horizon. Thus, objects more distant

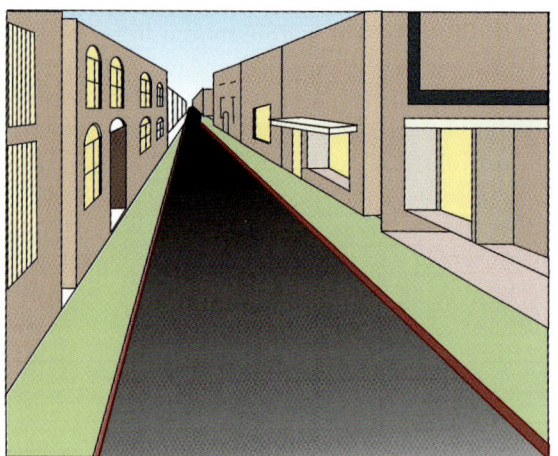

Fig. 4.13. *Drawing demonstrating the affect of linear perspective (vanishing point).*

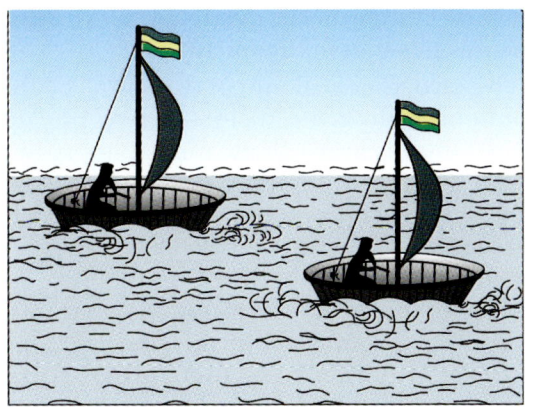

Fig. 4.15. *Drawing showing effect of distance from horizon in depth perception. Objects that are close to the horizon are perceived as being farther from the observer.*

from the observer will be higher in the visual field (Fig. 4.15).

6. Distribution of highlights, shadows, shades and light

Highlights and shadows provide a very important monocular clue for perception of depth. Since, sunlight comes from above, we have learned that the position of shadow is helpful in judging the raised and depressed area, that is the relative depth in objects. When there is a shadow on the lower portion of an object, the object appears to stick out in space. When

the shadow is above, the object appears to curve in.

A classic example of this is the picture of a pit in a wall with sunlight falling from above at a small angle against the wall. The upper portion of the pit will be filled with a dark shadow while the lower part is brightly illuminated. Turning the picture upside down, one no longer sees a pit but instead a distinct hump, the upper portion of which stands out brightly while its lower part casts a shadow (Fig. 4.16).

7. Aerial perspective

The influence of the atmosphere on contrast conditions and colours of more distant objects is referred to as aerial perspective. Objects appear less clear and acquire a more bluish tinge as the viewing distance increases. The colour change towards blue is particularly obvious, if one views the shadows of a mountain chain from some distance.

IV. INFLUENCE OF ACCOMMODATION AND CONVERGENCE ON DEPTH PERCEPTION

A given object at a given distance is imagined in a certain size on the retina. It would appear natural that the size of the retinal image determines the size in which the object is seen subjectively. This, however, is not the case. There is no doubt that the size in which an object is

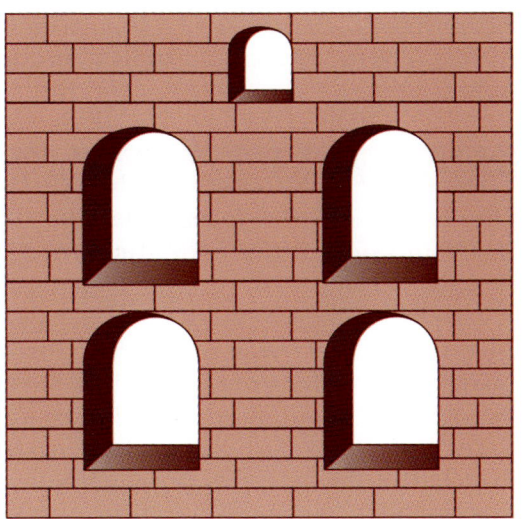
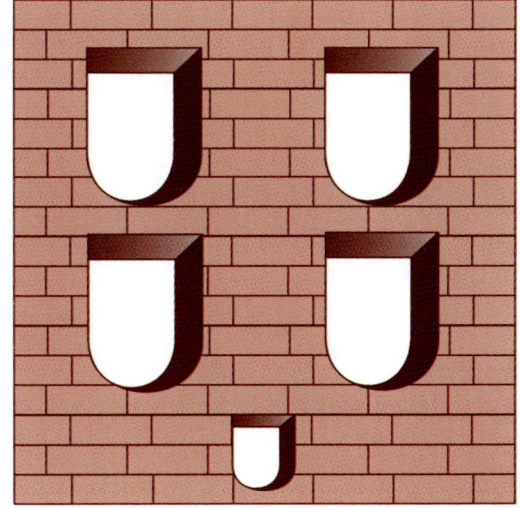

A   B

Fig. 4.16. *Drawing showing effect of highlight and shadows on depth perception: A, Upright picture; B, Same picture turned upside down.*

perceived can be changed mentally. The apparent increase in the size of an object that is brought closer to the eye does not correspond to the increase that might be expected on the basis of the enlargement of its retinal image. This effect has been attributed to the influence of accommodation and/or convergence, and in turn it was postulated that these functions contribute a clue for depth perception. There is no proof of this. However, experimental evidence points in the other direction that after a judgement of distance has been made, this then influences the apparent size of the object.

CONCLUSION

The impression of three-dimensionality imparted by these clues is a judgement, an interpretation. So false judgements are possible. Also these depend on past experience.

Monocular clues and binocular clues work hand in hand, one enhancing the effect of the other, but this is not always true. If one introduces into a stereogram confusing clues, i.e. monocular clues that conflict with stereoscopic clues, false observations can be made.

Some people are more responsive to stereoscopic clues, whereas others respond more readily to monocular clues.

Thus humans have two sets of clues for their orientation in space (depth perception). Monocular clues depend upon past experience and clues provided by fusion by disparate retinal images afford the direct perception of this relation on the basis of intrinsic physiologic arrangements.

INTEGRATION OF THE MOTOR AND SENSORY SYSTEM INTO BINOCULAR VISION

While it is convenient from a teaching point of view to separate the motor and sensory mechanisms of binocular vision, they are absolutely integrated in the visual process that we call binocular vision. The motor system aligns the foveae of the two eyes on the object of regard and maintains this fixation whether the subject or the object moves. It allows the field of vision to become the field of fixation. The sensory system is the feedback loop, which controls this motor alignment.

The processes of normal retinal correspondence allow the fusion of two physical retinal images into a single mental impression. When this fusion occurs, a new quality of the subjective visual process takes place and the perception of depth by parallax (stereopsis) results. The correspondence mechanism only allows for the relative localization of one object to another in physical space, and stereopsis represents the latitude that retinal correspondence allows and in which diplopia does not occur. The image perceived in depth is seen neither in the specific visual direction dictated by the right eye nor by the left eye but a visual direction corresponding to non-stimulated elements of the two eyes.

The mental process of absolute localization is essentially a compromise that not only requires decoding and analysis of retinal information, supplied by the correspondence mechanism, but that is also modified by other information from the efferent and afferent motor monitoring systems. This is best demonstrated by the patient with paralytic strabismus with normal retinal correspondence. The integration of the motor and sensory mechanisms in binocular vision represents a complex process, as will be seen in pathologic conditions affecting either one or both processes. The child with strabismus may show sensory adaptation to a motor anomaly or, may adapt to a sensory anomaly by changing motor response.

DEVELOPMENT OF BINOCULAR VISION

After having a workable knowledge about the psychophysical and sensory aspects of the binocular vision, it will be easier to understand development of this complex phenomenon. It is unequivocal that basic visual functions are innate and, therefore, present at birth. But their coordination, maturation and refinement take place during early postnatal period. Therefore, any obstacle during this period may cause abnormalities in the development of normal binocular vision. The subject matter on development of binocular vision includes:

- Prerequisites for development of binocular vision
- Eye at birth and normal postnatal development
- Maturation of binocular functions
- Neurophysiology of development
- Theories of development

PREREQUISITES FOR DEVELOPMENT OF BINOCULAR VISION

In order that simultaneous binocular vision be obtained, following conditions must be present:[53]

1. *Fixation.* There must be proper fixation with each eye. The muscles controlling the movements of each eye must function normally and turn both eyes in such a manner that the object of regard is fixated by corresponding retinae, i.e. the two foveae.

2. *Visual fields* of the two eyes must overlap to a large extent.

3. *Image* formed on each retina must be approximately similar, i.e. should be of the same size, shape, colour and intensity. This necessitates approximate equality in the optical apparatus of each eye.

4. *Common visual direction* must be there of two eyes, i.e. the retinae must possess physiologically corresponding points.

5. *Reflex activities* which produce fusional movements are very important. The eyes must be co-ordinated by this complex mechanism at all times so that retinal receptors which have a common visual direction will receive the same image at all times.

EYE AT BIRTH AND NORMAL POSTNATAL DEVELOPMENT

The anatomic development of the orbits and eyes is not completed at birth.

Orbits continue to change their size and shape throughout childhood into the teenage years, and the angle which their axes form with one another decreases from 50° at birth to 45° in later life. Thus, in adults, the medial wall of the two orbits are parallel to each other while the lateral wall diverge at 90°. At the same time, the interpupillary distance increases from an average of 45 mm at birth to about 58 to 66 mm

in adulthood. Accordingly, the convergence required to fixate an object at 33 cm distance increases from about 13 PD to about 19 PD. Angle lambda (λ) which is positive and may be as large as 10°, reduces to at least one-half of that amount during postnatal development.

Eyeballs also continue to grow. Growth of the globe is indicated by:

- *Change in length* from 17.5 mm at birth to 24 mm in adulthood.
- *Meridional fibres of the ciliary muscle* are completely formed at birth, but the circular portion continues to develop during the first one or two years of life.
- *Gross appearance of foveal cones changes* during the first a few months of life. Their fine structure, as revealed by electron microscopy, seems to be well developed.
- *Extraocular muscles*, although not of ultimate size, are fully functioning at birth.
- *Postural reflexes*, which are innate and unconditioned, are also functioning fully.

Bifoveal fixation does not exist at birth since binocular movements are not coordinated. The two eyes move more or less independent of each other. Fixation, therefore, is at first only monocular. The principal visual direction of the central fovea and the visual directions of the other retinal points relative to the principal direction are innate. Therefore, monocular fixation is present at birth, but it is poor. Furthermore, conscious fixation requires awareness of the presence of an object and then enough interest in the object to occupy an individual's attention for a certain length of time. The degree of mental activity necessary for this exceeds the capability of the newborn infant, and this is another reason why fixation is only rudimentary in the beginning.

At about 2 to 3 weeks of age, the infant begins to make movements of regard, turning his eyes to fixate an object. At 4 to 5 weeks of age, he can sustain monocular fixation of large near objects. Only after the age of 3 months the fixation become conscious rather than reflexive. Although the two eyes move independently at birth, aimless conjugate movements may occur. At about 6 weeks of age, fixation alternates rapidly between the two eyes, and a short time later the child begins to fixate binocularly and to perform conjugate pursuit movements, following persons or large near objects. Initially, the 3e pursuit movements are saccadic in character but become smooth and gliding between 3 and 5 months of age.

Disjugate vergence movements develop after conjugate movements. Convergence is demonstrable after 3 months of age and is stable at about 6 months.

Fusional movements occur at the same time, so that following an interruption of fusion, such as by introducing a prism before one eye, a corrective movement occurs to reestablish bifoveal fixation. Fusional movements are firmly established by the age of 1 year.

Visual acuity and fixation has always been considered to be very poor at birth. However, psychophysical and electrophysiologic research during recent years has established that visual acuity in infants develops much more rapidly than once thought, and that an infant's visual capacities are surprisingly rather well established shortly after birth, and that adult levels are reached at approximately 2 to 3 years of age.

This, of course, does not take into account the state of development of the interpretative mental functions but refers strictly to the resolving power of the visual system.

Visual development and estimated visual acuity

■ *At birth,* the fovea as well as lateral geniculate nucleus (LGN) is not developed, so an infant has peripheral vision only and can see to the sides but cannot focus the eyes straight ahead or smile back at the parents because of blurred central vision.[54,55] Visual acuity at birth is about 6/240 (Table 4.1).

■ *At about 6 weeks*, the child fixates peripherally which alternates rapidly. Vision is about 6/60 (Table 4.1)

■ *By 2 months of age,* LGN and its connections to the visual cortex in occipital lobe develop and the infant begins to follow moving objects.[55]

■ *By 3 months of age,* the fovea is fully developed. The fixation becomes central conscious rather than reflexive.[56] The child starts to focus on the parent's face, toys and responds. The infant responds better to high contrast images, bold colors and bright objects. Therefore, the parents should be advised to paint the baby's room in bright colours, decorate with contrasting shapes, handing brightly coloured toys over the crib, adding new furnishing to the room to retain interest, changing the direction of the crib frequently so that baby can see new furnishings. Even at night dim light should be kept on to help stimulating the baby's vision.

■ *At 6 months of age,* vision improves to 6/12 from 6/240 at birth (Table 4.1) as tested by visual evoked potential (VEP). However, on testing with optokinetic nystagmus (OKN) and preferential looking (PL) the visual acuity is reported about 6/30.[57,58] By the age of 6 months the hand–eye coordination also develops and the infant can now locate toys and tries to grasp them. So 6 months is the time when a detailed ophthalmological examination should be conducted for all infants to rule out gross refractive errors amblyopia, strabismus and a definitive treatment is started.

■ *By 1 year of age,* most children become emmetropic. At birth, all of the infants are born hypermetropic due to smaller axial length of eyeball.[59] Stimulation of retina by light results in growth of eyeball and resultant emmetropia by the age of 1 year.[60] The optic nerve is fully myelinated, the visual pathway is matured and the vision is about 6/6 to 6/9 by the age of 1 year.

■ *Age by which 6/6 vision* is achieved varies depending upon the test used as below:[61]
• *Optokinetic nystagmus (OKN):* 24–36 months
• *Preferential looking test (PLT):* 24–36 months
• *Visual evoked potential (VEP):* 6–12 months

MATURATION OF BINOCULAR FUNCTIONS
Development of fusion

Although basic visual functions are innate and, therefore, present at birth, other complex

Table 4.1 *Visual development and estimated visual acuity from birth to 6 years of age*

Age	Refractive status	Normal visual development	Estimated visual acuity		
			Optokinetic-nystagmus (OKN)	Preferential looking (Keelar PL cards)	Visual evoked potential
At birth	Hypermetropia	Pupillary light reflex present, fovea and lateral geniculate body not developed, no central fixation	————	6/300	6/240
1 month	Hypermetropia		6/120	6/200–6/90	6/120
2 months	Hypermetropia	Follow moving objects	6/60	6/90–6/60	6/60
3 months	Hypermetropia	Fovea developed, central fixation developed	6/36	6/90–6/60	6/36
6 months	Hypermetropia	Stereopsis developed up to 600 sec of arc (Firsby)	6/30	6/36–6/30	6/6–6/12
1 year	Emmetropia	Optic nerve myelination, complete visual differentiation of objects developed, stereopsis up to 210–170 sec of arc (Frisby)	6/18	6/24	6/6–6/9
18 months	Emmetropia	Visual acuty at adult level on paediatric acuity card, stereopsis developed up to 170–150 sec of arc (Frisby)	6/12	6/18	6/6
24 months	Emmetropia	Stereopsis developed up to 100–85 sec of arc (Frisby)	6/9	6/12	6/6
36 months	Emmetropia	Contrast sensitivity fully developed, stereopsis developed up to 85–55 sec of arc (Frisby)	6/6	6/6	6/6
Up to 5 years	Emmetropia	Stereopsis developed by 30–20 sec of arc (Frisby)	6/6	6/6	6/6
Up to 6 years	Emmetropia	Stereopsis developed up to 10–5 sec of arc (Frisby)	6/6	6/6	6/6

functions of binocular cooperation have to be learned before normal bifoveal single vision eventually is firmly established.

At birth, the eyes are not associated with each other, but act as two independent sense organs. The mechanisms necessary for binocular single vision are not completely developed. The foveas are not formed until the third month of life. As they develop, the stimulus to associate these areas is provided. By trial and error, the child learns that, when the image of an object is brought onto the two foveas simultaneously, the image is most detailed. For this reason alone, the visual axes are oriented in such a way that each fovea is directed at the object of regard.

Once this has become an established habit, the relative space perceptions of the child begin to take form. Objects to the right of fixation send images to retinal areas in the two eyes which have a common visual direction, i.e. to the right of fixation. The crossfiring of various sensory phenomena, such as touch with vision, eventually leads to an accurate determination of the child's space. An object seen so many degrees to the right of fixation is eventually interpreted in its correct position, and this is rewarded by checking accurately with the experiences of touch. Hence, by trial and error, and with tactile sensations the eyes become accurately associated with one another until gradually a normal child develops perception of space.

If the eyes are never allowed to become associated, as for example by a failure of development of one fovea or because of paralysis of an ocular muscle so that the two foveas cannot always be focussed together on the object of regard, the child never acquires binocular single vision and never learns to fuse the two images into one. Vision under these circumstances is always monocular and generally alternating; first one eye is used and then the other. The image of the eye which is not fixating the object is suppressed.

Development of stereopsis

▪ *Anatomic and physiologic factors necessary for depth perception* in the human being are either present at birth or develop shortly after birth so that, if the eyes are normal and the neuromuscular mechanism for moving the eyes is normal, depth perception will follow automatically.

▪ *Stereopsis seems to be in a class by itself* because it is claimed by some that there are persons with entirely normal eyes and neuromuscular apparatus who do not have depth perception by parallax when all other clues to depth are eliminated. As Ogle[46] has stated, "Stereopsis is a sensory phenomenon in its own right, with its own physiological mechanisms. It seems to be an all-or-none phenomenon, in that in a given person it is either present or not present. Training does not seem to develop stereopsis as such, but training may increase one's ability to discriminate depth differences just as the visual acuity may be slightly improved by training".

▪ *Age norms for stereoacuity* development and the tests used are depicted in Table 4.2.

NEUROPHYSIOLOGY OF DEVELOPMENT

▪ *The M and P cell neurophysiology.* Neuro-physiological animal studies have identified two specific pathways used to process visual information. These two pathways arise from different populations of retinal ganglion cells. Ganglion cell stimulation from a retinal image results in simultaneous parallel processing through these two different pathways. In the lateral geniculate nucleus, the nuclei can be divided into parvocelluar (P cells, or small cells) and magnocellular (M cells, or large cells). In the striate cortex, parvo- and magnorecipient

Table 4.2 *Age norms for stereoacuity and the tests used (measurements are all approximate)*

Age	Stereo (secs of arc)
Birth	——
One month	——
Three months	——
Six months	600 Frisby
Nine months	300 Frisby
One year	210 – 170 Frisby
18 months	170 – 150 Frisby
Two years	100 – 85 Frisby
Three years	85–55 Frisby
Four years	40–30 Frisby
Five years	30–20 Frisby
Six years	10–5 Frisby

(Adapted from A. Grounds by C. Rushen and L. Speedwell)

lamellae are segregated; however, there are interconnecting pathways, so information commingles. Parvocellular neurons are more sensitive to colour, high spatial frequencies, fine two-point discrimination, and fine stereopsis, and they project to areas of the central visual field and fovea. Magnocellular neurons, on the other hand, are sensitive to direction, motion, speed, flicker, gross binocular disparities, and gross stereopsis. Magnocellular neurons project to parafoveal and more peripheral retina. Magnocellular neurons are used for determining where, whereas parvocellular neurons examine static objects and determine what. Even though the two pathways are distinct, they overlap; and both systems interact to process visual information. From the striate cortex, information from M cells goes predominantly to parieto-occipital areas, while information from P cells goes to temporo-occipital areas.

- *Basic receptive field organisation of neurons and cortical architecture* are present since birth, although the retina and optic pathway are not completely developed.[62]

- *Properties of neurons in the visual cortex are markedly influenced by visual experience during the first a few postnatal months.* Neurophysiologic studies have demonstrated there specifically, these neural properties have been determined to involve binocularity, orientation specificity and disparity specificity.[63,64]

- *Excitatory connections of receptive fields* located in both retinae or retinotopic projections are largely present at birth. However, simultaneous occurrence of patterned visual input to both eyes during the development period is necessary to maintain their association.[63,64]

- *Plasticity during maturation stage* (i.e. in the neonatal visual system) is present to a great deal.[65, 66] This early plasticity seems to be vital for the formation of cells with closely matched receptive field properties in the two eyes, which is a necessary condition to form the substrate for stereoscopic vision. Patterned visual stimuli during stage of plasticity of visual system seem to act not only as a catalyst but also as directional stimuli in the consolidation, maintenance and

refinement of the neuronal connections in the visual cortex. A possible function of this plasticity in neuronal properties during early visual experience would be to allow the opportunity to match the properties of maximizing its capacity for analysis of the more important components of its environment. Also, the capacity to make modification in optimal disparity and preferred orientation would ensure that binocular cortical cells adapt similar receptive field positions and preferred orientations on the two retinae, which is a primary requirement for the probable role of these cells in binocular fusion and stereopsis. Thus, any disruption of the normal developmental conditions, such as a congenital or early strabismus or significantly subnormal vision in one eye (e.f. due to congenital cataract), will prevent the development of normal functional interrelationship and the loss of binocularity.

- *Maldevelopment of M versus P pathways secondary to strabismus or anisometropia and a blurred retinal image* is currrently being studied. Pattern deprivation amblyopia, which is a failure to develop fine two-point discrimination, is probably associated predominantly with abnormal P cell development. M cell development is also affected, especially if the retinal image disparity is quite large. M-neuron maldevelopment occurs predominantly in case of strabismus and may contribute to associated motor abnormalities such as latent nystagmus and asymmetrical horizontal smooth pursuit often seen in patients with congenital or infantile strabismus.

- *Postnatal morphological changes in the retina and retinal projections relative to the presence or absence of visual stimuli* are well-established. It has been observed that, in the lateral geniculate nucleus, neuronal cell growth is markedly reduced in the laminae with connection to visually deprived eye as compared with a nondeprived eye.[67, 68] The two types of retinal ganglion cells and geniculate cells seem to be differentially affected by visual deprivation. The large cells of the binocular segment are much more affected than either the large cells of the monocular segment or the small cells found mainly in the projection of the central area.[69]

■ *Orientation specificity and disparity specificity of cortical neurons* are also dependent on the visual experience in the early postnatal period. It has also been demonstrated experimentally.[70, 71]

THEORIES OF BINOCULAR VISION
Theory of correspondence and disparity

At present, this is the most widely accepted theory of binocular vision. Salient features of this theory are as follows:

- Corresponding elements of retina form the framework or zero system of binocular vision. Simultaneous stimulation of the corresponding points by one object transmits single visual impression with no depth quality.
- Simultaneous stimulation by two object points that differ in character, results in binocular rivalry.
- Diplopia occurs when disparate elements are stimulated by one object.
- Binocular single vision with stereopsis results, when the horizontal disparity remains within the limits of Panum's area.

■ *Neurophysiologic basis of correspondence theory:* Psychophysical data collected from human studies and neurophysiologic evidence collected from animal experimental studies of various researchers, Hubel and Wiesel being the pioneers,[72-74] have corroborated the correspondence theory. Till date following neurophysiological evidences are available:

- Approximately, 80% neurons of striate cortex are derived from each eye, 10% from the contralateral eye and 10% from the ipsilateral eye only. The two receptive fields of binocularly driven cortical cells are found to have corresponding location in the two retinae.[72-74]
- Of the binocularily driven cortical neurons, only 25% are stimulated equally well from each eye, while the remaining 75% show graded degrees of influence from the right or left eye (disparity sensitive binocular cells).[72-74]
- Stereopsis has been linked with horizontal disparity sensitive binocularly driven cortical neurons.[75]

- It has also been demonstrated that the distribution of cortical neurons (as mentioned above) is easily upset when animals are reared with experimental strabismus, anisometropia, or from vision deprivation by lid suture. This observation corroborates the fact that the properties of neurons in visual cortex are greatly influenced by the visual experience during the first a few postnatal months.[76,77]

Older theories of binocular vision

All the older theories of binocular vision have been abandoned. However, these are mentioned in brief, just to become familiar with the old concepts.

1. *Alternation theory of binocular vision.* This theory states that sensory fusion is perceptual unification of images perceived in corresponding locations in the two retinae. It assumes that corresponding retinal units are represented separately in the brain but that each of every pair is represented in consciousness by the same single unit. This conscious unit would receive the stimulus from only one retinal unit at a time, the other being excluded.[78]

This theory fails to explain many phenomena of binocular vision, particularly stereopsis.

2. *Projection theory of binocular vision.* This theory is based on the concept that the visual stimuli are exteriorized (projected to physical space) along the lines of directions.[79] This theory is not able to explain even the fundamental observation such as physiological diplopia and so abandoned.

3. *Motor theory.* This theory conceptualizes that the spatial orientation is obtained from the sensation derived from the movement of the head, conjugate movements of eyes and convergence. The eyes are made aware of their movements by muscle sense. It is this awareness that produces spatial localization. The sensations arising from the convergence effort determine whether one object is nearer or farther away than the others. This theory again fails to explain many sensory aspects of the binocular vision especially stereopsis.

4. *Theory of isomorphism.* This theory states that there exists a strict point-to-point relationship

between retina and cortex and strict comformity or isomorphism between the distribution of objects in space and cortical events form the basis of spatial orientation. Subjective visual directions as a property of the retinal-elements do not exist and that retinal correspondence cannot change.[80] However, it is interesting to point out that, there is no evidence for the physiologic rigidity of the retinocortical relationship or the convergence of the pathways on which this theory is based.

DISTURBANCES IN THE DEVELOPMENT OF BINOCULAR VISION

The time at which a lesion or defect in the visual system occurs is a most important factor with respect to the effect it will have on the disruption of existing functions and the prevention of further development. During the formative years, a neural pathway or neural function is maintained only through the stimulus of normal use. If this is disrupted, the involved structures will lose their functional capability. Naturally, if the disruption occurs before a certain function has become established, it will not be learned at all. Thus, the age of the child at the onset of a tropia is extremely significant in assessing the prognosis and deciding on the management. The earlier the deviation occurs, the less function will have developed and the easier will be disruption of existing functions. If it occurs between 18 months and 2 years of age, the prognosis for eventual bifoveal single vision is poor, whereas if it occurs at a later age, normal function may be regained with the adequate treatment. Anomalies in the development of binocular vision may be in the form of suppression, amblyopia, abnormal retinal correspondence.

Diplopia and confusion

■ *Diplopia* usually results from an acquired misalignment of the visual axes that causes an image to fall on the fovea of one eye and simultaneously on a nonfoveal point in the other eye. The object that falls on these non-corresponding points must be outside Panum's area to be seen double. In diplopia, the same object is seen as having two different locations in subjective space; the foveal image is always clearer than the nonfoveal image. The symptomatology of diplopia depends on the age at onset, duration, and subjective awareness. Visually immature children (less than about 6 or 7 years) rarely complain of diplopia. The younger the child, the greater the ability to suppress.

■ *Horror fusion* is an intractable diplopia in which there is an absence of central suppression. The angle of strabismus may be small or variable. Horror fusionis may occur in a number of clinical settings: for example, after fusion has been disrupted for a prolonged period, after head trauma, and rarely in long-standing squint. The management of these patients can be frustrating.

■ *Confusion,* like diplopia, is associated with ocular misalignment; however, confusion is very rare. Most adult patients with acquired ocular misalignment see double, i.e. two of the same image. Rarely, however, patients will describe the simultaneous perception of two different images superimposed on each other. Because the eyes are misaligned, dissimilar images fall on each corresponding fovea, and this, in a rare patient, will cause confusion rather than diplopia. In other words, objects that are physically separated in objective space are imaged on corresponding areas of the two retinas and are, therefore, seen as having the same location in subjective space.

Suppression

Suppression is an active cortical inhibition of the vision of one eye. Generally, it is supposed that the whole of one retinal function is extinguished in consciousness, but this is not usually so, and Burian[10] believes it is not generally the rule. Instead of total extinction, he considers that selective suppression in which only certain regions of one retina are suppressed take place more often. An example of this is the occurrence of suppression scotoma which can be demonstrated in the foveal area of some children with convergent strabismus. This scotoma disappears, however, in this eye when it is made to take up fixation alone, showing that the scotoma is purely a functional one and not due to any organic disease of the retina or visual pathways. Burian[10] believes that suppression may be selective also with regard to a specific retinal function; that is, the ability to resolve contours may be defective momentarily.

The suppression which occurs under conditions of strabismus, as just outlined, is facultative, i.e. occurs only under certain conditions. If the strabismus is not alternating, but is monocular with one eye remaining the fixation eye and the other constantly deviating, the suppression may become so constant and so deep that it persists. Then when the usually deviating eye is forced to take up fixation, the inhibition of its fovea remains, and the vision in this eye is defective. The suppression under these conditions is no longer facultative, but obligatory.[81] This obligatory suppression is called amblyopia.

Amblyopia

Amblyopia (functional amblyopia) by definition refers to a partial loss of sight in one or both eyes, in the absence of ophthalmoscopic and/or other marked objective signs. It results from psychical suppression of the retinal image. It may be anisometropic, strabismic or due to stimulus deprivation-amblyopia exanopsia (e.g. in a child with congenital cataract, severe ptosis). Amblyopia follows through a stage of suppression.

As just stated, suppression is a process of active inhibition, and at first it is probably always facultative, i.e. occurs only when both eyes whose visual axes are not in alignment are being used simultaneously. However, the degree to which facultative suppression can produce obligatory suppression or amblyopia probably depends upon the age of the child when one recalls that an infant is not born with fully developed eyes, anatomically or functionally. If suppression is induced in a very young infant, it probably can become obligatory in a much shorter period of time than if it starts in an older child. The amblyopia is therefore deeper and less easily broken up than when it begins later in life. This is in accord with clinical experience. Children whose strabismus begins early in life generally have more deep-seated amblyopia, if

the strabismus is monocular than those whose squint begins later. Further, it is said that, if suppression stops the development of foveal function before it has matured, normal vision never can be expected. It will be possible to restore only the function of the retina to the level to which it had developed before suppression set in.

Most of the evidence suggests that the site of interference in amblyopia is a block in the cortex and not a retinal activity. Most of the functions of the macula are intact in the presence of amblyopia, for example, dark adaptation and colour vision, but that form vision alone is affected.[82,83] In patients with amblyopia, the absolute threshold was found to be normal, both foveally and peripherally in cones and rods and in light-adaptation and dark-adaptation. The entire apparatus of light perception was found to be normal in these patients. The capacity for fixating and localizing illuminated points and areas on the central and peripheral retinae was also found to be normal. The capacity for discrimination of pattern fell as low as 2/200 or 2/400, without any loss of sensitivity to light. This shows that the apparatus for form vision is to some degree distinct from that involved in simple light perception.

Therefore, strabismic amblyopia, according to most authors, probably consists of cortical inhibition of the higher cortical function of pattern vision, without notable impairment of the lower cortical functions of simple light perception and spatial localization. Not all authors are satisfied with this concept that amblyopia is a selective inhibition of the form sense, as such, while all the other functions of the retina remain intact. The flicker fusion threshold of the foveal area of patients with amblyopia has been found to be considerably depressed as compared with values obtained from the surrounding retina and with the values obtained from the nonamblyopic eye in the same patients. However, the true nature of amblyopia is probably not known entirely. In addition to decreased visual acuity, there is some evidence which points to concomitant weakening of the power of central fixation. It is reported that only 20% of the subjects with amblyopia fixate along the central foveal axis of the poor eye when the good eye is occluded.[84] The shift from the true foveal axis to some outlying area increases with the increased depth of the amblyopia.

Abnormal retinal correspondence

Abnormal retinal correspondence (ARC) is an active cortical adjustment in the directional values of the two eyes which occurs in a child with early onset of squint (especially esotropia, occurring before 2 years of age). In this condition, the two foveae no longer have a common visual direction, and the fovea of one eye and a peripheral retinal element of the other eye acquire a common visual direction. This adaptation is brought about by an inherent desire for some form of binocular vision and to avoid diplopia and confusion that would otherwise take place. ARC is more common in esotropia than in exotropia. It is less common in vertical deviations and in true alternating squints with equal vision.

Types: ARC is of two types:
1. *Harmonious ARC* is present when the angle of anomaly (difference between the objective and subjective angle of the squint) equals the objective angle of squint.
2. *Unharmonious ARC* is present when the angle of anomaly is less than the objective angle of deviation.

- *Advantages of ARC* include:
- It gives the patient a form of binocular single vision.
- It tends to stabilize the angle of the deviation.
- The patient has a better visual judgement because he may have some binocular appreciation of depth.

- *Disadvantages of ARC* are:
- Once developed, it is extremely difficult to establish normal correspondence.
- Postoperatively, the angle of deviation may increase sometimes.

BINOCULAR VISION TESTS

TESTS FOR SIMULTANEOUS MACULAR PERCEPTION
See page 57 and Fig. 4.1A.

TESTS FOR FUSION
See page 58 and Fig. 4.1B.

TESTS FOR STEREOPSIS
Stereopsis tests are available in a variety of designs and produce a three-dimensional object in a variety of different ways. Most tests use simple geometrical shapes as test objects presented against a random patterned background. It seems to be unavoidable that stereo tests produce monocular clues of depth to some degree; precautions may need to be taken in the application of the tests to ensure that these clues are minimised.
- *For young children,* the Lang test and the Frisby screening test are designed to produce behavioural response. With these, the child attempts to reach out and grab the object. These tests may provide a result in some children as young as 6–12 months.
- *In older children,* a variety of tests are available.

Note. Various tests employed to test stereopsis must incorporate two essential features:
- The two eyes must be dissociated; that is, each eye must be presented with a separate field of view, and
- Each of the two fields or targets must contain elements imaged on corresponding retinal areas. The commonly employed tests are as follows:

Tests employed to check stereopsis can be grouped as below:
- Synaptophore or stereoscope tests
- Vectograph tests
- Random dot stereogram tests
- Simple motor task tests based on stereopsis

I. Synoptophore or stereoscope tests
See page 58, 138 and Fig. 4.1C.

II. Vectograph tests
A vectograph consists of polaroid material on which the two targets are imprinted so that each

target is polarized at 90° with respect to the other. The vectograph dissociates the eyes optically. With the use of properly oriented polaroid spectacles, each target is seen separately with the two eyes.

Titmus stereo test

The Titmus stereo test utilizes the principle of vectograph. This is perheaps the most familiar stereo test.

The three-dimensional polaroid vectograph which constitutes the Titmus test is basically made up of two plates in the form of a booklet (Fig. 4.17). To perform the test the plates are reviewed with polaroid glasses. The Titmus stereo test consists of three parts:

1. *The fly test.* The right side of the test booklet contains a large housefly to test gross stereopsis (threshold 3000 sec of arc). It is especially useful in young children. The subject is asked to pick up one of the wings of the fly. If the subject sees stereoscopically, he will reach above the plate. In the absence of gross stereopsis, the fly will appear as an ordinary flat photogrpah (Fig. 4.18).

2. *The animal test.* It is performed, if the gross stereopsis is present. This test consists of three rows of five animals each; one animal from each row is imaged disparately (thresholds 10, 200 and 400 sec of arc, respectively) (Fig. 4.17). And,

in each row, one of the animals correspondingly imaged in two eyes is printed heavily black (serves as a misleading clue). The subject is asked which one of the animals stands out. A subject without stereopsis will name the animal printed heavily (misleading clue); while in the presence of stereopsis he will name the disparately imaged animal.

3. *The circles test.* It consists of nine squares, each containing four circles arranged in the form of a lozenge (Fig. 4.17). Only one of the circles in each square is disparately imaged at random with threshold ranging from 800 to 40 sec of arc.

If the subject has passed other two tests, he is asked to 'push-down' the circle that stands out, beginning with the first set. When he makes mistakes or finds no circle to push down, the limit of his stereopsis is presumably reached.

Circle no. 5, equivalent to 100 sec of arc is considered to be lowest limit of fine central stereoacuity and is designated as the lowest limit of good stereoacuity.[85]

- ***Advantages.*** The Titmus test is simple and easy to perform and so is most widely used.

- ***Disadvantages***
1. Some of the circles of the Titmus test are selected by even stereoblind observers, because

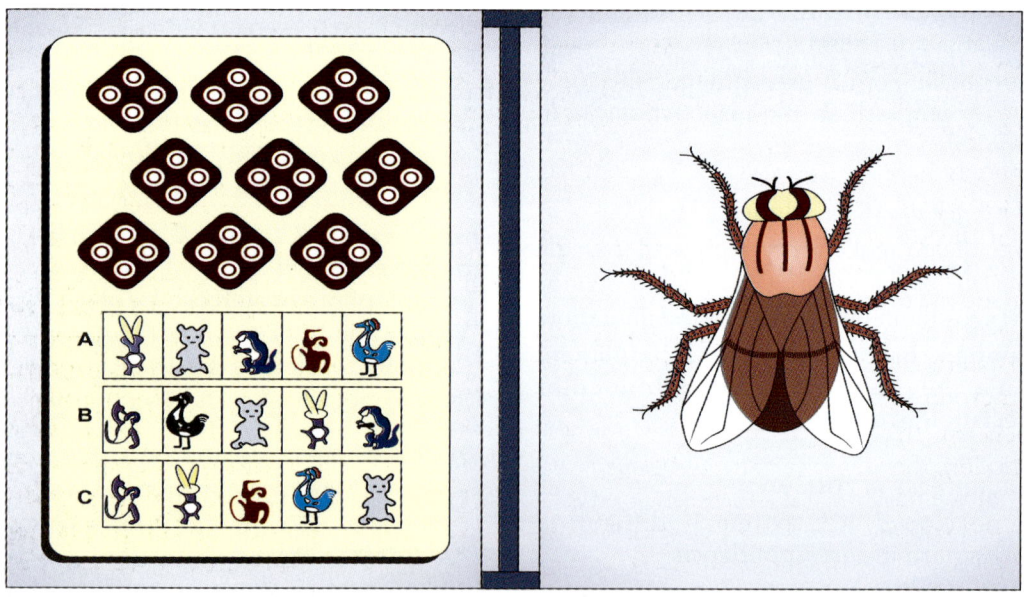

Fig. 4.17. *The Titmus stereo test.*

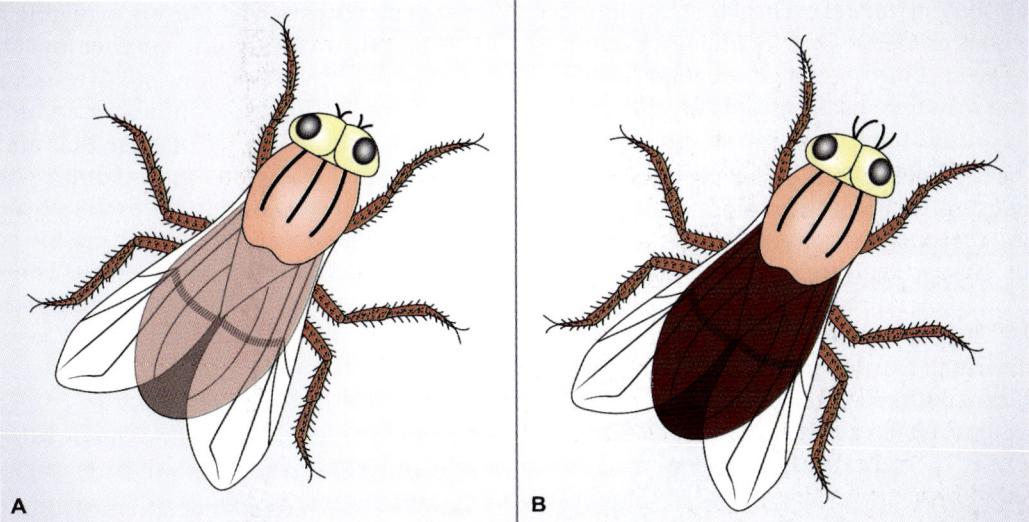

Fig. 4.18. *Titmus test using fly for gross stereopsis: A, No stereopsis; B, Stereopsis present.*

they look 'different' and not because they are seen stereoscopically.[86]

2. With the exception of the fine stereoacuity circles 5 to 9, this test often is unreliable in differentiating patients with amblyopia and heterotropia from those with normal vision.[87]

III. Random dot stereogram tests

The random dot stereogram tests are devoid of monocular clues and the patients cannot guess what the stereo figure is and where it is located on the test plate. So, this test provides truer measurement of stereopsis than the Titmus test.[88]

1. Random dot E-test (RDT). This test consists of three cards to be viewed with polaroid spectacles (Fig. 4.19).[89] One card is a bas relief model of the stereo test figure and is used to show the patient for what he should look (A). The second card contains the 'E' stereo figure with a random dot background (B). The third card is a stereoblank with an identical random dot background (C).

To perform this test (after showing the bas relief model), the two test cards are held 50 cm in front of the patient, who is asked to indicate which card contains the letter 'E'. The patient gives a 'pass' or 'fail' response. The stereoacuity, when present, can be quantitated by increasing the testing distance from the patient.

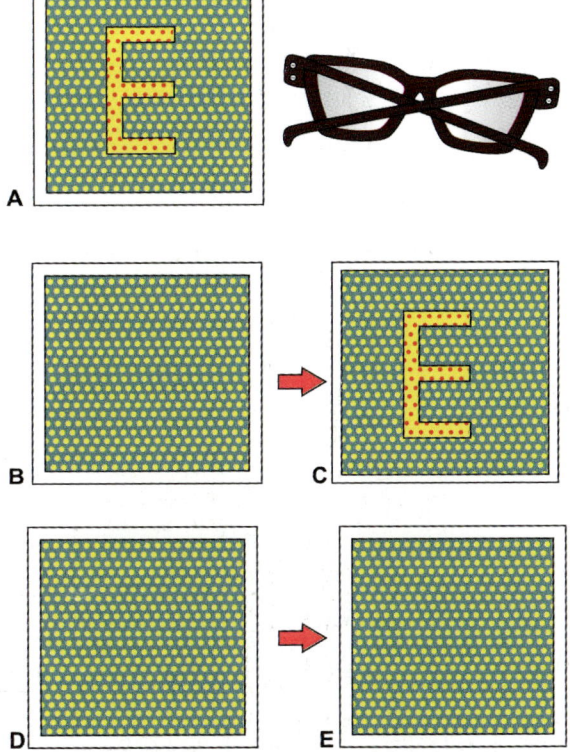

Fig. 4.19. *Random dot E-test: A, Bas relief model of stereo test figure; B, Random dot stereo figure seen without polaroid glasses; C, Random dot stereo figure as seen in the polaroid glasses—with stereopsis present; D and E, Stereo-blank card with random dot background as seen with (E) and without (D) polaroid glasses.*

2. TNO random dot test. The TNO random dot stereo test is graded to provide retinal disparities ranging from 15 to 480 sec of arc. It is based on the same principle as 'Random dot E-test', but has the advantage of eliciting quantitative responses without changing the testing distance.

It consists of a booklet containing seven plates. Each test plate consists of a stereogram in which various shapes (squares, dots, crosses) have been created by random dots in complementary colours. The plates contain two types of figures, the one which can be perceived when viewed binocularly with red green spectacles by normal subject having stereopsis (Fig. 4.20B). The second set of figures can be seen with and without the spectacles (Fig. 4.20A) even in the absence of stereopsis. The first three stereograms of the test booklet are used to establish the presence of gross stereopsis quickly, while the remaining four plates allow to quantitate the

level of stereopsis. TNO test is available in two versions one for adults and another for children.

3. Lang-test. This test consists of random dot stereogram with panographic presentation.[90,91] The stereoscopic images of a car, star and a cat (Fig. 4.21) embedded in random dots on the test card are seen disparately by each eye through the cylindrical lenses imprinted on the surface lamination of the test (Fig. 4.22). Therefore, polaroid glasses or red green spectacles are not required in this test; so especially useful in young children who refuse to wear glasses.

Lang test is available in two forms:

- *Lang I test,* which measures stereopsis at 550, 600 and 1200 seconds of arc and;
- *Lang II test,* which is finer and measures at 200, 400 600 seconds of arc.

To perform this test, the test card is held at a distance of 40 cm in front of the subject, who is asked to name or point to the shapes on the test card. The disparity of the car and star is 600 sec and of the cat 1200 sec of arc.[92]

4. Frisby test. In this test, stereogram consists of three plastic cards each containing four squares of small random shapes (Fig. 4.23). One of the squares in each plate contains a hidden circle which is seen disparately. The disparity is created by displacement of random shapes by the thickness of the plate. So, this test also does not require use of glasses. Thus, it is especially useful for young children who refuse to accept glasses.

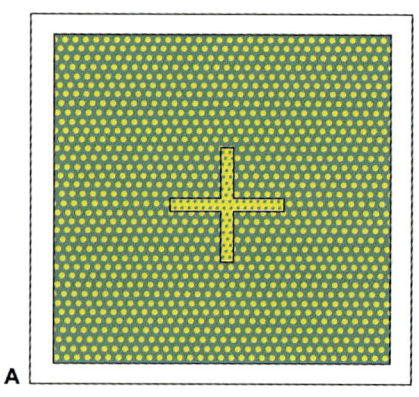
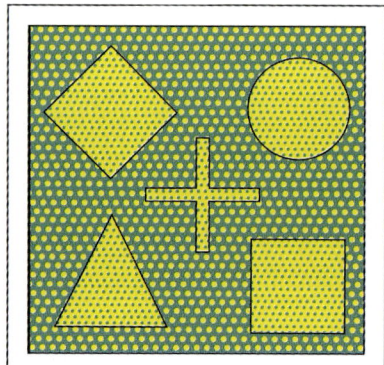

Fig. 4.20. *Figures in TNO test: A, Cross is seen with and without red-green spectacles; B, Four 'hidden shapes' which can be seen with red-green spectacles in the presence of stereopsis.*

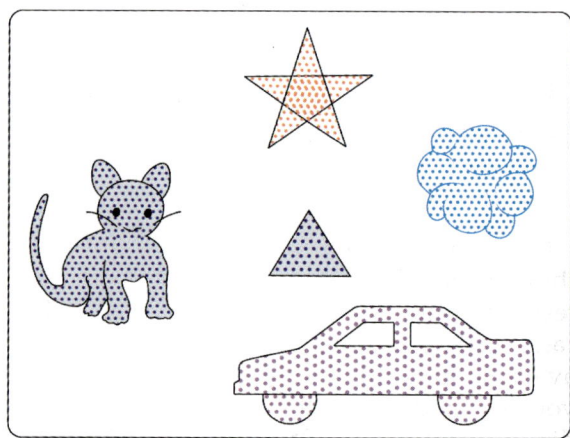

Fig. 4.21. *Stereoscopic images embedded in random dots of the Lang test stereogram.*

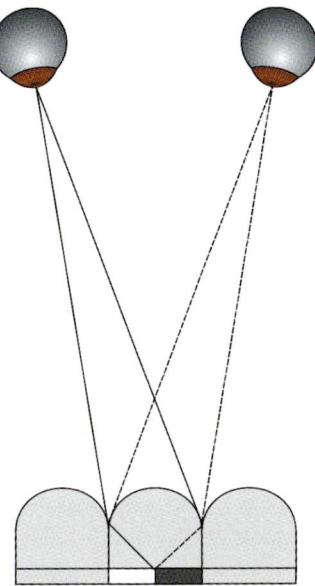

Fig. 4.22. Cylindrical gratings provide separate images for each eye (From Lang).[89]

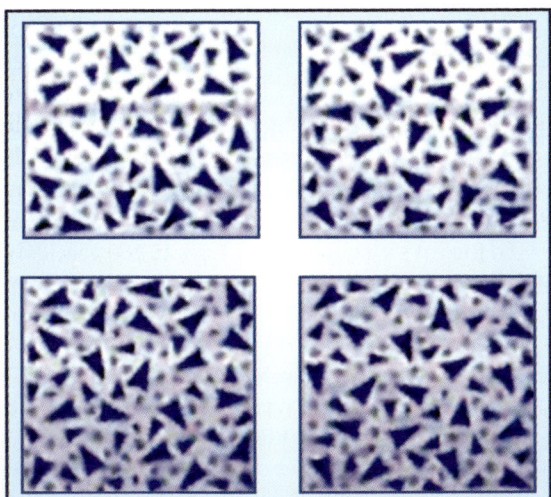

Fig. 4.23. The Frisby test.

looking responses can be observed to establish that stereopsis is present.

5. *Stereoscopic contours induced optokinetic nystagmus test*[87-88] and Television random dot stereo test[95] have recently been suggested to test stereopsis in infants. Such electronically generated stereopsis tests may become more relevant in view of the current emphasis on early diagnosis and treatment of strabismus in infants.

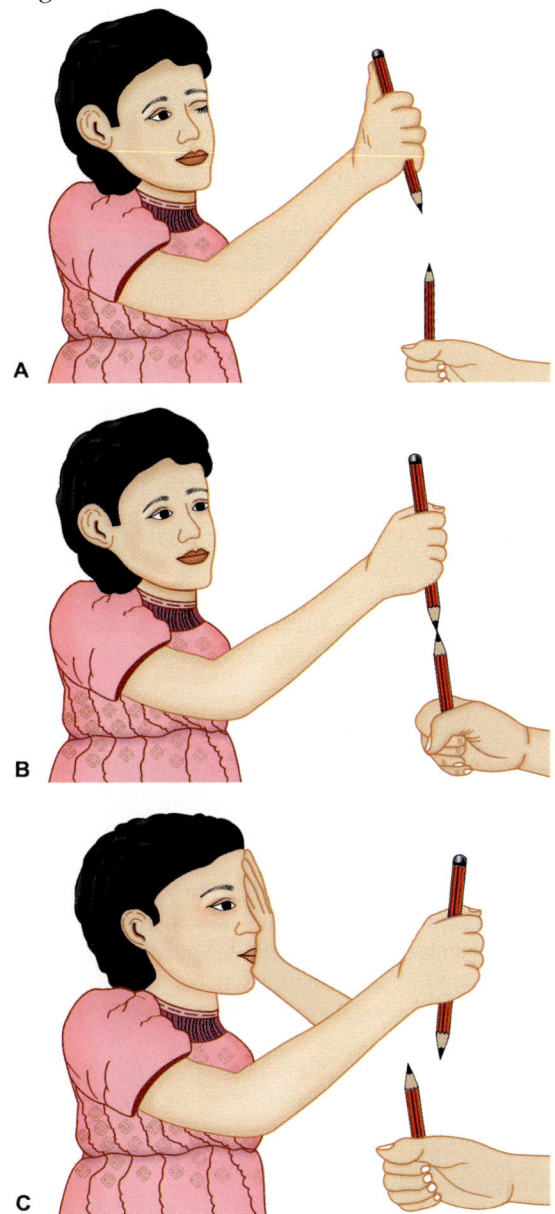

Fig. 4.24. Two-pencil test for stereopsis. For description see text.

Care must be taken to avoid monocular clues through parallax movements when using the test. The test can measure stereoacuity in the range 600–15 seconds of arc. The Frisby test is available in a screening version designed for younger children and infants. It presents a three-dimensional object field, together with a flat image side by side in a preferential looking format. In this case, a spontaneous pointing or

IV. Simple motor task test based on stereopsis

The two-pencil test

It is very simple primitive but an effective test for detecting presence or absence of gross stereopsis (threshold value 3000–5000 sec of arc).[92] Though known to even earlier ophthalmologists, it was popularized by Lang in 1975.[92]

To perform this test, examiner holds a pencil vertically in front of the patient, who is asked to touch its upper tip with the tip of the pencil held in his hand by one swift movement from above (Fig. 4.24A). Patient having stereopsis passes the test with both eyes open (Fig. 4.24B). Patients fail the test with one eye closed or when both eyes are open but stereopsis is absent (Fig. 4.24C).

REFERENCES

1. Romano PE, Romano JA. Fusion: a new classification and methods for determining the level of sensory binocular cooperation. Survey Ophthalmol 17:458, 1973.

2. Walls GL. The Vertebrate Eye. New York, Hafner, 1967.

3. Karten HJ, et al. Neural connections of the "visual Wulst"of the avian telencephalon. Experimental studies in the pigeon (Columba livia) and owl (Speotyto cunicularia), J Comp Neurol 150:253, 1973.

4. Pettigrew JD, Konishi M. Effect of monocular deprivation on binocular neurones in the owl's visual Wulst. Nature 264:753, 1976.

5. Pettigrew JD. Comparison of the retinotopic organization of the visual Wulst in nocturnal and diurnal raptors, with a note on the evolution of frontal vision. In: Cool SJ, Smith EL, III editors. Frontiers in visual science, New York, Spring er-Verlag New York, Inc., pp. 328-335, 1978.

6. Denny-Brown D, Fischer EG. Physiological aspects of visual perception. II, The subcortical vision direction of behavior. Arch Neurol 33:228, 1976.

7. Hering E: Vom Ortsinne der Netzhaut, Beitrage zur Physiologie, Leipzig, East Germany, Wilhelm Engelmann, pp. 9–80, 1861.

8. Hering E. Der Raumsinn und die Bewegungen der Augen. In Hermann, L., editor: Handbuch der Physiologie, Leipzig, Vogel, vol. 3/1, pp. 343–601, 1879. (Radde, c.A., translator: 1942, American Academy of Optometry.).

9. Howard IP and Templeton WB. Human spatial orientation, New York, 1966, John Wiley & Sons. Inc.

10. Burin H. Sensorial retinal relationship in concomitant strabismus. Tr Am. Ophth Soc. 43: 373, 1945.

11. Bagolini B. Anomalous correspondence: definition and diagnostic methods, Doc. Ophthalmol. 23:346, 1967.

12. Bielschowsky A. Lectures on motor anomalies. Hanover, 1940, Dartmauth college Publication.

13. A'guilonius F. Opticorum Libri Sex. Antwerp. Plantin, 1613.

14. Vieth GAU. Ueber die Richtung der Augen. Ann Phys 48:233–251, 1818.

15. Muller J. vom Gesichtsinn. In Handbuch der Physiologie des Menschen fur Vorlesungen. coblenz, Holscher, 1840.

16. Hering E. Beitrage zur Physiologie. Leipzig, W Engelman, 1864.

17. Hillebrand F. Die stabilitat der Raumwerte auf der Netzhaut. Z Psychol 5:1–59, 1893.

18. Ogle KN. Researches in Binocular Vision, Philadelphia, Sanders, 1950.

19. Panum PL. Physiologische Untersuchungen uber das Sehen mit zwei Augen. Kiel, Schwering, 1858.

20. Hering E. Beitrage zur Physiologie. Leipzig, W Engelman, 1864.

21. von Helmholtz H. Handbuch der Physiologische Optik: Hamburg, Voss, 1866.

22. Verhoeff FH. A new theory of binocular vision. Arch Ophthalmol 13:151-175, 1935.

23. Hubel DH, Wiesel TN. Receptive fields, binocular interaction and functional architecture in the cat's visual cortex. J Physiol 160:154, 1962.

24. Levelt WJM. On binocular rivalry, Soesterberg. The Netherlands, 1965, Institute for Perception RVD-TNO.

25. Panum PL. Physiolische Untersuchungen uber das Sehen mit zwei Augen, Kiel, 1858, Schwerssche Buchandlung, p. 52 ff.

26. Fechner G Th. Uber einige Verhaltnisse des binokularen Sehens, Abh. Sachs. Ges. Wiss. 7:337, 1861.

27. Helmholtz H von. In Southhall, P.C., editor: Helmholtz's treatise on physiological optics. English translation from third German edition, Ithaca, 1924, The Optical Society of America. Quoted from Dover reprint, New York, 1962, Dover Publicaions, Inc.

28. Hering E. Beitrage zur Physiologie, vol. 3, Leipzig 1864, Wilhelm Englemann, p. 182.

29. Fox R, Check R. Binocular fusion: A test of the suppression theory. Percept Psychophys 1:331-334, 1966.

30. Collyer SC, Bevan W. Objective measurement of dominance control in binocular rivalry. Percept psychophys 8:437–439, 1970.

31. Fox R, Check R. Detection of motion during binocular rivalry suppression. J. Exp. Psychol. 78:388–395,1968.

32. Wales R, Fox R. Increment detection thresholds during binocular rivalry suppression. Percept Psychophys 8:90–94, 1970.

33. Poggio CF, Fischer B. Binocular interaction and depth sensitivity of neurons in striate and prestriate cortex of the behaving rhesus monkey. J. Neurophysiol. 40:1392–1405, 1977.

34. Blake R, Fox R, McIntyre C. Stochastic properties of stabilized-image binocular rivalry alternations. J. Exp. Psychol. 88:327–332, 1971.

35. Barany EH, Hallden U. The influence of some central nervous system depressants on the reciprocal inhibition between the two retinas as manifested in retinal rivalry. Acta Psychol Scand 14:296–316, 1947.

36. Lack LC. The role of accommodation in the control of binocular rivalry. Percept Psychophys 10:38–42, 1971.

37. Levelt WJM. On binocular rivalry. Soesterberg. Institute for Perception, RVOTNO, 1965.

38. Cogan AL. Human binocular interaction, towards a neural model. Vision Res. 27:2139, 1988.

39. Wolfe JM, and Blake R. Monocular and binocular processes in human vision. In: Models of the cortex, Rose, D., and Dobson, V. (eds). New York, Wiley 1985, p. 192.

40. Julesz B. Binocular depth perception of computer generated patterns. Bell Syst Tech J 32:1125–1162, 1960.

41. Julesz B, Tyler CW. Neurontropy, an entropy-like measure of neural correlation, in binocular fusion and rivalry, Bio Cybernetics 23:25–32, 1976.

42. Tyler CW, Julesz B. The neural transfer characteristic (neurontropy) for binocular stochastic stimulation. Bio Cybernetics 23:33–37, 1976.

43. Wheatstone C. Contributions to the physiology of vision. Part the first. On some remarkable and hitherto unobserved phenomena of binocular vision, Phil. Trans. R. Soc. Lond 128:371, 1838.

44. Julesz B. Foundations of cyclop an perception, Chicago, 1970, University of Chicago Press.

45. Julesz B. Global stereopsis: cooperative phenomena in stereoscopic depth perception. In Held, R. et al, editors: Handbook of sensory physiology, Berlin, 1978 , Springer-Verlag, vol. 7, pp 215–256.

46. Ogle K. Present knowledge of stereoscopic vision. AMA Arch ophthalmol 6:770, 1958.

47. Burian HM: Stereopsis, Doc. Ophthalmol. 5–6: 169, 1951.

48. Joshua DE, Bishop PO. Binocular single vision and depth discrimination. Exp Brain Res 10:389–416,1970.

49. Pettigrew JD, Nikara T, Bishop PO. Binocular interaction of single units in cat striate cortex: stimulation by single moving slit. Exp Brain Res 6:391–410, 1968.

50. Von der Heydt R, Adorjani C, Hanny P, Baumgartner Q. Disparity sensitivity and receptive field incongruity of units in the cat striate cortex. Exp Brain Res 31:523–545, 1978.

51. Poggio CF, Fischer B. Binocular interaction and depth sensitivity of neurons in striate and p re striate cortex of the behaving rhesus monkey. J Neuro-physiol 40:1392–1405, 1977.

52. Blakemore C, Fiorentini A, Maffei L. A second neural mechanism of binocular depth discrimination. J Physiol 226:725–749, 1972.

53. Adler FH. Binocular vision in physiology of the eye. Clinical applications, 3rd ed. CV Moskey, St Lewis, 1959, page 739.

54. Garey LJ. Structural development of the visual system of man. Hum Neurobiol 1984; 3:75–80.

55. 15 Yuodelis C, Hendrickson A. A qualitative and quantitative analysis of the human fovea during development. Vision Res 1986; 26:847–55.

56. Saunders KJ, McCulloch DL, Shepherd AJ, Wil Emmetropisation following preterm birth. Br J 2002; 86:1035–40.

57. Madan A, Jan JE, Good WV. Visual development infants. Dev Med Child Neurol 2005; 47:276–80.

58. Birch EE, O'Connor AR. Preterm birth and visual de Semin Neonatol 2001; 6:487–97.

59. Scott R. Lambert, MDb, Anthony Kriss, PhD, Da FRCS. Delayed Visual Maturation : A Longitudinal and Electrophysiological Assessment. Ophthalmology 96:524–8

60. Smithers LG, Gibson RA, McPhee A, Makrides dose of docosahexaenoic acid in the neonatal perio visual acuity of preterm infants: results of a controlled trial. Am J Clin Nutr 2008; 88:1049–56.

61. Dobson V and Teller D. Visual acuity in human infants: a review and comparison of behavioral and electrophysiological studies, Vision Res. 18:1469, 1978.

62. Wiesel TN, Hubel DH. Ordered arrangement of orientation columns in monkeys lacking visual experience. J Comp Neurol 158:307–318, 1974.

63. Anker RL, Cragg BG. Development of the extrinsic connections of the visual cortex in the cat. J Comp Neurol 154:29–41, 1974.

64. Blakemore C, Van Sluyters RC. Innate and environmental factors in the development of the kitten's visual cortex. J Physiol 248:663–716 1975.

65. Wiesel TN, Hubel DH. Extent of recovery from the effects of visual deprivation in kittens. J Neurophysiol 28:1060–1072, 1965.

66. Blakemore C, Cooper GF– Development of the brain depends on the visual environment. Nature 228:447–478, 1970.

67. Wiesel TN, Hubel DH. Effects of visual deprivation on morphology and physiology of cells in the cat's lateral geniculate body. J Neurophysiol 26:978–993, 1963.

68. Garey LJ, Fisken RA, Powell TPA. Effects of experimental deafferentation on cells in the lateral geniculate nucleus of the cat. Brain Res 52:363–369, 1973.

69. Sherman SM, Hoffman KP, Stone J. Loss of a specific cell type from the dorsal lateral geniculate nucleus in visually deprived cats. J Neurophysiol 35:532–541, 1972.

70. Blakemore C, Mitchell DE. Environmental modification of the visual cortex and the neural basis of learning and memory. Nature 241:467–468, 1973.

71. Shlaer R: Shift in binocular disparity causes compensatory change in the cortical structure of kittens.; Science 173:638–641, 1971.

72. Hubel DH and Wiesel TN. Receptive fields of single neurons in the cat's striate cortex, J. Physiol. 148:574, 959.

73. Hubel DN and Wiesel TN. Receptive fields binocular interaction and functional architecture in the cat's visual cortex, J. Physiol. (Lond.) 160:106, 1962.

74. Hubel DH and Wiesel TN. Stereoscopic vision in macaque monkey, cells sensitive to binocular depth in area 18 of the macaque monkey cortex, Nature 225:41, 1970.

75. Barlow HB, Blakemore C, and Pettigrew JD: The normal mechanisms of binocular depth discrimination J. Physiol. (Lond). 193: 327, 1967.

76. Hubel DH, and Wiesel TN. Binocular interaction in straite cortex of kittens reared with artificial squint, J. Neurophysiol. 28:1041, 1965.

77. Hubel DH and Wiesel TN. The period of susceptibility to the physiological effect of unilateral eye closure in kittens, J.Pysiol. (Lond) 206:419, 1970.

78. Verhoeff FH. A new theory of binocular vision, Arch. Ophthalmol. 13:152, 1935.

79. Duane A. Projection and double vision: some new view points, Arch. Ophthalmol. 54: 233, 1925.

80. Linksz A. Physiology of the eye. In vision, vol. 2, New York, 1952, Grune and Strattonn, Inc.

81. Chavasse F. Worth's Squint, Philadelphia 1938, P. Blakiston's Son and Co. p 341.

82. Ludvigh E. A Hypothesis Concerning Amblyopia Ex Anopsia, Tr. New Erigland Ophth. Soc, Arch. Ophth. 43:397, 1950.

83. Wald S, and Burian H. The Dissociation of Form Vision and Light Perception in strabismic Amblyopia., Am. J. Ophth. 27: 950, 1944.

84. Brock F, and Givner I. Fixation Anomalies in Amblyopia AMA. Arch. Ophth. 47: 775, 1952.

85. Isomura Y, Awaya S. Studies on aniseikonia and binocular fusion with special reference to stereoacuity. Nippon Ganku Gakkai Zasshi; 84: 1619–28, 1980.

86. Kohler L and Stigmar G. Vision screening in four year old children, Acta Paediatr, Scand. 62: 17, 1973.

87. Simons K, and Reinecke RD. A reconsideration of amblyopia screening and stereopsis, Am. J. Ophthalmol 78: 707, 1974.

88. Julesz B. Foundations of cyclopean perception, Chicago, 1971, University of Chicago Press.

89. Reinecke R and Simons K. A new stereoscopic test for amblyopia secreening. Am. J. Ophthalmol. 78: 714, 1974.

90. Lang J. New stereotests. In Boschi MC and Frosini R, editors: Proceedings of the International Symposium on Strabismus, Florence, Italy, June 21-23, 1982, p. 177.

91. Lang J. A new stereotest, J Paediatr. Ophthalmol Strabismus 20:72, 1983.

92. LaRoche R and Noorden GK. Von: theoretical and practical evaluation of a simple stereotest (Abstract), Invest. Ophthalmol. Vis Sci. (Supp.) 22: 266, 1982.

93. Archer SM, Miller KK, and Helveston EM. Stereoscopic contours and optokinetic nystagmus in normal and stereoblind subjects, Vision Res. 27:841, 1987.

94. Fox R, Lehmkuhle S and Leguire LE. Stereoscopic contours induce optokinetic nystagmus, Vision Res. 18:1189, 1978.

95. Mizukami Y, Awaya S, Koizumi E, and Kamiya A. The investigation of stereoacuity in infants by the new TV random dot stereotest, Folia Ophthalmol. Jpn. 38:1182, 1987.

sight impairing disease of one eye, e.g. anisometropia, central chorioretinitis, etc.

5. **Consecutive heterotropia** is the term used to describe the deviation resulting from surgical overcorrection or spontaneous conversion of an esotropic eye into an exodeviation.

CLINICAL TYPES OF OCULAR DEVIATIONS

In day-to-day clinical practice, the ocular deviations are classified as below.

ESODEVIATIONS

A. *Esophoria (E or S)*
B. *Intermittent esotropia (E [T] or S [T])*
C. *Esotropia (ET or ST)*

I. *Concomitant esotropia*
1. *Infantile (congenital) esotropia*
2. *Accommodative esotropia*
    i. Refractive (normal AC/A ratio)
    ii. Non-refractive accommodative
        – *Hyperaccommodative (high AC/A ratio)*
        – *Hypoaccommodative (weak accommodation)*
    iii. *Mixed or partially accommodative*
3. *Non-accommodative esotropia*
    i. Acquired or late onset non-accommo-dative esotropia
        – *Basic esotropia*
        – *Convergence excess type*
        – *Divergence insufficiency type*
    ii. Acute concomitant esotropia
    iii. Microtropia
    iv. Nystagmus blockage syndrome
    v. Cyclic esotropia
    vi. Stress-induced esotropia
    vii. Esotropia in myopia
    viii. Esotropia due to spasm of near reflex
4. *Sensory esotropias*
5. *Consecutive esotropia*

II. *Incomitant esotropia*
1. *Paralytic esotropia*
    i. Lateral rectus paralysis
    ii. Divergence paralysis
    iii. Mobius syndrome

2. *A- and V-pattern esotropias*
3. *Special types of restrictive esotropia*
    i. Duane's retraction syndrome (with esotropia)
    ii. Thyroid myopathy
    iii. Medial orbital wall fracture
    iv. Strabismus fixsus
    v. Excessively resected medial rectus muscle

EXODEVIATIONS

A. Exophoria (X)
B. Intermittent exotropia (X [T])
C. Exotropia (XT)

I. *Concomitant exotropias*

1. *Primary exotropias*
    i. *Divergence excess type*
    ii. *Convergence insufficiency type*
    iii. *Basic exotropia*
    iv. *Pseudodivergence excess type*

2. *Sensory exotropia*
3. *Consecutive exotropia*

II. *Incomitant exotropias*
1. *Paralytic exotropias*
    i. *Isolated medial rectus paresis*
    ii. *Complete third nerve paralysis*
    iii. *Paralysis of convergence*

2. *A-, V- and X-pattern exotropias*
3. *Special types of restrictive exotropias*
    i. *Duane's retraction syndrome (with exotropia)*
    ii. *Craniofacial anomalies with divergent orbit.*
    iii. *Thyroid myopathy*
    iv. *Restriction due to trauma or excessive surgery*

VERTICAL DEVIATIONS

A. Hyperphoria (H)
B. Intermittent hypertropia [H (T)]
C. Hypertropia (HT)

I. *Comitant hypertropia*
1. Induced (refractive)
2. End result of long-standing paralytic deviation.

II. *Incomitant vertical deviations*
1. *Apparent oblique muscle dysfunction*
    i. Inferior oblique overaction (strabismus sursoadductorious) *now termed as* over elevation in adduction (OEA).

- *Primary OEA, or*
- *Secondary OEA.*

ii. Inferior oblique underaction, *now termed* as under-elevation in adduction (UEA).
- *Primary UEA, or*
- *Seconday UEA*

iii. Superior oblique overaction (strabismus deorsadductorious), *now termed* as over depression in adduction (ODA).
- *Primary ODA, or*
- *Seconday ODA.*

iv. Superior oblique underaction is now termed as under-depresson in adduction (UDA).
- *Primary UDA, or*
- *Secondary UDA.*

2. *Paretic vertical deviations*
- Congenital unilateral superior oblique paresis.
- Non-congenital superior oblique paresis.
- Bilateral superior oblique paresis.
- Monocular elevation deficiency (MED), (old name: Double elevator palsy).
- Monocular depression deficiency (MDD); (old name: Double depressor palsy).
- Superior rectus paresis (isolated).
- Inferior rectus paresis (isolated).
- Skew deviation.

3. *Restrictive vertical deviations*
a. Restrictive vertical deviations due to misdirected muscle force
   i. *Congenital cranial dysinnervation disorders (CCDDs) primarily affecting vertical ocular motility:*
      - *Congenital fibrosis of extraocular muscles (CFEOMs)*

   ii. *Iatrogenic displacement of inferior oblique muscle after its anteriorization.*

b. Restrictive vertical deviations due to mechanical restrictions
   i. *Tight extraocular muscles*
   ii. *Restrictive vertical deviation due to structural adhesions (induced adhesive syndromes)*
   iii. *Restrictive vertical deviation due to orbital mass lesions.*

III. *Dissociated vertical deviations (DVD)*
1. Monocular DVD
2. Binocular or alternating DVD

CYCLODEVIATIONS

A. Cyclophorias
1. Incyclophoria
2. Excyclophoria

B. Intermittent cyclotropias
1. Intermittent incyclotropia
2. Intermittent excyclotropia

C. Cyclotropias
1. *Incyclotropia*
   i. Inferior oblique paralysis
   ii. Inferior rectus paralysis
2. *Excyclotropias*
   i. Superior oblique paralysis
   ii. Superior rectus paralysis

SYMBOLS USED FOR PHORIAS AND TROPIAS

In medical charts and orthoptic record, the deviations are usually indicated by the symbols. Though, variations may exist between different squint clinics, the symbols listed in Table 5.1 are fairly uniformly used as abbreviations for different types of deviations.

Table 5.1 *Symbols used for ocular deviations*

| Deviation | Phoria | | Tropia | | | |
| | Distance | Near | Distance | | Near | |
			Constant	Intermittent	Constant	Intermittent
Eso	E	E^1	ET	E (T)	ET^1	$E(T)^1$
Exo	X	X^1	XT	X(T)	XT^1	$X(T)^1$
Right hyper	RH	RH^1	RHT	RH(T)	RHT^1	$RH(T)^1$
Left hyper	LH	LH^1	LHT	LH(T)	LHT^1	$LH(T)^1$

ETIOLOGY OF STRABISMUS: AN OVERVIEW

Etiology of strabismus varies in different clinical varities and has been described there and then. Further, etiology of strabismus is still illusive or only presumptive in many cases. As a general concept, causes of acquired paralytic strabismus (which is usually acute in onset) are comparatively better defined and different from the causes of non-paralytic types of strabismus, and are described (page 285).

In general terms, the development of a non-paralytic strabismus is the result of an abnormality of one or more of the many factors which are concerned in the establishment of normal binocular vision. As we know, the binocular vision and coordination of ocular movements are not present since birth but are acquired in the early childhood. The process starts after birth and is, by and large, completed by the age of 5–6 years. Therefore, any obstacle to the development of these processes may result in concomitant strabismus. Basically, there is no difference between the causes leading to a heterophoria and those resulting in a heterotropia. Rather, it is a matter of degree to which the interference disrupts a given function. If the interference is minor, the resulting defect may be compensated during binocular vision so that only a latent deviation (heterophoria) results. If it is more severe, a manifest strabismus may be the result.

The general etiological factors which play role in the development of strabismus can be discussed as under:

- Obstacles in the development of normal binocular vision and co-ordination.
- Role of heredity.
- Influence of age on the development of strabismus.
- Development of squint in a blind eye.

OBSTACLES IN THE DEVELOPMENT OF NORMAL BINOCULAR VISION AND CO-ORDINATION

Prerequisites for development of normal binocular vision and binocular coordination include the following:

- *Normal optical media* to produce an image on the retina of each eye.

- *Binocular similar images* (in size and sharpness) should be formed so that fusion can occur.
- *Normal visual pathway* from retinal receptors to visual centres in the brain is required for a normal visual perception.
- *Brain centres must fuse* the input from both eyes into a unified single perception.
- *The neural pathway* from the various oculo-motor centres to the extraocular muscles must function properly.
- *The extraocular muscle function* should be normal and symmetrical in two eyes.
- *The binocular co-ordination of eye movement* must be such that the fixation object is imaged in the centre of each fovea.
- *Retinal correspondence* must be normal.

Thus, malfunction of any of the above factors can be an obstacle for the development of normal binocular vision and binocular co-ordination resulting in strabismus. These obstacles can be arranged into three groups namely: Sensory, motor and central.

1. Sensory obstacles

These are the factors which hinder the formation of a clear image in one eye and include the following:

- Uncorrected refractive errors
- Prolonged use of incorrect spectacles
- Anisometropia
- Opacities in the media such as corneal opacities, lenticular opacities and vitreous opacities
- Prolonged covering of one eye with a bandage or eye shade
- Severe unilateral congenital ptosis
- Prolonged use of one eye as with watch-maker's eye-glass
- Diseases of macula, e.g. central chorioretinitis.
- Optic atrophy

2. Motor obstacles

These factors hinder the maintenance of the two eyes in the correct positional relationship in primary gaze and/or during different ocular movements. A few such factors are:

- Congenital abnormalities of the size and shape of orbit.

- Abnormalities of extraocular muscles such as faulty insertion, faulty innervation, mild paresis, underdevelopment, overdevelopment and muscle slips.
- Abnormalities of fascial structures such as check ligaments, intermuscular membranes, connections between the fascial muscle sleeves where two muscles cross, etc. may also lead to deviation.
- Abnormalities of accommodation, convergence and AC/A ratio play an important role in ocular deviations.

3. Central obstacles

These may be in the form of:

- Deficient development of fusion faculty.
- Abnormalities of cortical control of ocular *movements* as occur in mental trauma, and hyperexcitability of the central nervous system during teething.
- Purposive use of the convergence reflex initiated in the motor area of frontal cortex may also play a role in the development of strabismus. This occurs classically in the voluntary squint which may be produced as a temporary phenomenon in most normal individuals; but in children it may be more sustained often as a result of some psychological upset.

ROLE OF HEREDITY

It is unequivocal that the incidence of strabismus is higher in certain families than in general population and that heredity plays a definite role in the occurrence of this disorder. However, this role cannot be defined as a distinct genetic pattern of strabismus; but certain defects such as a refractive error, usually a high degree of hypermetropia, which in turn may cause strabismus are genetically transmitted.

INFLUENCE OF AGE ON THE DEVELOPMENT OF STRABISMUS

The age of the patient, at the time, when the strabismogenic factors become operative, plays an important role in the determination of the strabismus. In a younger patient, the immature binocular reflex may be unable to withstand even small obstacles which mitigate against the fulfilment of full binocular function, whereas in an older patient, the more mature binocular reflexes may be able to overcome quite formidable obstacles. Chavasse stated that a very slight and transient paresis in adult patients with well-developed binocular vision may cause only heterophoria but in an infant it may be sufficient to severe the slighter bonds which associate the two eyes.

DEVELOPMENT OF STRABISMUS IN A BLIND EYE

It has been reported that if the loss of vision in one eye occurs in the first a few months of life, there may occur, sensory esotropia or exotropia, and after this till childhood, usually there occurs sensory esotropia. Occurrence of poor vision in adulthood due to any reason tends to cause a sensory exotropia. However, Sidkaro and von Noorden have reported that:

- *Up to 5 years* of age, there are almost equal chances of getting sensory esotropia and exotropia.
- *After 5 years*, definitely there are more chances of developing sensory exotropia.

Note. The exact mechanism of development of sensory heterotropia is not known, however, some views have been put forward (*see* page 238).

BIBLIOGRAPHY

1. Bielschowsky A: Lectures on motor anomalies. Hanover NH, 1943 (reprinted 1956). Dartmouth College Publications.
2. Bredemeyer, HG, and Bullock K: Orthoptics: theory and practice, St Louis. 1968. Mosby - Year Book Inc, p.86.
3. Broendstrup, P: The squinting position of weak-sighted eyes, Acta Ophthalmol 20:386, 1944.
4. Chavasse, FB: Worth's squint or the binocular reflexes and the treatment of strabismus, ed. 7, Philadelphia, 1939, P Blakiston's Sons & Co., Inc.
5. Duane, A: A new classification of the motor anomalies of the eyes based upon physiological principles together with their symptoms, diagnosis and treatment, reprinted from Ann. Ophthalmol Otolaryngol, October, 1896, and edited by White, JW, nd.
6. Keiner, GBJ: New viewpoints on the origin of squint. The Hague, 1951, Martinus Nijoff's ND.

7. Lancaster, WB: "Terminology," with extended comments on the position of rest and fixation. In Allen, JH, editor: Strabismus ophthalmic symposium I, St. Louis, 1950, Mosby -Year Book, Inc.

8. Lyle, TK, and Wybar, KC: Lyle and Jackson's practical orthoptics in the treatment of squint (and other anomalies of binocular vision), ed. 5, Springfield, III, 1967, Charles C Thomas, Publisher.

9. Paul, TO, and Hardage, LK: The heritability of strabismus, Ophthalmic Genet. 15:1, 1994.

10. Scobee, RG: Anatomic factors in the etiology of heterotropia, Am. J. Ophthalmol. 31:781, 1948.

11. Worth, C: Squint, its causes, pathology and treatment, ed. 6, London, 1929, Bailliere, Tindall and Cox.

Chapter

6

Evaluation of a Case of Strabismus and Orthoptic Instruments including Computer-Based Orthoptic Programs

EVALUATION OF A CASE OF STRABISMUS

To avoid repetition, the subject of evaluation is discussed even before the clinical description of different varieties of the squint. Though the list of tests is exhaustive, all of these may not be required in every case. An experienced strabismologist chooses a set of tests to be performed in a particular patient.

Main components of evaluation of a case of strabismus are:

I. *History, vision evaluation and prelimary examination*
- History
- Vision evaluation
- Prelimary examination

II. *Motor evaluation*
- *Head posture evaluation*
- *Evaluation for ocualr deviation*
  - Cover tests
  - Corneal reflex tests
  - Subjective tests for measurement of deviation
  - Measurement for cyclodeviation
- *Assessment for ocular movements*
  - Evaluation of duction
  - Evaluation of version
  - Evaluation of vergence
- Assessment of accommodation, and AC/A ratio
- Assessment for extraocular muscle paresis

III. *Sensory evaluation*
- Tests for fusion,
- Tests for binocularity and diplopia
- Tests for fixation
- Tests for status of retinal correspondance
- Tests for suppression and amblyopia
- Tests for stereopsis.

In general, for a systematic evaluation, following approach may be adopted.

HISTORY, VISION EVALUATION AND PRELIMINARY EXAMINATION

HISTORY

A detailed and meticulous history taking before beginning the examination is very important in the management of a case of squint. A complete history taken should contain the following information.

1. *Age of the patient*

2. *History of present illness.* Information about deviation of eye should include:
- Time when first noticed. It is desirable to document the age of onset of deviation or symptoms. All available old photographs of the child are invaluable for this purpose.
- Onset, sudden or gradual.
- Constant or intermittent deviation.
- Unilateral or alternating deviation.
- If alternating, which eye more frequently fixates (dominating eye).
- Alleged cause, if any, such as trauma, illness, psychologic disturbance, change in occupation, increase in close work, etc.

- Abnormal head posture (ask to demonstrate).
- Associated symptoms such as diplopia, blurred vision, headache, asthenopia.
- Any histroy of closing or covering one eye in bright light indicates intermittent squint.

3. *Birth history.* It is specially important in cases of childhood onset deviations. Enquiry should be made regarding:
- Problems during pregnancy and
- Problems during delivery

4. *Family history.* History regarding any of the following disorders in grandparents, parents, siblings or even in uncles, aunts and cousins is important;
- Strabismus
- Refractive errors
- Lazy eye
- Other ocular defects

5. *Past history*
- General ill health
- Any systemic disease
- Any ocular defect

6. *History of previous treatment*
  a. *Optical treatment*
   - *When and how long?*
   - *Were glasses worn constantly?*
   - *Effect of glasses on the deviation.*
   - *Date of last refraction.*
  b. *Orthoptic treatment.*
   - *Occlusion.* Type, when, how long, effect on vision.
   - *Exercises.* When, type, how long, effect on deviation.
  c. *Surgical treatment*
   - *When performed?*
   - *Eye operated: Right, left or both.*
   - *Muscle touched. Medial, lateral or both (if known).*
   - *Patient's/parents' opinion about the result of surgery.*

VISION EVALUATION

Testing of visual acuity of each eye separately is critical in evaluation of any patient with strabismus. Visual acuity should be tested without glasses and with glasses (if worn); and for near and distance vision.

Methods of testing visual acuity in infants, preschool age children and in schoolage children as well as adults have been described in Chapter 3 (page 40–51). However, for a ready reference, these are enumerated below.

Methods of estimating visual acuity in infants
1. Fixation behaviour test
2. Preferential looking test
3. Optokinetic nystagmus
4. Visually evoked response
5. CSM method

Methods of estimating visual acuity in preschool-age children
1. Marble game test
2. Hand chart
3. Illiterate E-game test
4. Allen's preschool vision test
5. Sheridan-Gardiner test

Methods of estimating visual acuity in schoolage children and adults
1. Snellen's test types
2. E-chart
3. Landolt's broken-C chart

Visual acuity in patients with nystagmus. In patients with nystagmus, visual acuity may be better with both eyes open than with one eye occluded. In order to assess this situation, it may be helpful to place a +5.00D sphere lens in front of the eye not being tested, and then reverse this in order to test the other eye.

PRELIMINARY EXAMINATION

Inspection

Large degree squint (convergent or divergent) is obvious on inspection.

Epicanthus, when observed in infants, may be the cause of pseudoesotropia.

Facial asymmetries may also create the impression of pseudostrabismus especially hypertropia.

Abnormal head posture (AHP) when present, becomes obvious during initial inspection of the patient. Infact observation for AHP should always be made without any instructions to the patient, otherwise a lot of information may be lost after the patient becomes concious of being examined. As described in detail on page 288, observation should be made for all the three components of head posture, i.e.
- *Chin* elevation or depression (vertical component),
- *Face turn* to right or left (horizontal component), and
- *Head tilt* to right or left shoulder (torsional component)

Interpupillary distance (IPD) should also be inspected and measured. Unusually, narrow IPD may be the cause of pseudoesotropia and an exceptionally wide IPD may be a cause of pseudoexotropia.

Inspection during pen light examination may sometimes erroneously reveal strabismus owing to presence of a large angle kappa. A large positive angle kappa may be a cause of pseudoexotropia and a large negative angle kappa may be a cause of pseudoesotropia. For details of angle kappa and its measurement, *see* page 188.

Pupillary Reactions

Light reflexes may be abnormal in patients with sensory deviations due to diseases of retina and optic nerve.

Media and Fundus Examination

It may reveal associated diseases of the ocular media, retina or optic nerve.

Refraction

It is most important, because a refractive error may be responsible for the symptoms of the patient or for the deviation itself. Though, mentioned in the beginning, in practice, refraction is performed after complete squint check-up. Preferably, refraction should be performed under full cycloplegia especially in children. The commonly used cycloplegics are as follows:

1. *Atropine* is indicated in children below the age of 7 years. It is used as 1% ointment thrice daily for 3 consecutive days before performing retinoscopy. Its effect lasts for 10–20 days.

2. *Homatropine* is used as 2% drops. One drop is often instilled every 10 minutes for 6 times and the retinoscopy is performed after 1 to 2 hours. Its effect lasts for 24–28 hours. It is used for most of the hypermetropic individuals between 7 and 35 years of age.

3. *Cyclopentolate* is a short-acting cycloplegic. Its effects last for 6 to 18 hours. It is used as 1% eyedrops in patients between 7 and 35 years. One drop of cyclopentolate is instilled every 10 minutes for 3 times (Havener's recommended dose) and the retinoscopy is performed 1 to 1½ hours later after estimating the residual accommodation, which should not exceed one dioptre.

MOTOR EVALUATION

EVALUATION FOR OCULAR DEVIATION

COVER TESTS
Prerequisites for cover tests

- Patient should be co-operative enough to fixate a target.
- Should have sufficient vision to see the target.
- Should have central fixation in both eyes.
- Latent nystagmus should not be present.

Methods of cover tests

The cover tests should be performed with and without glasses at distance (6 m) and at near (33 cm). The patient is asked to fixate a 6/12 visual acuity symbol or any object that keeps patient's attention, such as a small picture or a toy (especially in small children), with one eye. This is to prevent the use of accommodation, when torch light is used (which is a common practice). The other eye is then covered with the help of an occluder or palm of the hand. The interpretations are made as described below.

Direct cover test

Aim. *To confirm the presence of a manifest squint.*
Procedure. To perform this test, patient is first asked to fixate (Fig. 6.1) a point with both eyes open. The normal looking eye is covered while observing the movement of the uncovered eye. In the presence of manifest squint, the uncovered eye will move in the opposite direction to take fixation. For example, when an exotropia is present, the eye taking up fixation will move towards nose and in the presence of esotropia, it will move towards the temple.

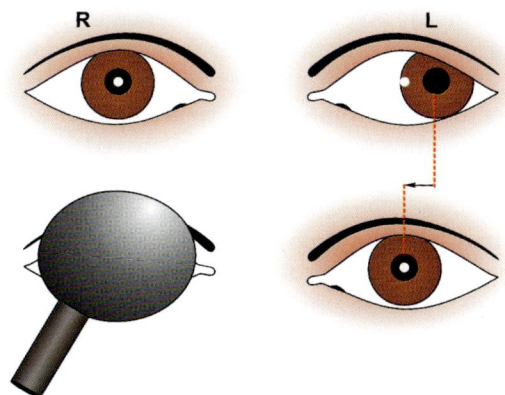

Fig. 6.1 *Direct cover test depicting left exotropia.*

No movement of the uncovered eye on covering the seemingly fixating eye indicates any of the following:

- No squint (pseudostrabismus)
- Gross eccentric fixation (there may be very small or no movement of redress in the uncovered deviated eye)
- No vision in the deviated uncovered eye.

Cover-uncover test

Aim. *To establish the presence and type of heterophoria (latent deviation).*
Procedure (Fig. 6.2). It is performed, when direct cover test has established that no manifest deviation is present. To perform it, one eye is covered with an occluder and the other is made

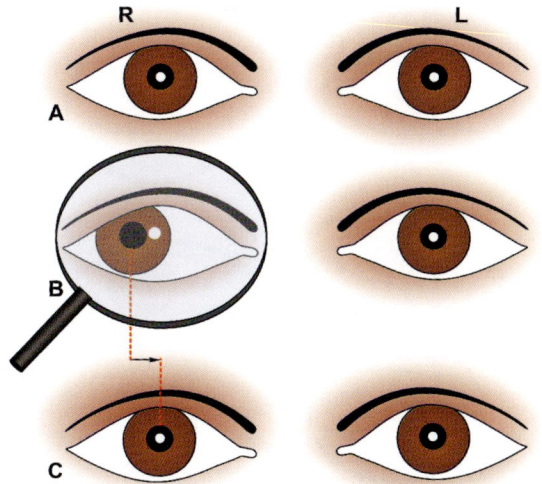

Fig. 6.2 *Cover-uncover test depicting exophoria. Note orthophoria in primary position (A) and immediate inward movement of right eye on removal of the cover (B and C).*

to fixate an object. In the presence of heterophoria, the eye under cover will deviate (since covering one eye of a patient with normal binocular vision interrupts fusion). After a few seconds, the cover is quickly removed and the movement of the eye (which was under cover) is observed. Direction of the movement of the eyeball tells the type of heterophoria (e.g. the eyeball will move towards the nose in the presence of exophoria and towards the temple in the presence of esophoria) and the speed of movement tells whether recovery is slow or rapid.

Alternate cover test

Aim. To *establish whether the squint is unilateral or alternate* and also to *differentiate concomitant squint from paralytic squint* (where secondary deviation is greater than primary deviation).

Procedure (Fig. 6.3). To perform this test, patient is asked to fixate an object alternately with each eye. It is important to place occluder alternately in front of each eye several times to dissociate the eyes and to maximize the deviation. Further, the occluder should be quickly transferred from one eye to other to prevent fusion from occurring. Observations made are as follows:

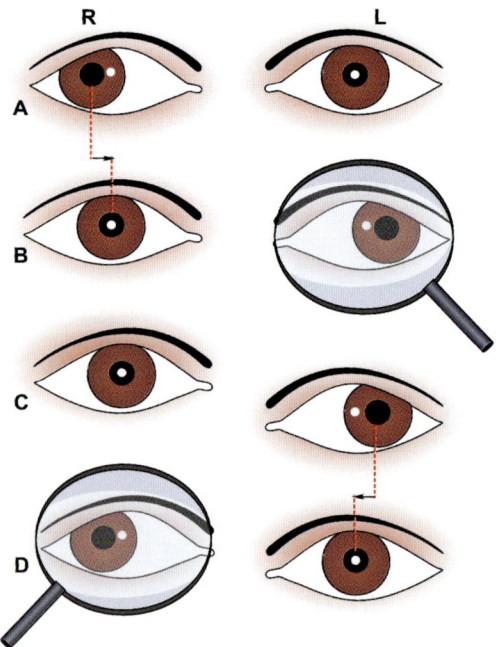

Fig. 6.3 *Alternate cover test depicting alternate exotropia.*

In the presence of an alternate squint, either eye fixates and the opposite eye under cover deviates and maintains the position of deviation on removing the cover; but in the presence of a unilateral squint, after removal of the cover, always the normal looking eye takes up fixation and the squinting eye deviates.

To differentiate concomitant squint from paralytic squint, observation about the degree of deviation in the eye under cover is made while performing the alternate cover test. In concomitant squint, primary deviation is equal to secondary deviation (deviation of the normal eye under cover); while in paralytic squint, secondary deviation is much more than the primary deviation.

Limitations of cover tests

Following deviations may be either overlooked or cannot possibly be diagnosed with cover tests:

- A small heterophoria
- A small angle esotropia (of less than 5^Δ)
- A microtropia
- A monofixation syndrome
- A cyclodeviation

QUANTITATIVE MEASUREMENT OF ANGLE OF DEVIATION

Various methods for quantitative measurement of angle of deviation can be grouped as under:

Objective tests for heterotropia
- Hirschberg corneal reflex test
- Prism and cover test (prism bar cover test)
- Prism reflex test (Krimsky's corneal reflex test)
- Synoptophore test
- Perimeter method

Subjective tests for heterotropia
- Maddox rod test
- Synoptophore test
- Diplopia test
- Hess/Lees screen test

Objective tests for heterophoria
- Prism and cover test

Subjective tests for heterophoria
- Maddox rod test
- Maddox wing test
- Double prism test

Tests based on corneal reflex

- Hirschberg corneal reflex test
- Prism and cover test (prism bar cover test)
- Prism reflex test (Krimsky's corneal reflex test)
- Perimeter method
- Synoptophore method
- Bruckner test

Dissimilar image tests

- Maddox rod test for heterophoria or hetero-tropia
- Double Maddox rod test for cyclodeviations
- Red glass test

Dissimilar target tests

- Major amblyoscope test
- Lancaster red-green projection test
- Hess screen test

Bruckner pupillary red reflex test

This is a screening test and does not measure the size of deviation. It is performed with the help of a direct ophthalmoscope. Patient is made to look into the light and examiner compares the brightness of pupillary red reflex of both eyes obtained simultaneously,

- *In orthophoria*, the Bruckner red reflex is symmetric in the two eyes.
- *In strabismus*, the reflex is brighter in the deviated eye.
- *In ocular pathologic conditions* such as large anisometropia, gross retinal pathology, large retinal detachment, media opacities (corneal, lenticular or vitreal), the red reflex is altered in the affected eye.

Hirschberg corneal reflex test

It is a rough but handy method to estimate the angle of manifest squint. In this test, patient is asked to fixate at a point light held at a distance of 33 cm and the deviation of corneal reflex from the centre of pupil is noted in the squinting eye. Hirschberg reported that each 1 mm decent-ration of corneal reflex corresponds to 7° (14$^\Delta$) of deviation of the visual axis. Thus, roughly the angle of squint is 15° and 45°, when the corneal light reflex falls on the border of pupil and limbus, respectively (Fig. 6.4).

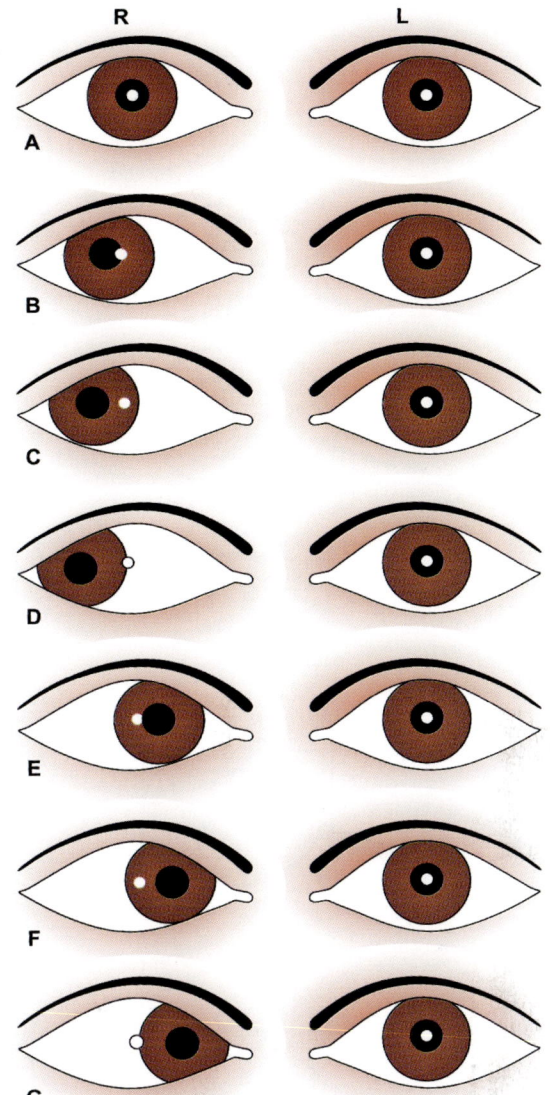

Fig. 6.4 *Hirschberg corneal reflex test depicting ortho-position (A), right exotropia (B:15°, C:30°, D:45°) and right esotropia (E:15°, F:30°, G:45°).*

Prism and alternate cover test
(prism bar cover test, i.e. PBCT)

In practice, this test is most popular and a simple method of measuring the angle of deviation objectively in various diagnostic positions of gaze.

Prisms of increasing strength with apex towards the deviation are placed in front of one eye and the patient is asked to fixate a target with the other eye. For large deviations, a loose prism of

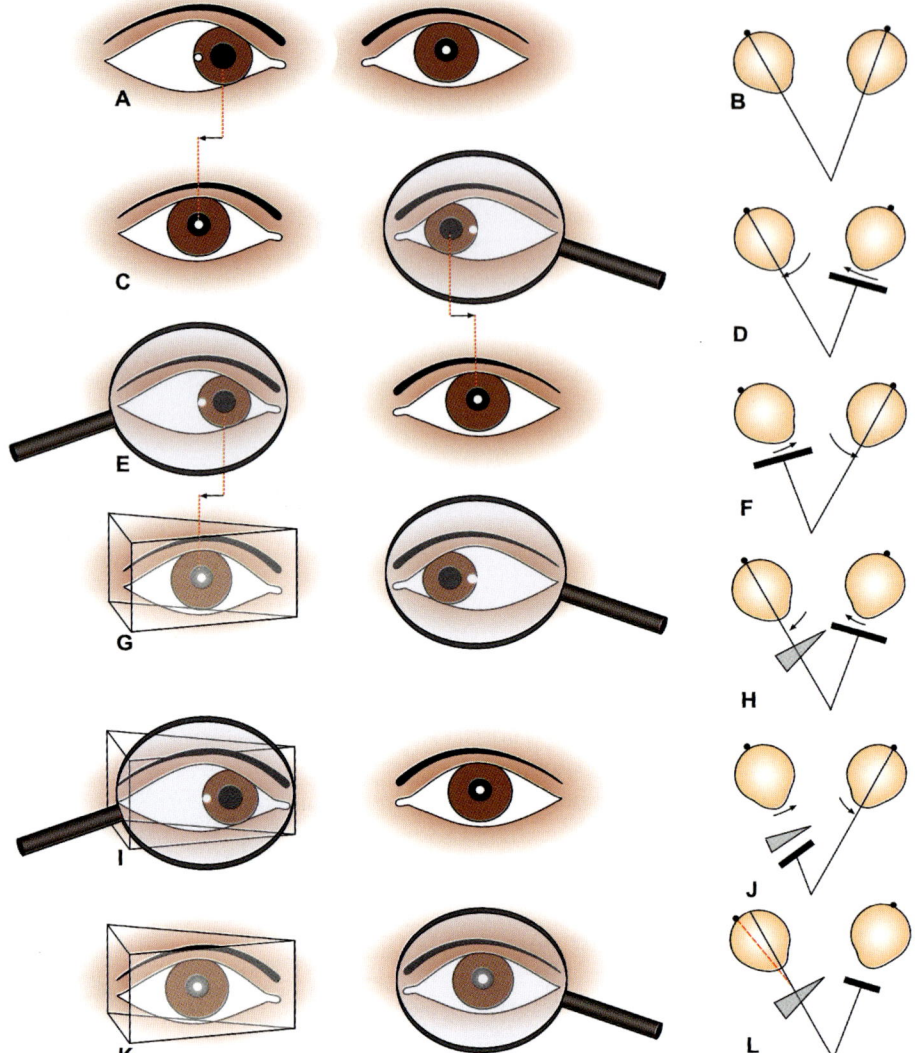

Fig. 6.5 *Prism and cover test with its optical principle. A, right esotropia; B, image of the object fixated by left eye is projected on major half of retina of the right eye; C and D, when left eye is covered, right eye moves outwards to take over fixation and under the cover left eye performs an inward movement of equal amplitude following Hering's law of equal innervation; E and F, when cover is transferred to right eye, the left eye moves outwards to takeover fixation and under the cover right eye performs an inward movement; G and H, a prism base-out is held before the right eye and cover is transferred to the left eye. There is still outward movement of the right eye when taking over fixation; I and J, cover is again transferred and a prism of greater power is held before the right eye; K and L, transfer of cover to the left eye does not show any outward movement of the right eye indicating that it is the end point of the prism and cover test. At this juncture, prism of sufficient power offsets the nasal displacement and the right eye will no longer change its position when left eye is covered. The power of this prism equals the deviation.*

30 or 45 prism dioptre is placed in front of one eye and the prism bar is used in front of the other eye.

- *When horizontal and vertical deviations co-exist,* the prisms are placed horizontally in front of one eye and vertically in front of the other eye.

- *Alternate cover test* is then performed till there is no recovery movement of the eye under cover (Fig. 6.5). This will tell the amount of deviation in prism dioptres.

Both heterophoria as well as heterotropia can be measured objectively by this method.

Test should be performed for distance and near fixation. An accommodative target should be used for near fixation distances.

Test should be performed, preferably in all the nine diagnostic positions of gaze. In Boyce-Smith deviometer (Fig. 6.6), nine prefixed retroilluminated slides (accommodative targets) positioned 35° from the primary position are used to perform cover and prism test in diagnostic positions of gaze.

One great advantage of using a deviometer is that the prism and cover test can be performed in diagnostic positions under exactly the same conditions on different occasions and thus permit meaningful comparison of test results (e.g. preoperative and postoperative).

Comparison of prism and cover test performed in primary position, straight up position and straight down position is very useful in detecting the 'A', 'V' and 'X' pattern heterotropias.

Test should be repeated by holding the prism and occluder before the other eye to detect any difference between right and left fixation, which would indicate incomitance.

Uses of prism and cover test

A carefully performed PBCT can provide following useful information:

1. *Nature of deviation* of esotropia (basic or convergence excess or divergence insufficiency type) and exotropia (basic or convergence insufficiency or divergence excess type) can be known from the results of near and distance measurements.

2. *Accommodative element of deviation* can be known from measuring deviation for far and near with and without glasses (including bifocals, if any).

3. *Incomitance*, if any, can be detected by performing the test in 9 cardinal positions of gaze.

4. *A-V patterns* can be detected by measuring the deviation in upgaze of 25° and downgaze of 35°.

5. *Primary versus secondary deviation* can be detected by measuring the deviation with right and left eye fixating alternately.

6. *Divergence excess versus simulated divergence excess exotropia* can be differentiated by measuring the deviation before and after prolonged occlusion.

Limitations of prism and cover test

- Since, this test requires an accurate fixation, so it cannot be performed, if the deviating eye is blind or has gross eccentric fixation.
- The optical qualities of the prisms also limit the test accuracy. The stronger the prism, the greater the error.
- The spectacle lenses with power more than ±5D introduce a significant artifact in measurement of deviation. Plus lenses decrease and minus lenses increase the measured deviation.
- The presence of manifest as well as latent nystagmus hinders the accurate measurements by prism and cover test.
- Test accuracy is also limited by the minimum movement of redress that the examiner can detect with naked eye.

Prism reflex test (Krimsky's corneal reflex test)

Prism reflex test first described by *Krimsky* has become universally accepted as a practical method of estimating the size of the angle of

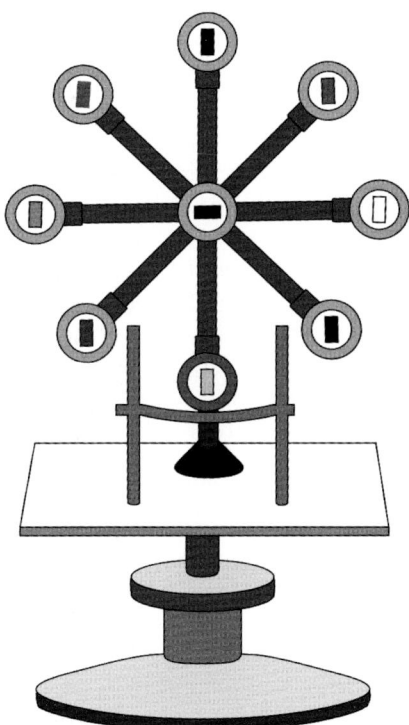

Fig. 6.6 *The Boyce-Smith deviometer.*

squint in patients with a blind or deeply amblyopic eye with or without eccentric fixation.

To perform the test, patient is asked to fixate on a point light and prisms of increasing strength (with apex towards the direction of manifest squint) are placed in front of the normal fixating eye till the corneal reflex is centered in the squinting eye (Fig. 6.7). The power of prism required to centre the light reflex in the squinting eye equals the amount of squint in prism dioptres. To avoid errors from parallax, the examiner must observe the corneal reflex with one eye by sitting directly in front of the deviating eye while keeping his other eye closed.

In an alternative method, prism of increasing power can be placed in front of the deviating eye until the corneal reflexion is centred. However, since the observation of the corneal reflexion through prisms is difficult, therefore, the method described above is preferred.

Advantages of Krimsky's test
• Since the test requires only that the patient fixate the light, being entirely objective otherwise, it is useful in testing small children.
• It is quicker to perform than the prism cover test.
• It can be used in patients in whom the deviating eye has a low visual acuity or has lost central fixation.

Limitations of the Krimsky's test
• Since the angle kappa is included in the measurement, the test is inaccurate.
• It is impossible to perform the test for distance fixation, since the position of the examiner's head required to obtain an accurate observation prevents the patient from seeing the fixation light.

Simultaneous prism cover test

Aim. The aim of this test is to measure only the tropia without dissociating the phoria.

This special cover test is used to measure the tropia component of patient with small tropia <10 PD and a larger phoria (i.e. monofixation syndrome). It is not useful for larger tropia (>10 PD), which does not permit fusion and, therefore, does not have an associated phoria.

Procedure. This test is performed as below:
• *Hirschberg corneal reflex test* is performed to estimate the approximate size of tropia (Fig 6.8A).
• *Simultaneous prism cover test* is then performed by placing the prism of the size of tropia in front of deviating eye and an occluder in front of the fixating eye (Fig. 6.8B). The power of prism with which the deviated eye does not show refixation shift equals the tropia.

Note. For patients with monofixation syndrome, the amount of tropia is measured with simultaneous prism cover test and the total angle (tropia plus phoria) is measured with the alternate prism cover test.

Perimeter method

Patient is asked to fixate at O-mark on the arc perimeter with normal eye and a flash light is moved along its arc till the corneal reflexion is

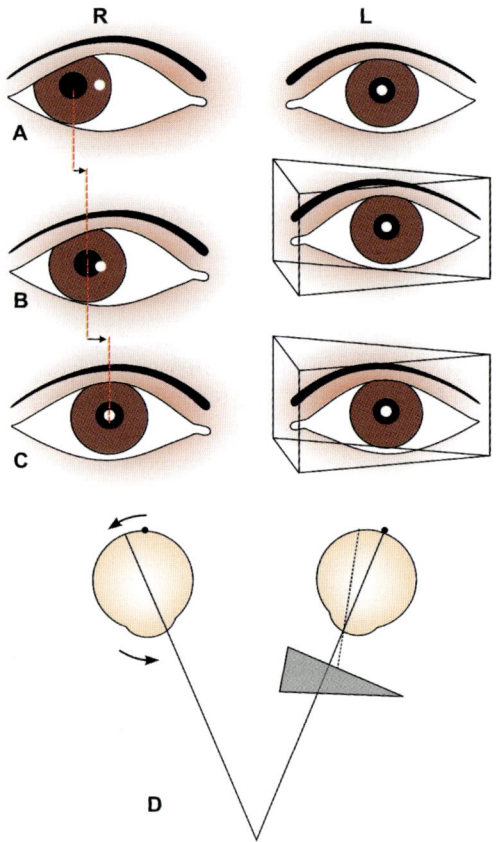

Fig. 6.7 *The Krimsky's corneal reflex test.* A, *right exotropia;* B *and* C, *prism base-in of increasing powers are placed in front of the fixing left eye till the corneal reflex centres in the right eye (C);* D, *optical principle of the prism reflex test.*

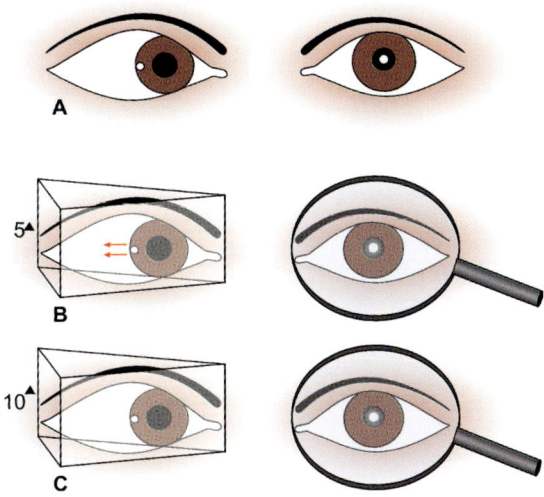

Fig. 6.8 *Simultaneous cover test: Hirschberg test depicting small esotropia (A). Simultaneous placement of prism on the esotropic eye and occluder on the fixing eye will show fixing movement in the esotropic eye when the power of prism is less (B) and no movement when the power of prism is equal to the degree of tropia (C).*

centred in the pupil of the squinting eye. This point on perimeter gives the angle of manifest squint in degrees.

This method, used in the past, is not popular nowadays.

Maddox rod test

It is a subjective test, based on the principle of diplopia, which can be employed to measure both heterophoria as well as heterotropia. The

Maddox rod consists of a series of parallel glass cylinders of higher power (usually of red colour) set together in a metallic disc (Fig. 6.9A). The Maddox rod produces a linear image of a point light. When viewed through the rod, the line image is formed perpendicular to the axis of the cylinders.

Measurement of heterotropia

The patient is asked to fix on a point light in the centre of a Maddox tangent scale (Fig. 6.9B) or any point light at a distance of 6 metres. The Maddox rod is placed before one eye with axis of the rod parallel to the axis of deviation (Fig. 6.10). Thus, for measuring a horizontal deviation, the rod is placed in such a way that the patient sees a vertical line of light (Fig. 6.10A). Depending upon the type of deviation, the red vertical line will be seen either to the right or to the left of fixation light. The number on Maddox tangent scale where the red line falls will be the amount of deviation in degrees. Alternatively, prisms of successively increasing power (with apex towards the deviation) are placed in front of the rod until the patient sees the line passing through the fixation light. This gives the amount of heterotropia in prism dioptres. The test should always be repeated with the Maddox rod in front of the other eye, so that deviation during right fixation and left fixation can be compared, and any discrepancy, if there, can be noted. Such an endeavour, specially gives information about:

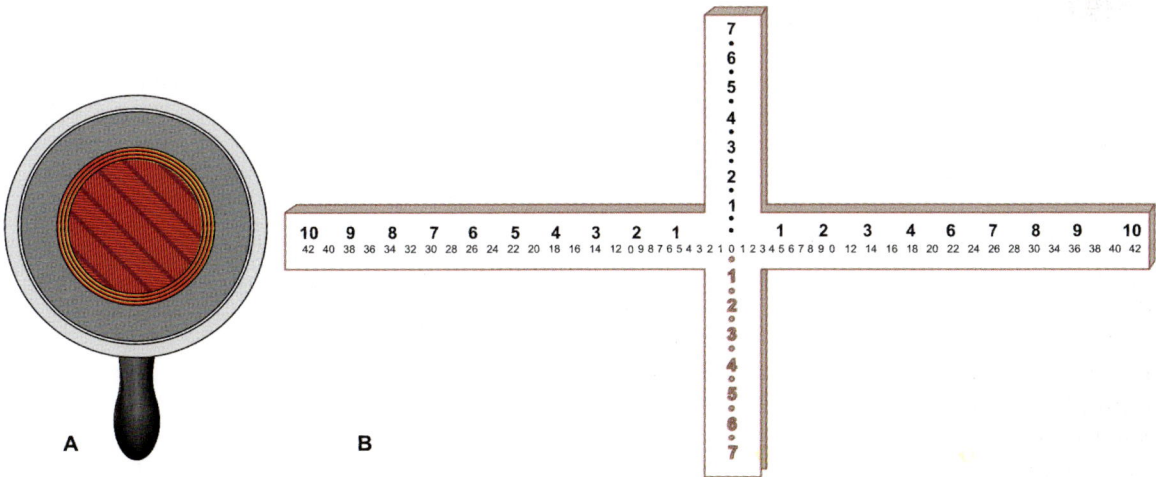

Fig. 6.9 A, *Maddox rod*; B, *Maddox tangent scale.*

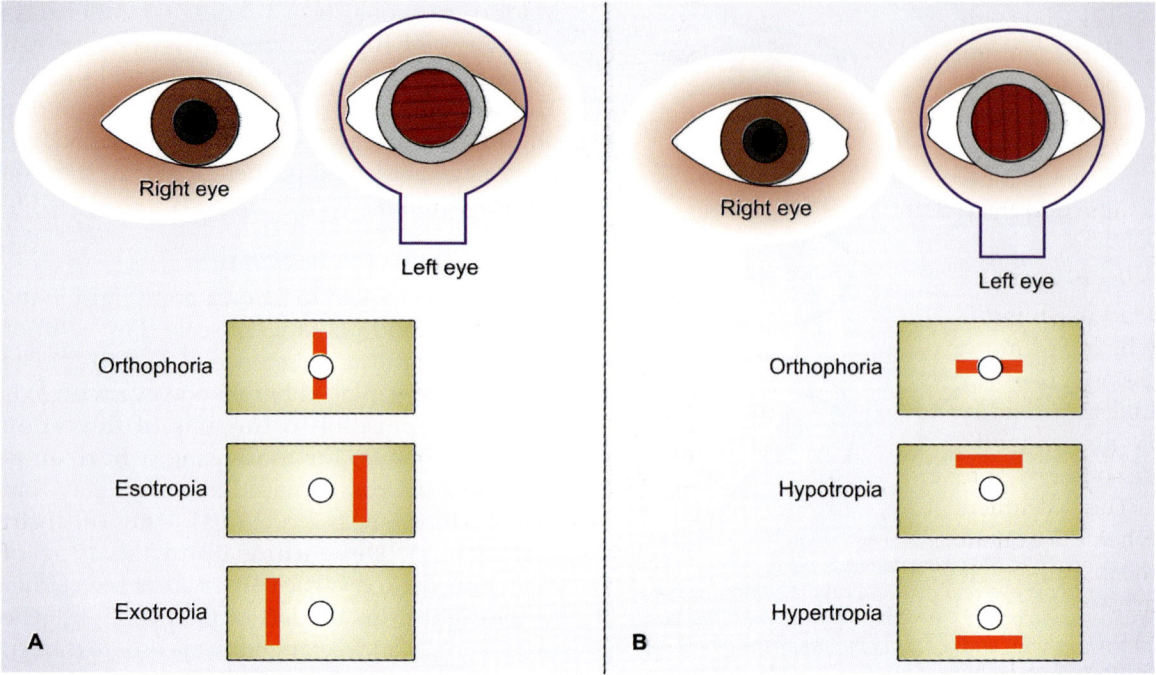

Fig. 6.10 *Maddox rod test for horizontal (A) and vertical (B) heterotropia.*

- Primary and secondary deviations in the presence of paralytic element.
- Any change in retinal correspondence with the change in fixation.
- Presence of dissociated vertical deviations may be discovered.

Maddox rod test in conjunction with the Maddox tangent scale can be performed successfully in co-operative children as young as 3 to 4 years of age. Such children should be asked to go to the scale and put their finger on the place where they saw the line rather than asked to tell the number from a distance.

In case of vertical deviation, the Maddox rod is rotated so that the line is seen horizontally (Fig. 6.10B) and the deviation is measured directly from the tangent scale or by using prism base-up or base-down depending upon the direction of deviation (apex of prism is kept towards deviation). To measure a cyclotropia, the patient is asked to turn the Maddox rod around the anteroposterior axis, until he/she has the impression that the line is horizontal. The amount of cyclotropia in degrees can be read from the trial frame.

Measurement of heterophoria

To measure heterophoria, the Maddox rod test is performed exactly in a similar manner as performed to measure the heterotropia with the following one exception:

In heterophoria, an occluder is placed before the Maddox rod and while the patient fixates the light source with his/her other eye, the occluder is removed only for a second and the necessary enquiries are made. After making necessary adjustments of the prism, the occluder is again removed for a second. The procedure is repeated till the patient sees red line and point light as superimposed.

The use of a cover is necessary in a phoria, because, if both the fixation light and red line are seen continuously, there will be a constant change in the degree of deviation and the red line will never achieve a steady position relative to the fixation light.

Limitations of the maddox rod test

1. It can be performed, only if there is no suppression under the test conditions.

relaxing or increasing the accommodative effort or in cases of a variable angle of deviation.

Problems which may come across while performing this test are as follows:

1. Suppression may prevent the patient from superimposing the pictures. In such cases, simultaneous macular perception or simultaneous paramacular perception slides can be used. The larger the image formed on the retina, the less likely it is to be suppressed.

2. The patient may never succeed in putting the lion in the cage, and it may suddenly be seen on the other side of the cage (in an uncrossed or homonymous position in divergent deviations and in a crossed or heteronymous position in convergent deviations). In such cases, the crossing point is considered to be the subjective angle.

3. It must be realized that the measurement obtained by the subjective method is only the true angle of deviation, if normal retinal correspondence is present.

Measurement of cyclodeviation with synoptophore

There is no way to carry out an objective measurement of a cyclodeviation. The subjective measurement can be performed as follows.

Simultaneous perception slides are used. The slide with lion is kept in front of the right eye and that with cage is kept in front of the left eye. The patient is asked to look at each one in turn and is asked whether the cage appears level. In the presence of cyclodeviation, the cage appears tilted. In incyclotropia, the cage's left-hand side is seen lower than the right-hand side. This is corrected by wheel rotating the slide towards the patient. In the presence of excyclotropia, the cage's right-hand side appears lower than the left-hand side. This can be corrected by wheel-rotating the slide away from the patient (towards the examiner). The amount of deviation is read in degrees from the scale located on the slideholder of the instrument. It should be remembered that the tilt of the image is in the direction opposite to the tilt of the eye.

Double prism test

Double prism test consists of two prisms which are mounted base to base. It is used to elicit cyclophorias. To perform this test the, double prism is placed before one eye in such a manner that the junction of the two bases intersects the pupil and is horizontal. Then the patient is asked to look at a horizontal line against an empty background which does not offer any fusional stimuli and inferences drawn are as follows:

- Patient will see two parallel lines with the eye having double prism in front of it, i.e. one line displaced above and the other displaced below with respect to the single line seen by the other eye.
- In the absence of any cyclophoria, all three lines will be parallel.
- If a cyclophoria is present, the single line will have an angle relative to the other two lines as follows:
  – In incyclophoria, the line or lines seen by the right eye will be tilted towards right and those seen by left eye will be tilted towards left.
  – In excyclophoria, the line or lines seen by the right eye will be tilted towards left and those seen by left eye will be tilted towards right.

Haploscopic tests

Tests based on the haploscopic principle to measure the deviation include Lancaster red-green test, Hess and Lees screen tests. These tests are very useful for measuring incomitant strabismus in patients with diplopia (*see* page 121–126).

ASSESSMENT OF OCULAR MOVEMENTS

ASSESSMENT OF DUCTIONS

1. *Duction test.* Ductions are monocular movements and are measured at near distance. When examining ductions, one eye is covered and the fellow eye fixates a spotlight which is moved to bring the fixating eye to the farthest possible position, in all the cardinal directions of gaze. For interpretation of the observations, following methods are in vogue:

i. In most frequent practice, the examiner observes whether *movement lags or is excessive* in any direction. If no lags are noticed, the ductions are recorded as full; if lags are noticed, the muscle and the eye involved are indicated. Usually, a subjective assessment is made on scale of 7 points (+3 to −3) or 9 points (+4 to −4). Further, a note is also made of the occurrence of any nystagmoid movements in the presence of full ductions.

ii. Judging the *normalcy of adduction and abduction in relation to fixed points.* Following useful guidelines have been suggested:

- In maximal adduction, *an imaginary vertical line through the lower lacrimal punctum should coincide with a boundary line between the inner one-third and the outer two-thirds of the cornea* (Fig. 6.15A).

  − *In excessive adduction, more cornea is hidden* (Fig. 6.15B).
  − *In defective adduction, more cornea is visible. Some of the sclera may also be visible* (Fig. 6.15C).

- *In maximal abduction,* the lateral limbus touches the outer canthus (Fig. 6.15D).
  − *In excessive abduction, some of the cornea is hidden under the outer canthus* (Fig. 6.15E).
  − *In defective abduction, some of the sclera is visible between the outer canthus and the limbus* (Fig. 6.15F).

2. *Kestenbaum's limbus test of motility.* The duction movements are measured with the help of a transparent ruler as follows:

- *Adduction* is measured by noting a difference between the position of the temporal limbus in primary position and maximum adduction.
- *Abduction* is measured by noting a difference between the position of the nasal limbus in primary position and maximum abduction.
- Similarly, *elevation* and *depression* are measured with respect to inferior limbus and superior limbus, respectively.
- Normal values reported are:

  − Adduction : 10 mm
  − Abduction : 10 mm
  − Elevation : 5–7 mm
  − Depression : 10 mm

3. *Subjective perimeter method of measuring ductions.* In this method, to measure the amplitude of duction movements, the patient's head is placed into the chin rest of a perimeter in such a way that the eye to be examined is in the centre of the perimeter arc or perimeter hemisphere. The other eye is occluded and the

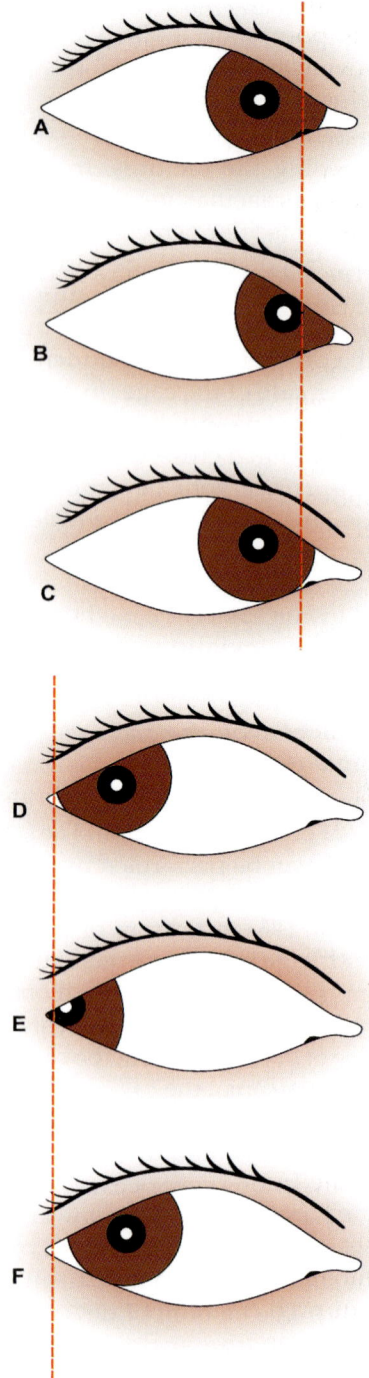

Fig. 6.15 *Judgement of adduction* (A, B, C) *in relation to lower punctum and abduction* (D, E, F) *in relation to lateral canthus. For explanation see text.*

patient is asked to fixate and follow the perimeter target that is moved from the centre of the field to periphery. He/she is instructed to indicate, when he/she can no longer see the target. This point indicates the limit of the duction movement in that particular direction. Normal values reported by this method are:

– Adduction : 50°
– Abduction : 50°
– Depression : 50°
– Elevation   : 40°

4. *Objective perimeter method or corneal reflex method of measuring ductions.* The amplitude of duction movements can be checked somewhat more objectively by using corneal light reflex. In this method, after closing one eye, patient is asked to turn his/her eye maximally in a given direction. Then the examiner moves a small flash light along the arc of the perimeter until the reflex from the patient's cornea appears to be centred in the pupil. The examiner views it with one eye from the position of flash light. This point gives the limit of the particular duction movement.

Note: It is important to be aware of the fact that, in practice, the measurement of ductions is not of much value in the investigation of strabismus, since only a small fraction of the fibres of a muscle need to function in order to rotate the eye to the limits of its field of duction. A defect in the amplitude of duction occurs, only when almost complete paresis of a muscle occurs. Therefore, a partial paresis usually cannot be diagnosed on testing ductions.

ASSESSMENT OF VERSIONS

In general, study of versions is more important factor than the study of ductions, when deciding on which muscle or muscles to operate.

Further, the investigation of versions is of greatest importance in patients with non-comitant strabismus, because comparison of the extent of movement of the two eyes relative to each other during a version is the most sensitive test to detect underfunction of a muscle.

1. Version test

It is performed at approximately 15 inches. The patient is asked to hold his head straight and still and to make eye movements on command or to follow a fixation light in all the cardinal directions of gaze. The fixation light should be kept at such a distance that one can always observe the corneal reflections in both eyes. The following observations should be made on version test.

- For excessive or defective movements in any direction.
- To detect underaction of one muscle and overaction of its contralateral synergist.
- To detect overaction of one muscle without underaction of its contralateral synergist.
- To note any retraction of the globe and narrowing of palpebral fissure in certain direction of gaze (as seen in Duane's retraction syndrome).
- To detect the overaction of inferior and superior obliques.

Clinically, the overaction of oblique muscles can be graded by following methods:

i. *Depending upon the vertical deviations,* the overactions of obliques is graded as:

a. *Mild overaction*—when vertical deviation (e.g. hypertropia in inferior oblique overaction) is appreciated only in sursumadduction.

b. *Moderate overaction*—when vertical deviation is appreciable on adduction itself.

c. *Severe overaction*—when hypertropia is seen in primary position.

ii. *Depending on the angle, the adducting eye makes with the horizontal line* as it elevates and abducts (if overacting) on lateral version to the opposite side, the overaction of inferior oblique is graded as shown in Fig. 6.16.

Similarly, the overaction of superior oblique also can be graded by observing the angle the adducting eye makes with the horizontal line as it depresses and abducts.

2. Perimeteric method of measuring versions

The amplitude of versions can be measured on the perimeter in the same way as ductions except that the patient fixates and follows the test object with both eyes until he/she sees it double or until it moves too far out for him/her to follow.

In general, such a measurement of the absolute amplitude of versions is of little practical value.

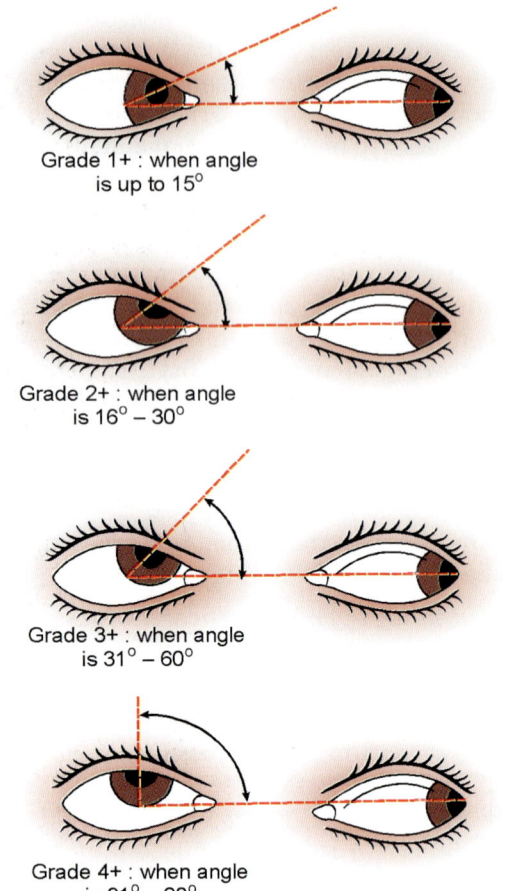

Grade 1+ : when angle
is up to 15°

Grade 2+ : when angle
is 16° – 30°

Grade 3+ : when angle
is 31° – 60°

Grade 4+ : when angle
is 61° – 90°

Fig. 6.16 *Grading of inferior oblique overaction depending on the angle adducting eye makes with horizontal line.*

MEASUREMENT OF VERGENCES

The status of motor fusion is assessed by measuring the vergences, i.e. the fusional amplitudes. In the presence of heterophoria or an intermittent heterotropia, the fusional amplitudes can be measured both by the prism method or synoptophore method. While, in a patient with heterotropia, only the synopto-phore method is useful, since fusion in casual gaze is necessary for testing with prism method. Fusional divergence is measured from the subject's phoria position, whereas relative divergence is measured from the position of fusional demand, i.e. the orthoposition.

Testing of fusional amplitudes with prism method

The test can be performed using a prism bar or a rotatory prism (Risley prism) or single prism.

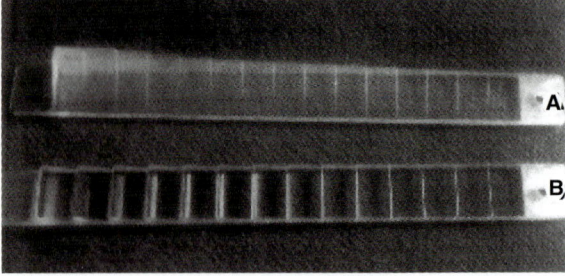

Fig. 6.17 *Prism bars, horizontal (A) and vertical (B).*

A prism bar consists of a series of prisms of increasing strength (Fig. 6.17). It is held by the examiner in front of one of the patient's eyes and merely needs to be moved higher or lower to bring a stronger or weaker prism into the line of sight.

Amplitudes of divergence are measured first and those of convergence second.

Measurement of amplitude of divergence

To perform the test for distance, patient is asked to fixate the 6/12 symbol at 6 metres and the prism bar is used with the prism base directed in BI in front of the one eye (preferably the non-dominant one). By progressively increasing the amount of base in prism power, the eyes are diverged to the limit of bifoveal single vision, i.e. up to the point, when the patient just appreciates diplopia. This point is the end point of the test and is called the *break point*. Its reading is recorded. At this point, the power of the prism is decreased slowly, until he/she again fuses. This point called as the *recovery point* is also noted.

To measure the amplitude of divergence for near, the above test is repeated at 33 cm. The end point and the recovery point are recorded. But unlike the test for distance, the end point for the near test is blur point, i.e. the maximum amount of base-in (BI) prism power after which the patient's vision is blurred. The mechanism of blurring of vision is as follows:

The retinal disparity produced by the use of base-in prism evokes fusional divergence that maintains bifoveal single vision until its amplitude is exhausted. At this point, the patient, who is accommodating during near vision, can produce further divergence and maintain single vision longer, if he/she relaxes his/her accommodation, because this simultaneously decreases the amount of accommodative, convergence present. But, due to relaxation of accommodation, the near object becomes blurred.

Measurement of amplitude of convergence

To perform the test for near, patient is asked to fixate 6/12 symbol at 33 cm and the bar is used with prism base directed out (BO). By progressively increasing the amount of BO prism power, the eyes are converged to the limit of bifoveal single vision, i.e. up to the point, when the patient just appreciates diplopia. This point is the end point, of the test and is called the *break point*. Its reading is recorded. At this point, the power of the prism is decreased slowly until he/she again fuses. This point, called the *recovery point*, is also recorded. Theoretically, before the break point, there will be a blur point because after the exhaustion of the fusional convergence patient starts using his/her accommodative convergence to avoid diplopia. This, however, can only be done by accommodating in excess of the requirements for the given distance (pseudomyopia) and consequently the image is blurred. Therefore, it is important to record the *blur point* in order to know what kind of fusional amplitudes are measured.

To perform the test for distance, the same procedure is repeated at 6 m and the blur point, break point and recovery point are recorded.

An example of a recording of fusional amplitudes as tested with the prism bar:

Distance : Diverged to 12ᐃ BI/recovered at 9ᐃ BI
Converged to 32ᐃ BO/recovered at 21ᐃ BO
Blurred at 12ᐃ BO

Near : Diverged to 14ᐃ BI/recovered at 9ᐃ BI
Converged to 36ᐃ BO/recovered at 24ᐃ BO
Blurred at 18ᐃ BO

Synoptophore method of measuring fusional amplitudes

To begin with, the objective angle of deviation is determined using simultaneous macular perception slides. Then, the second-grade fusion slides (similar targets with control marks for each eye) are introduced and if the patient fuses these targets and sees them as one with both control marks, the examiner blocks the arms at the objective angle. Then, first the amplitude of divergence and second the amplitude of convergence are measured as below.

To measure the divergence, the arms of the synoptophore are slowly diverged and the patient is instructed to report occurrence of diplopia or the disappearance of one or the other control mark of the picture (suppression). This point—the *break point*—is recorded and the arms of the synoptophore are slowly converged (i.e. brought to less divergent position) and the *recovery point*, where fusion occurs, is noted.

To measure the convergence, the arms of the synoptophore are further converged slowly till the fusion breaks and the *break point* is noted. Then, the arms are moved back into a less convergent position until fusion is regained and the *recovery point* is noted.

To measure the amplitude of vergences for near with synoptophore, a –3.0 DS lens is placed before each eye. In order to see clearly with –3.0DS lens, the subject has to overcome these lenses by accommodating as if he/she was fixating an object at a distance of 33 cm. To simulate the orthoposition for near fixation, the synoptophore tubes have to be set according to the convergence requirement for a point 33 cm distant which, in prism dioptres, is three times the patient's interpupillary distance in centimetres.

The procedure of testing for near is the same as for distance.

Normal values of vergences are as follows:

Vergence	Distance (6 m)	Near (33 cm)
Convergence	14–20ᐃ	35–40ᐃ
Divergence	5–8ᐃ	15–20ᐃ
Vertical vergence	2–4ᐃ	2–4ᐃ
Incyclovergence	10–12°	10–12°
Excyclovergence	10–12°	10–12°

An example of recording of fusional amplitudes as tested with the synoptophore:

Distance:

- *30ᐃ ET, objectively and subjectively.*
- *First- and second-grade fusion at angle.*
- *Convergence to 42ᐃ BO/recovery at 32ᐃ BO.*
- *Divergence to 12ᐃ BO/recovery at 20ᐃ BO.*

Near (with –3.0 D):
- *44^Δ ET objectively and subjectively*
- *First- and second-grade fusion at angle.*
- *Convergence to 56^Δ BO/recovery at 44^Δ BO.*
- *No divergence past angle, suppression OD.*

Measurement of near point of convergence

The near point of convergence (NPC) is the closest point at which an object can be seen single during bifoveal vision. In other words, it is the point at which the two foveal lines of sight intersect, when maximum convergence is exerted.

The NPC practically measures all types of convergence; since an object actually approaches the eyes during testing. That is, the test for NPC simultaneously stimulates fusional, accommodative and proximal convergence and during the last phase, if the patient is co-operative, there will be a strong voluntary effort to converge.

Instruments. Near point of convergence can be measured simply with the help of a graded plastic rule placed at the outer canthus and a fixation target (e.g. tip of a sharp pencil) moved towards the eye; or by use of specially designed rule such as RAF rule (Fig. 6.18), Livingstone binocular gauge (described on page 139) and Prince rule. These specially designed instruments basically consist of a bar or rule made from plastic, metal or wood on which a rider with the test chart can be moved back and forth (fixation target). At one end of the bar is a wing-like support that fits over the nose and rests against the lower orbital margins during the measurement. In Prince rule, the bar is 24 inches long and 1/2 inch square that has different markings on each of its four sides. One side is divided into centimetres (to be used for measurement of NPC and NPA), the second one into inches, and the third one into dioptres (for NPA in dioptres), and the age is indicated in years on the fourth side. The sliding target contains targets for measuring NPA and NPC.

Procedure. For measurement of convergence, a dot or a vertical line may be used as the target. It is advanced towards the patient at, or slightly below the eye level, until the patient has converged maximally and cannot sustain single bifoveal fixation as the target is brought closer. At this break point, the subject's non-dominant eye will diverge *(objective test)* and patient may appreciate diplopia *(subjective test)*. The distance from the canthus to this point is read on the rule and the NPC is recorded in mm or cm. Some of the near point rules have the zero point of their scales at the so-called spectacle point (i.e. 27 mm in front of the baseline). Therefore, with such instruments, 27 mm must be added to the distance that is read off the scale.

Normal values. The normal values of NPC vary considerably among different persons and even in different examinations of the same person. In normal adults, its average value is 70 mm (7 cm) with a range between 50 and 100 mm (5 to 10 cm). A distance closer than 5 cm is excessive, however, in children it may be as close as tip of the nose. NPC further away than 10 cm is defective or remote. In patients with convergence insufficiency (CI), it may be as remote as 25 or 30 cm or more.

Measurement of maintenance of convergence

The ability of the eyes to maintain convergence after the patient has been able to converge his/her eyes to a near vision can be tested by the inappropriately named test—*the drop convergence test*. In this test, after bringing the fixation target into reading distance, patient is asked to maintain convergence at this point and the fixation object is dropped suddenly. Some patients are better able than others to keep their eyes converged in the absence of a fixation object.

ASSESSMENT OF ACCOMMODATION AND AC/A RATIO

ASSESSMENT OF ACCOMMODATION

As we know, accommodation is a unique mechanism, by which our eyes can even focus

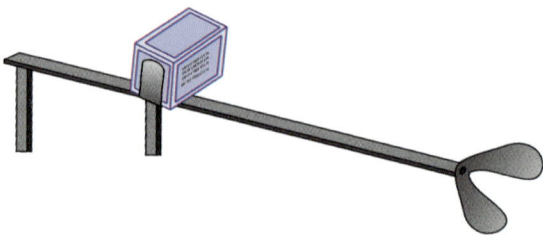

Fig. 6.18 *RAF rule.*

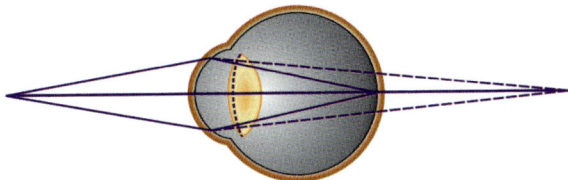

Fig. 6.19 *Effect of accommodation on divergent rays entering the eye.*

the diverging rays coming from a near object on the retina in a bid to see clearly (Fig. 6.19). Assessment of accommodation is of great diagnostic value in cases of incomitant strabismus of non-paralytic origin. Assessment of *amplitude of accommodation* (the difference between the dioptric power needed to focus at near point 'P' and far point 'R', i.e. A = P – R) in practice can be made either by measurement of near point of accommodation (NPA) or by use of minus lenses as below.

Measurement of near point of accommodation

The near point of accommodation (NPA) is the closest point at which small objects can be seen clearly. It is also called 'near point' or 'punctum proximum'.

NPA is measured using a near point rule such as RAF rule (Fig. 6.18) or Prince rule. The description of such a rule has been given in the discussion on the measurement of the near point of convergence.

To determine the NPA, a sliding target with 6/9 letters, numbers or fine lines is moved from or towards the eye until closest point is found at which it still can be seen clearly. During the examination, the patient has to wear his/her full optical refractive correction. The NPA is determined first for each eye separately and then for both eyes together. The NPA is measured in centimetres marked on one side of the instrument bar. The side of bar marked in dioptres will indicate the amplitude of accommodation in dioptres. The third side of the bar shows the age corresponding the accommodation. For example, if the patient reports that the point appears blurred at 25 cm, the dioptric markings will show +4.0 D and the age 40 years.

If, while measuring the NPA, the patient's amplitude of accommodation is found so low that his/her near point is beyond the length of the instrument, plus lenses are added to his/her correction until the near point is brought within range. The dioptric power of these additional lenses is then deducted from the measured values of amplitude of accommo-dation. Conversely, in young patients with very high accommodative power, minus lenses may be added to his/her distance correction to move his/her near point away from his/her eyes. The dioptric power of those minus lenses is then added to the measured value of amplitude of accommodation.

Measurement of amplitude of accommodation using minus lenses

This test is also performed first for each eye separately and then for both eyes together and during examination patient has to wear his/her full refractive correction. The patient is asked to fixate 6/60 symbol at a distance of 6 metres and minus lenses of progressively increasing power are added before the eye till he/she can see the target clearly. The power of this minus lens is equivalent to the amplitude of accommodation in dioptres.

ASSESSMENT OF ACCOMMODATIVE CONVERGENCE/ACCOMMODATION (AC/A) RATIO

The AC/A ratio is the relationship between accommodative convergence (AC), expressed in prism dioptres ($^\Delta$) and accommodation (A), expressed in lens dioptres (D). This relationship is linear one and is thought to be relatively stable throughout life. The normal AC/A ratio is about 3 to 5 prism dioptres for one dioptre of accommodation. The concept of AC/A ratio was first clearly defined by Fry who later with Haines introduced the abbreviation AC/A ratio.

Methods of measurement of AC/A ratio

1. *Heterophoria method.* To measure AC/A ratio, in this method, the deviation is measured with full optical correction at 6 metres distance and at 33 cm distance in prism dioptres, and IPD is measured in centimetres. Then the AC/A ratio is calculated from the following formula:

$$AC/A = IPD + \frac{^\Delta n - ^\Delta d}{d}, \text{ where;}$$

IPD = Interpupillary distance in centimetres

$^\Delta n$ = Deviation at 33 cm or 3 dioptres distance in prism dioptres

$^\Delta d$ = Deviation at 6 metres distance in prism dioptres

d = The fixation distance at near in dioptres

Note: Esodeviations are denoted by positive (+) and exodeviations by negative (–) sign.

For example, if IPD = 6 cm, $^\Delta n = 9^\Delta$ exophoria and $^\Delta d = 3^\Delta$ exophoria, then

$$AC/A = 6 + \frac{-9 - (3)}{3}$$
$$= 4^\Delta/D$$

2. Gradient method. This method is based on the fact that for a given fixation distance, minus lenses placed before the eyes increase the requirement for accommodation and plus lenses relax accommodation. Further, it is assumed that –1.0D lens produces an equivalent of 1.0D of accommodation, whereas +1.0D lens relaxis accommodation by 1.0D.

In practice, original deviation is found at near while the patient wears his/her optical correction and then with additional +3.0D lens and the calculations for AC/A ratio are made as follows:

$$AC/A = \frac{^\Delta L - ^\Delta O}{D}, \text{ where}$$

$^\Delta L$ = Deviation with additional lenses.

$^\Delta O$ = Original deviation without additional lenses.

D = Dioptric power of the additional lenses.

For example, if original deviation ($^\Delta O$) = 2^Δ esophoria, deviation with additional lenses ($^\Delta L$) = 10^Δ exophoria and the power of additional lenses (D) used is +3D, then:

$$AC/A = \frac{2 - (-10)}{3} = 4^\Delta/D$$

Alternatively, the patient's original distance phoria ($^\Delta O$) is determined while he/she wears full optical correction. A –3.0D lens is then placed before his/her eyes and the distance deviation ($^\Delta L$) is measured once more. The AC/A is calculated as above.

The gradient method is inaccurate because it does not take into account the patient's interpupillary distance (IPD).

3. Clinical distance-near-relationship method. This is a very simple method in which AC/A ratio is known by substracting distance deviation (D) at 6 metres from the near deviation (N) measured at 33 cm; i.e: AC/A = N – D. For examples:

i. In a patient with esotropia (ET) of 40 PD at near and 20 PD at distance, the AC/A ratio
= 40 – 20 = 20D PD.

ii. In a patient with distance orthophoria and near exotropia (XT) 15 PD the AC/A = –15 – 0 = –15PD

The results are interpreted as below:
- Up to 10 PD of N – D is normal.
- >10 PD of N – D is high AC/A ratio and
- <10 PD of N – D difference is less AC/A ratio.

4. Fixation disparity method. In this method, AC/A ratio is indirectly derived from the fixation disparity induced either by forced convergence by use of prism or by altering the accommodative stimulus by use of optical lenses. Because of its complexity, this test is not performed in routine clinical practice.

5. Haploscopic methods. In haploscopy, the visual fields of the two eyes are differentiated and a separate target is presented to each eye. Hering's original instrument was designed primarily for studying the AC/A ratio. In practice, this method is no more used. However, the haploscopic devices, such as the major amblyoscope, are of fundamental importance for the study of the sensorimotor co-operation of the eyes.

ASSESSMENT FOR EXTRAOCULAR MUSCLE PARESIS

When paresis of one or more extraocular muscles is suspected as cause of squint, in addition to the duction test and version test, following tests should also be performed:

- Abnormal head posture examination
- Diplopia charting

- Quantitative measurement of extraocular muscle actions
- Field of binocular fixation
- Bielschowsky phenomenon test
- Bielschowsky three-step test

I. ABNORMAL HEAD POSTURE EXAMINATION

Note the abnormal head posture, if any and examine its components in detail (*see* page 288–291).

II. DIPLOPIA CHARTING

Plotting of diplopia fields is indicated in patients complaining of confusion or double vision. The test is easy to perform provided the patient is co-operative. To perform the diplopia charting, patient is asked to wear red-green diplopia charting goggles; red glass being in front of the right eye and green in front of the left eye. The patient is made to sit with his/her head straight in a semidark room and is shown a fine linear light from a distance of 4 ft. The light is moved from primary position into all of the other eight directions of gaze. For each direction, patient is asked to comment on the position, brightness and separation between the red and green images. From the patient's comments, the examiner notes the following points:

- Whether horizontal diplopia is homonymous or heteronymous.
- Whether the image seen by right eye (red image) is higher or lower than the image seen by the left eye (green image) or vice versa.
- In which direction of gaze, separation between red and green images is greatest.
- Whether there are any directions in which fusion is present.

In a modified test of Franchchetti, instead of red green goggles, a red Maddox rod is placed in front of right eye and white Maddox rod in front of the left eye and the patient fixates on a spotlight which is seen as vertical red line with right eye and vertical white line with left eye.

Diplopia charts of patients with paresis of different extraocular muscles are shown in Figs 12.13 and 12.14.

Disadvantages of diplopia plotting test
- This test is only qualitative, therefore, it is not possible to comment on the minor changes of the improvement or deterioration from the records of different dates in the same patient.
- The test requires intelligent patient, especially to comment where the separation is maximum.
- It is not possible to perform the test in colour blind patients.
- This test is not of use in congenital palsies and those of long-standing onset, because due to deep suppression diplopia cannot be elicited.

III. QUANTITATIVE MEASUREMENT OF ACTIONS OF EXTRAOCULAR MUSCLES

The quantitative measurement of actions of extraocular muscles is essential to comment about the paretic muscles and the pathological sequelae of the paralysis, viz. overaction, contracture and secondary inhibitional palsy.

The tests employed for quantitative measurements of ocular movements are based on haploscopy. The haploscopic tests are based on the principle described by Burian that in the presence of normal retinal correspondence, the two test objects presented to the two eyes will be superimposed, if they stimulate the foveae of the two eyes, irrespective of the position of the two eyes (Fig. 6.20).

Commonly used haploscopic tests to have a graphic record of the relative power of extraocular muscles in all directions of gaze include:
- Lancaster red-green test,
- Hess screen test, and
- Lees screen test.

1. Lancaster red-green test

The Lancaster red-green test is a haploscopic test. It utilizes a Lancaster red-green screen which is window-shade type of screen that can be rolled up when not in use. The screen contains horizontal and vertical lines forming squares of 7 cm (Fig. 6.21). All the squares are of the same size and the tangential error is not taken into account. While performing the test, the patient's eyes should be in level with the centre zero mark, and he/she can be seated at either 1 or 2 metres. At 2 metres, each square subtends an angle of $2° = 3.5^\Delta$; at 1 metre it subtends an angle of $4° = 7^\Delta$. The patient is given a red-green reversible goggles (e.g. red glass in front of right

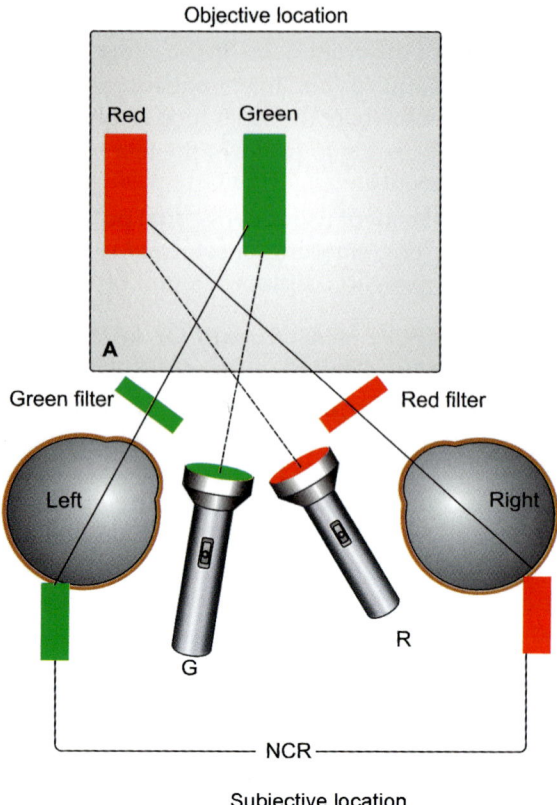

Objective location

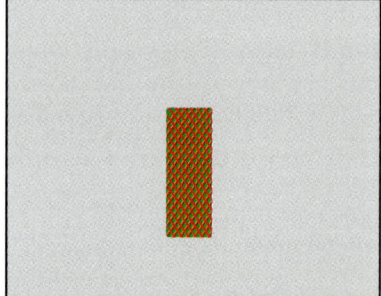

Subjective location

Fig. 6.20 *Burian's principle of haploscopic tests. Note, the right eye is esotropic and two different objects (red and green) presented to the two eyes (A) are stimulating the foveas and are thus subjectively localized as superimposed over each other (B).*

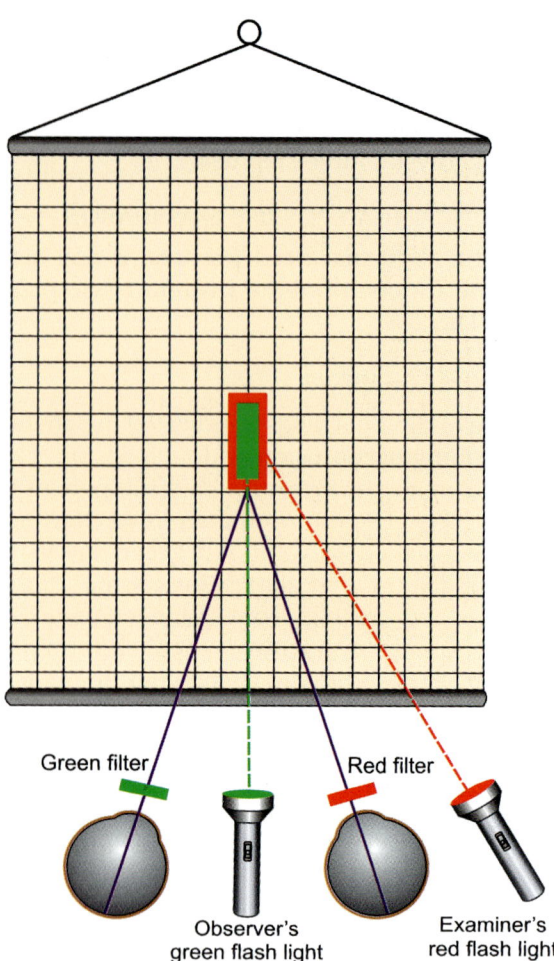

Fig. 6.21 *Lancaster red-green test.*

eye and green glass in front of left eye) and green flashlight that projects a linear image. The examiner has a similar red flash light and projects the red streak of light on the zero mark on the screen. The patient is asked to superimpose his/her green light on the examiner's red light. This is then repeated in all cardinal directions of gaze. The distance between the streaks of light represents the measurement of the objective deviation provided retinal correspondence is normal. The results are plotted on a chart that is an exact replica of the screen. Since the projected image is a line, the patient's response may indicate the presence of cyclotropia, when his/her streak is tilted. This test is most useful in patients with ocular paralysis and least useful in patients with heterophoria or intermittent heterotropias.

2. Hess screen test

Principle
The Hess screen test is based on the haploscopic principle. It utilizes the Hering's law of equal innervation, which states that in all voluntary

movements of the eye, equal and simultaneous innervation flows from the brain to the muscles of both eyes concerned in the respective direction of gaze (yoke muscles).

Prerequisites

Patient should have:

1. Full understanding about what he/she is supposed to do, since the test is purely subjective.
2. Good vision in both eyes.
3. Central fixation.
4. Normal retinal correspondence.

Discription of conventional Hess screen

Original Hess screen consisted of a single tangent screen made up of a black cloth 3 ft wide × 3½ ft long, marked by a series of horizontal and vertical red lines (Fig. 6.22). The distance between each line subtends a visual angle of 5°. Fixation points are indicated at the centre of the screen and at the intersections of the 15° and 30° lines by red dots. Thus, the red dots form an inner square of 8 dots along the 15° lines and an outer square of 16 dots along the 30° lines. The inner square represents the 8 cardinal directions

of gaze and the outer square the extreme directions of gaze. In the original Hess screen, indicator consists of a knot tying three green cords together to form the letter Y. The end of central vertical green cord is fastened to a movable black rod 50 cm long. The ends of the other two green cords, forming upper two limbs of the letter Y, are kept taut by black threads that pass through loops to small weights at corresponding upper corners of the screen. This arrangement enables the patient to move the indicator freely and smoothly over the whole surface of the screen in all directions.

Modified wooden Hess screen. One of the modifications of the original Hess screen is a wooden screen with small red lights forming the fixation points (Fig. 6.23) and a green dot light projecter as the indicator. Presently, it is more commonly in use.

Procedure Hess screen test

The patient wears red-green goggles and sits 50 cm from the commonly used modified wooden Hess screen. The patient now sees the fixation points (red light) with one eye and the indicator (green light of projector) with the other eye. The patient is asked to superimpose the indicator successively on each of the fixation points, and the relative position of the eyes is plotted for each of these directions of gaze on a chart which is replica of the Hess screen.

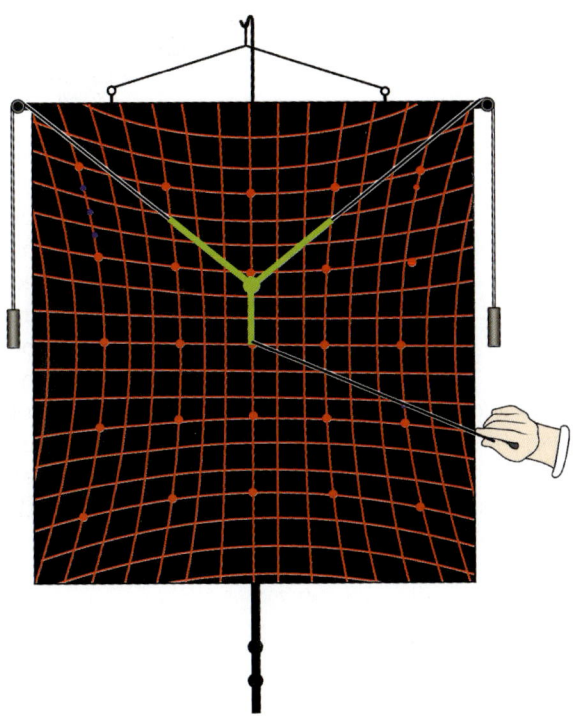

Fig. 6.22 *The Hess screen.*

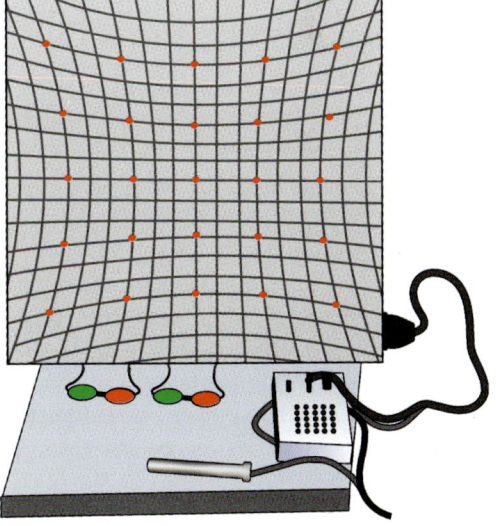

Fig. 6.23 *Modified Hess screen.*

Digital Hess screen

Digital or the PC Hess screen provides the clinician, a new computer-based tool for assessing patients suffering from paralytic strabismus, using image manipulation technology and software technology. It is designed to run on any computer operating under Windows, with a 19″ (or larger) monitor. When the program is run for the first time, the user is required to calibrate the size of the screen (by measuring the dimensions of a box displayed on the screen) and to enter the preferred viewing distance (usually 25–50 cm). It provides integration function of diagnosis of strabismus, data record and analyze.

Key features

- Rapid and accurate assessment of the size and direction of phoria/tropia
- Results plotted in conventional Hess screen format allow the clinician to establish whether a deviation is concomitant or incomitant and which muscle is affected.
- A variety of analytical tools to help the clinician form a diagnosis
- Built in database allows results to be archived for future reference
- Results can be printed or pasted into referral letters and reports
- Runs on a standard PC
- Voice instructions, possible.

Operating methods

Digital Hess screen is a computer program which is designed to run on any computer. Steps of use are as below:

- *Patient wears red and green goggles* and is positioned in front of the computer screen at the appropriate distance (Fig. 6.24A).
- *Room lights are extinguished and a red and a blue circle are displayed on the screen* (the right eye sees the red circle and the left the blue). Initially the red circle is placed in the top left of the screen and the patient is instructed to move the blue circle using the mouse until it appears to be centred on the red circle.
- *As the eyes are dissociated,* any deviation in this direction of gaze will result in a misalignment

of the circles (Fig. 6.24B). This is repeated for either 9 or 25 directions of gaze (depending on the option selected). The colour of the circles is then reversed and measurements repeated with the left eye fixating. The nine point test takes approximately 4 minutes to complete.

- *Results are then displayed* in the conventional format on the screen.
- *Multiple plots can be superimposed* to assess longitudinal changes and the exact amplitude of any deviation can be displayed at any point on the chart (Fig. 6.25).

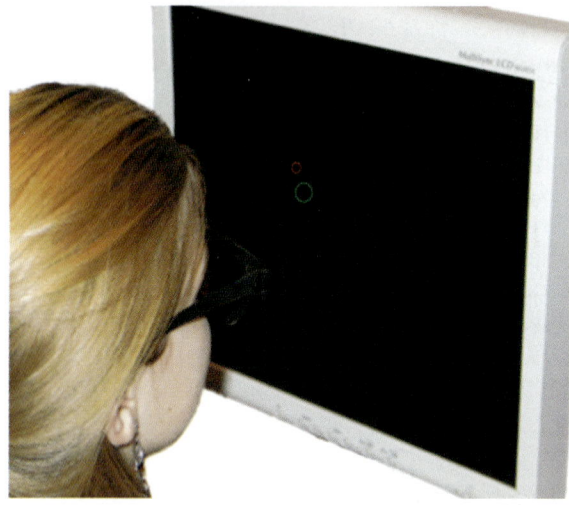

Fig. 6.24A *Patient is seated in front of a PC Hess screen after wearing red and green goggles.*

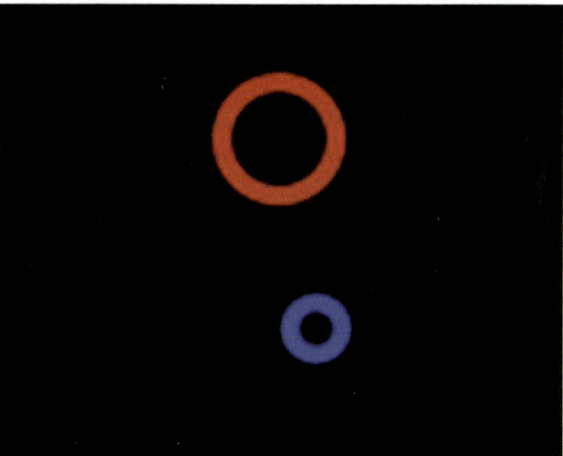

Fig. 6.24B *Misalignment of the circles seen due to any deviation in the direction of gaze.*

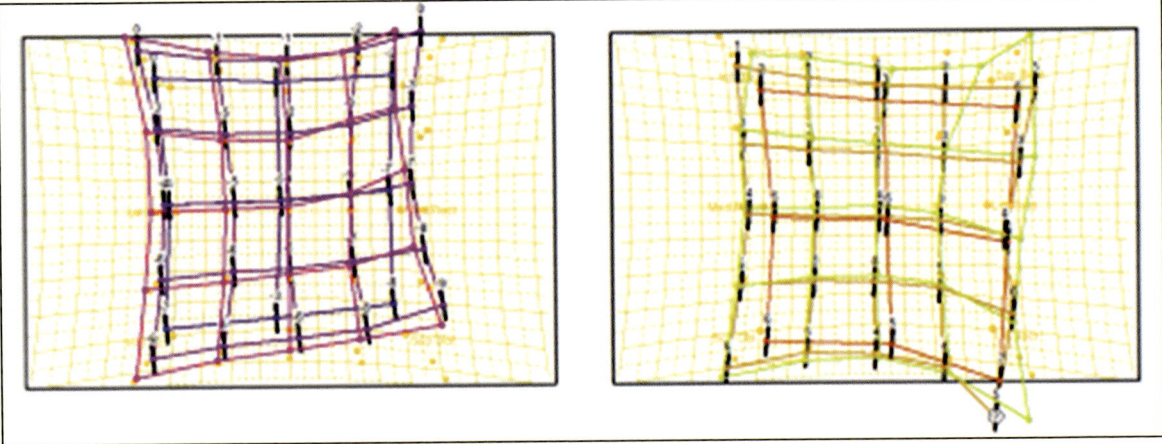

Fig. 6.25 *Hess screen plots superimposed to assess longitudinal changes and the exact amplitude of any deviation.*

- *A number of analytical tools can then be applied to the data to help the clinician establish a diagnosis. For example, the program will automatically calculate the relative areas of the plots for the left and right eyes, helping the clinician to determine which eye has a palsied muscle and providing an index for monitoring the progression of an incomitant deviation.*

3. Lees screen test

Lees screen, also known as the Hess-Lees screen, is another modification of the original Hess screen. The Hess-Lees screen (Fig. 6.26) consists of two tangent screens made of white translucent material placed at a right angle with a plane mirror bisecting this right angle and dissociating the fields of the two eyes. The tangent pattern similar to the original Hess screen printed in black dots (fixation points) on a white background is placed just behind both the translucent screens, and is seen only when the translucent screens are illuminated for performing the test.

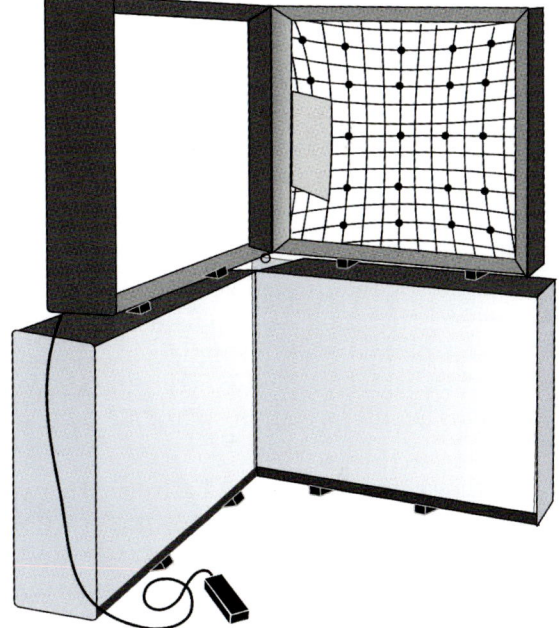

Fig. 6.26 *Lees screen.*

Procedure

To perform the test with right eye fixing, the patient sits facing the left tangent screen at 50 cm from it with his/her forehead leaning against the central vertical rim of the mirror. The line bisecting the mirror horizontally lies in the same plane as the centre of the horizontals of the tangent screens. Patient's pupils are levelled with this horizontal line by an adjustable chin rest. The patient is given a pointer with a ring at its tip. The examiner has another pointer with a small disc at its tip, half the diameter of the patient's pointer. The right screen is illuminated and left screen is kept non-illuminated. The patient's right eye vision is intercepted by the mirror, in which he/she sees the right screen projected forward as a virtual image that appears to be superimposed upon the left screen.

The patient's left eye sees the left screen directly (he/she is facing that screen) but cannot see the right screen, situated laterally. The examiner now places his pointer on the zero (central) point of the right screen. Its image that appears to be superimposed on the left screen is seen by the patient's right eye. Patient is asked to super-impose his/her pointer on the examiner's pointer with his/her left hand on the left screen. By means of a foot pedal, the left screen is illuminated for 1–2 seconds so that the examiner can plot on the diagnostic Hess chart the precise location of the patient's pointer on the left screen. The 8 dots of the inner square are then plotted in sequence and, wherever necessary, this is followed by the plotting of the 16 dots of the outer square.

To perform the test with left eye fixing, patient sits facing the right screen which is kept unilluminated while looking with his/her left eye into the mirror, where he/she sees the virtual image of the left (illuminated) screen. The procedure described above is then repeated.

Diagnostic interpretation of the Hess chart

The diagnostic interpretation of the Hess chart is done by comparing the two fields, i.e. one, of the left eye plotted while the right eye fixing and other, of the right eye plotted while the left eye is fixing. The interpretation should be done as follows:

1. *Compression of the space* between the two plotted fixation points indicates underaction of a muscle acting in that direction.

2. *Expansion of the space* between the two plotted fixation points indicates overaction of the muscle acting in that direction.

3. *Smaller field belongs to the eye* with the paretic muscle (Fig. 6.27A).

4. *Non-affected eye shows the larger field* expressing the overaction of the contralateral synergist (Fig. 6.27B).

5. *Fields of similar shape and size are suggestive of comitant deviation*, while the fields of dissimilar shape and size indicate incomitance.

6. *In the smaller field, the greatest displacement (compression) away from the normal cardinal direction* will indicate the paretic muscle

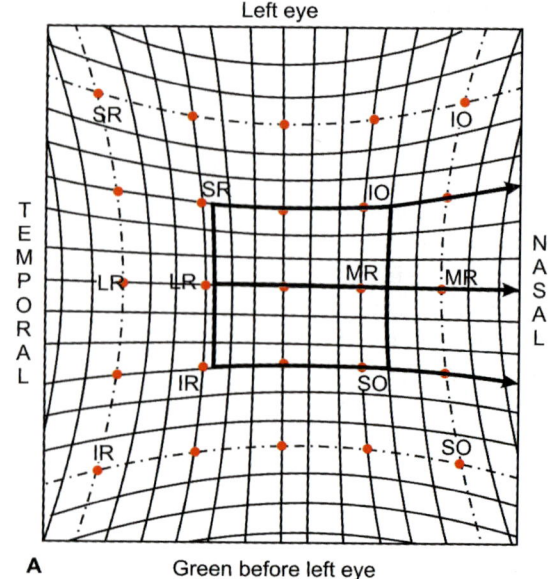

A   Green before left eye

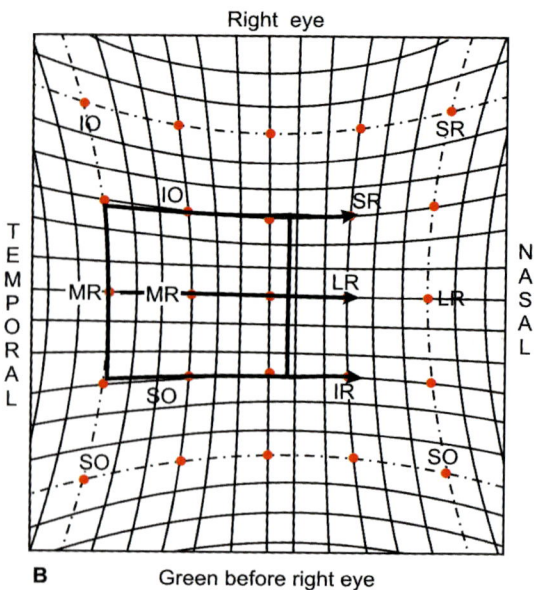

B   Green before right eye

Fig. 6.27 *Hess chart of a patient with right lateral rectus palsy.*

(underaction). In many cases, displacement in the direction of the field of the antagonist (due to contracture) may also be seen.

7. *In greater field, the greatest displacement (expansion) away from the normal cardinal direction* will indicate the overacting muscle (contralateral synergistic or yoke muscle of the paretic muscle). In many cases (especially in those of long duration), there may also be displacement

of the field away from the direction of the antagonist of this muscle (due to inhibitional palsy of the contralateral antagonist).

IV. FIELD OF BINOCULAR FIXATION

It should be tested in patients with incomitant squint, where applicable, i.e. if patient has some field of binocular single vision. The area of binocular single vision is opposite to the direction in which ocular motility is impaired. In general, the field of binocular fixation represents the extreme limits of conjugate movement of the eyes in all directions in the absence of any movement of the head.

Procedure

The test is performed on the perimeter using a central chin rest. The patient fixates a small (3.5 mm) movable white target in the primary position, which is then moved along the arc until diplopia results or it goes out of the fixation limits. This point is recorded. The arc is then moved on successively in 15° steps and the test repeated for each position until the whole field has been examined. Normal field of fixation is shown in Fig. 6.28.

If the patient has diplopia in central position fixation, the target is moved in the periphery till the target becomes single or the target goes out

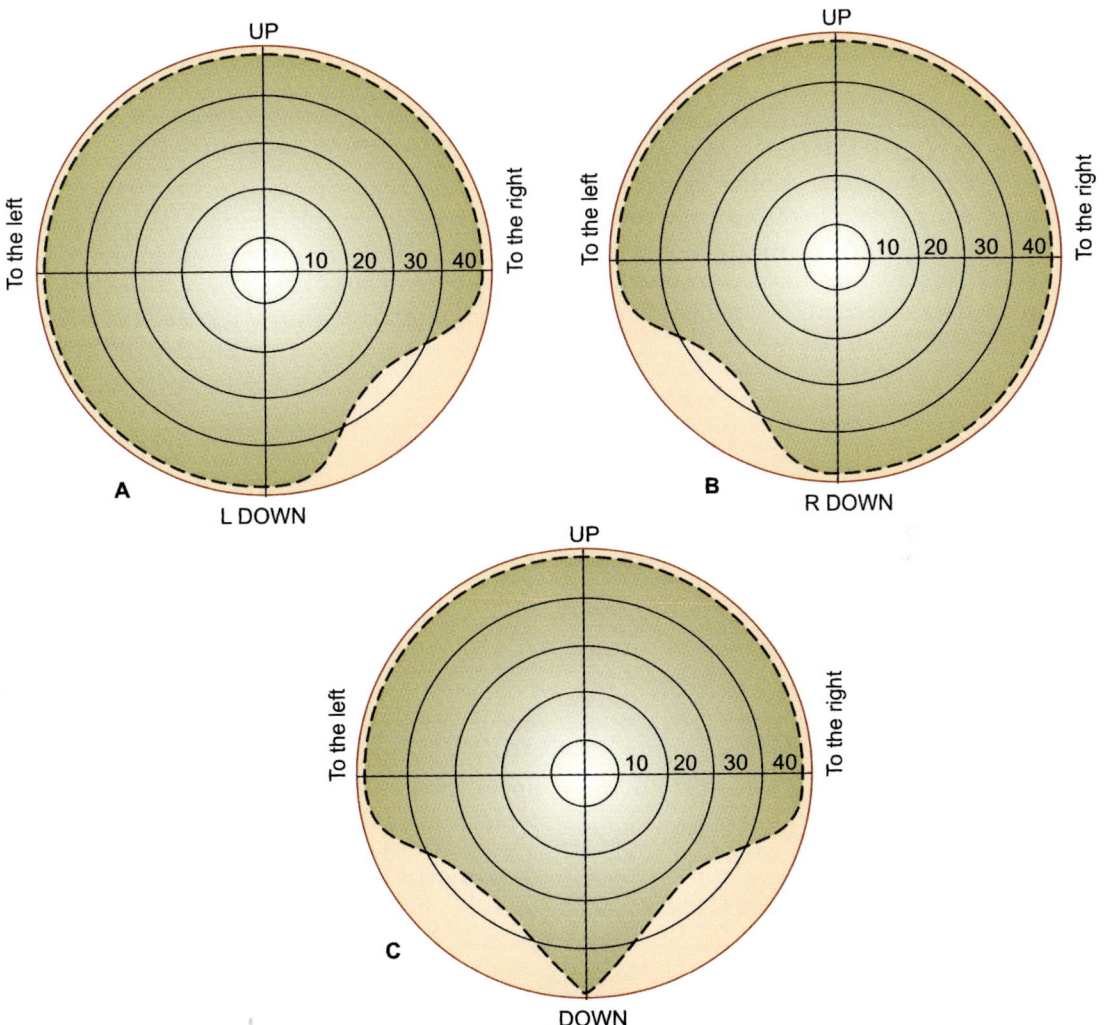

Fig. 6.28 *Field of fixation: A, left eye; B, right eye and C, binocular.*

of fixation point. The record of binocular field of fixation is completed as above.

The diplopia as well as binocular fixation is better appreciated, when the test is performed using red and green goggles in front of the eyes and a movable spot of white light as target. In the area of binocular single fixation, the target spotlight will appear as mixture of red and green, and when binocular fixation is lost it will appear red or green.

It is standard to shade the area of binocular single vision after plotting on the chart. In the presence of suppression, the test can be performed with filters, but this may diminish the fusional response. In general terms, the field of binocular fixation is more or less circular with a radius of about 45–50° from the fixation point in the primary position, except below when it is restricted on either side by the nose (Fig. 6.33C).

In a patient with paresis of an extraocular muscle, it may be helpful to record a patient's successive fields of binocular fixation on the same chart, thus making it easy to observe the clinical cause of the condition. As an example, Fig. 6.29 shows field of binocular fixation before and after operation (on the same chart) in a patient having 3rd nerve palsy of 2 years duration.

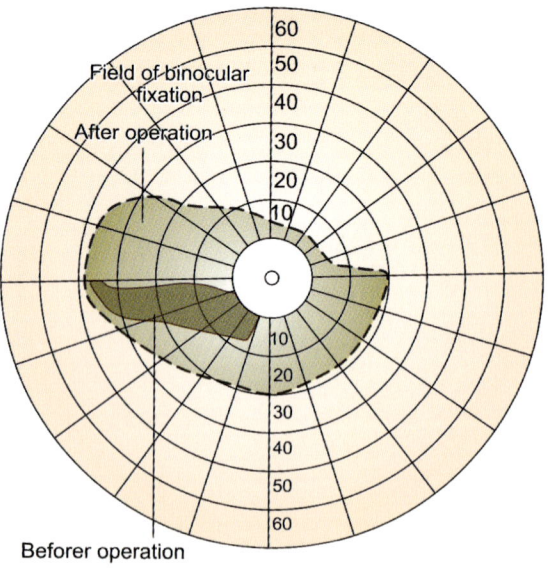

Fig. 6.29 *Field of binocular fixation before and after extraocular muscles surgery in a patient with third nerve palsy.*

V. BIELSCHOWSKY'S PHENOMENON TEST

This test is performed for confirming the diagnosis of alternating sursumduction suspected on alternating cover test. The eye under cover deviates upwards and extorts. When the cover is removed, the eye slowly rotates downward to return to its previous position.

To perform the Bielschowsky phenomenon test, patient is asked to fixate a spotlight with one eye and the other eye is covered by an occluder. It is observed that the eye under cover moves up and extorts. Then, a filter is held before the fixating eye, keeping a watch on the eye under cover, which moves downward and intorts. This influence of changing the light stimulus in the fixating eye on the deviation of the covered eye is known as the Bielschowsky phenomenon. Its presence confirms the diagnosis of alternating sursumduction made on alternate cover test.

VI. BIELSCHOWSKY'S HEAD TILT TEST

This test was originally recommended by Bielschowsky to differentiate between superior oblique palsy in one eye and superior rectus palsy in the contralateral side. The modified *three-step technique of Bielschowsky's head tilt test* is used for the diagnosis of paretic vertical recti and oblique muscles. For details, *see* pages 293–297.

SENSORY EVALUATION: ASSESSMENT FOR BINOCULAR CO-OPERATION AND SENSORY ANOMALIES

Normal binocular single vision consists of three grades: Simultaneous perception, fusion and stereopsis. It is maintained with central fixation and normal retinal correspondence.

There are variety of sensory adoptations that occur in response to clinical situations that disrupt binocular vision. The devlopement of a specific type of sensory adaptation depends on when (age of the patients) the sensory anomaly occurred and the severity and type of binocular disruption.

Visually mature patients may develop following sensory adaptations:

- Diplopia,
- Confusion, or
- Rivalry

Visually immature patients may develop following sensory adaptations:

- Monofixation syndrome,
- Anomalous retinal correspondence (ARC), or
- Large regional suppression

Amblyopia, not actually a sensory adaptation may occur as a consequence of suppression. Sensory adaptations and amblyopia are described in details on page 177–201.

Tests for binocular co-operation and sensory anomalies are as given below.

A. TESTS FOR FIXATION BEHAVIOUR

Fixation behaviour should be tested in each patient with strabismus having vision less than 6/6 Snellen's. It can be tested with the help of a visuscope (page 140) or fixation star of the ophthalmoscope. Patient is asked to cover one eye and fix the star with the other eye. Fixation may be *centric (normal on the fovea) or eccentric* (which may be unsteady, parafoveal, paramacular, centrocaecal, paracaecal or temporal; Fig. 6.30). The preliminary checking of fixation should be done without dilating the pupil, since this would be an obstacle to the pursuit of the rest of the diagnostic tests. However, in the end, pupils should be dilated and fixation test repeated along with the detailed fundus examination.

A steady central foveal fixation is a good prognostic sign. An unsteady but central foveal fixation indicates a possibility of good vision with conventional occlusion while a steady paramacular or peripheral eccentric fixation indicates a poor prognosis.

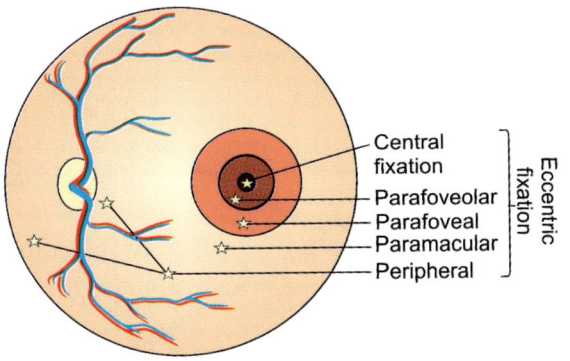

Fig. 6.30 *Types of fixation.*

B. TESTS FOR THE STATE OF RETINAL CORRESPONDENCE

Assessment for the state of retinal correspondence is neccessary only in the presence of a constant manifest deviation. It is absolutely essential to know the state of monocular fixation, whether it is eccentric or central, so that this can be taken into account, when evaluating the results of the various tests.

In the absence of normal retinal correspondence (NRC), a patient with strabismus may develop anomalous retinal correspondence (ARC). ARC is an unstable secondary adaptation of sensory interaction between the two eyes that has developed under conditions of everyday stimulation and exists under these conditions.

The tests employed to evaluate state of retinal correspondence are described here in decreasing order of their similarity to normal circumstances.

1. Striated glass test *(Bagolini test)*

This test, performed with the Bagolini striated glasses, is closest to everyday visual conditions. The eyes are not dissociated during the test and can be observed by the examiner.

Bagolini's striated glasses (sometimes referred to as lenses) are in fact glass plates without refractive power. The glass plates contain extremely fine parallel striations on the surface. When looking through them, a spotlight appears as a fine streak of light perpendicular to the striations. The principle basically is the same as for the Maddox rod except that the patient can actually see through Bagolini's glasses. The glasses are mounted so that they can be inserted into a trial frame. Marks on the glass indicate the direction of the streak seen by the patient.

Procedure to perform the test (Fig. 6.31). Preferably the test should be performed in a room with subdued light. The test is performed for distance (6 metres) as well as near (33 cm). Patient is instructed to fixate on a spotlight. The striated glasses are placed in a trial frame with their axis oriented respectively at 45° and 135°, so that a normal subject would see two streaks of light forming a × intersecting at the spotlight (Fig. 6.31A). In a patient with strabismus, one of the following observations may be made:

1. A patient with a constant tropia having normal retinal correspondence (NRC) with no demonstrable suppression will experience

diplopia, i.e. will see two spotlights each one crossed by one streak of light (Fig. 6.31B). According to the deviation, they will be seen either in crossed or in uncrossed diplopia.

2. In the presence of suppression of one eye, the patient will see the spotlight crossed by the line in front of the non-suppressing eye only (Fig. 6.31C).

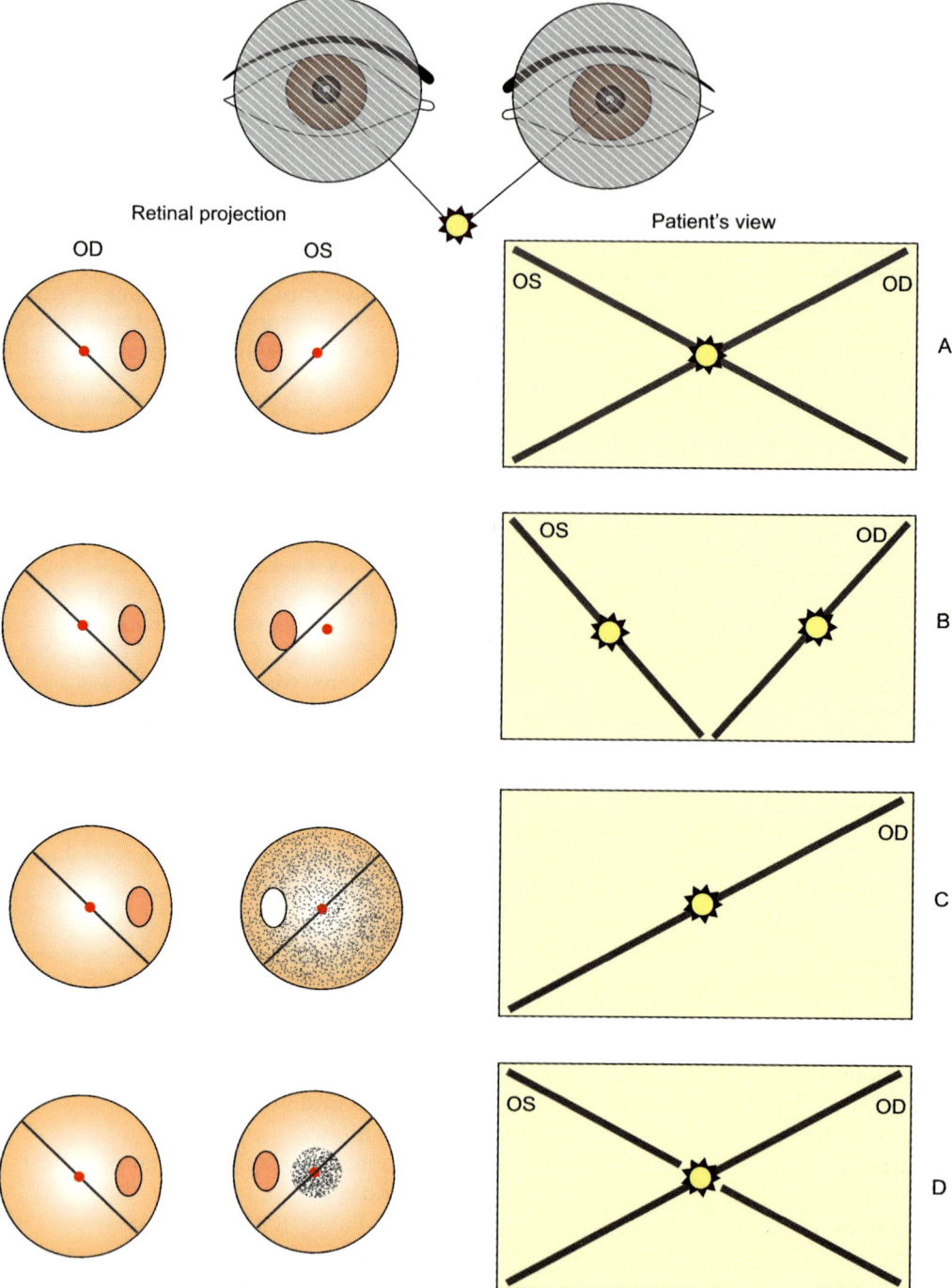

Fig. 6.31 *Bagolini's striated glass test (for explanation see text).*

3. A patient with harmonious anomalous retinal correspondence will see a perfect cross, as seen by a normal person (Fig. 6.31A), but the cover test will show the presence of a tropia.

4. Two streaks, but only one crossing through the centre of the light (the other one being displaced away from the light with a portion of it missing), indicate a suppression area with either normal retinal correspondence or unharmonious ARC (Fig. 6.31D).

5. In the presence of a small angle tropia, if the patient sees a perfect cross as seen by a normal person (Fig. 6.31A), and there is no movement on cover test, NRC is indicated (although there may be lack of bifoveal fixation). Parks records such cases as having 'unknown retinal correspondence'.

Advantages of Bagolini's test
- This test is closest to the everyday visual conditions, i.e. there is minimal interference with normal visual condition since the patient can see with both eyes.
- It is a simple and easy test both for the patient and the examiner. Even a child can describe exactly what he sees.
- The test can be performed for any fixation distance.
- Since the eyes are not dissociated during the test, these can be observed by the examiner.

Disadvantages
- The test is only qualitative since the angle of anomaly cannot be measured.
- Small angles of anomaly may be overlooked.

2. Diplopia test

To perform this test, patient's deviation is first determined objectively and the diplopia test is then performed under the same conditions (i.e. same fixation distance and refractive correction) to permit comparison. In the diplopia test, the patient fixates a spotlight on the centre of a tangent scale through a red filter and the deviating eye is uncovered. To begin with, each eye is covered alternately, so as to show him, that the fixation light and the tangent scale or screen is seen with one eye and red spot of light with the other eye. When both eyes are uncovered, the patient may see one or two lights as follows:

- When the patient sees one red light and one white light, it indicates either normal retinal correspondence or unharmonious ARC (if the separation of the images is not compatible with the angle of deviation).
- When the patient sees only one red light, it indicates suppression of the deviating eye.
- When the patient sees a mixture of red and white or a light red light, it indicates probability of harmonious ARC.

Advantages
The test is very simple and can be performed in children of average intelligence who are as young as 4 years of age.

Disadvantages
It is difficult to differentiate between fusion of the images and suppression of the deviating eye, since even in binocular vision, the fixating eye will be dominant and the image will tend to appear red.

3. Prism bar and red filter test

To perform this test, patient is asked to fixate a spotlight at 6 metres distance and a prism bar cover test is carried out with prism bar in front of the fixating eye, till the deviation is neutralized. The prism bar reading at this point equals the objective angle of squint. A red filter is then placed in front of the deviating eye and the patient is asked to describe what he/she sees. The various possibilities are as below:

1. Patient may suppress one eye, i.e. he/she does not see red light or a mixture of red and white light. This makes the test useless.

2. In the presence of normal retinal correspondence (i.e. when the foveae have a common visual direction), the patient may see the light as a blend of red and white.

3. In the presence of ARC, i.e. when the foveae have different visual directions, the patient will see two lights, a white and a red one. In a patient with esodeviation, the diplopia will be crossed and with exodeviation uncrossed (paradoxical diplopia).

4. To measure the angle of anomaly, in the presence of ARC, the prism bar is now moved slowly (decreasing the base-out strength for esodeviations or the base-in strength in

exodeviations) until the diplopia disappears or until the type of diplopia is reversed. The prism bar value at this point equals the subjective angle of squint. The difference between the objective and subjective angles represents the angle of anomaly.

4. Synoptophore test

To detect ARC by synoptophore method, *objective and subjective angles* of the squint are measured using dissimilar slides (e.g. lion and the cage) as discribed on page 112, respectively, and the results are interpreted as below:

1. If the objective and subjective angles of the squint coincide, normal retinal correspondence (NRC) is present.

2. If the objective angle is greater than subjective angle, the anomalous retinal correspondence (ARC) is present; and the difference between these angles is called the angle of anomaly, when the angle of anomaly is equal to the objective angle, i.e. when subjective angle is zero, the ARC is harmonious. In unharmonious ARC, angle of anomaly is smaller than the objective angle.

5. Worth's four-dot test

For this test, patient wears red-green goggles with red lens in front of the right eye and green lens in front of the left eye and views a box with four lights—one red, two green and one white (Fig. 6.32A). Since the lights are of the colours complementary to those of the filters before the patient's eye, he/she can see the red light only through the red filter and the two green lights only through the green filter. The white light can be seen with both eyes.

Depending upon the patient's observation, the results are interpreted as below:

1. If the patient sees all the four lights (one red, two green and one white or red or green or mixture of red and green) in the absence of manifest squint, he/she has normal binocular single vision (Fig. 6.32A).

2. With abnormal retinal correspondence (ARC), patient sees all the four lights as above even in the presence of a manifest squint (Fig. 6.32B).

3. If the patient sees only two red lights, he/she has left suppression (Fig. 6.32C).

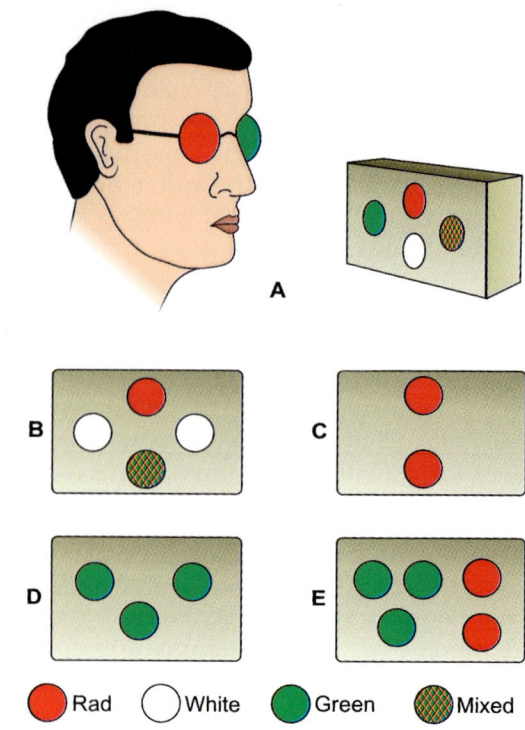

Fig. 6.32 *Worth's four-dot test.*

4. If the patient sees only three green lights, he/she has right suppression (Fig. 6.32D).

5. When the patient sees three green lights and two red lights alternately, it indicates presence of alternating suppression.

6. If the patient sees five lights (2 red and 3 green), he has diplopia (Fig. 6.32E).

6. Bielschowsky's after image test

In this test, patient's right fovea is stimulated with a vertical bright light and left fovea with a horizontal bright light (Fig. 6.33A) for 15 seconds each and the patient is asked to draw the position of after images. Perception of the after images is easiest, when the patient closes his/her eyes or when he/she looks at a blank screen. *The results are interpreted as below:*

1. A patient with normal retinal correspondence will draw a cross (Fig. 6.33B).

2. A right esotropic patient with ARC will draw vertical image to the left of horizontal image (Fig. 6.33C).

3. A right exotropic patient with ARC will draw vertical image to the right of horizontal (Fig. 6.33D).

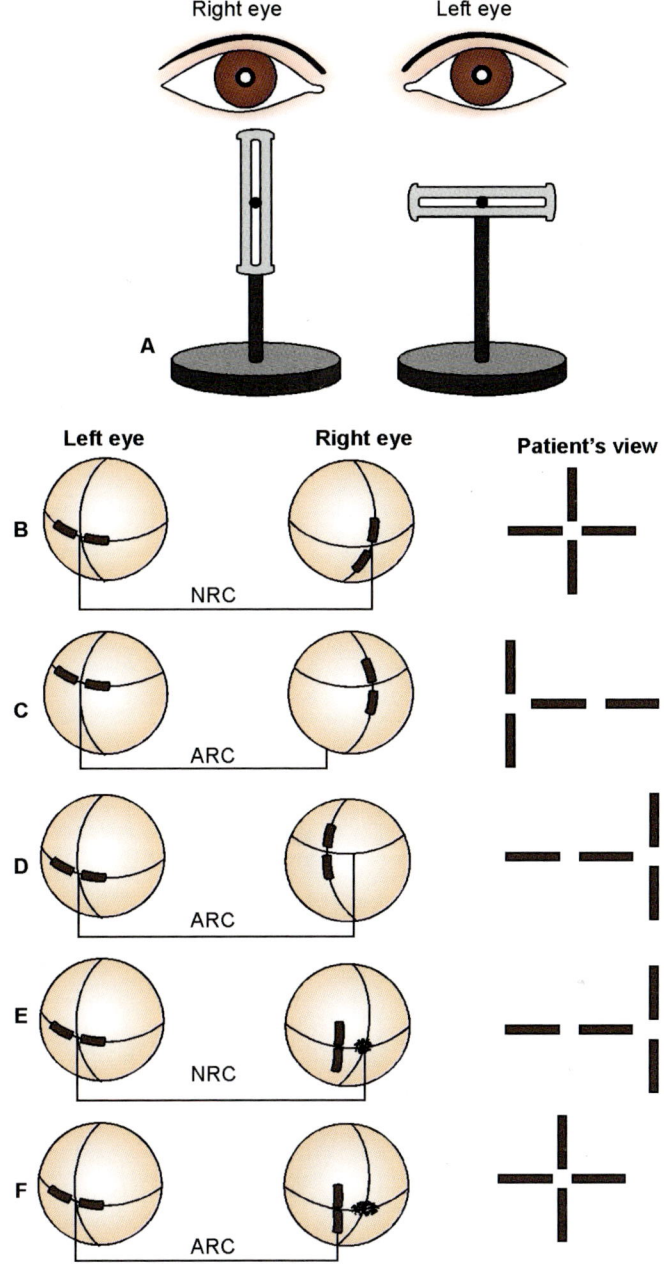

Fig. 6.33 *Bielschowsky's after image test (for explanation, see text).*

4. A response showing the images in a crossed position in exotropia (Fig. 6.33E) and in an uncrossed position in esotropia (Fig. 6.33F) indicates the presence of paradoxic diplopia in the presence of ARC with eccentric fixation.

5. The patient may draw only vertical image (in left suppression) or only horizontal image (in right suppression). In alternate suppression, patient sees vertical and horizontal lines alternately.

Disadvantages

1. The after image test is the most unphysiologic of all the tests for ARC, since an after image and a normal visual stimulation are so different that they cannot even be compared.

2. Small children do not understand what they should observe.

7. Cupper's binocular visuscope test

In this test, the patient sits 5 metres away from a Maddox scale and is asked to fixate the light on the centre of scale with fixing eye and the examiner looks the images of the visuscope on the retina of patient's deviated eye. Since it may be difficult for the examiner to look through the visuscope without blocking the patient's view of the fixation object, i.e. the patient is asked to fixate through a plane mirror or prism (which changes the direction of fixation) (Fig. 6.34A).

The examiner projects the star of the visuscope on the patient's fovea and asks the patient to tell its position on the Maddox scale in respect to the central fixation light. The results are interpreted as below:

1. In the presence of normal retinal correspondence, the patient sees star superimposed on the fixation light (Fig. 6.34B).
2. In the presence of ARC, patient sees star to the right or left of the fixation light depending

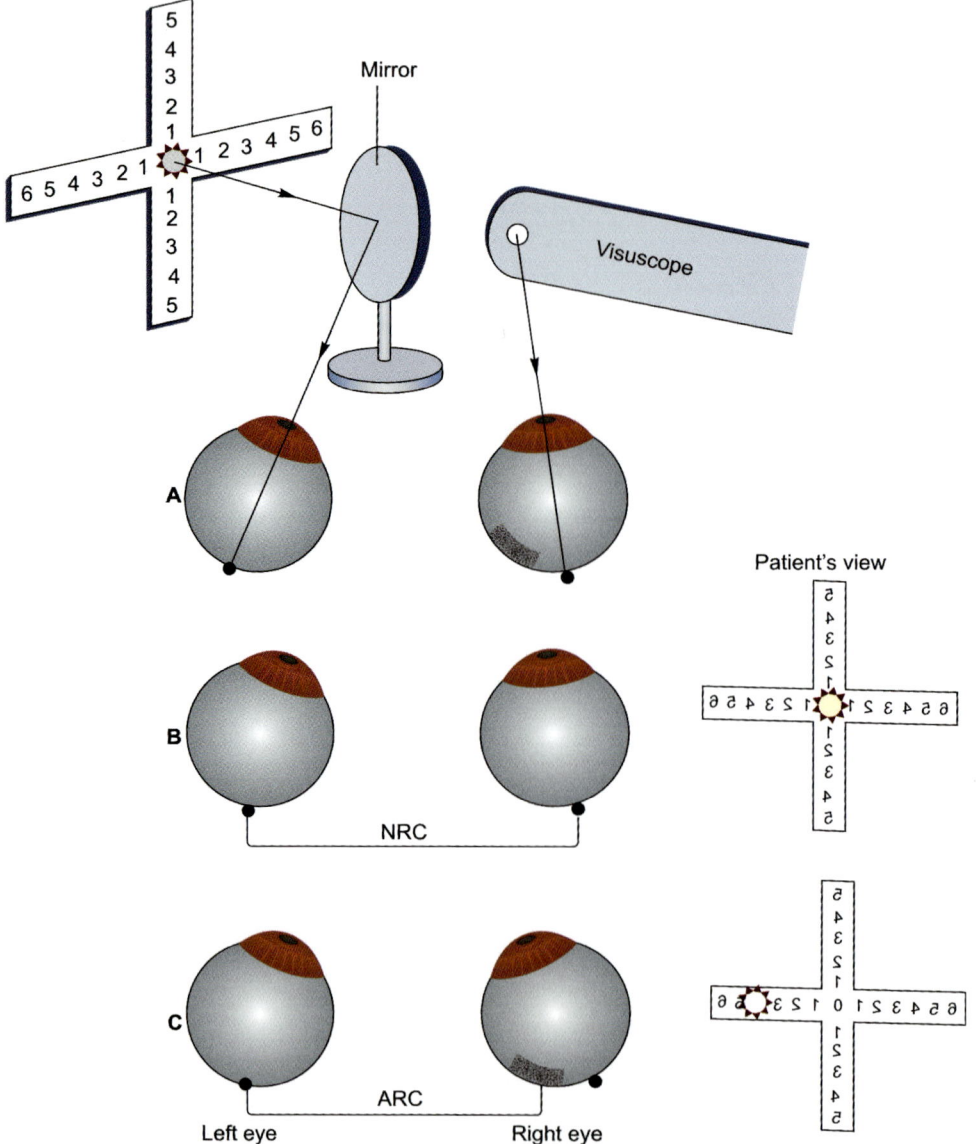

Fig. 6.34 *Cupper's binocular visuscope test (for explanation, see text).*

upon the deviation. The number on the Maddox scale coinciding with the star gives the angle of anomaly (Fig. 6.34C).

After the presence of ARC is established, the examiner moves the visuscope until the star and the fixation light coincide, and at this point, the examiner notes the position of the star on the patient's retina. This peripheral point on the retina of the patient's deviated eye has acquired a common visual direction with the fovea of the dominant eye. This point is not always the same as the one used for eccentric fixation. In other words, the angle of anomaly is not always identical with the distance between the fovea and the retinal point used for fixation.

Disadvantages
The binocular visuscope test is difficult to perform with young children.

Evaluation of tests for retinal correspondence

A great disparity between the results of various tests performed for evaluation of state of retinal correspondence is reported in the literature. In general, as stated earlier, the tests that interfere least with the ordinary conditions of seeing (e.g. Bagolini's test) show more ARC response and the tests which cause most dissociating conditions (e.g. after image test) show less ARC response.

C. ASSESSMENT FOR GRADES OF BINOCULAR SINGLE VISION

Assessment for grades of binocular single vision (BSV) is essential, since its achievement is the ultimate goal in the management of a case with strabismus. As stated earlier, the three grades of BSV include simultaneous perception (first grade), fusion (second grade) and stereopsis (third grade). Various tests employed to assess the state of BSV have been described on page 58.

D. TESTS TO ASSESS SUPPRESSION AND AMBLYOPIA

See pages 171 and 186.

ORTHOPTIC INSTRUMENTS

GENERAL CONSIDERATIONS

Uses

The orthoptic instruments are required for diagnostic, therapeutic or both purposes.

A. *Diagnostic uses of orthoptic instruments*
1. Measurement of angle of deviation (subjective and objective).
2. Measurement of range of fusion.
3. Measurement of accommodative convergence/accommodation (AC/A) ratio.
4. To know the sensory status of binocular vision and to detect the sensory anomalies such as suppression, amblyopia and ARC.
5. To evaluate for stereoacuity.
6. To evaluate the motor status of binocular vision.

B. *Therapeutic uses of orthoptic instruments*
1. Exercises to improve the fusional range.
2. Exercises to improve the relative convergence or relative accommodation.
3. Anti-suppression exercises.
4. Amblyopia therapy.

Working principle of orthoptic instruments

Working of most orthoptic instruments is based on the fact that they either allow or detect the dissociation of fusion of binocular vision.

The common modes by which an orthoptic instrument can cause dissociation of two eyes are as follows:

1. Use of septum so that each eye sees the different half of the field, as in Maddox wing, diploscope, Remy separator, cheiroscope and pigeon-cantonnet stereoscope.
2. Use of two tubes, one in front of each eye as in synoptophore.
3. Use of red and green complimentary glasses one in front of each eye.
4. Use of polaroide glasses.
5. Use of striations as in Bagolini's glasses.
6. Use of cylinderical lenses as in Maddox rod.

Types of orthoptic instruments

- Conventional, i.e. non-computerised orthoptic equipment, and
- Computerised orthoptic programs *see* page 149.

CONVENTIONAL (NON-COMPUTERISED) ORTHOPTIC INSTRUMENTS

Like any other branch of science, the science of orthoptic and strabismus is also advancing and changing fast. With time, certain instruments have become obsolete and some have become less important. For example, even synoptophore is no more considered an essential equipment for orthoptic set-up. However, its persence do adds grace to the orthoptic clinic. Description of certain instruments which are used only for diagnostic purposes has been given along with the diagnostic tests under the evaluation of a case of strabismus.

A few other important orthoptic instruments which have not been described elsewhere will be described in this section. Orthoptic instruments can be grouped as below:

I. Essential orthoptic instruments

The bare minimum equipment required for the clinical work of a patient with strabismus are:
1. A refraction trial set with prism of 1–8 D
2. Snellen's vision chart and single letter E-chart.
3. Prism bars, horizontal and vertical (page 116)
4. Loose prism set
5. Fixation targets, for near and distance
6. Occluders
7. Bagolini's striated lenses (pages 129)
8. Red and green goggles
9. Maddox rods (page 109)
10. Direct ophthalmoscope
11. Transparent foot ruler

II. Desirable orthoptic instruments

These instruments, when present, add grace and completeness to the orthoptic clinic. These include:
1. Synoptophore
2. Random dot stereo test (page 85)
3. Hess screen (page 123)
4. RAF rule (page 118)
5. Worth four dot test (page 132)
6. Indirect ophthalmoscope
7. Spielman's occluder

III. Additional orthoptic instruments

There is no limit to additional orthoptic instruments. Additional orthoptic instruments can be grouped as below.

Priority additional orthoptic instruments
1. Haidinger brushes and after images attachment for synoptophore.

2. Teller acuity cards with screen
3. Optokinetic nystagmus drum
4. VER and electronystagmography
5. System perimeter
6. Camera for documentation

Non-priority additional orthoptic instruments
1. Livingston binocular gauge
2. Remy separator
3. Reading bars
4. Cheiroscope
5. Neutral density filters and graded density bar
6. Maddox wing (page 111)

IV. Orthoptic instruments not used presently

1. Bishop-Harman diaphragm
2. Stereoscope (Holmes, Keystone)
3. Projectoscope
4. Visuscope
5. Euthyscope
6. Co-ordinator
7. CAM vision stimulator
8. Pigeon-Cantonnet stereoscope
9. Tibbs binocular trainer
10. Diploscope

SYNOPTOPHORE

Synoptophore (major amblyoscope) is a haploscopic device. Though not an essential instrument but its presence is most desirable in an orthoptic clinic. It essentially consists of two tubes, having a right-angled bend, mounted on a base having a chin rest and a forehead rest (Fig. 6.35). Each tube contains a light source for

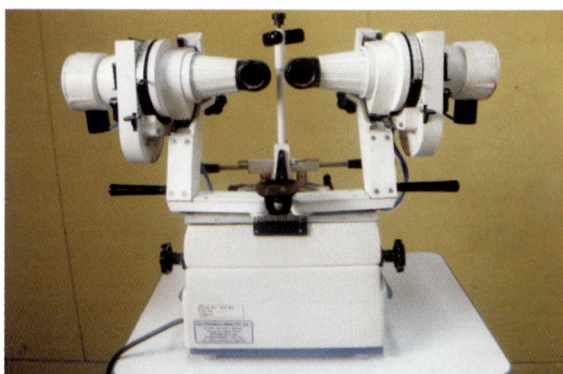

Fig. 6.35 *Synoptophore.*

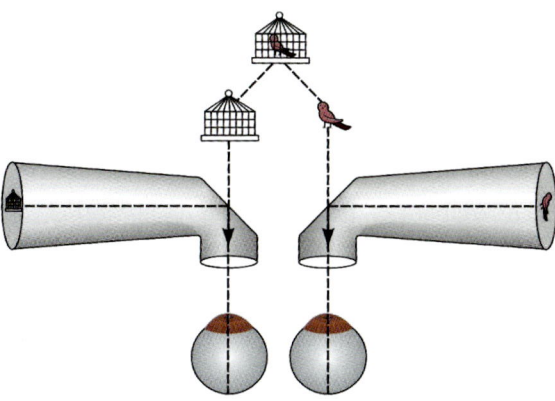

Fig. 6.36 *Optical principle of synoptophore.*

illumination of slides and a slide carrier at the outer end, a reflecting mirror at the right-angled bend and an eyepiece of +6.5D at the inner end (Fig. 6.36). The two tubes can be converged, diverged and moved vertically separately or together by means of knobs. The tubes can also be adjusted to the patient's interpupillary distance. Each slide carrier can be rotated to adjust for any torsion. The horizontal, vertical and torsional positions of each tube with regard to normal zero position can be read on scales in either degrees or prism dioptres.

The graduations from the zero mark inward represent base-out prisms or degrees of convergence (+), while those from the zero mark outward represent base-in prisms or degrees of divergence (−).

Light switches permit the simultaneous or alternate illumination of the tubes, useful for performing the cover tests.

Synoptophore slides

The pair of slides used to perform various diagnostic and therapeutic purposes include the following.

1. *Simultaneous perception slides.* Two dissimilar slides, such as one having picture of a bird and the other of the cage, constitute a pair of simultaneous perception slides (Fig. 6.37A). Each slide is presented separately to each eye. Ideally, the pictures should not have overlapping contour since this will induce suppression. These slides are graded by their size into three groups:

a. *Simultaneous foveal perception (SFP) slides.* This pair consists of small sized pictures, the images of which do not exceed the size of the fovea.

b. *Simultaneous macular perception (SMP) slides.* The pictures in this pair of slides are slightly larger than those on the SFP slides.

c. *Simultaneous paramacular perception (SPP) slides.* These slides have the largest pictures and form images that extend into paramacular areas.

(*Note:* As a routine, if possible, the smallest slides should be used. However, the larger slides may be required in the presence of suppression or amblyopia).

2. *Fusion slides.* Fusion slides consist of two similar pictures, each of which is incomplete in one small detail. For example, there are two rabbits each lacking either a tail or a bunch of flowers. If fusion is present, one complete rabbit with tail and holding a bunch of flowers will be

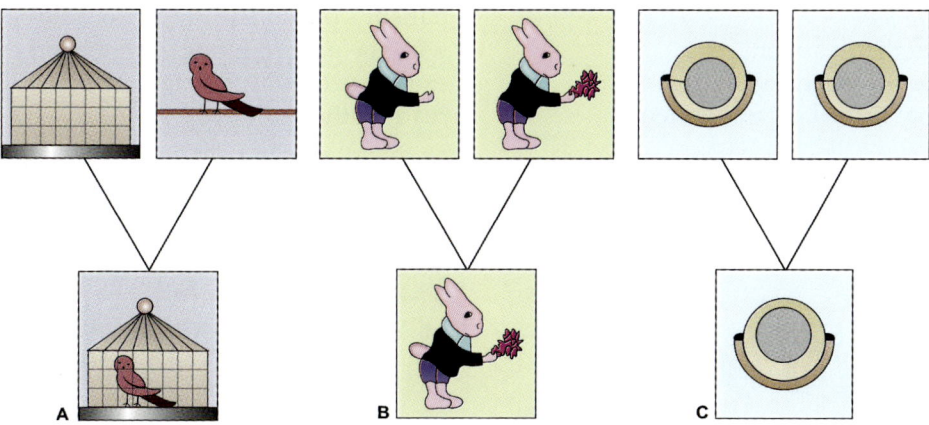

A   B   C

Fig. 6.37 *Synoptophore slides for simultaneous perception (A), fusion (B) and stereopsis (C).*

seen (Fig. 6.37B). In the presence of suppression, either tail or bunch of flowers will be missing in the respective eye.

*Grading.*The fusion slides are also graded according to the size in the same way as the simultaneous perception slides.

3. *Stereoscopic slides*. Stereoscopic slides consist of two pictures of the same object which have been taken from slightly different angles, i.e. the picture for one eye is in part dissimilar from that for the other eye. These dissimilar parts are imaged on disparate retinal areas in the two eyes and, when the entire picture is fused, the disparity gives rise to the perception of stereopsis of the dissimilar portions (Fig. 6.37C).

Uses of synoptophore

Diagnostic uses

1. Measurement of the objective and subjective angles of deviation (page 112).
2. Measurement of the primary and secondary deviations.
3. Measurement of deviation in cardinal directions of gaze.
4. Measurement of interpupillary distance (IPD)
5. To investigate the state of retinal correspondence (page 129).
6. Estimation of grades of binocular vision (page 57).
7. To estimate presence and type of suppression (page 168).
8. Measurement of range of fusion or vergence (page 116).
9. Measurement of angle kappa.

Therapeutic uses

It is used in the treatment of:
1. Suppression (page 168).
2. Abnormal retinal correspondence.

3. Eccentric fixation.
4. Accommodative esotropia (dissociation training).
5. Heterophorias and intermittent heterotropias (improvement of fusional amplitude).

Measurement of anlge kappa with synoptophore

To measure the angle kappa with synoptophore, a special slide is placed in front of the eye under observation. This slide consists of a row of numbers and letters (4 3 2 1 0 A B C D) and animal pictures (for small children and illiterate patients) placed at 1° intervals (Fig. 6.38). The patient is asked to focus on the '0' mark while the examiner looks for the corneal reflex. If the corneal reflex is on the nasal side of centre of pupil, the angle is positive; if it is on the temporal side, it is negative. The patient is then asked to look in turn either one letter or one number until the reflex is centred. The degree of deviation corresponding to the letter or number is then recorded. For example, if the left eye is being tested and the corneal reflex is centred, when the patient looks at the number 3, the patient has 3° negative angle kappa in the left eye.

Measurement of interpupillary distance with synoptophore

To measure the IPD, arms of the synoptophore are placed at zero and the patient is instructed to look at the centre of the picture in the right hand tube with his/her right eye. The examiner, with his right eye closed, aligns the central white line which is on the mirror unit of the tube, with the reflection of the light on the centre of the patient's pupil. The same procedure is repeated with the patient fixing with the left eye and the examiner closing his right eye. The IPD is then read on the millimetre scale.

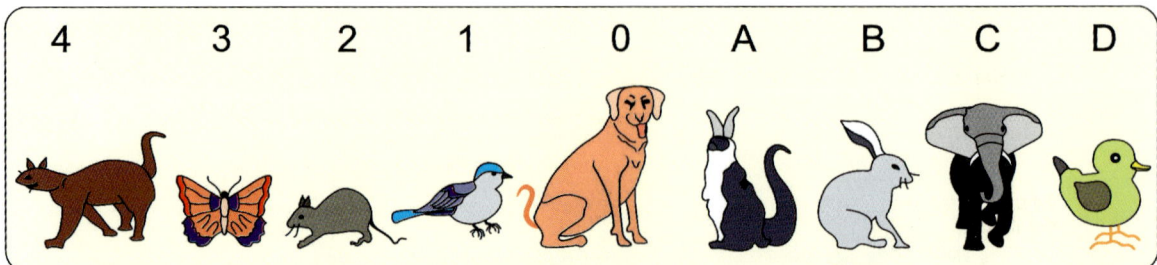

Fig. 6.38 *Synoptophore slide for measurement of angle kappa.*

Digital synoptophore

Digital synaptophore, introduced recently, is likely to soon replace the currently used electric synoptophore for sensory and motor assessment of strabismus patients as well as measurement of the angle of deviation.

Features of digital synaptophore

Digital Synoptophore (Fig. 6.39) comprising of a computer controlled display device consists of both hardware and software components:

Hardware component consists of various subunits as described below:

- *Computer system* with colour monitor.
- *Screen divider*. An opaque vertical screen divider, to divide the display screen into 2 equal right and left halves.
- *Input device* to move the generated screen targets, such as mouse, trackball, etc.
- *Two tubes* to carry the images from the display screen to each eye separately which contain a lens system and eyepieces assembly with adjustable interpupillary distance.
- *Adjustable chin-rest and head-rest* for stabilizing the patients head.

Software component consists of various computer programs designed for various orthoptic test.

Procedure

Before examination, the interpupillary distance (IPD) for the patient must be first measured in millimetres. The distance between the eyepieces is then set according to this measurement. The patient places his chin on the chin-rest and his forehead against the headrest. The chin-rest is adjusted in such a way that the eye level is at the centre of screen vertically.

Uses

It is used to perform the following tests on patients with strabismus:

- Simultaneous perception (foveal, macular and paramacular)
- Fusion
- Stereopsis
- Assessing retinal correspondence
- After image testing
- Measure the angle of deviation
- Orthoptic exercises

LIVINGSTON BINOCULAR GAUGE

Livingston binocular gauge (Fig. 6.40) is an apparatus used for the measurement of convergence and accommodation. Basically, it consists of a 36 cm long wooden ruler marked

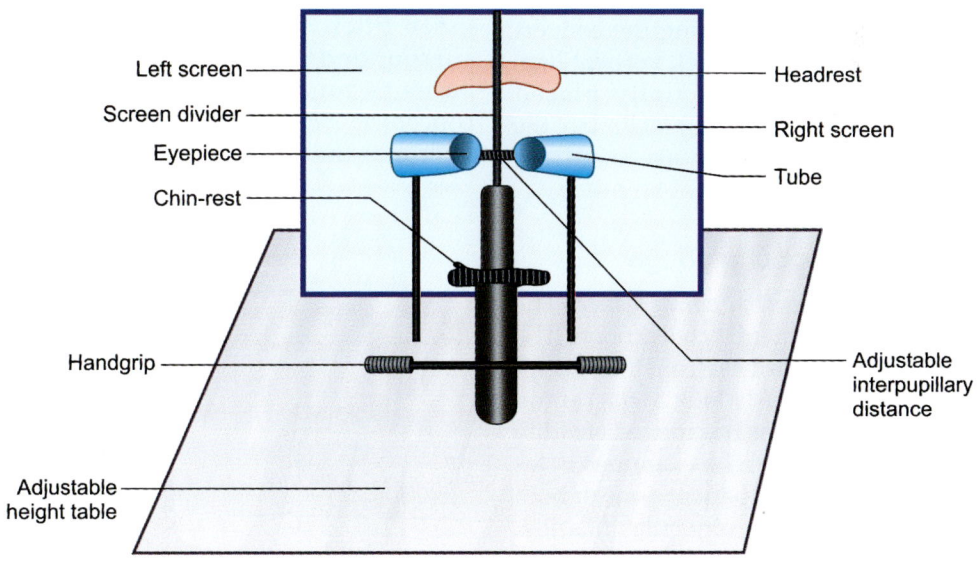

Fig 6.39 *Hardware component of digital synoptophore*

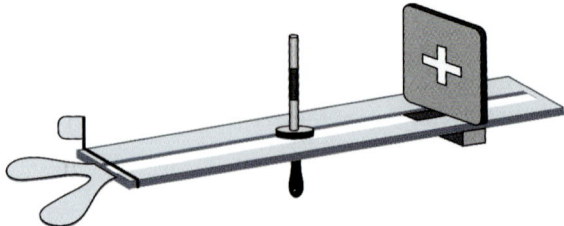

Fig. 6.40 *Livingston binocular gauge.*

in centimetres and half-centimetres. In the centre of this ruler, from 6 cm mark to 21 cm mark, there is a slot into which is present a slidable convergence rod (white vertical rod, the centre third of which is painted black). One end of this ruler is so designed that when in position, it straddles the patient's nose and rests upon his/her cheek bones. At this facial end of the ruler, a detachable occluder is attached which can be used to occlude either eye while measuring uniocular accommodation. In this position, the markings on the ruler indicate distance from the anterior surface of cornea. At the other end of the ruler, there is a box-like attachment which can slide towards the eye. This box-shaped attachment is 6 cm wide and has a cross-like opening (cut in the surface facing the patient) through which the back surface of the box consisting of a white rectangular card with a central black vertical line (opposite the vertical limb of the cross-opening) is seen. The black vertical line is used for measuring the convergence. On either side of the black vertical line, there are three black horizontally placed letters—ALT, opposite the horizontal limb of the cross-opening. These letters are used for measuring accommodation.

Uses of livingston binocular gauge

1. *Measurement of objective convergence.* The ruler is fitted on the patient's cheek bone. The convergence rod is kept farthest from the patient, who is asked to continuously look at the central black section of the rod which is moved steadily towards the patient's eyes. The examiner notes the scale reading, where the patient's one or both eyes diverge on the loss of binocular fixation. Normally, the objective convergence varies between 6 and 10 cm in young adults.

2. *Measurement of subjective convergence.* After fitting the ruler on the patient's face, the central convergence rod is removed and the box-like attachment is kept farthest from the patient. The patient is asked to look at the black vertical line placed in the centre of vertical limb of cross-opening while the box is slid towards the patient's face. The point where the patient observes that the line has moved slightly to the right or to the left or has become double is noted on the scale. This reading gives the measurement of subjective convergence. The normal value of subjective convergence is less than 20 cm, but is almost invariably greater than that of objective convergence.

3. *Measurement of accommodation.* The instrument is used in the same way as used for measuring subjective convergence; except that now the patient is asked to look at the letters placed corresponding to the horizontal limb of the cross opening of the box-like attachment. The point where the patient reports blurring of the letters gives the reading of his/her near point (punctum proximum).

VISUSCOPE

It is an instrument similar to ophthalmoscope (Fig. 6.41) which is used to examine the fixation pattern of patients during monocular vision. It was designed by Cupper. With the help of this instrument, examiner projects a disc with a green filter having a star in the centre and surrounded by concentric rings on to the patient's fundus. The distance between the concentric rings is ½°. The patient is asked to look into the star after occluding the eye not

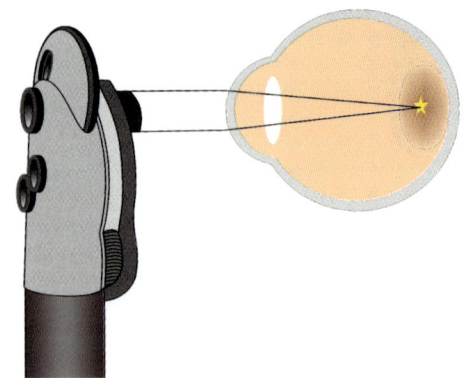

Fig. 6.41 *Examination of fixation pattern with visuscope.*

being examined. Normally, the foveolar reflex of the patient coincides with the star if the fixation is central. In the presence of eccentric fixation, the star, will not coincide with the foveolar reflex and can be anywhere on either the nasal or temporal retina or above or below the fovea (Fig. 6.20). The degree of eccentricity may be known from the concentric ring with which the star coincides.

EUTHYSCOPE

Euthyscope is a modified form of ophthalmoscope (Fig. 6.41) which is used in pleoptics for the re-education of the fovea that has lost its principal visual direction in eccentric fixation.

This instrument projects an approximately 30° wide beam of light in the centre of which an opaque 3° or 5° disc can be moved to cause a black dot. This serves to shield the fovea during the exposure of the surrounding retina. Since the light intensity used is moderate, the peripheral retina is not dazzled but only stimulated enough to produce an after image. A green filter disc enables the examiner to locate the fovea without dazzling the patient's retina. Since pleoptic treatment is now obsolete, so this instrument is also not used in the modern orthoptic clinics.

DIPLOSCOPE

The diploscope consists of a 25 cm long metal shaft supported by a handle having face-piece at one end and a card holder at the other end. Depending upon the model, the face-piece can rest on the nose (Fig. 6.42), the cheek bones, or the upper lid. The card holder contains a card with white background. On this card are printed letters DOG, with a green sqaure placed centrally above the O and a red square centrally below the O. About 6.5 cm in front and parallel to the card holder is mounted a metal septum which is perforated by four holes, each 8 mm in diameter. The two holes are situated horizontally 15 mm apart from each other and at an equal distance from the centre of the septum. The other two holes situated vertically, one below the horizontal left-hand hole and other above the horizontal right-hand hole.

When in use, the septum dissociates the two eyes in such a way that each eye can see only two of the three letters on the white card and only one of the two-coloured squares. The left eye sees the letters OG and the lower red square, while the right eye sees the letters DO and upper green square (Fig. 6.43).

Uses

1. Suppression and the presence or lack of binocular vision can be detected. With normal retinal correspondence and bifoveal fixation, when the two images of O are fused, the patient will see three holes with the word DOG in them (Fig. 6.43).

2. The main use of the instrument is to exercise for relative convergence, when binocular single vision is present. To perform exercise, patient is asked to move his/her eyes in relation to septum and card at four different positions (described below). As the patient does so, he/she sees a change in the relative position of the letters and colours as perceived by each eye simul-taneously. This movement of letters into a definite pattern is utilized in training the patient to appreciate and control the position to which his/her eyes are directed. Thus, it teaches the patient to switch easily from distant to near fixation and vice versa improving the fusional amplitudes which are essential for a comfortable binocular single vision.

Procedure

The four positions of fixation and the various kinds of physiological diplopia, when practising with the diploscope, are as follows (Fig. 6.43).

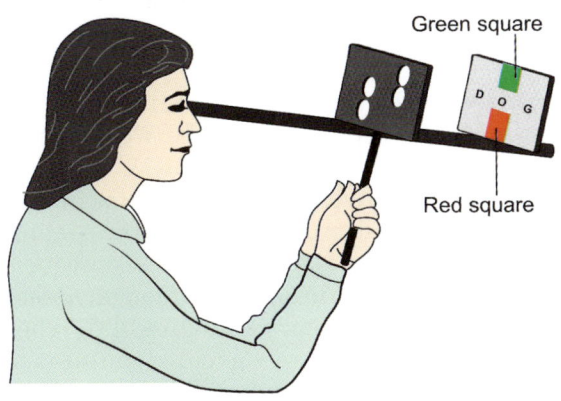

Green square

Red square

Fig. 6.42 *Diploscope.*

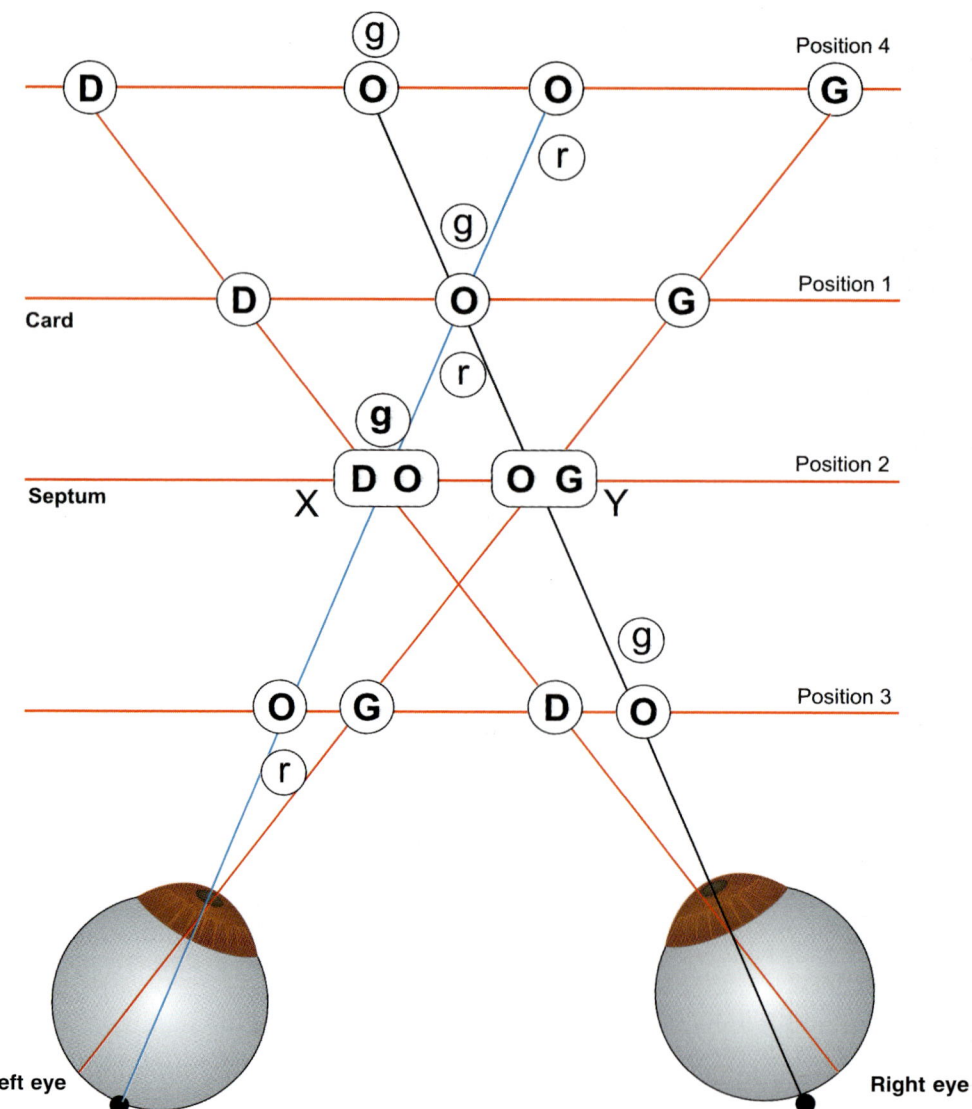

Fig. 6.43 *Principle of diploscope and observations made by the patient while in use at positions 1, 2, 3 and 4 (for explanation, see text).*

Position 1. The point of fixation is central letter O on the card. In this position, letter D falls on a point temporal to the fovea in the right eye and is projected to the left of O, while G falls on point temporal to the fovea in the left eye and is projected to the right of O. Thus, the letters DO are seen with the right eye and the letters OG with the left eye and in the presence of binocular single vision patient will perceive three holes with the word DOG in them.

Position 2. The second point of fixation is the centre of metal septum midway between the two horizontally placed holes (Fig. 6.43). When the patient's eyes converge on this point, the images of O no longer fall on both foveas, but on a retinal element nasal to the fovea in each eye. Consequently, the O will be seen in uncrossed (homonymous) diplopia and the patient sees DO and OG. When the patient will exert a greater amount of convergence, he/she may see only DG, because the D and O and the G and O will overlap.

Position 3. The point of fixation is tip of a pencil or other object held midway between the septum and his/her eyes. When the patient's eyes converge on this point, the images of both D and O in the right eye and G and O in the left eye fall on a retinal element nasal to fovea in each eye and thus will be projected temporally, and the patient will see OGDO on the card.

Position 4. The point of fixation is an object (such as a picture on the wall) situated beyond the printed card. When the patient fixates at this distant point, the images of D and O and G and O fall on retinal element temporal to fovea in each eye and thus will be projected nasally, and the patient will see D O O G.

Note: The aim of exercise with diploscope is to teach the patient to obtain and maintain all four positions with ease so that effortless convergence and divergence is fully established. It is advisable to practise for 2 to 3 minutes for 2 to 3 times a day. Position four is quite useful in improving the fusional divergence (fusional negative convergence).

REMY SEPARATOR

Remy separator is a simple instrument which consists of a septum with a handle having a transparent slide holder at one end and a nose-piece at other end (Fig. 6.44). The patient resting the septum on his/her nose is instructed to look through the slides at an object beyond them. If his/her eyes are properly focused for the distant object, the picture of the slides (such as a star and a circle) will be imaged one on each fovea

and will be seen superimposed by the patient (Fig. 6.45).

Uses. The instrument is designed in such a way that when used properly, it teaches the patient to relax his/her convergence and strengthen the fusional divergence.

READING BARS

Reading bars are simple devices used to train the patient for subjectively controlling the maintenance of binocular vision.

Principle. All reading bars are based on the principle of physiologic diplopia.

Common reading bars include thumb bar reader, zig-zag bar reader, the Mayan bar reader, the Jaual grid, Tibb's physiologic diplopia reader.

Method. By introducing a bar between the patient's eyes and the reading material, the patient is made aware of physiologic diplopia (Fig. 6.46). As the patient reads the print binocularly, he/she perceives the bar in crossed diplopia, each image of bar hiding on position of the print from one eye, but not the other, so that the print can be read normally. Maintaining the correct position of his/her eyes despite this obstacle will strengthen the binocular vision of the patient. This is a very useful and simple home exercise.

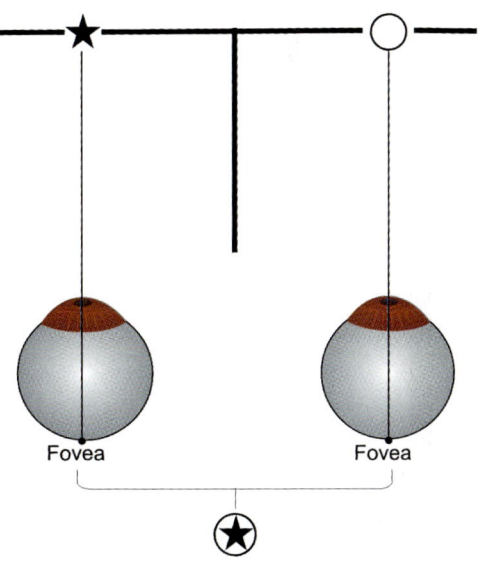

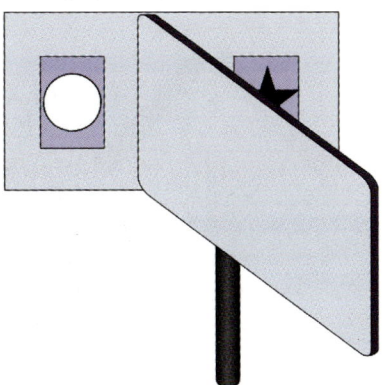

Fig. 6.44 *Remy separator.*

Fig. 6.45 *Optical principle of Remy separator.*

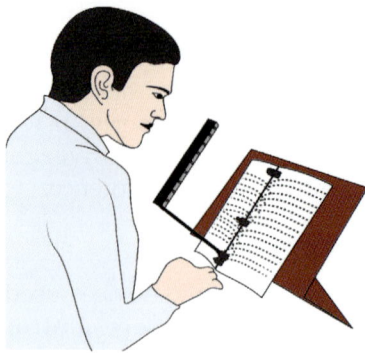

Fig. 6.46 *Zig-zag bar reader in use.*

CHEIROSCOPE

The cheiroscope (Fig. 6.47) is an instrument for anti-suppression exercises. It consists of a working base, a picture carrier to one side, a headrest containing a pair of +7.0D spherical lenses, and an obliquely placed septum extending from the centre point between the lenses to the base of the picture carrier. A plane mirror is attached to the septum on the side where the picture is located. The distance between lenses and the working base is 14 cm, which is the focal length of each lens and the eyes are consequently focused for distance. Most cheiroscope models may be turned around so that the mirror is in front of the right or left eye, depending upon which eye is required to fixate.

Uses. The instrument can be used in cases of heterophorias, intermittent tropias, or small tropias (in the latter, prisms to neutralize the deviation have to be taped over the eyepiece).

Procedure. The picture to be copied is placed in the picture carrier and a sheet of paper on the base of the instrument. The patient should look with his/her fixating eye into the mirror and with the suppressing one on the paper. He/she is instructed to trace the picture (which has black outlines) on the paper using a pencil (a red-coloured pencil is very helpful, especially in the beginning). Steady fixation of the picture should be stressed to prevent rapid alternation, which can be suspected, if the patient's drawing is either smaller or larger than the picutre or if parts of the picture are missing.

TIBB'S BINOCULAR TRAINER

The Tibb's binocular trainer (Fig. 6.48) is a haploscopic instrument designed for home use. However, in offices where a major amblyoscope is not available, it can also be used as a diagnostic instrument. It consists of three parts: A middle septum and two wingboards that fold together like a book. The middle septum has a mirror on both sides so that it can be used with either eye fixating. Each of the wingboards has a vertical scale of 20$^\Delta$ base-up and base-down and a horizontal scale of 40$^\Delta$-base in and base-out. Four cards (target carriers) come with the instrument and consist of peripheral, macular, and foveal superimposition and fusion pictures.

Uses. It can be used for both diagnosis and treatment of suppression and abnormal retinal correspondence and for increasing fusional amplitudes.

Procedure. One wingboard is placed so that it rests along the table at a slight angle to it. The vertical wingboard is to the right side, when the

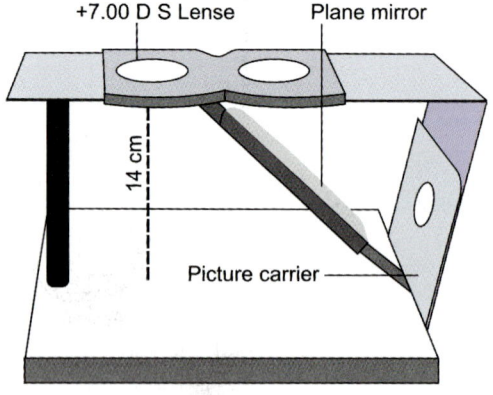

Fig. 6.47 *Cheiroscope.*

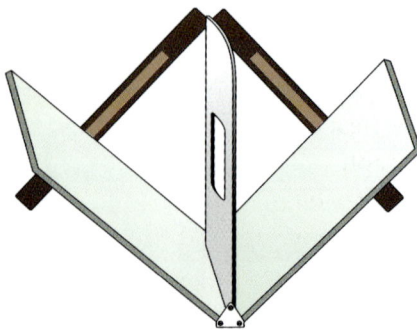

Fig. 6.48 *Tibb's binocular trainer. Direct cover test depicting left exotropia.*

right eye is the fixating one; it is to the left side, when the left eye is fixating. The patient places the bridge of his/her nose against the curved part of the septum so that his/her visual axis is perpendicular to the table. His/her head should not be tilted.

One target carrier (such as the dog) is taped on the vertical wingboard so the zero mark shows in the window. This target is seen in the mirror. The patient places another target on the horizontal wingboard (such as the cage for superimposition or another dog for fusion) and moves it until the two images are superimposed. This target is not viewed in the mirror.

COMPUTER-BASED ORTHOPTIC PROGRAMS AND INSTRUMENTS

Computer-based orthoptic programs have brought a revolutionary change in the diagnosis and management of orthoptic disorders. Computer-based orthoptic practice includes:

- Computerised orthoptic-diagnostic programs for sensory as well as motor evaluation, and
- Computer-based orthoptic therapy programs for vision therapy, and neurovision therapy.

Recently many computer based systems have been developed for orthoptic practice which are either only diagnostic, or therapeutic, or combined diagnostic and therapeutic programs. Some of these are listed below:

I. *Computer-based diagnostic programs*
- Electronic vision testing programs.
- Optodrum [Software for optokinetic drum (OKN)].
- Digital Hess chart and diplopia chart
- BVA (Binocular Vision Assessment Program)
- PTS (perceptual therapy system)
- ReadAlyzer eye movement recording system
- TOVA (test of variable attention)
- Visagraph

II. *Computer-based therapeutic programs*
- Vision therapy programs
- Neurovision therapy programs.

III. *Computer-based combined diagnostic and therapeutic systems*
- TRYe vision therapy software

- Computer orthoptics programe by HTS INC solutions.
- Computer orthoptics.

I. COMPUTERIZED ORTHOPTIC DIAGNOSTIC PROGRAMS AND INSTRUMENTS

Several applications are available for smart-phones, tablets, laptop, and PCs that reproduce many eye tests. These can be used by optometrists, ophthalmologists and some programs by the patients also. Computer orthoptics includes complex monocular and binocular stimuli, which allow automatic testing and measurement of the following skills: Oculomotor (pursuits and saccades); fusional ranges; phorias; motor fields; fixation disparities, suppressions; retinal correspondence; accommodative facility; stereopsis, visual memory and aniseikonia.

Some common such programs are described briefly.

Electronic vision testing programs. Electronic charts are available for far as well as near vision testing. Few examples are:
- Chart Pro (*www.eyechartprotoapp.com*)
- Optos' chart remote (*blog.optos.com/index.php/ optos.chart.remote.ipad.app*)
- Vision Test (*https://itunes.apple.com/ca/app/ vision-test/id380288414?mt=8 or https:// play.google.com/store/apps/details? id=com.threesidedcube.visiondroid*)
- With sight Book (*www.digisight.net/patients/ vision_testing*)
- AAPOS Vision Screening App.(*www.aapos.org/ ahp/aapos_vision_screening_app*) has optotype for both adults and children, and can be used by anyone including healthcare workers.

Optodrum. The Optodrum (www.linsay.com/ Linsay_associates_Medical/Optodrum.html) is a good alternative to the expensive and bulky optokinetic drum for adults and children. It even has a version for the iPad that uses its camera to record a video of the patient's eye movement while looking at moving patterns.

BVA is a stand-alone binocular vision screening program. It is capable of automatic testing of heterophorias, fusional range, saccades, pursuits, accommodation, suppressions, fixation disparities and an asthenopia survey.

PTS test. Computerized perceptual therapy system allows automatic testing for speed of information processing, visual sequential processing, visual simultaneous processing.

ReadAlyzer eye movement recording system. This system allows fixations, regressions, fixation duration, reading speed, cross correlation between right and left eye, play-back of recorded eye movements.

TOVA (test of variables attention). It assesses ADD, ADHD and impulsivity.

Visagraph an eye movement recording system is capable of computerized recordings of reading eye movements, saccades and fixations.

Digital Hess screen *See* page 123.

Digital syneptophore Described on page 139.

II. COMPUTER-BASED VISION THERAPY AND NEUROVISION THERAPY PROGRAMS

VISION THERAPY PROGRAMS

Vision therapy is effective for:
• Eliminating amblyopia
• Breaking suppressions
• Improving oculomotor skills
• Improving visual memory
• Improving accommodative facility
• Altering retinal correspondence; increasing fusional ranges; and/or treating strabismus.

The gamepad and mouse allow the patient's therapy responses to alter the target demands. The Computer Orthoptics graphics are instantly moved, rotated or changed to create any base-in base-out disparity. A few computer-based orthoptic programs are mentioned below.

Computer vergence system (CVS)

This program uses random dot stereograms to form pictures that require bi-foveal fixation to stimulate the vergence system. The program gradually increases the amount of vergence required to appreciate the stereogram picture and can monitor progression on line. This may be used as part of the home therapy program and the results of the computer program are often followed by an eye care professional with print outs that can be brought in to the office visit. A maintenance program consists of activities that preserve the patient's present level of function and/or prevent regression of that function. Maintenance begins when the therapeutic goals of a treatment plan have been achieved, or when no additional functional progress is apparent or expected to occur.

Perceptual visual tracking program (PVT)

This program is designed to improve specific tracking deficits that are often found in persons. Perceptual visual tracking skills are basic to all aspects of reading and other academic areas. Improvement in tracking is often accompanied by improvement in reading, spelling, attention, and speed of working. PVT contains a variety of visual tracking programs that have been clinically proven. They are game-like in nature so that improvement takes place almost effortlessly. Individuals of all ages from five years up can benefit from PVT. It is a sophisticated yet user-friendly computer application that will run on almost any personal computer.

Vision builder: Computer vision training

A home vision training program designed to treat both binocular vision disorders such as convergence problems (i.e. eye-teaming problems), accommodation problems (i.e. non-refractive focusing difficulties), suppression (i.e. "lazy eye") and eye-tracking difficulties, as well as visual perceptual or visual information processing difficulties that can impact on a student's learning by limiting their ability to understand and remember what they see.

Eyeport @ Vision Training System

Has revolutionized the way people look at their vision. To read more comfortably, learn more easily, work less painfully, and play sports more effortlessly, people everywhere are doing daily eye exercises with the EYEPORT.

Eyelights

Target the weaker functioning side of the brain via the non-dominant eye. Light stimulation directly to the non-dominant brain causes an excitatory barrage to travel to the mesencephalon, the most metabolic area of the brain, where an increase in cellular activity takes place.

The excitatory barrage travels also to the parietal, temporal, and occipital lobes of the brain, while collateral fibers lead to the pineal gland, pituitary gland, and hypothalamus.

AmbP iNet Program

An amblyopia hand-eye coordination program which uses principles of operant conditioning and behavior modification to appropriately alter stimuli characteristics to improve visual acuity (Fig. 6.49A&B).

- Patients begin therapy with targets that are easily seen and become progressively smaller as therapy progresses. Correct responses are reinforced with subsequent reduction in the size of the stimuli. Therapy is directed to improve resolving ability with concomitant use of hand-eye coordination tasks. Therapy can be preformed monocularly or monocularly in a binocular field (Fig. 6.50A&B).

- The AmbP iNet programme provides a cumulative graph depicting each session's performance. The computer denotes date, time, duration and denotes when the patient has performed the assigned tasks as well as if they were performed correctly.

PTS II iNET. It is a home-based computerized perceptual therapy program that has been designed to address a variety of visual perceptual information processing domains, including simultaneous processing, sequential processing, speed-of-information processing, visual temporal processing, and rapid auto-matized naming,

- Dyslexia
- Ordinary reading disability

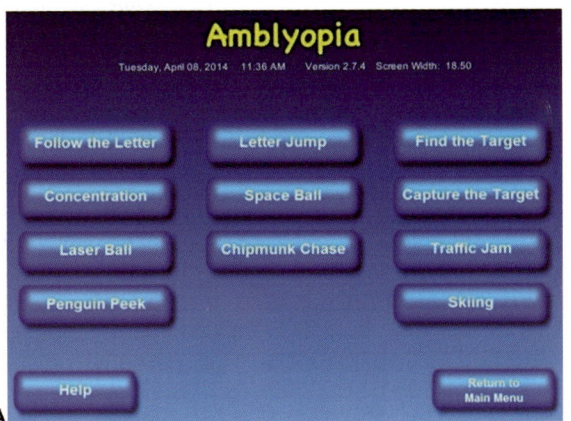
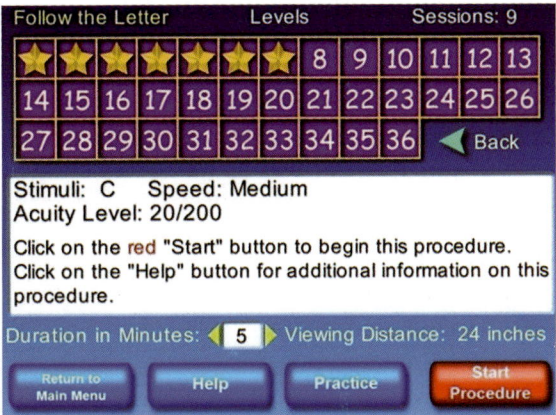

Fig. 6.49A and B *AmbP iNet program.*

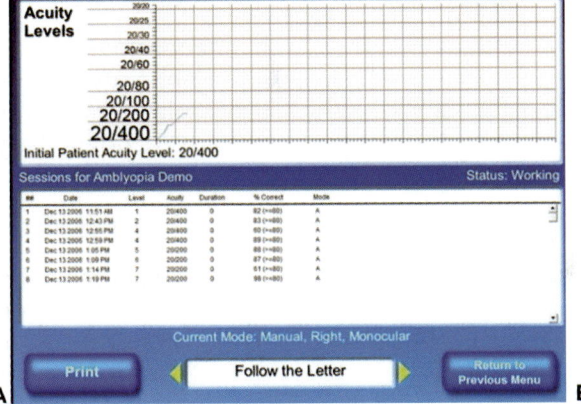
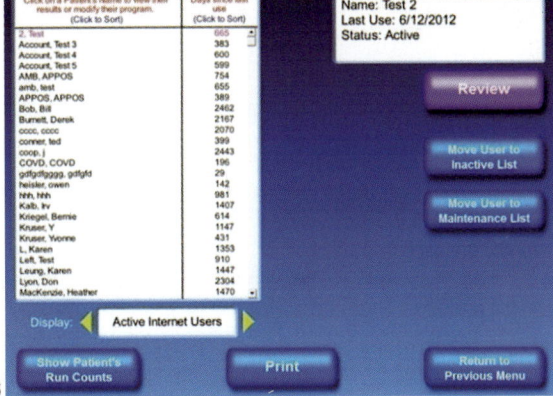

Fig. 6.50A and B *Protocol of therapy with AmbP iNet program.*

- Word decoding difficulty
- Problems in reading comprehension
- Spelling problems
- Memory disorders
- Laterality-directionality deficits
- Slow speed of information processing
- Non-verbal learning disability
- Mathematics difficulty
- Above average intelligence but not achieving up to potential
- Acquired brain injury with perceptual-cognitive deficits
- Attention disorders
- Diagnosis of perceptual/visual information processing deficits (Fig. 6.51A&B).

Therapy procedure. PTS II iNet presents the patient with a grid that shows the different difficulty levels for each procedure. Each time the patient meets or exceeds a therapy goal they receive a gold star. The program gives the patient verbal reinforcement. It prompts them to "Get Ready" before a stimulus is presented. PTS II iNet also verbally reinforces correct and incorrect responses. For example, it will encourage them by saying "Good Job" after they input a correct response.

Dynamic reader. The dynamic reader is a home Vision Training program designed to improve reading eye movements and thus reading fluency and comprehension.

ADR iNet. Moving text, standard, and whole line dynamic reading

Brainware safari. Therapy for 14 cognitive skills in six areas.

Play attention. Improves attention.

Sanet vision untegrator. Procedures for saccadic trainer, tactile feedback, hand speed function, "visual search" saccadic, metronome, tachisto-scope functions.

Sub iNet. Addresses subitizing deficits to improve math skills.

Track and read. Twelve therapy procedures for developing saccadic eye movements, span of recognition, and visual sequential memory skills.

NEUROVISION THERAPY PROGRAMS

1. Revital vision. Concept of neurovision therapy is based on the visual plasticity, which is the ability of the visual system to change its responses in order to adapt to the changes in the visual input. Revital vision is a pereptual Learning therapy program developed by "Revital Vision Technology". Perceptual learning is an alternative treatment option which modifies visual function in adult amblyopia. The perceptual learning therapy program (Revital Vision) is a non-invasive software-based patient-specific, interactive perceptual learning tool based on visual stimulation. It facilitates neural connections at the cortical level through a computerized training regimen using Gabor patches to improve contrast sensitivity and visual acuity. The term perceptual learning describes a process whereby practicing certain visual tasks leads to an improvement in visual

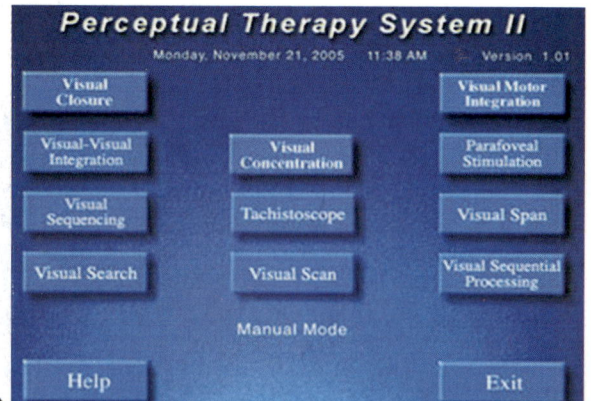
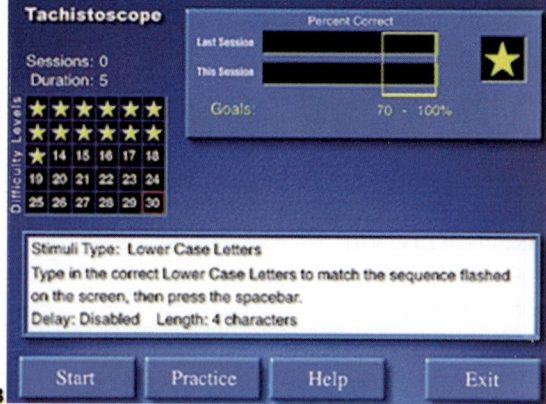

Fig. 6.51A and B *Diagnosis of perceptual/visual information processing deficit.*

performance. As visual perception depends on both the optical input received from the eye and the neural processing of that input in the visual cortex, Revital vision technology improves quality of vision (visual acuity and contrast sensitivity) by enhancing neural processing in the primary visual cortex.

The typical building blocks of the visual stimulus in the field of visual neuroscience are:

• Gabor patch,
• Neuronal lateral interactions,
• Brain (neural plasticity), and
• Perceptual learning.

Effects of revital vision–perceptual learning. Neurovision technology (Revital) is formed around proprietary algorithms and has proved successful in the following ways:

• Improvement of lateral interactions in amblyopia
• Improvement of CSF in amblyopia
• Improvement of CSF in non-amblyopic groups
• Improvement of VA
• Transfer to improvement of binocular vision.

2. Neurovision rehabilitator used for those with brain injury is useful as ocular vestibular integrator, visual motor enhancer, visuomotor integrator, dynamic ocular motor processing, fixation anomalies.

III. COMPUTER-BASED COMBINED DIAGNOSTIC AND THERAPEUTIC PROGRAMS

1. TrYe (Train your eyes) vision therapy software
TrYe (Train your eyes) vision therapy software has been designed and developed by 'Digital Works Technology Private Ltd', using the domain expertise of 'Sankra Nethralya, Chennai, India'. This program has the ability to run on multiple platforms, such as PC, Laptop, Mobile and Tablet.

Uses of TrYe software include:
• *Binocular vision assessment,* and thus addresses to the binocular vision dysfunctions. Binocular vision assessment programme in TrYe is based on aperant conditioning using random dot stereograms (RDS) as targets. RDS targets are devoid of monocular cues and have been recommended for fusional vergence testing and training.
• *'Office vision therapy'* (TrYe-Doctor's module) program for dysfunctions of binocular vision, accommodation and ocular motor system.
• *Home based vision therapy program* (TrYe-Patient's module) for vision therapy at home.

2. Computer orthoptics program by HTS INC solutions™. HTS iNet/Computer Vergence System (CVS) is a sophisticated yet easy-to-use vergence exercise computer application that the patients can run on Windows and Mac computers. It encourages and motivates patients by continuously evaluating their progress and making the exercises more challenging whenever the goals are achieved.

To assure compliance, CVS uses random-dot stereograms. Each exercise requires bifovial fixation for correct responses. The responses required are a simple choice of four arrows keys; up, down, left or right. The results of each exercise session are documented as the program notes the date, duration and vergence demand of each exercise. All results are available for your review via the Internet. The HTS iNet program is fully automated and easy to use. *Procedures* include:

• Pursuits
• Saccades
• Base-in/base-out vergence
• Auto Slide Vergence
• Jump ductions
• Base-up/base-down vergence
• Accommodative rock

3. Computer orthoptics. It includes both orthoptic therapy and diagnostic procedure:

• *Therapy procedures* include smooth vergence, rotations, jump ductions, multiple choice vergence, accommodative rock, pursuits, saccades, visual memory, cheiroscope and amblyopia therapy procedures.
• *Diagnostic procedures* for heterophobia, fusional ranges, accommodative facility, pursuits, saccades, Worth 4 dot, motor field, fixation disparity, visual memory, aniseikonia.

BIBLIOGRAPHY

1. American Academy of Pediatrics. Learning Disabilities, Dyslexia, and Vision: A Subject Review. Pediatrics 1998; 102(5):1217–1219A statement of reaffirmation for this policy was published on August 1, 2008.

2. Bagolini B: Tecnica per l'esame della visione binoculare sensa introduzione di elementi dissocianti: "test del vetro striato," Boll. Ocul. 37:195, 1958.

3. Bielschowsky A: Application of the afterimage test in the investigation of squint. Am J Ophthalmol 20:408, 1937.

4. Bielschowsky A: Lectures on motro anomalies. Hanover, NH, 1943 (reprinted 1956), Dartmouth College Publications.

5. Birch E, Shimojo S, and Held R: Preferential-looking assessment of fusion and stereopsis in infants aged 1–6 months. Invest. Ophthalmol Vis Sci. 26: 366, 1985.

6. Bixenmann WW and Noorden, GK von: Apparent foveal displacement in normal subjects and in cyclotropia. Ophthalmologica 89:58, 1982.

7. Brown HW: The cover test. In Allen, JH, editor: Strabismus ophthalmic symposium, II, St Louis, 1958. Mosby - year Book, Inc., p. 225.

8. Capobianco NM: the subjective measurement of the near point of convergence and its significance in the diagnosis of convergence insufficiency. Am Orthopt J 2:40, 1952.

9. Carniglia P, Cooper J. Vergence Adaptation in Esotropia. Opt Vis Sci, 69 (4): 308–313, 1992.

10. Convergence Insufficiency Treatment Trial Study Group. Randomized clinical trial of treatments for symptomatic convergence insufficiency in children. Arch Ophthalmol 2008 Oct;126(10): 1336–49.

11. Cooper J, Burns C, Cotter S, Daum KM, Griffin JR, Scheiman M. Optometric Clinical Guideline: Care of the patient with accommodative or vergence dysfunction. Am. Optom. Ass. 1998.

12. Cooper J, Citron M. Microcomputer Produced Anaglyphs for Evaluation and Therapy of Binocular Anomalies. Journal of the American Optometric Association, 65: 185–188, 1983.

13. Cooper J, Ciuffreda KJ, Carniglia PE, Zinn KM, Tannen B. Orthoptic Treatment and Eye Movement Recordings in Guillain-Barre Syndrome. A case report. Neuro-ophthalmology 15(5):249–256, 1995.

14. Cooper J, Duckman R. Convergence Insufficiency: Diagnosis and Treatment. Journal of the American Optometric Association, 49(6):, 1978.

15. Cooper J, Feldman J, Eichler R. Relative Strength of Central and Peripheral Fusion as a Function of Stimulus Parameters. Opt. Vis Sci, 69: 1992.

16. Cooper J, Feldman J, Janus S, Appleman W, Appel S, Horn D. Pupillary Dilation andFunduscopy with 1% Hydroamphetamine Plus 0.25% Tropicamide (Paremyd) Versus Tropicamide (0.5% Or 1%) as a Function of Iris and Skin Pigmentation, and Age. J Am Opt Ass. 67(11): 669–75, 1996.

17. Cooper J, Feldman J, Pasner K. Intermittent Exotropia: Stimulus Characteristics Affect Tests for Retinal Correspondence and Suppression. Bin Vis & Eye Mus Qtly. 15(2):131–140, 2000

18. Cooper J, Feldman J. Operant Conditioning and the Assessment of Stereopsis in Young Children. American Journal of Optometry & Physiological Optics, 55(8): 532–542, 1978.

19. Cooper J, Feldman J. Random Dot Stereogram Performance by Strabismic, Amblyopic and Ocular Pathology Patients in an Operant Discrimination Task. American Journal of Optometry & Physiological Optics, 55(9): 599–609, 1978.

20. Cooper J, Feldman J. Operant Conditioning of Fusional Convergence Ranges Using Random Dot Stereograms. American Journal of Optometry & Physiological Optics, 57(4): 205-213, 1980.

21. Cooper J, Feldman JM, Selenow A, Fair R, Bucciero F, MacDonald D, Levy M. Reduction of Asthenopia Following Accommodative Facility Training. Am J OptomPhysiol Opt. 64, 30–436, 1987.

22. Cooper J, Medow N. Correspondence: Sensory Status in Intermittent Exotropia. Bin Vis Eye MusSurg Qtly. 9:11–12, 1994.

23. Cooper J, Medow N. Intermittent Exotropia of the Divergence Excess Type: Basic and Divergence Excess Type (Major Review). Bin Vis Eye MusSurg Qtly 8:187–222, 1993.

24. Cooper J, Record CD. Suppression and Retinal Correspondence in Intermittent Exotropia. Brit J Ophth. 700: 673–676, 1986.

25. Cooper J, Selenow A, Ciuffreda J, Feldman J, Faverty J, Hokoda S. Reduction of Asthenopia in Patients with Convergence Insufficiency Following FusionalVergence Training. Am J Opt Physl Opt, 60: 982–989,1983.

26. Cooper J. "Diagnosis and Remediation of Accommodative Anomalies", Chapter in Clinical Diagnosis of Optometric Problem Ed: John Amos Butterworth Publications, 1987.

27. Cooper J. Review of Computerized Orthoptics with Specific Regard to Convergence Insufficiency. Am. J. of Optom. and Phys. Optics. 65(6): 455–463, 1988.

28. Crone RA, Everhard-Halm Y: Cyclofusion. In Moore S, Mein J (eds): Orthoptics: Past, Present, and Future. New York, Stratton Intercontinental, 1976, p 409.

29. Dell Osso LF Daroff RB: Eye movement characteristic and recording techniques. In Glaser JL (ed): Neuro-ophthalmology. Hagerstown MD Harper and Row, 1978, p 187.

30. Duke-Elder S, Wybar K: System of Ophthalmology. In Duke-Elder S (ed): Ocular Motility and Strabismus, vol 6. St Louis, Mosby, 1973.

31. Eskridge, JB: Perrigin, DM and Leach, NE: the Hirschberg test: correlation with corneal radius and axial length Optom Vis Sci 67: 243, 1990.

32. Feldman J, Cooper J, Carniglia P, Schiff FM, Sheete TN. Comparison of Fusional Ranges Measured by Risley Prisms, Vectograms, and Computer Orthoptics, Optom and Vis Sci 66(6): 375–382, 1989.

33. Feldman J, Cooper J, Reinstein F, Swiatoca J. Asthenopia Induced by Computer-Generated FusionalVergence Targets. Opt Vis Sci, 69: 710–716, 1992.

34. Fink, WH: The vergence test - an evaluation of the various techniques Am J Ophthalmol 31: 48, 1948.

35. Hardesty, HH: Diagnosis of paretic vertical rotators. Am J Ophthalmol 56: 818, 1963.

36. Jampolsky, A: The prism test for strabismus screening J Pediatr Ophthalmol 1:30, 1964.

37. Lyle, TK, and Wybar, KC: Lyle and Jackson's practical orthoptics in the treatment of squint (and other anomalies of binocular vision), ed. 5, London, 1967, HK Lewis and Company Ltd.; also Spring field, III, 1967, Carles C Thomas, Publisher.

38. Noorden GK von: Atlas of Strabismus. St Louis. Mosby, 1977.

39. Noorden, GK von: Infantile esotropia: a continuing riddle (Scobee Lecture). Am Orthopt J 34:52, 1984.

40. Pickwell LD: Eye movements during the cover test. Br J Ophthalmol 28:23, 1973.

41. Robinson GL, Foreman PJ. Scotopic sensitivity/Irlen Syndrome and the use of coloured filters: a long-term placebo controlled and masked study of reading achievement and perception of ability. Perceptual and Motor Skills1999August;89(1):83–113.

42. Romano, PE, and Noorden, GK von: Limitations of cover test in detecting strabismus. Am J Ophthalmol 77:10, 1971.

43. Rubin ML: Optics for Clinicians Gainesville, Fl, Triad, 1974.

44. Ruttum, M and Noorden, GK von: the Bagolini striated lens test for cyclotropia Doc Ophthalmol. 58:131, 1984.

45. Scheiman M, Mitchell GL, Cotter S, Cooper J, Kulp M, Rouse M, Borsting E, London R, Wensveen J; Convergence Insufficiency Treatment Trial Study Group. A randomized clinical trial of treatments for convergence insufficiency in children. Arch Ophthalmol. 2005 Jan; 123(1):14–24.

46. Schnider C, Ciuffreda K, Cooper J, and Kruger P. Accommodation Dynamics in Divergence Excess Exotropia. Investigative Ophthalmology, 25: 414–418, 1984.

47. Ziring PR, et al. Learning Disabilities, Dyslexia, and Vision: A Subject Review (RE9825). American Academy of Pediatrics Policy Statement Volume 102, No 5 November 1998, 1217–1219.

Chapter

7

Anomalies of Convergence, Divergence and Accommodation

CONVERGENCE

Convergence is a disjugate movement in which both eyes rotate inward so that the lines of sight intersect in front of the eyes. It allows bifoveal single vision to be maintained at any fixation distance. Convergence remains more or less same throughout life. It does not deteriorate with increasing age, unlike accommodation, but may deteriorate under certain abnormal circumstances. The power of convergence can be increased by exercises.

TYPES OF CONVERGENCE

Convergence is a very complex process. It may be voluntary or reflex.

I. Voluntary convergence

It is that amount of convergence of visual axes that can be produced at will. It is not a part of normal convergence movement as it occurs in everyday vision. Voluntary convergence is thus a separate phenomenon from the reflex convergence involved in normal visual activities; and that not every one is capable of doing or learning this.

Comedians learn to invoke voluntary convergence to cross their eyes. Some patients learn to use voluntary convergence to produce convergence nystagmus.

II. Reflex convergence

It is the convergence of visual axes which is not under complete voluntary control. Reflex convergence has four components: Tonic, fusional, accommodative and proximal convergence.

1. *Tonic convergence*

It is that part of reflex convergence which results from some inherent innervational tone of the extraocular muscles, when the patient is awake. It is the sum of excitatory and inhibitory influences from different sources such as cortical centres, subcortical centres and vestibular organs. It is independent of fusion or object proximity. This is a form of proprioceptive eye position control that keeps the eye converged even after one eye is occluded for a while. It is very important in determining the position of a person's eyes, i.e. under the influence of tonic convergence, the eye position will be more convergent than before, but from an absolute point of view, it will still be divergent. Tonic convergence is most prominent in childhood and decreases with age. The emotional energy level of the individual may affect tonic convergence. It disappears under deep general anaesthesia and after patching one eye for 30 to 60 minutes.

2. *Fusional convergence*

Fusional convergence, also called positive fusional convergence, is the convergence that is produced to ensure that similar retinal images are projected onto corresponding retinal areas. It occurs without a change in refractive state of the eye and is initiated by a bitemporal retinal image disparity. In other words, fusional convergence implies a responsiveness to disparate stimuli lying outside the Panum's fusional area. It is not a voluntary process, but one of the *optomotor reflexes* and thus forms a kind of fusion reflex or motor fusion. Fusional vergence, in general, forms an important mechanism for the achievement of bifoveal single vision. And that a fusional vergence may be a convergence, a divergence or a vertical vergence movement.

Fusional convergence is the most important type of convergence in the study of motor anomalies. It has been found that the amplitude of fusional convergence is greater, when attention is directed between the two disparate retinal images than when the attention is directed at only one of the two images. The normal fusional convergence amplitude for distance is about 18 D and for near it is 35 D. Fusional convergence helps to control exophoria (latent divergent squint). The fusional convergence may be decreased by fatigue or illness, converting a phoria into a tropia. The amplitude of fusional convergence can be improved by orthoptic exercises.

3. *Accommodative convergence*

It is that component of convergence which occurs, when the eyes accommodate, or when a nerve impulse to accommodate is discharged to the eyes. Thus, the stimulus for accommodative convergence is blurred retinal images rather than the retinal disparity that stimulates fusional convergence. In contradiction to fusional convergence, accommodative convergence is not dependent on binocular vision and occurs even if one eye is occluded. Patients with one blind eye still show convergence of the eyes, when accommodating on near objects. In fact, the accommodative convergence is a part of the *triad of synkinetic near reflex complex.* Other two components of this neurosynkinesis being accommodation and miosis. The quantitative relationship between the accommodative convergence and accommodation is expressed as the AC/A ratio. This relationship is a linear one and is thought to be relatively stable throughout life. In it, the accommodative convergence is measured in prism dioptres and the accommodation in lens dioptres. The AC/A ratio, therefore, is expressed as so many prism dioptres per one dioptre of accommodation. The normal AC/A ratio is about 3 to 5 prism dioptres for one dioptre of accommodation.

The fact that AC/A ratio remains almost normal in presbyopic persons, indicates that it is the stimulus for the accommodation that evokes the response of accommodative convergence rather than the amount of accommodation that actually takes place. The majority of myopes have a high AC/A ratio and hypermetropes have a low AC/A ratio as compared with the emmetropes. However, there is no correlation between the degree of myopia, hypermetropia and the magnitude of AC/A ratio. The pupillary distance must also be considered in the determination of the AC/A ratio, since the convergence requirement for an individual with a wide interpupillary distance is greater than for a patient with a narrow interpupillary distance looking at the same fixation distance.

Abnormalities of the AC/A ratio are very important causes of strabismus. A high AC/A ratio may cause excessive convergence and produce a convergent squint (esotropia) during accommodation on a near object. A low AC/A ratio may cause a divergent squint (exotropia), when the patient looks at a near object.

4. *Proximal convergence*

Proximal convergence, also known as instrument convergence, is that component of reflex convergence which is induced by the proximity of the object of regard or the awareness of the proximity of a near object. It appears to be initiated by psychological factors, since it occurs also when a subject just believes that he/she is looking at a near object although he/she actually is not. For example, while using the haploscope optically set at infinity, proximal convergence is often induced.

There exists a linear relationship between proximal convergence and the changes in fixation distance, similar to accommodative convergence. Here the change in fixation distance is expressed as changes in the vergence of light, i.e. in dioptres. Thus a change in fixation from infinity to 1 metre is a change of 1D; as is a change from 1 metre to 0.5 metre. It has been found that for about each dioptre of change of fixation distance, an approximate change of 1.5^Δ occurs in proximal convergence.

ANGLE OF CONVERGENCE

It refers to the angle that is formed between the primary lines of sight during convergence (Fig. 7.1A). Its size depends on the fixation distance, becoming smaller with increasing distance of fixation object (Fig. 7.1B) and on the interpupillary distance (IPD), becoming larger with increasing IPD (Fig. 7.1C).

The effect of IPD on the angle of convergence is usually negligible and so practically not taken into consideration while measuring the convergence angle. Convergence angle can be measured in metre angles or in prism dioptres.

Metre angle

One metre angle convergence is exerted by each eye, when the eyes are directed to an object at a distance of one metre of the meridian line between the two eyes (Fig. 7.2). The convergence exerted in metre angle (ma) by each eye is inversely proportional to the distance in metres the object is infront of the eyes, i.e. it would be 0.5 ma at 2 metres and 2 ma at half metre (Fig. 7.2).

In an emmetropic eye, the number of dioptres of accommodation required to see an object clearly is equal to the number of metre angles through which each eye must converge to see the object singly. Thus, one dioptre of accommodation is associated with one metre angle of convergence of each eye.

Convergence in prism dioptres

When a converging prism (base out) is placed in front of the eye, it will deviate the rays of light entering the eyeball outwards and will tend to produce diplopia. To maintain a binocular single vision, the eye will turn inwards (converged) through a corresponding degree (Fig. 7.3). The convergence required to see singly an object placed at one metre distance from the eyes with a prism of one dioptre placed in front of one eye is called one prism dioptre convergence. It has

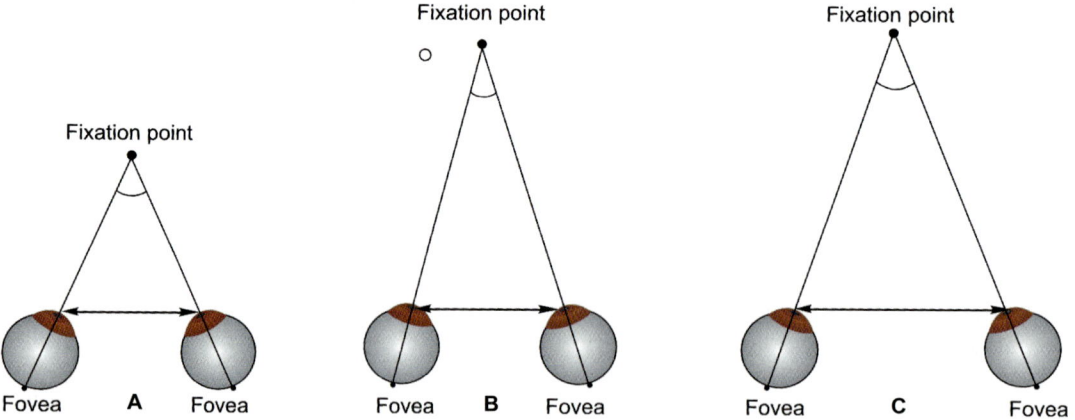

Fig. 7.1 *Angle of convergence (A) which becomes smaller with increasing fixation distance (B), and becomes larger with increasing interpupillary distance (C).*

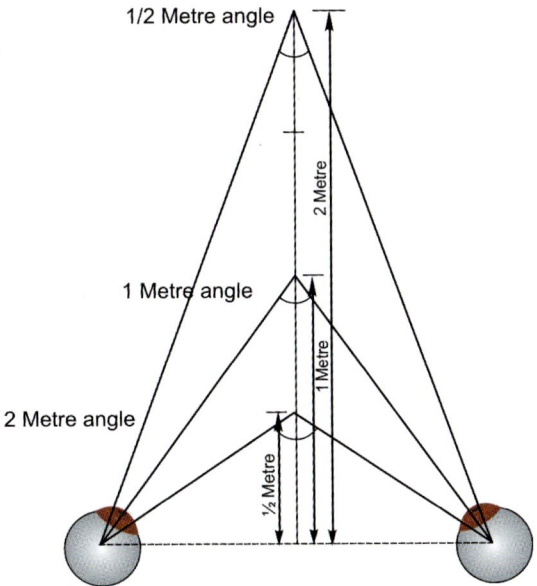

Fig. 7.2 *Convergence in metre angles.*

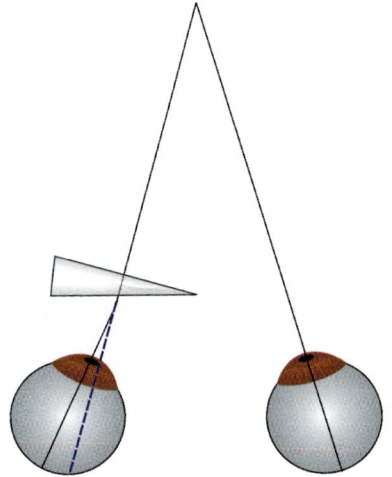

Fig. 7.3 *Convergence in prism dioptres.*

been estimated that roughly 1 metre angle convergence is equal to 3^Δ convergence.

NEAR POINT, FAR POINT, RANGE AND AMPLITUDE OF CONVERGENCE

Near point of convergence (NPC) is the closest point at which an object can be seen singly during bifoveal vision. In other words, it is the point at which the two foveal lines of sight intersect, when maximum convergence is exerted. It is always closer than the near point of accommodation and is usually less than 8 cm.

Far point of convergence refers to relative position of the eyes when they are completely at rest. It is usually infinity. At rest, eyes may be in slight divergence and so the far point of convergence may be in negative (behind the eyes).

Range of convergence is the distance between far point of convergence and near point of convergence. The part of the range of convergence between the eye and infinity is called *positive convergence,* and the part beyond infinity, i.e. behind the eye (when eyes are in slight divergence) is called *negative convergence or divergence.*

Amplitude of convergence refers to difference in the convergence power exerted to maintain the eye in a position of rest and in a position of maximum convergence.

Measurement of Amplitude of Convergence and Near Point of Convergence

See pages 117 and 118 respectively.

ACCOMMODATIVE CONVERGENCE/ ACCOMMODATION (AC/A) RATIO

See page 119.

ANOMALIES OF CONVERGENCE

CONVERGENCE INSUFFICIENCY

Convergence insufficiency is the inability to obtain and/or maintain adequate binocular convergence for any length of time without undue effort. It is the most common cause of ocular asthenopic symptoms.

Etiology

1. *Primary or idiopathic.* In many cases, exact etiology of the convergence insufficiency is not known. It may be associated with a wide inter-pupillary distance and delayed or inadequate functional development. General debility, psychological instability, over work and worry may be the precipitating factors.

2. *Refractive errors.* Convergence insufficiency may be associated with uncorrected high hypermetropia and myopia. Diseases of accommodative convergence mechanism result in convergence insufficiency in such patients as follows:

- High hypermetropes (more than 5D) usually make no effort to accommodate and thus there is deficient accommodative convergence as well.
- *Myopes* may not need accommodation and thus lack accommodative convergence.
- Patients who have worn too full a plus spherical correction may also exert less accommodation and thus less accommodative convergence.

3. *Presbyopia.* With the advent of presbyopia, near point of eye recedes and so there is less use of convergence. Neglect of presbyopia may lead to fixation of this anomaly.

On the other hand, patients may also develop convergence insufficiency with the first time use of presbyopic correction. This has been explained by the fact that the relief of sustained accommodative effort afforded by the use of presbyopic correction causes a decrease of accommodative convergence.

4. *Muscular imbalances.* Extraocular muscular imbalances in the form of exophoria, intermittent exotropia and vertical muscle imbalances, if neglected for a long time may be associated with convergence insufficiency.

5. *Consecutive convergence insufficiency* may occur following either recession of medial recti or resection of lateral recti muscles.

Clinical features

Convergence insufficiency becomes a clinical problem in children with increased school work, prolonged periods of reading, desk workers and percision workers. It is usually not a problem in farm and manual labour workers.

Symptoms of convergence insufficiency are similar to that of heterophoria and in general the term *asthenopia* is used to denote the symptom complex. Unsuitability of the glasses is the most frequent complaint of patients using glasses and having asthenopic symptoms. Such patients change their refractionist and glasses frequently without any satisfaction. Asthenopic symptoms may be grouped as given below.

1. *Symptoms of muscular fatigue*

These result due to continuous use of the neuromuscular power and are usually marked with near work. These include:

- *Eye strain and a sensation* of tension in and around the globes is a common complaint of such patients.
- *Headache and eye ache* after prolonged use of eyes especially for near work, which are relieved, when the eyes are closed for a while. Some patients may show even migrainous tendencies.
- *Difficulty in changing the focus* from distant to near objects.
- *Itching, burning and soreness* of eyes and even hyperaemia of the nasal half of the conjunctiva may occur after prolonged close work.

2. *Symptoms due to failure to maintain binocular vision*

- *Blurred near vision* and crowding of words while reading.
- *Intermittent crossed diplopia* for near vision under conditions of fatigue is not uncommon.
- *Characteristically, one eye will be closed* or covered while reading to obtain relief from visual fatigue.

Diagnosis

Diagnosis of convergence insufficiency is confirmed by:

1. *Remote near point of convergence (NPC).* Convergence insufficiency is said to exist, if NPC is more than 10 cm from the baseline.

2. *Decreased fusional convergence for near.* When measured on synoptophore, the convergence insufficiency is said to exist, if there is difficulty in attaining 30° of convergence.

3. *Prism convergence* is low but prism divergence is normal.

4. *Exophoria* at near with orthophoria at distance may occur. However, convergence insufficiency may be associated with orthophoria and even exophoria.

5. *Near point of accommodation* (NPA) is normal and corresponds to the age of the patient. However, measurement of NPA is essential in each case to diagnose and manage patients suffering from a combined insufficiency of convergence and accommodation. Further, rarely accommodative spasm may occur, if voluntary accommodation and convergence are stimulated in an effort to overcome the convergence insufficiency.

Differential diagnosis

Convergence insufficiency needs to be differentiated from the following conditions presenting with almost similar symptoms.

1. *Convergence insufficiency versus convergence paralysis*

- In convergence paralysis, there is total lack of ability to overcome any amount of base-out prism; while in convergence insufficiency several dioptres of convergence amplitude can be demonstrated.

- On receiving a convergence impulse, a patient with convergence paralysis will show pupillary constriction but inability to converge; in a patient with convergence insufficiency, pupillary constriction will occur while converging on an approaching target, followed by dilation of the pupil, when convergence can no longer be maintained.

2. *Convergence insufficiency versus accommodative effort syndrome*

- Usually an exophoria at near is associated with convergence insufficiency, while patients with accommodative effort syndrome have esophoria.

- Convergence insufficiency is helped by the −3D test, which compensates for the lack of good fusional convergence; while a patient with accommodative effort syndrome breaks into a tropia during this test.

- Plus lenses will worsen the convergence insufficiency due to relaxation of accommodative convergence, while they will improve the symptoms in the accommodative effort syndrome for the same reason.

Treatment

Convergence insufficiency has an excellent prognosis in the majority of cases. *Children* are treated, when fusional vergences are poor and the patient is showing signs of becoming exotropic. *Adults* with this condition receive treatment only in the presence of symptoms. *Treatment* of convergence insufficiency includes: optical treatment, orthoptic treatment, prismotherapy and surgery.

1. *Optical treatment*

Proper refraction should be carried out and the correct glasses should be prescribed for any associated refractive error. Myopes are given full correction and hypermetropes undercorrection to stimulate their accommodation which will simultaneously stimulate convergence. In adults above the age of 40 years, proper presbyopic correction should also be done.

2. *Orthoptic treatment*

Aim of orthoptic exercises is to improve the binocular convergence and to increase the amplitude of fusional convergence. *'Vision therapy'*. The term used for orthoptic treatment includes:

A. *Conventional or non-computerised excercises for:*
   - In-office vision therapy, and
   - Home vision therapy
B. *Computerised orthoptic excercises for:*
   - In-office vision therapy, and
   - Home vision therapy

Note. Conventional, i.e. non-computerised excercises are described here. For computerised exercises *see* page 146.

Conventional or non-computerised exercises

Orthoptic treatment for convergence insufficiency is by and large same as for exophoria and includes the following exercises:

(a) *Exercises to improve near point of convergence*
   i. *Advancement exercises* (*see* page 215).
   ii. *Jump convergence exercises* (*see* page 215).

(b) *Exercises to increase amplitude of fusional convergence*
   i. *Convergence exercises with prisms* (*see* page 214).
   ii. *Convergence exercisess using synoptophore* (*see* page 214).
   iii. *Exercises using convergence card.* Convergence card consists of dots on either side; so also known as physiologic dot card. On one side of the card, dots are coloured red and on the other side blue. Dots identical in size are in the same place on each side of the card and these are of three sizes—large, medium and small.

To perform the exercise, the card is put in front of the patient's eyes with one end of the card resting on his/her nose, with the large dots farthest away, so that he/she will see the red dots with one eye and the blue with the other eye. The patient is instructed to look at the large dots and to see them fused or blended together, then the middle dots and finally the smallest ones. The patient must be aware of heteronymous physiologic diplopia on those dots between his/her eyes and the fused ones; and homonymous physiologic diplopia on those beyond the fused one.

With the use of convergence card, there is a great deal of retinal rivalry. If the patient is unable to do the exercises as instructed above, it may be easier for him/her, if the three dots are connected with a black line on both sides of the card (Fig. 7.4). Now, when fixating on the large size dots, he/she should see the lines as ∨. When he/she is able to fuse the large dots easily, he/she may then fixate on the middle size dots and see the black lines as X. Lastly, he/she should fixate the small size dots and see the black lines as ∨.

iv. *Physiologic diplopia exercise using stereogram in the uncrossed position* (*see* page 214).

v. *Convergence exercise using diploscope* (*see* page 141).

(c) *Training of voluntary convergence*
It is very helpful, if the patient is intelligent and co-operative. It aims at developing the control of the position of eyes. Patient is made to understand physiological diplopia which he/she practices. If a finger is brought in the field of vision while the patient is fixing a distant light, there will appear two fingers. Now, if the patient fixes at the finger, then there will appear two lights at the distance. While the finger is moved

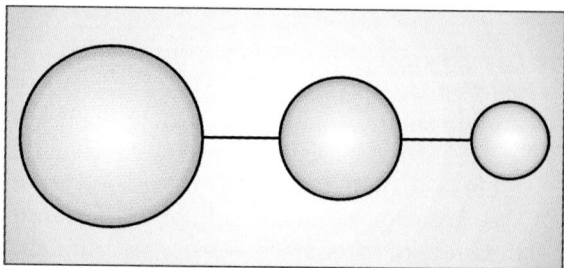

Fig. 7.4 *Convergence card.*

to and fro, the distance between the lights increases or decreases. Patient is asked to maintain the two lights apart as long as possible. The finger may again be brought in, if the two lights become single as soon as the finger is removed. This exercise is completed, when the patient is able to double the lights without the aid of the finger. Development of voluntary convergence goes a long way in relieving symptoms.

(d) *Relaxation exercises*
Relaxation using relative negative convergence may be carried out after the treatment by any of the following methods:

  i. Stereogram in crossed position (*see* page 214).
 ii. Divergence with prisms (*see* page 213).
iii. Synoptophore exercises (*see* page 214).

Criteria for good orthoptic management
- Patient should be symptom free.
- There should be good binocular convergence.
- Voluntary convergence should be possible easily.
- Patient should have good fusional reserves.

3. Prismotherapy
When all the exhaustive orthoptic exercises fail, then prismotherapy may be tried to relieve symptoms.
- *Base in prism* reading glasses or bifocals with prism in the lower segment are useful as relieving prisms.
- *Relieving prisms and bifocals* in young age should be avoided.

4. Surgical Treatment
As a last resort, when all other measures fail, especially when convergence insufficiency is associated with a large exophoria at near vision, medial rectus muscle resection can be performed in one or both eyes. In some cases, exophoria at near fixation tends to recur.

Convergence insufficiency treatment trial
Convergence insufficiency treatment trial (CITT) was conducted to compare three forms of vision therapy with office-based placebo therapy:
- *Office-based vision therapy with a trained therapist along with home reinforcement.* Children in this

group came to the office once per week for a 60-minute therapy session with a trained therapist. During these sessions, the children worked on 4–6 procedures designed to improve the ability to converge the eyes. The children in this group also did home therapy for 15 minutes, 5 days per week to practice the procedures learned during the office visits.

- *Home-based pencil push-ups therapy.* In this group, the child had to follow a small letter on a pencil as the pencil was moved toward the bridge of his nose. His goal was to keep the letter clear and single, but to stop if the letter became double. The child was told to try and get the pencil closer and closer to the bridge of his nose each day. This was practiced for 15 minutes, 5 days per week.
- *Home-based computer vision therapy and pencil push-ups.* In this group, the child was given complex exercises using a computer program plus pencil push-ups.
- *Office-based placebo therapy.* This group was given placebo vision activities designed to simulate office-based therapy.

CITT concluded that office-based vision therapy with a trained therapist plus at-home reinforcement was most effective in treating CI in children 9 to 17 years old.

CONVERGENCE INSUFFICIENCY ASSOCIATED WITH ACCOMMODATIVE INSUFFICIENCY

Convergence insufficiency in some patients may be secondary to accommodation insufficiency. Therefore, before treating the patient for a functional convergence insufficiency, it is important to rule out associated accommodation insufficiency.

Etiology

Secondary convergence insufficiency associated with primary accommodation insufficiency has been reported to occur in following conditions:
1. Early Adie's syndrome
2. Sequelae to head trauma, particularly posterior occipital or whiplash injury.
3. Subclinical viral encephalopathies.
4. Infectious mononucleosis
5. Diphtheria
6. As a conversion reaction.

Clinical features

1. Symptoms of the patients are similar to those of functional convergence insufficiency.
2. Near point of convergence (NPC) is reduced.
3. Near point of accommodation (NPA) is reduced drastically.
4. Accommodative convergence/accommodation (AC/A) ratio may be low or even absent.

Treatment

1. *Orthoptic exercises* alone are usually not much effective. Exercises need to be combined with reading glasses.

2. *Plus lenses for reading and base-in prism* is the treatment of choice. The reading spectacle prescription should be titrated according to patients need. The minimal power necessary to achieve comfortable vision should be prescribed. Fresnel membrane prisms glued on glass lenses in the lower segment of bifocals may be useful, since a frequent change may be necessary before the final adjustment is made. Alternatively, two piece executive bifocals with decentered plus lenses for prism power in the lower half may be prescribed.

3. *Surgery* is usually not indicated for this condition. However, it has been reported that resection of both medial rectus muscles followed by prescription of bifocal adds may be helpful in untreatable cases.

CONVERGENCE PARALYSIS

Convergence paralysis refers to a total lack of ability to overcome any amount of base-out prisms. It is an uncommon entity and should not be confused with functional convergence insufficiency which is very common.

Etiology

Convergence paralysis occurs secondary to some organic diseases of the brain in the region of corpora quadrigemina or the nucleus of third cranial nerve. The organic brain lesions reported to be associated with convergence paralysis are as follows:

- Head injury
- Encephalitis

- Disseminated sclerosis
- Tabes dorsalis
- Narcolepsy
- Tumours

Clinical features

Convergence paralysis is characterized by following features:

1. *Convergence* is completely absent. There is acute onset of convergence failure.
2. *Exotropia* and *crossed diplopia* occur on attempted near fixation only.
3. *Adduction* is normal.
4. *Accommodation* is usually normal. But in some cases it may be reduced or even absent.

Parinaud's syndrome refers to convergence paralysis associated with vertical gaze paralysis.

Pretectum-posterior commissure syndrome (dorsal midbrain syndrome) which is commonly caused by tumour in the pineal region includes:

- Convergence paralysis
- Vertical gaze paralysis
- Pupillary areflexia to light with light near dissociation.
- Bilateral fourth nerve paralysis may be present sometimes.
- Lid retraction may also occur in some patients.

Diagnosis

Bielschowsky's criteria for diagnosis of the convergence paralysis include: (1) evidence of intracranial disease, (2) history of sudden onset of crossed horizontal diplopia at near fixation, (3) reproducible findings on subsequent exami-nations and (4) preservation of accommodation and pupillary reaction on attempts to converge.

Differential diagnosis

Convergence paralysis can be differentiated from functional convergence insufficiency by use of base-out prisms. A patient with convergence paralysis will immediately have diplopia, while in convergence insufficiency several dioptres of convergence amplitude can be demonstrated.

Treatment

1. *Base-in prisms* are prescribed at near to alleviate the diplopia at near.
2. *Plus lenses with base-in prisms* may be required in patients having weakness of accommodation.
3. *Occlusion of one eye* at near may be indicated in patients where it is not possible to restore comfortable single binocular vision.
4. Eye muscle surgery is contraindicated in this condition.

■ CONVERGENCE SPASM

Convergence spasm refers to a condition characterized by intermittent episodes of maximal convergence usually associated with spasm of accommodation.

Etiology

1. Functional causes. It has been reported that in most of the cases, convergence spasm is functional in origin. It occurs in patients with hysteria or neurosis.

2. Organic causes. Rarely convergence spasm may be secondary to some underlying organic lesion. It has been reported to occur after head trauma, encephalitis, tabes, pituitary adenomas, posterior fossa neurofibroma and Arnold-Chiari malformation.

Clinical features

In most of the cases, the condition is episodic. In between the attacks, patients are normal. During the episode of convergence spasm, a patient may exhibit following clinical features:

1. *Extreme convergence.* Eyes may be fixed in a position of extreme convergence resembling bilateral abducens palsy.

2. *Homonymous diplopia* may be experienced. Patient may give history of intermittent diplopia.

3. *Blurring of vision.* During the attack, patient may have blurred vision for near due to associated spasm of accommodation. Patient may come with a complaint of difficulty in reading.

4. *Miosis.* Pupils usually become miotic, as a part of near reflex.

5. *Induced myopia* to the tune of 6D (confirmed by retinoscopy) has been reported due to

associated spasm of accommodation. Thus, during the attack, patient may also have a reduced distance visual acuity.

Psychiatric examination may reveal the underlying hysteria and neurosis in many cases.

Management

Neurological evaluation. Organic lesions are a rare cause of spasm of convergence; however, each patient should undergo detailed neurological evaluation to rule out associated condition, if any.

Treatment of functional spasm of convergence includes:
1. *Prolonged atropinization with plus lenses* in lower segment of bifocals for near work may be required to break the cycle.
2. *Alternate monocular occlusion* may be considered as an alternative to atropinization.
3. *Psychiatric work-up and therapy* is useful as a long-term measure.

DIVERGENCE

As mentioned earlier, divergence refers to disjugate but symmetrical and simultaneous outward rotation of the two eyes from a given position. It is unknown whether *voluntary divergence* exists. Certainly, it is possible to relax one's convergence voluntarily and to produce in this way a more divergent position of the eyes. Thus, from clinical point of view, the only significant form of divergence is fusional divergence.

Fusional divergence

Fusional divergence, also called negative fusional convergence, is the divergence that is produced (like the positive fusional convergence) to ensure that similar retinal images are projected onto corresponding retinal points of two eyes. It occurs without a change in refractive state of eye and is initiated by a *binasal retinal image disparity*. In other words, fusional divergence implies a responsiveness to disparate stimuli lying outside of Panum's fusional area. Similar to fusional convergence, it is a kind of optomotor reflex.

When fusional divergence amplitudes are measured with a prism bar, the normal range is 4D to 6D at distance and 8D to 12D at near. As discussed earlier, in the case of fusional convergence, the end point of the amplitude (i.e. the point of maximal convergence) is marked by an identical phenomenon, that is, blurring of vision both for distance and near. However, in fusional divergence, the end point of amplitude differs in character for near (blurring of vision) and distance (double vision) as follows:

- *End point of amplitude of fusional divergence for distance:* Beyond the maximal limit of fusional divergence, there occurs diplopia (end point).
- *End point of amplitude of fusional divergence for near:* In near vision, as we know, the eyes are accommodated and also converged. Under these circumstances, when measuring the amplitude of fusional divergence beyond the limits of maximal fusional divergence the accommodative convergence is relaxed to prevent retinal disparity. But along with the relaxation of accommodative convergence, the accommodation is also relaxed resulting in blurring of vision (end point).

Measurement of amplitude of divergence

See page 116.

ANOMALIES OF DIVERGENCE

DIVERGENCE INSUFFICIENCY

Divergence insufficiency is not synonymous with divergence paralysis, but is a separate clinical entity.

Etiology

Exact etiology is not known. It has been assumed that perhaps in divergence insufficiency, a pre-existing esophoria at distance fixation caused by an anomalous position of rest becomes manifest.

Clinical features

Characteristic features are as follows:
1. *Esodeviation.* Intermittent or constant eso-deviation is much larger at distance than near. Usually, patients maintain the fusion at near. Esodeviation is comitant in all fields of gaze.

2. *Ductions and versions* are normal in all the directions.
3. *Fusional divergence* is markedly reduced both at distance and near fixation.
4. *Absence of any neurologic disease* (e.g. divergence paralysis).

Treatment

1. *Prismotherapy.* Divergence insufficiency is a self-limiting condition. However, to alleviate the patient of symptoms, *prism base-out* is prescribed to provide comfortable single vision at distance. Prism power is decreased stepwise in months and ultimately discarded.
2. *Surgical treatment.* In the form of resection of both lateral rectus muscles is indicated, rarely when the prismotherapy fails.

DIVERGENCE PARALYSIS

Divergence paralysis is a rare entity characterized by a sudden onset esotropia at distance fixation and a homonymous diplopia.

Etiology

Divergence paralysis may be associated with a head trauma or other neurologic diseases such as encephalitis, tabes, disseminated sclerosis, vascular disorder, neoplasm and raised intracranial pressure.

Clinical features

Clinical features of divergence paralysis are similar to divergence insufficiency except that it is of sudden onset and usually associated with some organic neurologic diseases.

Differential diagnosis

1. *Unilateral or bilateral sixth nerve palsy.* Clinically, a paralysis of fusional divergence is differentiated from the bilateral sixth cranial nerve paralysis by the fact that in the former, at a given distance, the deviation is comitant and that the distance between the double images remains the same irrespective of the position of the object of regard, as it is moved laterally in the radius of a circle with the patient at the centre. This observation indicates that perhaps a separate *divergent centre exists.* However, still no specific midbrain or central nervous system centre has been proved to be divergence centre that abduction is completely normal bilaterally.
2. *Convergence spasm* may also be confused with divergence paralysis because in both the conditions patients have uncrossed diplopia at distance fixation. However, in convergence spasm visual acuity is reduced due to induced myopia and the divergence fusional range is normal.

Management

A thorough neurologic work-up is required for any associated disease. However, divergence paralysis has no localizing significance for the neurologist. Further, despite the association of neurologic diseases, mostly divergence paralysis is self-limiting and disappears within 5 to 6 months. During this period, *prismotherapy* as described for divergence insufficiency is required. Bilateral lateral rectus resection may be indicated in some cases where divergence paralysis persists beyond 6 months.

ACQUIRED MOTOR FUSION DEFICIENCY

Acquired motor fusion deficiency refers to a combined deficiency of the fusional convergence and fusional divergence.

Etiology

It has been assumed that, perhaps, a midbrain lesion accounts for the acquired motor fusion deficiency. The lesions reported to be associated with this rare entity are as follows:
- Closed head trauma
- Cerebrovascular accidents
- Intracranial tumours
- Brain surgery

Clinical features

1. *Asthenopia.* Most patients complain of severe asthenopic symptoms.
2. *Diplopia* is usually intractable and variable, i.e. may be crossed at one moment and uncrossed at another.
3. *Fusional amplitudes* (convergence as well as divergence) are either markedly decreased or completely absent.
4. *Sensory fusion and stereopsis* are intact during the brief moments and that such patients may be able to superimpose the double images.
5. *Accommodation range* may be decreased.

Differential diagnosis

Acquired motor fusion deficiency needs to be differentiated from following conditions:

1. *Combined convergence and accommodation deficiency* (*see* page 159).

2. *Motor fusion deficiency* in adults due to prolonged unilateral use of the eye as seen with unilateral cataract or untreated unilateral aphakia.

3. *Malingering:* Some patients may malinger for diplopia-like acquired motor fusion deficiency following work-related trauma to get compensation. Measurement of fusional amplitudes with a rotatory prism helps in differentiating the two conditions.

Treatment

Treatment of this condition is usually frustrating. Prisms cannot be employed because of frequent adjustments for near and distance. The only way to get relief from symptoms is unilateral occlusion. Infrequently, a spontaneous recovery may occur.

ACCOMMODATION

ACCOMMODATION AND RELATED TERMS

Accommodation

As we know that in an emmetropic eye, parallel rays of light coming from infinity are brought to focus on the retina, with accommodation at rest. Our eyes have been provided with a unique mechanism by which we can even focus the diverging rays coming from a near object on the retina in a bid to see clearly (Fig. 7.5). This mechanism is called accommodation. In it, there occurs increase in the power of the crystalline lens.

Far point, near point, range and amplitude of accommodation

The nearest point at which small objects can be seen clearly is called near point or *punctum proximum* and the distant (farthest) point is called far point or *punctum remotum*. The distance between the near point and the far point is called *range of accommodation*. The difference between the dioptric power needed to focus at near point (P) and to focus at far point (R) is called *amplitude of accommodation* (A). Thus, A = P – R.

Far point and near point of the eye vary with the static refraction of the eye. In hypermetropic eye, far point is virtual and lies behind the eye, while in myopic eye, it is real and lies in front of the eye (Fig. 7.6). In an emmetropic eye, far point is at infinity and near point varies with age; being about 7 cm at age of 10 years, 25 cm at the age of 40 years and 33 cm at the age of 45 years. Thus the amount that the eye can alter its refraction is greatest in childhood and slowly decreases until it is lost in middle age. Amplitude of accommodation in dioptres as function of the age, as studied by Duane is depicted in Fig. 7.7.

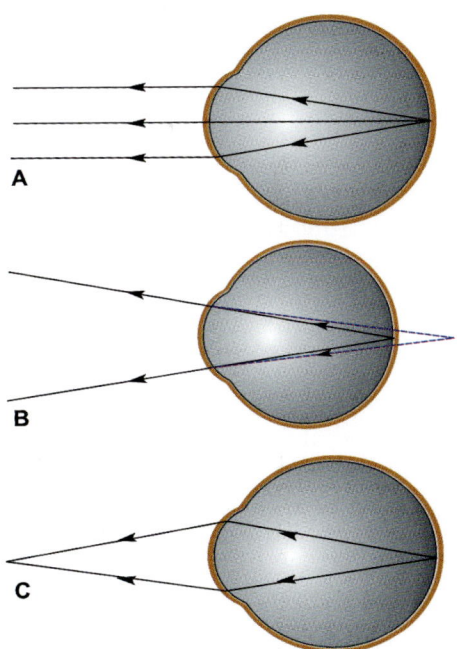

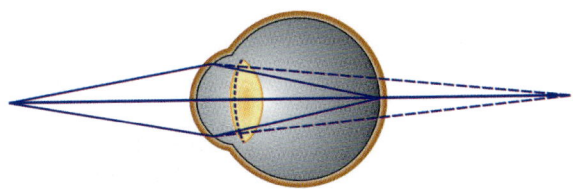

Fig. 7.5 *Effect of accommodation on divergent rays entering the eye.*

Fig. 7.6 *Far point in emmetropic eye (A), hypermetropic eye (B), and myopic eye (C),*

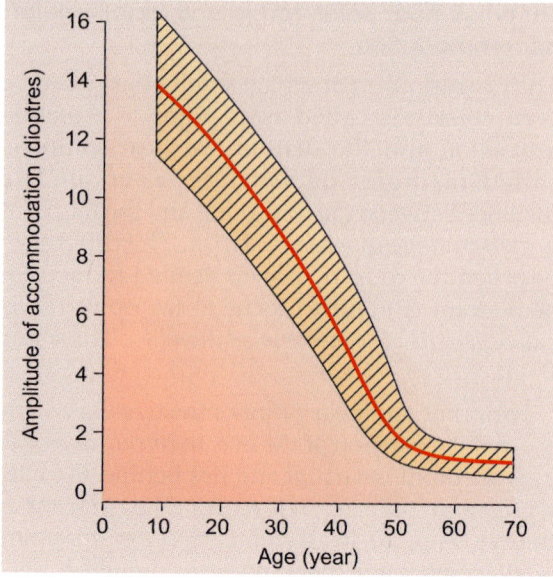

Fig. 7.7 *Decrease in the amplitude of accommodation with age in human (from Duane A : Arch Ophthalmol 54: 566–587, 1925).*

ASSESSMENT OF ACCOMMODATION

See page 118.

AGE-RELATED CHANGES IN ACCOMMODATION

As discussed earlier, in an emmetropic eye, far point is infinity and near point changes with age, being about 7 cm at the age of 10 years, 25 cm at the age of 40 years, 33 cm at the age of 45 years and about 50 cm at the age of 50 years. Therefore, at the age of 10 years, amplitude of accommodation (A) = 100/7 (dioptric power needed to see clearly at near point) – I/a (dioptric power needed to see clearly at far point); i.e. A (at age 10) = 14 dioptres. Similarly, A at age 40 years = (100/25 – I/a) = 4 dioptres; at age 45 years, A = 3 dioptres and at 50 years = 2 dioptres. Since, we usually keep the book at about 25 cm, so we can read comfortably up to the age of 40 years and after that the near point recedes beyond the normal reading or working range. This condition of failing near vision due to related decrease in the amplitude of accommodation or increase in the near point (punctum proximum) is called presbyopia.

ANOMALIES OF ACCOMMODATION

Anomalies of accommodation are not uncommon. These include:

I. *Deficient or decreased accommodation*
  1. Presbyopia (physiological deficiency of accommodation).
  2. Insufficiency of accommodation (pathological deficiency of accommodation).
  3. Paralysis of accommodation

II. *Excessive accommodation or spasm of accommodation*

INSUFFICIENCY OF ACCOMMODATION

The term insufficiency of accommodation is used, when the accommodative power is significantly less than the normal physiological limits for the patient's age. Therefore, it should not be confused with presbyopia in which the physiological insufficieny of accommodation is normal for the patient's age.

Causes

1. Premature sclerosis of lens.
2. Weakness of ciliary muscle due to systemic causes of muscle fatigue such as debilitating illness, anaemia, toxaemia, malnutrition, diabetes mellitus, pregnancy stress and so on.
3. Weakness of ciliary muscle associated with primary open angle glaucoma.

Clinical features

All the symptoms of presbyopia are present, but those of asthenopia are more prominent than those of blurring of vision.

Treatment

1. The treatment is essentially that of the systemic causes.
2. *Near vision spectacles* in the form of weakest convex lens which allows adequate vision should be given till the power of accommodation improves.
3. *Accommodation exercises* help in recovery, if the underlying debility has passed.

PARALYSIS OF ACCOMMODATION

Paralysis of accommodation, also known as cycloplegia, refers to complete absence of accommodation.

Causes

1. *Drug-induced cycloplegia* results due to the effect of atropine, homatropine or other parasympatholytic drugs.
2. *Internal ophthalmoplegia* (paralysis of ciliary muscle and sphincter pupillae) may result from neuritis associated with diphtheria, syphilis, diabetes, alcoholism, cerebral or meningeal diseases.
3. *Paralysis of accommodation as a component of complete third nerve paralysis* may occur due to intracranial or orbital causes. The lesions may be traumatic, inflammatory or neoplastic in nature.

Clinical features

1. *Blurring of near vision.* It is the main complaint in previously emmetropic or hypermetropic patients. Blurring of near vision may not be marked in myopic patients.
2. *Photophobia* (glare) due to accompanying dilatation of pupil (mydriasis) is usually associated with blurring of near vision.
3. Examination reveals, abnormal receding of near point and markedly decreased range of accommodation.

Treatment

1. Self-recovery occurs in drug-induced paralysis and in diphtheric cases (once the systemic disease is treated).
2. Dark glasses are effective in reducing the glare.
3. Convex lenses for near vision may be prescribed, if the paralysis is permanent.

SPASM OF ACCOMMODATION

Spasm of accommodation refers to exertion of abnormally excessive accommodation.

Causes

1. *Drug-induced spasm* of accommodation is known to occur after the use of strong miotics such as echothiophate and DEP.
2. *Spontaneous spasm* of accommodation is occasionally found in children who attempt to compensate for a refractive anomaly that impairs their vision. It usually occurs, when the eyes are used for excessive near work in unfavourable circumstances such as bad illumination, bad reading position, lowered vitality, state of neurosis, mental stress or anxiety.

Clinical features

1. Defective vision due to induced myopia.
2. Asthenopic symptoms are more marked than the visual symptoms.

Diagnosis

Diagnosis is made with refraction under atropine.

Treatment

1. Relaxation of ciliary muscle by atropine for a few weeks and prohibition of near work allow prompt recovery from spasm of accommodation.
2. Correction of associated causative factors, prevent recurrence.

BIBLIOGRAPHY

1. Convergence Insufficiency Treatment Trial (CITT) Study, Group. "The convergence insufficiency treatment trial: design, methods, and baseline data.". *Ophthalmic epidemiology.* 2008;15 (1): 24–36.
2. Cooper J, Duckman R. Convergence insufficiency: incidence, diagnosis, and treatment. J Am Optom Assoc 1978; 49:673-80.
3. Cooper J. Accommodative dysfunction. In: Amos JF, ed. Diagnosis and management in vision care. Boston: Butterworths, 1987:431–59.
4. Daum KM. Divergence excess: characteristics and results of treatment with orthoptics. Ophthalmic Physiol Opt 1984; 4:15–24.
5. Duane A: Studies in monocular and binocolar accommodation with their clinical applications. Am J Ophthalmol 1922;5:865.
6. GK. Van Norden, "Anomalies of convergence and divergence," in Binocular Vision and Ocular Motility, G. K. Von Norden, Ed., Mosby, 4th edition, 1990.
7. Goss, DA. Ocular accommodation, convergence, and fixation disparity: a manual of clinical analysis, 2nd ed. Newton, MA: Butterworth-Heinemann, 1995:14.
8. MattiWestman; M. Johanna Liinamaa. "Relief of asthenopic symptoms with orthoptic exercises in convergence insufficiency is achieved in both adults and children". *Journal of Optometry.* 2012;5 (2). pp. 62–67.

9. Morgan MW Jr. Relationship between accommodation and convergence. AMA Arch Ophthalmol 1952;47:745–759.

10. Rutstein RP, Daum KM, Amos JF. Accommodative spasm: a review of 17 cases. J Am OptomAssoc 1988; 59:527-38.

11. Scheiman M, Mitchell GL, Cotter S, Cooper J, Kulp M, Rouse M, Borsting E, London R, Wensveen J, Convergence Insufficiency Treatment Trial Study Group (Jan 2005). "A randomized clinical trial of treatments for convergence insufficiency in children". *Arch Ophthalmol*. 123 (1): 14–24.

12. Scheiman M, Mitchell GL, Cotter S, Kulp MT, Cooper J, Rouse M, Borsting E, London R, Wensveen J. "A randomized clinical trial of vision therapy/orthoptics versus pencil pushups for the treatment of convergence insufficiency in young adults". *Optom Vis Sci*. 2005; 82 (7): 583–95.

13. Wilson ME, Saunders RA, Berland JE. Dissociated horizontal deviation and accommodative esotropia: treatment options when an eso- and an exodeviation co-exist. *Journal of Pediatric Ophthalmology and Strabismus*. 1995;32(4):228–230.

Adaptations to Strabismus and Amblyopia

INTRODUCTION

When the visual functions are normally developed, the individual possesses a binocular single vision, which implies a point-to-point normal correspondence of two retinae with foveas being the principal corresponding point. With the occurrence of strabismus, the alignment of the corresponding retinal points is disturbed. Consequently, the fixation point is imaged in the centre of the fovea of the non-deviating eye and some extrafoveal (peripheral retinal) point in the deviated eye. This results in diplopia and confusion.

- *Diplopia* occurs due to formation of image on dissimilar points of the two retinae (Fig. 8.1) and

- *Confusion* occurs due to formation of image of two different objects on the corresponding points of the two retinae (Fig. 8.2).

- *To escape the disabling and troublesome situation* created by diplopia and confusion, the strabismic patients (below the age of 7–9 years; with immature visual system) develop certain adaptations which allow them to have a comfortable single vision. Older patients who develop strabismus for the first time suffer from diplopia and confusion for a long time till they learn to ignore (psychological adaptation).

Adaptations to strabismus. To avoid repetition, adaptations to strabismus are being discussed

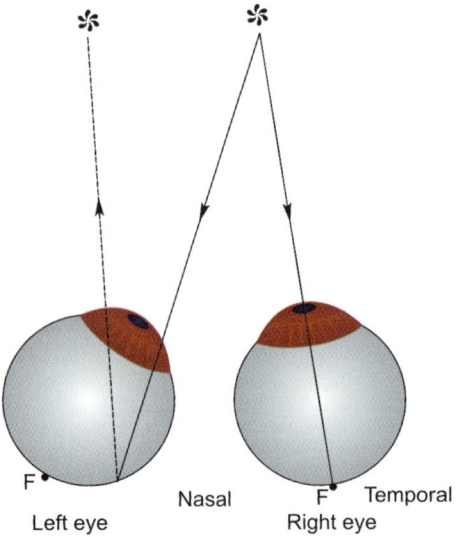

Fig. 8.1 *Diplopia due to formation of image on dissimilar points of the two retinae.*

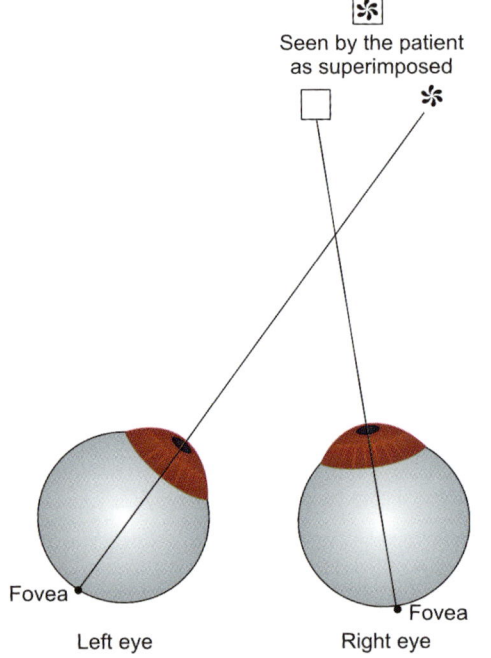

Fig. 8.2 *Confusion due to formation of image of two different objects on the corresponding points of two retinae.*

before the clinical description of different varieties of strabismus. Adaptations to strabismus include the following:

Sensory adaptations
• Monofixation syndrome
• Suppression
• Anomalous retinal correspondence (ARC)

Note. Amblyopia, not actually a sensory adaptation, may occur as a consequence of suppression, and so is described in this chapter. The term strabismic amblyopia is used for the amblyopia seen in patients with unilateral constant squint.

Motor adaptations
• Compensatory head posture
• Blind spot syndrome and mechanism

Psychological adaptations
• Ignoring

SENSORY ADAPTATIONS

A sensory adaptation may be defined as the manner in which a patient makes sensory adjustments to an interruption in the normal binocular single vision caused by the occurrence of squint. In other words, sensory adaptations are nature's way out of trouble but at the cost of binocular single vision. Sensory adaptations are more frequent in patients with strabismus of childhood onset as compared to the patients with strabismus of adult onset.

Sensory adaptations include the following:

• Suppression
• Monofixation syndrome
• Amblyopia (not actually an adaptation but a consequence of suppression)
• Anomalous retinal correspondence (ARC)

SUPPRESSION

Suppression may be defined as a temporary active cortical inhibition of the image of an object formed on the retina of the squinting eye. This phenomenon occurs (to avoid diplopia and/or confusion) only during binocular vision (i.e. with both eyes open). However, when the fixating eye is covered, the squinting eye fixates, i.e. suppression disappears (Fig. 8.3).

TYPES OF SUPPRESSION

Suppression has been variously classified:

I. *Depending upon the etiopathogenesis*

1. Physiological suppression

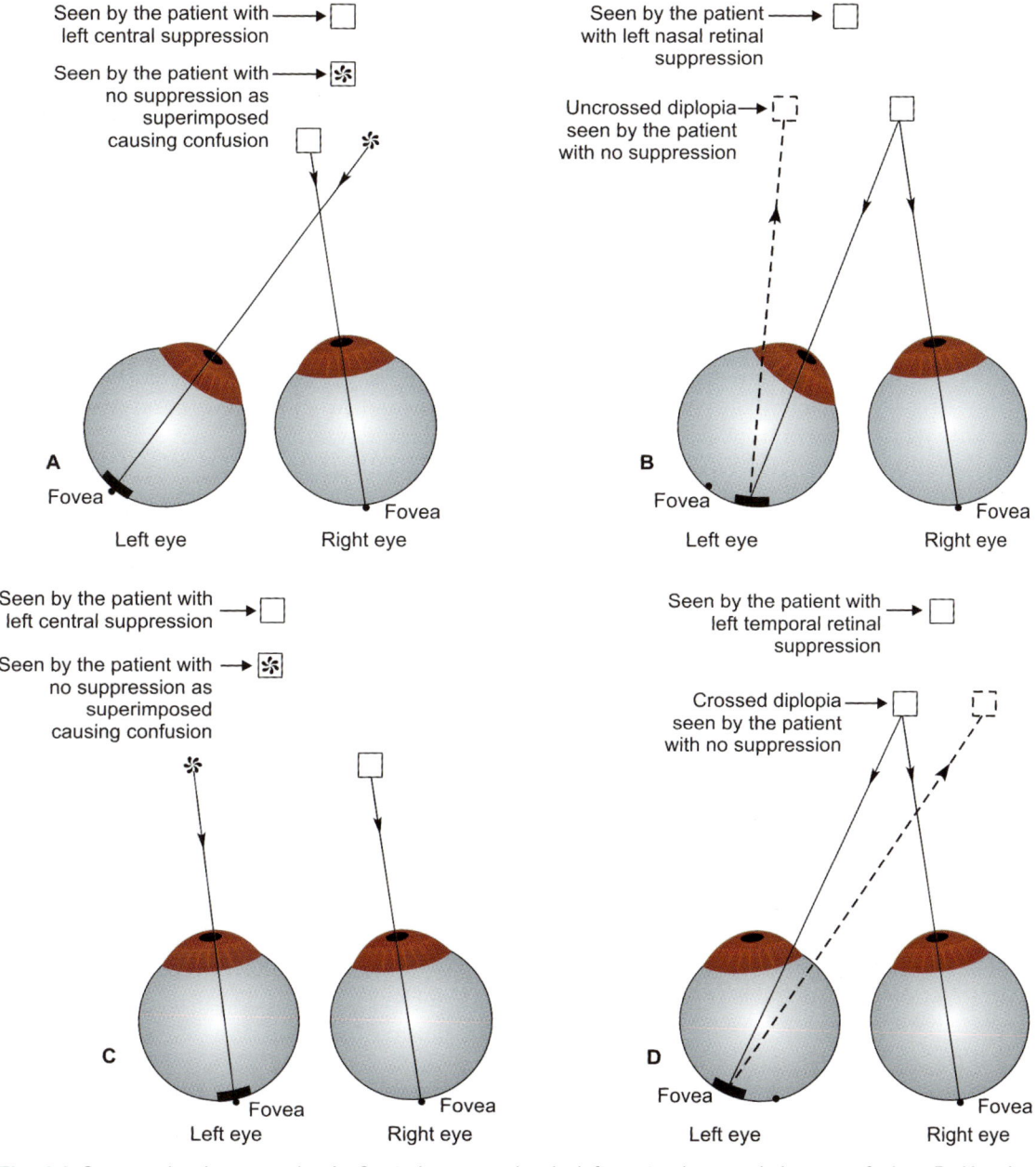

Fig. 8.3 Suppression in esotropia: A, Central suppression in left esotropic eye obviates confusion; B, Nasal retinal suppression scotoma obviates diplopia. Suppression in exotropia: C, suppression scotoma in left fovea obviates confusion; and D, Temporal retinal scotoma obviates diplope; *Suppression in left esotropic eye during binocular vision.*

2. Pathological (abnormal) suppression. It is further of two types:

 a. Facultative suppression

 b. Obligatory suppression

II. *Depending upon the retinal area where image is suppressed*

1. Foveal suppression
2. Macular suppression
3. Peripheral suppression
4. Large regional suppression

III. *Depending upon the constancy*
1. Intermittent suppression
2. Constant suppression

IV. *Depending upon the eye involved*
1. Monocular suppression
2. Alternating suppression

Physiological suppression

Physiological suppression refers to the suppression present in everyday life of every individual having normal binocular single vision. It occurs due to retinal rivalry and to avoid physiological diplopia. As a matter of fact, the physiological suppression is very helpful in everyday life, since it allows greater concentration on the object of interest. The specific examples of physiological suppression in everyday life while using one eye with both eyes open are as follows:

• While using monocular microscope, the image of the other is suppressed.
• A watchmaker keeps both eyes open but normally suppresses one eye while viewing the delicate parts of a watch through a monocular magnifying instrument with the other eye.
• While looking down the barrel of a rifle with the dominant eye, the person may suppress his nondominant eye.

Pathological suppression

It refers to the suppression of the image of one eye that occurs to avoid diplopia and/or confusion. It occurs in patients with strabismus and anisometropia. It can be described as:

• Facultative versus obligatory suppression, and
• Central versus peripheral suppression

Facultative versus obligatory suppression

Facultative suppression. It occurs to avoid diplopia and/or confusion under conditions of binocular vision but ceases, when the fixating or the dominant eye is covered. It may occur under following situations:

• Latent squint
• Intermittent squint
• Alternating squint (there is alternate suppression)
• Manifest deviations of recent onset with normal retinal correspondence.

Obligatory suppression. It refers to constant suppression of the image from one eye which occurs under all conditions and remains even when the fixating or dominant eye is covered. Obligatory suppression in the long run leads to amblyopia and decreased visual acuity in the affected eye.

Central versus peripheral suppression

Central suppression occurs to suppress the image formed at the fovea of the deviating eye to avoid confusion (Fig. 8.3A and C).

Peripheral suppression, i.e. suppression of the image formed at some peripheral area of the retina of the deviating eye that corresponds to the image falling on the fovea of the fixating occurs to prevent diplopia (Fig. 8.3B and D).

Size and shape of suppression scotoma

Size and shape of suppression scotoma are different in esotropia as compared with an exotropia.

• *In esotropia*, a small round scotoma involving nasal retinal area corresponding to the fovea of fixating eye is produced (Fig. 8.3B). Rarely this scotoma can be bit larger.
• *In exotropia*, a comparatively much larger scotoma occurs on temporal retina of the deviated eye (Fig. 8.3D). This is explained by the fact that intermittent exotropia, slowly increases in size and so is the area of suppression scotoma.

PATHOGENESIS

Mechanism of suppression

Retinal rivalry, i.e. struggle for dominance of each eye is considered a prerequisite to suppression. Retinal rivalry is a situation that occurs when dissimilar objects are presented to the two eyes. That is, two complete images of the dissimilar objects are not seen. In an area of the field, part of one image predominates while the corresponding part of the second image is suppressed as shown in Fig. 8.4. This condition is constantly changing and the different parts of the image are suppressed in turn.

Burian popularized the concept that suppression is merely an exaggeration of the same process which is involved in blocking out certain

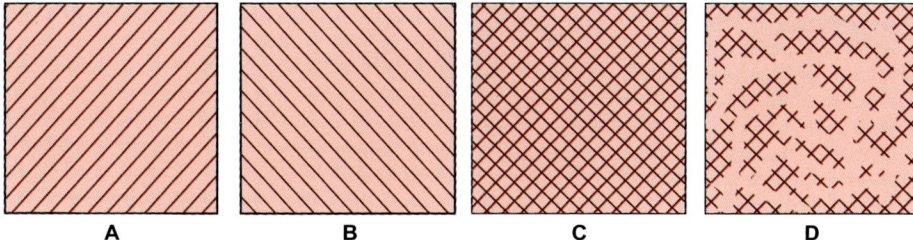

Fig. 8.4 *Retinal rivalry occurring due to dissimilar objects being present to the left* (A) *and the right* (B) *eyes. Patient will not see the picture as shown in* (C) *but will see as shown in* (D) *due to suppression.*

parts of the image seen by each eye in binocular rivalry. However, Smith and coworkers concluded that though the retinal rivalry may be an important phase in the development of the strabismic suppression, but the suppression and the retinal rivalry are mediated by different mechanisms.

Present knowledge is far from complete to authentically designate the primary seat of the suppressive mechanism. However, most studies implicate the cortex as being the probable seat of suppression, since normal ERG with reduction in the amplitude of the VER has been reported in patients with suppression. Results of some of the electrophysiological and psychophysiological studies are mentioned in the discussion of amblyopia.

Selective suppression. Burian believes that suppression may be selective even with regard to a specific retinal function; that is, the ability to resolve only contours may be defective momentarily.

Suppression pattern usually corresponds with the deviation pattern, i.e. suppression is intermittent in patients with intermittent squint, monocular and constant in patients with uniocular constant deviation and it is alternating in patients with alternating squint.

TESTS FOR SUPPRESSION

Tests for detection of suppression

1. Worth's four-dot test. This test can be employed to diagnose the suppression involving the peripheral retina. As described in detail on page 131, the patients having left suppression will see only two red lights and that having right suppression will see only three green lights

(Fig. 6.32). In the presence of alternate suppression, patients will see alternately two red lights and three green lights.

Disadvantages. Worth's four-dot test is not a very useful test for suppression because of the following reasons:

- It does not detect foveal suppression.
- Since the eyes are easily dissociated with red-green glasses, a patient with unstable but functionally useful binocular vision may exhibit a suppression response with this test.
- In a patient having ARC, a normal fusion response (the patient sees all four dots in a rectangular arrangement) occurs even in the presence of suppression.

2. The 4D base-out prism test (Fig. 8.5). This test popularized by Jampolsky is performed for detection of small angle heterotropias and the presence of central suppression scotoma.

Technique. To perform this test, patient fixates a penlight (Fig. 8.5A). Then a 4D prism is placed with base-out in front of the right eye and the examiner observes the presence of a biphasic corrective movement of the left eye (Fig. 8.5B and C). This is absent in the presence of a central suppression scotoma (Fig. 8.5D).

Mechanism of biphasic corrective movements can be explained as below:

- The prism displaces the image towards its base, in other words, from the fovea of the right eye towards a point on the temporal half of the retina (4D or 2° away from the fovea). The relaxation movement of the right eye will elicit conjugate movements of both eyes to the left (levoversion), if the right eye has no foveal suppression (Fig. 8.5B).
- This displaces the image in the left eye from the fovea to the temporal retina and thus the

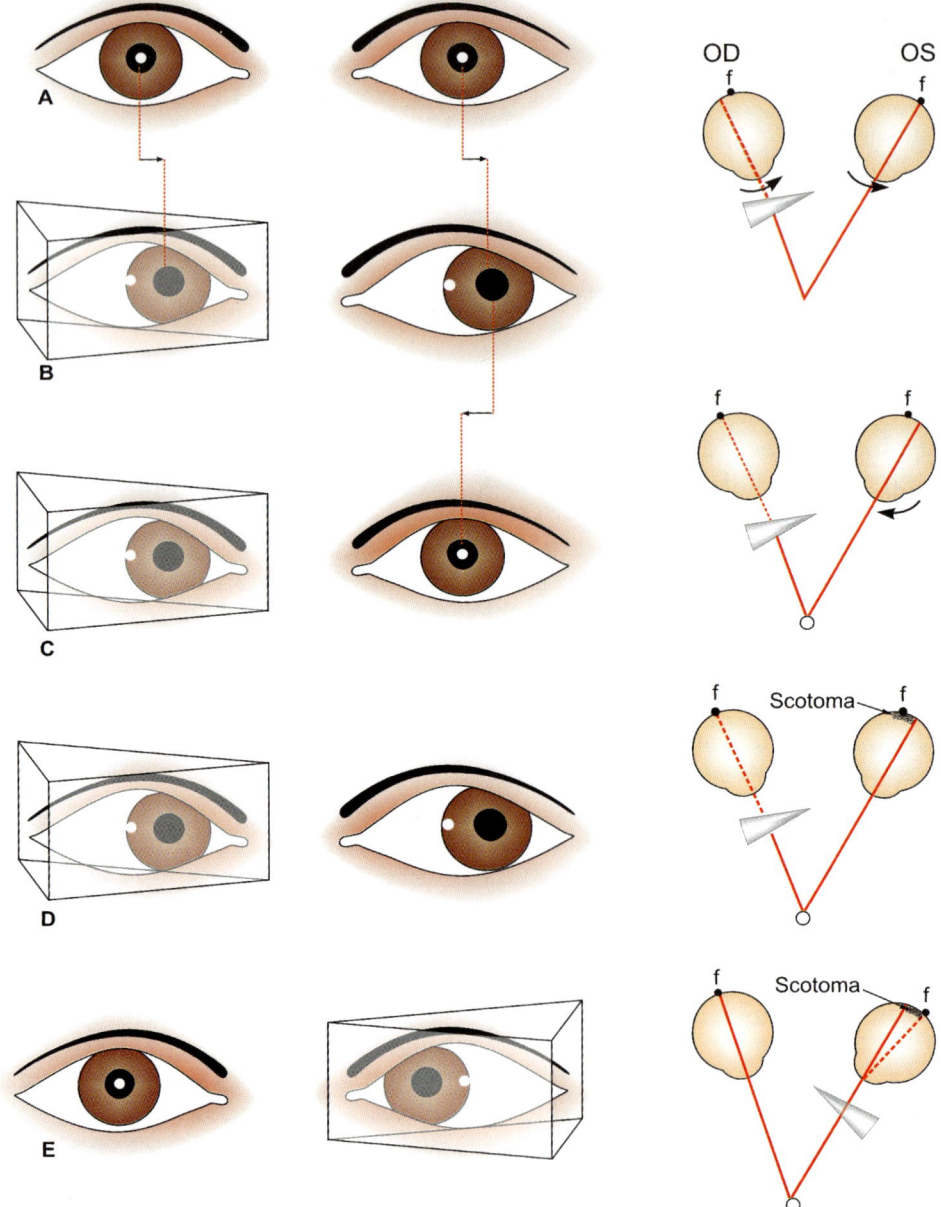

Fig. 8.5 *The 4D base-out prism test with its optical principle (for explanation, see text).*

left eye now makes a fusional movement in the opposite direction, if no foveal suppression is present (Fig. 8.5C). In the presence of central suppression scotomal this will be absent (Fig. 8.5D)

• The test should be repeated with prism over the left eye (Fig. 8.5E) and observation for a biphasic corrective movement in the right eye should be made.

3. **Diplopia test or red glass test.** *See* page 131.

4. **Bagolini's striated glass test.** A foveal (central) suppression scotoma in orthotropic patient or a fixation point scotoma in the presence of microtropia can be detected with Bagolini's striated glass test. As described on page 129 and shown in Fig. 6.31, a patient with fixation point suppression will see a central interruption of the light streak.

5. Visual acuity test with Project-O-Chart slide of American optical. It is a very effective test to detect foveal suppression in patients with microtropia or in patients with subnormal binocular vision after surgical correction of essential infantile esotropia. In this test, visual acuity of each eye is measured under binocular conditions with the Project-O-Chart slide of American optical. Presence of decreased visual acuity in one eye that is not present, when the eye is tested under monocular conditions indicates the foveal suppression.

6. Synoptophore test. Suppression can be diagnosed with the use of simultaneous perception slides (e.g. a cage and a lion) as well as fusion slides (e.g. identical pictures of a rabbit, one having a candle and the other having flower). When simultaneous perception slides are used, normally patient should see the lion in the cage. In the presence of suppression, patient sees either lion or cage.

To begin with, simultaneous foveal perception (SFP) slides are used. When foveal suppression is present, the simultaneous macular perception (SMP) slides are used. In the presence of macular suppression, simultaneous paramacular perception (SPP) slides are used and observations are made. While using fusion slides, if the patient sees a rabbit with both the candle and flower, it indicates normal binocular single vision. In the presence of suppression, either the candle or the flower is absent. The fusion pictures are graded according to the size in the same way as the simultaneous perception pictures.

Suppression scotoma can be mapped out, at least in the horizontal meridian with synoptophore. One arm of the instrument is rotated, and the points are noted at which the target carried by the moving arm disappears and reappears.

Test for measurement of depth of suppression

Depth of suppression is not equal in all the patients. The degree to which facultative suppression can produce obligatory suppression probably depends upon the age of the child, when facultative suppression begins. The deeper the suppression, more difficult it is to overcome.

Depth of suppression can be measured with the help of red filter ladder (Fig. 8.6) which contains a series of red filters of increasing density. The red filter ladder usually consists of gelatine fibres, beginning with one layer and increasing to six or eight layers. The more the layers, the darker the filter.

To measure the depth of suppression, the patient is asked to fixate a small light, and the filters in increasing density are placed in front of the fixating eye till the patient sees double lights. Some patients see double with a filter made of single layer; while the others require filters of three or more layers depending upon the depth of suppression. The greater the number of layers needed, the deeper is the suppression.

TREATMENT OF SUPPRESSION

Indications

The role of antisuppression orthoptic therapy is controversial, since it is not clear whether patients treated by antisuppression orthoptic therapy gain better functional results than others who receive passive treatment such as alternating occlusion or no treatment at all. Further, in some cases, antisuppression therapy may cause either intractable diplopia or confusion as suppression disappears.

In general, suppression should be treated only when one expects to achieve bifoveal single vision. The suitable cases for suppression therapy are:

1. *Patients with intermittent tropias* in whom fusion is present, when the deviation is controlled, are the most suitable cases. In intermittent tropias, the suppression is more superficial than in constant deviation and is, therefore, less difficult to disrupt.

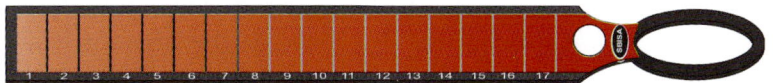

Fig. 8.6 *Red filter ladder used for measuring depth of suppression.*

2. *Patients with convergence insufficiency* and suppression are also suitable candidates for therapy. They should perform antisuppression exercises in conjunction with convergence exercises.

3. *Patients with constant tropias* in whom fusion ability can be demonstrated during examination, usually are those in whom the deviation occurred after about 2½ years of age.

4. *Patients with fully corrected accommodative esotropia* who continue to have an intermittent deviation with suppression, should receive suppression therapy. In such cases, antisuppression exercises should be combined with divergence exercises to increase fusional divergence amplitude.

5. *Postsurgical patients with slight under correction* who are suppressing and thereby inhibiting the potential for fusion also need antisuppression exercises.

Methods of treatment

In fact, therapy for suppression involves the treatment of the strabismus as a whole which includes:

- **Proper refractive correction** wherever indicated to render both eyes emmetropic.
- **Occlusion therapy** to permit equal and alternate use of each eye and to overcome any amblyopia which may be present.
- **Alignment of the visual axes** to permit simultaneous stimulation of corresponding retinal elements by the same object.
- **Antisuppression orthoptic exercises** may be needed before and/or after the surgical therapy of strabismus.

Antisuppression orthoptic exercises

Antisuppression orthoptic exercises are undertaken stepwise to overcome the tendency of the image from one eye to suppress the images from other eye, when both eyes are open. Ideally, the steps involved in antisuppression orthoptic exercises are as follows:

- *First step* is to make the patient *aware of diplopia.*
- *Second step* is to make the patient learn to hold fixation with either eye, always seeing the blurred image from the deviated eye off to the side (*simultaneous perception*). However, if the

deviation is sufficiently large, surgical alignment should be considered first.

- *Third step* is to make the patient learn *fusion* on both an instrument and in free space.
- *Fourth step* is to improve the *fusional amplitude.*

(A) Diplopia exercises

The aim is to make the patient aware of physiological diplopia in heterophoria and intermittent tropia and of diplopia in heterotropia.

1. *Awareness of physiological diplopia.* Awareness of physiological diplopia is an effective means of treating suppression in patients with phorias, intermittent tropias and phorias recently converted from tropias by surgery and/or orthoptics. Patients should be taught to experience both homonymous and heteronymous physiological diplopia (as described below). This will stimulate both the nasal and temporal elements of the retina and thus will help the patient to overcome suppression over the entire retina.

I. *Awareness of homonymous (uncrossed) diplopia.* Patient is asked to make note of light situated about 6 metres from him/her while fixating a light held 33 cm directly in front of his/her nose. While doing so, by practice, patient will learn to see one light at near (33 cm) and two lights at distance (6 metres) simultaneously. Now, if the orthoptist slowly covers and uncovers his/her right eye several times with an occluder, the patient should recognize that the right light at distance intermittently disappears. Similarly, if the left eye is covered, the left light at distance disappears. Thus, patient experiences homonymous (uncrossed) diplopia, due to bilateral nasal retinal stimulation by the distant light while patient is fixating on near light (Fig. 8.7).

II. *Awareness of heteronymous (crossed) diplopia.* Patient is asked to make a note of light held 33 cm in front of his/her nose while fixating a light situated 6 metres away. While doing so, by practice, patient will learn to see one light at distance and two lights at near simultaneously.

Now, if the orthoptist slowly covers and uncovers patient's right eye several times with an occluder, the patient should recognize that

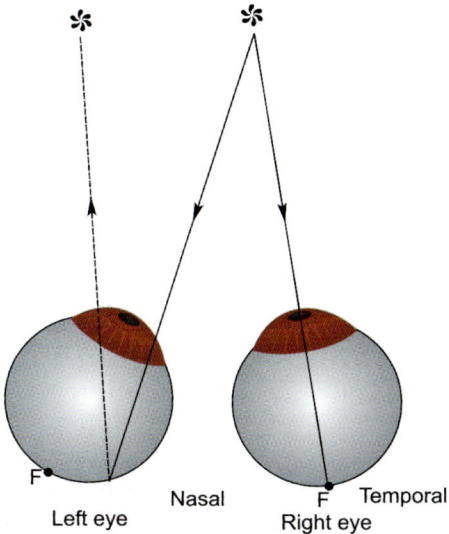

Fig. 8.7 *Homonymous (uncrossed) diplopia.*

the left light situated at near intermittently disappears. Similarly, if the left eye is covered, the right light at near disappears. Thus the patient experiences heteronymous (crossed) diplopia due to bilateral temporal retinal stimulation by the near light while patient is fixating at distant light (Fig. 8.8).

III. Exercises utilizing physiological diplopia

i. Framing. Framing is a good home exercise based on physiological diplopia. Patient is asked to make note of a pencil held at 15 cm in front of his/her nose while fixating at a distant object in

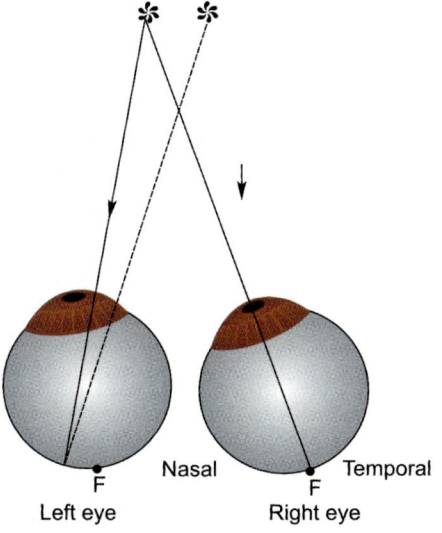

Fig. 8.8 *Heteronymous (crossed) diplopia.*

the room (Fig. 8.9A). Patient should see two pencils and one distant object (awareness of heteronymous diplopia) (Fig. 8.9B). Now the patient is asked to move the pencil away from his/her nose. During this procedure, patient will note that two pencils are moving closer to each other. Similarly, when the pencil is moved towards the nose, its two images will be seen moving farther apart from each other. Once the patient learns this, he/she is asked to fix at different distant objects in the room and move the pencil backward or forward so that the distant object is framed between the two pencils, i.e. the object is centred with pencils touching its each side (Fig. 8.9C).

ii. Bar reading. Bar reading exercise is also based on the principle of awareness of crossed physiological diplopia. Patient is asked to hold bar (thumb, finger, pencil or any other bar) about 5–6 cm from his/her nose and asked to read a print kept at about 33 cm from his/her eyes (Fig. 6.43). As the patient reads the print binocularly, he/she perceives the bar in crossed diplopia, each image of the bar hiding a portion of the print from one eye, but not the other, so that patient can read the print normally. Such a practice of maintaining the correct position of his/her eyes despite the obstacle will strengthen the binocular vision of the patient. However, till suppression is present, he/she will see only one bar, which will hide some of the print and thus continuous reading will be impossible. So, the patient will either shift his/her head or move the bar to see the print.

The better way to eradicate suppression with this exercise is to start the patient with a few large letters on a card. Slowly the amount of letters on a line may be increased and the size of the letters decreased as the suppression disappears until he/she can easily read a page of small print.

2. Diplopia exercises with coloured filters. These exercises are based on the fact that a patient with strabismus suppresses similar images in contrast to normal person who tends to suppress dissimilar images. In this exercise, patient is asked to fixate a white light and a red filter is placed in front of one eye and a green filter in front of the other eye. The dissimilar images produced by the filters are sufficient to

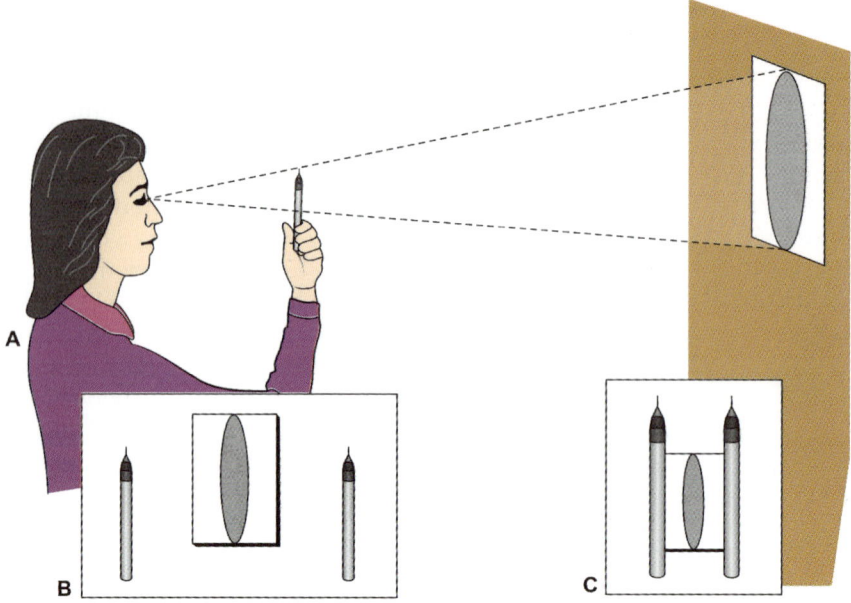

Fig. 8.9 *Framing — a home exercise for suppression (for explanation, see text).*

overcome suppression in most instances and produce diplopia. After the diplopia is evoked, patient is asked to look alternately from one image to the other. During this process, first one filter and then the other is removed in an attempt to have the patient notice diplopia without the help of filters. When patient is able to do so, the fixation light is exchanged for another fixation object which is a less intense stimulus. In this way, patient should be taught diplopia during both near and distance fixations.

3. *Diplopia exercise with prisms.* In this orthoptic exercise, a vertical prism (base up or down) sufficient enough to displace the image outside the suppression scotoma is placed in front of one eye. Consequently, the patient will have diplopia. Gradually, the prism power is reduced until finally the patient has diplopia without any vertical displacement of one image. Once the patient learns to perceive diplopia without prism, the fixation light is then replaced by a less intense stimulus. In this way, patient should be taught diplopia during both near and distance fixations.

(B) *Exercises with use of red filter*

1. *To treat suppression at near,* a red filter is placed over the dominant eye and patient

(depending upon his/her age and interest) is asked to do any of the following exercises:
• Colour, trace or draw with a red pencil matching the red filter.
• Little girls may follow red design drawn on a white cloth with a needle and a light red or pink thread.
• Children can draw lines with a red pencil using the number-to-number games in their colouring books.
• Children can also select red beads for a necklace
• The boys can play ping-pong with a red ball.

2. *To treat suppression at distance,* patient may be asked to watch colour television with the red filter over the dominant eye.

(C) *Exercises with major amblyoscope*

1. *Macular massage.* This exercise stimulates the retina of deviated eye. It is accomplished by moving the visual target on the major amblyo-scope back and forth across the suppression scotoma (macular massage) as below:

The major amblyoscope tubes having slides of paramacular simultaneous perception are locked at the patient's objective angle. While he/she looks constantly straight ahead, the tubes are moved rapidly from side to side over a large arc. Since they are at the objective angle, the images moving over the retina will always stimulate normally corresponding areas. In the periphery, they will be superimposed. When approaching the suppression area, however, one picture will disappear or the two will separate. The excursion of the tubes is gradually reduced until eventually the patient can maintain superim-position while looking at the pictures, when tubes are held still.

2. *Crossing technique.* A pair of paramacular simultaneous perception slides is put in the tubes of major amblyoscope. Patient is asked to fixate the target viewed by the dominant eye, while the target in front of the suppressed eye is moved in from the periphery of the field towards the suppression scotoma. It will disappear, when it reaches the suppressed area and reappear on the other side after the entire scotoma has been crossed. This back and forth movement of the target across the suppression area is continued until this area has decreased to such an extent that the patient can simultaneously perceive both targets and can superimpose the two images. In normal correspondence, peripheral size targets may be used first followed by macular and foveal size targets.

3. *Chasing technique.* It is a technique of subjective exercise using the smallest simultaneous perception slides that the patient can superimpose. The two arms of the major amblyoscope are loosened and the patient is asked to hold the handle of the tube in front of the suppressed eye. The examiner moves the picture tube that is in front of the fixating eye in a random position. The patient is asked to chase it and superimpose the two pictures by moving the other tube. This chasing technique is exercised repeatedly. As the patient's performance improves, increasingly smaller pictures are used until he/she can superimpose the foveal slides.

(D) Exercises with cheiroscope

The cheiroscope is a very good instrument for antisuppression training. For details *see* page 144.

(E) Exercises with Tibb's binocular trainer

Tibb's binocular trainer is an excellent instrument for antisuppression exercise, especially for home. For details *see* page 144.

MONOFIXATION SYNDROME

Definition and causes

Monofixation syndrome, also known as Park's syndrome, is the term coined by Marshal Park for the sensory adaptation occurring in patients with microtropia (angle of strabismus <10 PD).

Other clinical situations associated with monofixation syndrome are:
- Anisometropic amblyopia, unilateral astigmatism and
- Unilateral partial cataract.

Characteristic features

It is characterized by absence of bifoveal fusion (unilateral central suppression) with the presence of peripheral fusion.
- *Central suppression* in the microtropic eye occurs because the central retina has small receptive field and high spatial resolution potential, so relatively small difference in image clarity or retinal image position are recognized. Patients with monofixation syndrome usually have stereo acuity in the range of 30 to 70 seconds of arc and the central scotoma measures between 2° and 5°.
- *Peripheral fusion* is maintained because in the peripheral field slight interocular image differences are not detected since the peripheral retina has large receptive field and relatively low spatial resolution. Small retinal image discrepancies between fellow eyes are, therefore, not disruptive in the peripheral fields and so peripheral fusion is maintained.

AMBLYOPIA

Amblyopia, by definition refers to, a partial loss of sight in one or both eyes, caused by abnormal visual development secondary to abnormal visual stimulation in the absence of ophthalmoscopic or other marked objective signs. Literally speaking, amblyopia is a spectrum of visual loss, ranging from missing a few letters on the 20/20 lines to hand motion vision.

However, for practical purposes, amblyopia is labelled, when there is at least two Snellen lines difference in the visual acuity between the eyes. Amblyopia occurring in a patient with strabismus is not a sensory adaptation per se, but the consequence of suppression which is a sensory adaptation.

CLASSIFICATION AND TERMINOLOGY

The self-explanatory terms used for amblyopia in present day orthoptic practice are as follows:

1. Strabismic amblyopia. The term strabismic amblyopia is used for the amblyopia seen in those patients with unilateral constant squint who strongly favour one eye for fixation from birth to 6 years of age. Peak age for development of fixation preference in strabismic children is about 1 year (range 9 months to 24 years).

Strabismic amblyopia is a common form of amblyopia and typically shows following features that are uncommon in other forms of amblyopia:

- *Grating acuity* is often considerably less reduced than the Snellen's acuity. This is because forms seen by the affected eye are in a twisted or distorted manner that interfere more with letter recognition than with the simpler task of determining whether a grating is present or not.
- *Neutral density filter effect,* i.e. when illumination is decreased, the acuity of an eye with strabismic amblyopia does not decline further while it does so in organic amblyopia.
- *Laterality,* strabismic amblyopia is always unilateral and is caused by an active inhibition within the retinocortical pathways of visual input originating in the fovea of the deviating eye. Strabismic amblyopia follows through a stage of suppression, giving rise to the term suppression amblyopia.
- *Type of strabismus.* Strabismic amblyopia is seen far more often in esotropes than the exotropes. This might be related to the fact that in esotropia, the fovea of the deviating eye has to compete with the strong temporal hemifield of the fellow eye; while in exotropia, the fovea of the deviating eye has to compete with the weaker contralateral nasal hemifield.
- *Strabismic amblyopia occurs very rarely in patients with hypertropia,* as they usually manage to maintain fusion in some positions of gaze with an anomalous head posture.
- *Patients with alterante strabismus do not have amblyopia* but they do have abnormal binocular function.

2. Stimulus (visual) deprivation amblyopia. It is caused by those conditions wherein one eye is prevented from seeing early in life. Such conditions would include:

- Monocular congenital or traumatic cataract
- Complete ptosis
- Corneal opacity and
- Prolonged patching of the normal eye for treatment of amblyopia (occlusion amblyopia).

Constant monocular occlusion of the visual axis for more than a weak per year of life places a child at significant risk for the development of stimulus deprivation amblyopia until about 5–6 years of age.

Deprivation amblyopia is characterized by following features:

- It is the least common but most damaging and difficult to treat form of amblyopia.
- Amblyopic visual loss resulting from unilateral deprivation is worse than that produced by bilateral deprivation of similar degree. This is because of the fact that in the unilateral deprivation, interocular effects add to the direct developmental impact of severe image degradation.

Bilateral deprivational amblyopia may develop in small children with bilateral media opacities, e.g.:

- Bilateral congenital cataract
- Bilateral corneal opacities (Peter's anomaly)
- Bilateral vitreous haemorrhage

3. Refractive amblyopia occurs due to consistent defocus of the retinal image in one or both eyes due to presence of refractive error. It can be of following subtypes:

- *Anisometropic amblyopia.* The term anisometropic amblyopia refers to the amblyopia occurring in an eye having higher degree of refractive error than the fellow eye.
- *Anisohypermetropic versus anisomyopic amblyopia.* It has been reported that amblyopia is more common and is of a higher degree in patients with anisohypermetropia than in those

with anisomyopia. Even 1.5 to 2 dioptre hyperopic anisometropia may cause amblyopia while up to 3 dioptre myopic anisometropia usually does not cause amblyopia. However, unilateral high myopia (–6D or more) often results in severe amblyopia. It has been presumed that both the forms, vision deprivation as well as the abnormal binocular interaction that is caused by unequal foveal images in the two eyes, might be playing role in the development of anisometropic amblyopia.

Strabismus is frequently associated with anisometropia. In such cases whether amblyopia occurs due to anisometropia or strabismus or both is very difficult to determine.

• *Meridional amblyopia.* This refers to amblyopia occurring in patients with uncorrected astigmatic refractive error due to selective visual deprivation for visual stimuli of a certain spatial orientation. Thus, meridional amblyopia is a selective amblyopia for a specific visual meridian. 1.25D of arriso astigmatism may cause amblyopia.

• *Isoametropic amblyopia.* Isoametropic amblyopia is bilateral amblyopia occurring in children with bilateral uncorrected high refractive error. Hyperopia of more than +5.0D and myopia in excess of –10.0D have a risk of inducing bilateral amblyopia. Such amblyopia is usually of milder form. It is supposed to result from the effect of blurred retinal images alone (pattern vision deprivation). Bilateral meridional amblyopia is caused by bilateral astigmatism. Significant meridional amblyopia occurs with astigmatism greater than –2.5D.

PATHOGENESIS AND PATHOPHYSIOLOGY OF AMBLYOPIA

Despite an enormous research in this field, pathogenesis and pathophysiology of amblyopia is still not elucidated fully. However, the clinical features and laboratory findings in eyes with amblyopia permit certain conclusions for understanding the nature of the processes underlying amblyopia and its treatment. Psychophysical studies in human strabismic, anisometropic and visual deprivation amblyopia show differences between the function of the fovea versus the retinal periphery. Further, there

are also differences in the severity and reversibility of the various types of amblyopia. However, the most pertinent factual knowledge about the changes occurring in amblyopia which has been obtained through experimental studies (electrophysiologic and histopathologic) in kittens suggests that the structural and functional involvement of the afferent visual pathway in different forms of amblyopia is the same as is the sensitive period during which amblyopia occurs, regardless of the etiology. Therefore, on the basis of this recent neurophysiologic reasearch, largely done in experimental animals, it has been postulated that the basic amblyogenic mechanisms are—light deprivation, foveal form vision deprivation, abnormal binocular interaction and active cortical inhibition.

The initial development of amblyopia from any cause rarely occurs in children older than about 5–6 years. However, once amblyopia has developed and has been treated with therapy, it may recur until about 9–11 years of age.

Pathophysiology of amblyopia thus can be discussed under following headings:
• Amblyogenic factors,
• Role of retina in the development of amblyopia, and
• Active cortical inhibition

[A] AMBLYOGENIC FACTORS

The basic mechanisms responsible for amblyopia, which have been recognized on the basis of neurophysiologic research, largely done in experimental animals, are as follows:

• Deprivation of form vision
• Light deprivation
• Abnormal binocular interaction

1. Deprivation of form vision

• *Monocular deprivation of form vision* during the critical period of visual development results in amblyopia of the deprived eye. Since the deprived eye becomes dominated by the normal eye so a *competitive amblyopia* of profound intensity develops. Monocular visual deprivation works as an amblyogenic factor in strabismic, anisometropic, stimulus deprivation ambloypia.
• *Binocular deprivation of form vision* during the critical period of visual development results

in bilateral deprivational amblyopia. Since in binocular deprivation, the binocular interaction is not disrupted so a competitive amblyopia is not superimposed; so the resultant amblyopia not so severe as in unilateral deprivation. Binocular deprivation plays the role of amblyogenic factor in children with bilateral cataract, ametropia and bilateral high refractive errors.

2. Light deprivation

Light deprivation works as an amblyogenic factor in children with unilateral as well as bilateral complete cataracts.

3. Abnormal binocular interaction

Abnormal binocular interaction is highly amblyogenic. It produces a profound amblyopia due to a competition amblyopia. Abnormal binocular interaction plays the role of amblyogenic factor in children with strabismic, anisometropic and unilateral stimulus deprivation amblyopia.

Thus, the amblyogenic factors for different types of amblyopia are same. However, their contribution to each may vary and so is the severity of amblyopia (Table 8.1).

Neurophysiological basis of role of amblyogenic factors

The above conclusions about the role of various amblyogenic mechanisms have been drawn from the various experimental studies done in cat, kitten and monkey. A few key studies to understand the neurophysiologic basis of normal binocular vision and amblyopia are described briefly here.

Neurophysiologic basis of normal binocular vision

Hubel and Wiesel are pioneers in the neurophysiologic studies of binocular vision. They have concluded that in normal cat or kitten:

• Approximately 80% neurons of striate cortex are derived from each eye, 10% from the contralateral eye and 10% from the ipsilateral eye only. The two receptive fields of binocularly driven cortical cells are found to have corresponding location in the two retinae.

• Of the binocularly driven cortical neurons, only 25% are stimulated equally well from each eye, while the remaining 75% show graded degree of influence from the right or left eye (disparity sensitive binocular cells). Stereopsis has been linked with horizontal disparity sensitive binocularly driven cortical neurons.

• It has been reported that at birth (i.e. without previous visual experience or training) the visual system of kittens gives responses which are in no way different from those obtained in adult cats. From this, the conclusion was drawn that the basis for visual recognition and binocular interaction is already fully developed at birth. The immaturity of visually dependent behaviour in young animals, such as the lack of pursuit movements, therefore, cannot be explained by incomplete development but must be due to other factors, possibly lack of interpretation/visuomotor cooperation.

Types of amblyopia	Amblyogenic factors			
	Light deprivation	Deprivation of form vision	Abnormal binocular interaction	Severity of amblyopia
• Stimulus deprivation amblyopia				
– Unilateral (e.g. cataract)	+	+	+	+ + +
– Bilateral (e.g. cataract)	+	+	–	+ +
• Strabismic amblyopia	–	+	+	+ +
• Anisometropic amblyopia	–	+	+	+ +
• Ametropic amblyopia	–	+	–	+

Table 8.1 *Role of amblyogenic factors in different types of amblyopia*

- To understand the pathophysiologic mechanisms concerned with binocular vision and development of amblyopia, the visual pathway carrying visual sensations from the retina to visual cortex have been classified in X, Y and W-system (Fig. 8.10) as follows:

X-system. The fibres from the retinal ganglion cells carrying the sustained response to visual stimuli are found in the X-cell system—the medium velocity system. The X-system is associated with central form vision and, therefore, central visual acuity. Cells of this system project only to the lateral geniculate nucleus.

Y-system. The fibres from the retinal ganglion cells carrying a transient response are in the Y-cell, or fast system. The Y-system is associated with the peripheral retina and is concerned with the location of objects in space, which enables fixation movements to be made. This system projects to both the lateral geniculate nuclei and superior colliculus.

W-cell system (slow system). It is believed to be the pursuit system. It projects only to superior colliculus.

Neurophysiologic studies in experimental and clinical amblyopia

Neurophysiology of amblyopia is a complex mechanism and its understanding is far from complete. Some of the observations made from the study of experimental modification of visual experience in animals and laboratory testing of amblyopic human beings are given below.

Monocular deprivation studies

Methods. Monocular deprivation was produced in experimental animals (kitten and monkey) by suturing the eyelids of one eye during the critical period of development.

Observations are as below:
- Deprived eye developed amblyopia, probably because this eye was dominated by the normal eye due to the interruption in binocular co-operation.
- Changes observed in visual system neuron functions were as follows:
  - In the lateral geniculate body, cells in those layers receiving input from the deprived eye showed a profound shrinkage. Larger cells shrank more than the smaller ones.
  - Cells of primary visual cortex either lost their innate ability to respond to stimulation or showed significant functional deficiency.

It has been reported that there occurs a selective reduction in the number of cortical cells driven by Y-input from retina, suggesting that perhaps visual deprivation selectively involves the Y-system.

Note. Similar experiments in adult animals did not reveal such changes.

Conclusions. These studies indicate that uniocular visual deprivation produces amblyopia by changes in the visual system neurons. It has also been concluded that deprivation during the

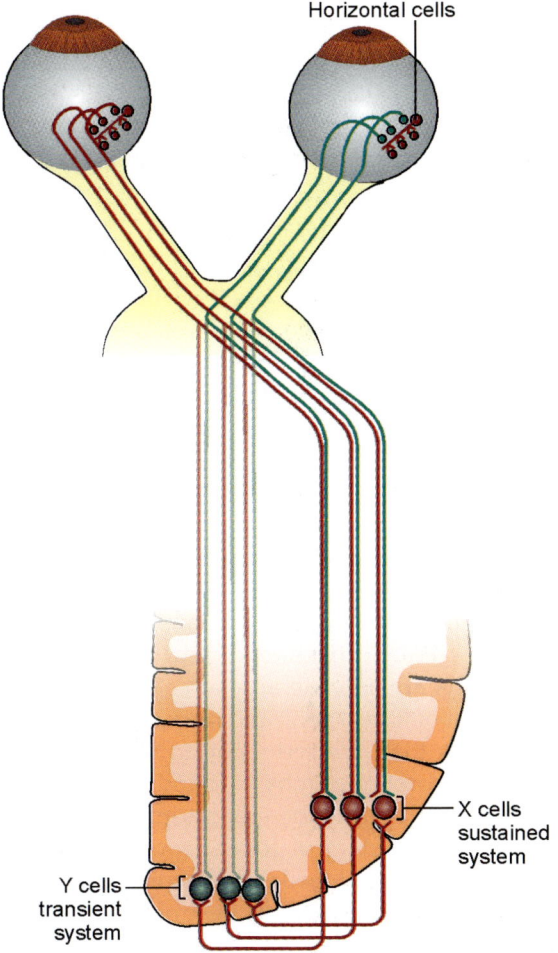

Horizontal cells

X cells sustained system

Y cells transient system

Fig. 8.10 *X, Y and W-system of cells in the visual cortex.*

early part of critical period of development is more deleterious than at a later stage. This experimental work of uniocular deprivation closely resembles the clinical situation of unilateral cataract, severe congenital ptosis or corneal opacity producing profound amblyopia.

Binocular deprivation studies

Technique. Binocular visual deprivation was made by bilateral tarsorrhaphy in kittens and monkeys during sensitive period of development and also in visually mature animals and following *observations* made were as below:

- A mild bilateral amblyopia occurred in infant animals due to visual deprivation. Perhaps amblyopia was mild due to the fact that the competition amblyopia was not superimposed since the binocular interaction was not abnormal in binocular equal deprivation.
- Changes observed in visual system neuron functions were as follows:
  - Cell shrinkage produced in lateral geniculate body was less than that produced in uniocular deprivation.
  - There occurred a decrease in the specific responsiveness of cells and an increase in number of cells that respond sluggishly or abnormally. In addition, there were many cells that did not respond at all.
  - The number of Y-cells was reduced by 307%.
  - It was postulated that in binocular deprivation, there may be a competition for synaptic space in the cortex between the X-cells and the more disadvantaged Y-cells.

Conclusions. The amblyopia produced by binocular deprivation was less severe than that produced by uniocular deprivation, owing to the fact that binocular interaction was not abnormal. This work closely resembles the clinical situations of bilateral amblyopia seen in children with bilateral cataract and also to some extent the ametropic amblyopia.

Experimental strabismus amblyopic

In monkeys made artificially strabismic, by disinserting lateral or medial rectus, only the binocular portion of the lateral geniculate body showed cell shrinkage, while in visually deprived monkeys, both the monocular and binocular portions of the lateral geniculate nucleus showed shrinkage. Thus, two different neural mechanisms appear to underlie the deprivational and strabismic amblyopia. However, it has been postulated that visual deprivation (since central fixation is not used in strabismus), abnormal binocular interaction and active cortical inhibition similar to that occurs, in suppression, all play a role in the amblyopia associated with strabismus. While this seems reasonable intuitively and laboratory findings suggest this, but definitive proof is still lacking.

Exprerimental anisometropic amblyopia

Experimental anisometropic amblyopia was produced in primates by putting high plus convex lens in one eye and/or atropine. Observations made were as below:

- *Visual cortex cells* of striate cortex layer IV and outside layer IV (driven by the involved eye and a fraction of binocular driven cells) had reduced contrast sensitivity.
- *Lateral geniculate body* showed anatomical changes in the form of diminution of cell size limited only to the parvicellular layers that subserve high spatial frequency.

[B] ROLE OF RETINA IN DEVELOPMENT OF AMBLYOPIA

There is some evidence that the retina itself is abnormal in amblyopia. Whether retinal abnormality is the effect or cause of amblyopia is debatable. The views have differed, if retinal threshold and sensitivity have been affected in amblyopia. It is, however, widely believed and proved experimentally that there is a decreased sensitivity of foveal cones in amblyopia. Even flicker fusion threshold and differential thresholds are considerably affected. However, reduction of foveal cone and retinal sensitivity is much less than the reduction in visual acuity. Also electroretinography is found to be normal in amblyopic eyes. It, therefore, is improbable that a functional defect of foveal cones would be responsible for reduced visual acuity. However, amblyopic eye is not at its best under photopic condition than under mesopic conditions. In fact it has been observed that there is a quicker dark adaptation in such eyes suggesting takeover of rod functions from decreased retinal foveal cones. It is, therefore, logical to believe that reduced inputs from the rods and cones in the affected eye cause certain neurophysiological changes, transmitted aberrantly to the CNS which triggers the onset of amblyopia. The vicious circle continues, till the process is reversed. It may become irreversible in later stages.

That retinal sensitivity is related to onset of amblyopia is further proved by the fact that eyes which had relatively poor sensitivity, responded to amblyopia treatment better than those which had better retinal thresholds. Perhaps a different mechanism is also responsible, i.e. a central suppression exists in amblyopia.

[C] ACTIVE CORTICAL INHIBITION

The neurophysiologic research points out that visual deprivation and active cortical inhibition are the two fundamental mechanisms for the development of amblyopia. The role of active cortical inhibition is evidenced by following studies.

1. *Physiologic evidence.* In one study, in experimental animals, deprivation amblyopia was produced in one eye. After 5 months of deprivation, these animals, were divided into two groups. In group-I animals the normal eye was enucleated, while in group-II, the normal was retained and following observations were made:

In group-I animals (with normal eye enucleated), the amblyopic eye was found to drive 31% of the visual cortex cells. While in group-II animals, in which normal eye was retained, only 6% of the visual cortex cells were driven by the amblyopic eye. In other words, after removal of the normal eye, the deprived eye showed marked capacity for recovery indicating thereby that perhaps the normal eye may be responsible for an active cortical inhibition in unilateral amblyopia.

2. *Pharmacologic evidence.* It has been ascertained that under normal circumstances, most of the excitatory synapses in the visual cortex are cholinergic. Further, it has also been reported that the visual cortex is inhibited by the gamma aminobutyric acid (GABA)—an inhibitory neurotransmitter. The assumption that perhaps in amblyopia, active cortical inhibition might be mediated by GABA led the researchers to perform certain experiments.

Duffy et al. produced deprivation amblyopia in kittens and studied the effects of some anti-GABA agents. Following observations were made by them:

– *Intravenous injection of biculline* (an anti-GABA agent) led to stimulation of 60% visual cortex cells which were otherwise unresponsive due to deprivation amblyopia. However, convulsions were noted as a complication of this drug.

– *Intravenous injection of naloxone,* another anti-GABA agent, also restored binocular inputs in the visual cortex cells which were otherwise unresponsive due to deprivation amblyopia.

Kasamatsu and Pettigrew produced depletion of brain catecholamines by using 6-hydroxy-dopamine and norepinephrine and observed a failure of ocular dominance shift after monocular occlusion in kittens.

The above studies provide a pharmacologic evidence of the role of active cortical inhibition in the amblyopia. However, further studies will reveal as to where we stand in understanding the pathological basis of onset of amblyopia.

CLINICAL CHARACTERISTICS AND LABORATORY FINDINGS IN AMBLYOPIA

1. Visual acuity. Amblyopia, by definition, refers to a partial loss of sight in one or both eyes in the absence of ophthalmoscopic and other marked objective signs. It has been recommended that a difference of two lines on a visual acuity chart should be there to diagnose amblyopia. However, strictly speaking, any difference between the two eyes especially in strabismic amblyopia should be considered significant.

Certain clinical characteristics associated with visual acuity in patients with amblyopia are as follows:

i. *Recognition acuity* (Snellen's or similar charts) is more affected than the resolution acuity (Teller's chart or VER) and the detection acuity (Catford drum test or Bailey-Hall cereal test).

ii. *Snellen's acuity and grating acuity* are affected equally in anisometropic amblyopia whereas in strabismic amblyopia, the grating acuity is affected to half the extent of Snellen's acuity. Thus, strabismic amblyopia is under-estimated on grating test.

iii. *Effect of neutral density filter.* It has been reported that when visual acuity is tested with a neutral density filter placed in front of the affected eye, the visual acuity improves by one or two lines in patients with developmental amblyopia; while in patients with organic amblyopia, the visual acuity decreases by two to three lines. Therefore, the *neutral density filter test* has been recommended to differentiate between developmental amblyopia and organic amblyopia.

The neutral density filter test is based on the fact that under photopic conditions, visual acuity of amblyopic eye is less than that under scotopic conditions. Since the neutral density filter, when placed in front of an eye, produces a state of scotopic conditions, the vision of amblyopic eye improves.

iv. *Crowding phenomenon.* Crowding pheno-menon, also known as *separation difficulty,* refers to the inability of an amblyopic eye to distinguish letters (or other symbols) crowded together. Therefore, the vision in an amblyopic eye is better, when tested with isolated optotypes than when tested with line or Snellen's acuity charts having rows of letters. In other words, single optotype visual acuity is better than linear visual acuity. The larger the discrepancy between the linear and single letter acuity, the poorer the prognosis.

Crowding phenomenon is the result of contour-interaction between the neighbouring test targets because of decreased lateral inhibition in amblyopia.

2. Fixation pattern. Amblyopia may be associated with central fixation, eccentric viewing or eccentric fixation. In a normal eye, three characteristics of foveolar area, which appear to be responsible for maintaining the fixation reflex central, are:

a. Peak visual acuity in the foveolar region,
b. A principal occulocentric direction of straight ahead, and
c. A retinomotor value of zero.

Amblyopia with central fixation. In amblyopia with foveolar fixation, the foveola has preserved the principal visual direction and its zero retinomotor value. Amblyopia is secondary to a central suppression scotoma.

Amblyopia with eccentric viewing. In amblyopia with eccentric viewing, patients prefer to view with an extrafoveal point bacause of the deep suppression scotoma, but the fovea has still not lost its principal visual direction. In eccentric viewing, patients look past the object they have been asked to fix. This can be demonstrated during visuscopic examination of a co-operative patient, who will tell the examiner that he/she is aware of the fact that he/she has to look over to one side to see the star clearly and when he/she looks straight ahead the fixation target appears blurred. The examiner can also observe that in eccentric viewing, patient will place the image of fixation target first on the fovea and then immediately from the fovea on to the paramacular retinal elements.

Amblyopia with eccentric fixation. In amblyopia with eccentric fixation, the fovea has lost its principal visual direction, its retinal motor value is no longer zero and an extrafoveal point is now the bearer of these properties. Patients report that they are looking straight at an object stimulating non-foveolar retinal area. If the image of an object is placed on the patient's fovea (by means of an instrument), this object is sensed as being in some other direction than straight ahead.

Types of eccentric fixation. Depending upon the retinal area with which the eyes appear to fixate, the eccentric fixation may be of following types (Fig. 8.11):

• *Parafoveolar*—just outside the foveal reflex.
• *Parafoveal*—outside but close to foveal wall.
• *Paramacular*—on or just outside the rim of the macula. Many workers have now abandoned the use of this term because of vague ophthal-moscopic definition of the macula.
• *Peripheral*—outside the macula, anywhere between the macula and extreme retinal periphery.

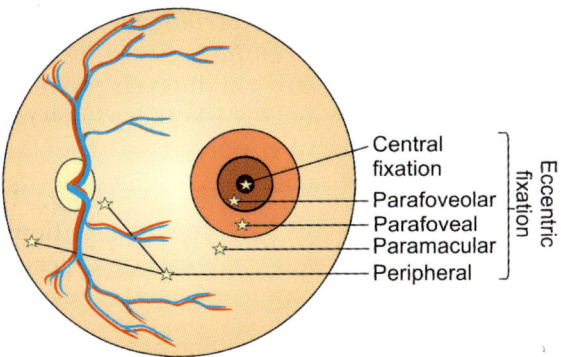

Fig. 8.11 *Types of fixation pattern.*

Steady versus wandering fixation. Central as well as eccentric fixation may be steady or wandering. Wandering fixation, which occurs only upon covering the sound eye, must be distinguished from the monocular, spontaneous, pendular and vertical oscillations that are occasionally found in deeply amblyopic eyes. This condition has been designated as the *Heimann-Bielschowsky phenomenon.* It is clinically similar to other forms of monocular nystagmus that may occur in connection with posterior fossa or brainstem disorders.

Paradoxical eccentric fixations. Ordinarily, there develop nasal eccentricity in esotropic and temporal eccentricity in exotropic patients. However, sometimes the eccentric fixation may be paradoxical, i.e. reverse of the expected situation. In other words, there may be nasal eccentricity in exotropic and temporal eccentricity in esotropic patients. Such a situation can occur under following circumstances:
- Following surgical overcorrection of the deviation.
- In patients with spontaneous reversal of the deviation.
- Following prolonged occlusion of the sound eye in amblyopia.
- With no obvious cause (rarely).

3. Absolute central scotoma. Monocular scotometry on visual field charting may plot an absolute central scotoma. Visual field charting for this purpose should never be done binocularly, otherwise, a facultative binocular suppression scotoma (present only with binocular viewing) may be mistaken as the absolute central scotoma. The scotometry may

not be possible in amblyopic, patients with unsteady fixation.

4. Localization of an object of regard. Localization of an object of regard is normal in patients having amblyopia with central as well as eccentric fixation. However, in patients having amblyopia with eccentric viewing, localization of an object of regard is faulty.

5. Colour vision. Colour vision anomalies may occur in patients with amblyopia only if visual acuity is markedly reduced below 6/36. Anomalous colour vision in such cases has been related to peripheral eccentric fixation, i.e. a peripheral retinal area is being used for fixation rather than foveola.

6. Light perception. There occurs a dissociation of the form vision and light perception in amblyopia, since form vision is abnormal (especially under photopic condition) while absolute light threshold is found to be normal. However, differential threshold (i.e. how much brighter the test field must be than its surrounding so that a difference is perceived) is elevated in amblyopia.

7. Pupillary light reflexes. Generally speaking, pupillary light reflex is normal in amblyopes. However, rarely in patients with a deep amblyopia, an afferent pupillary defect may occur. It has been suggested that perhaps the afferent pupillary defect may result from synaptic inhibition in the retina, since this pathway does not reach the geniculate body.

8. Light and dark adaptation. Usually, dark adaptation is not abnormal in amblyopes, though a significant difference in adaptation between amblyopic and normal eyes has been found in the region of Kohlrausch's bend (the kink or bend in the adaptation curve normally produced by increased sensitivity of the rods).

9. Critical flicker frequency (CFF). It has been reported that in amblyopia, central CFF tends to approach the CFF of peripheral retina or of rod mechanism. It has also been reported that CFF is significantly faster in amblyopic eyes that fixated eccentrically than in those with foveal fixation. Some workers have reported that examination of CFF with a simple apparatus is a useful tool to distinguish reduced visual acuity in maculopathies from amblyopia, since in the former the thresholds are below normal.

10. Electroretinography (ERG) and electro-oculography (EOG). An enormous data is available on ERG studies in amblyopia, however, till date it has not been definitely answered whether ERG is normal or abnormal in amblyopia. Many studies report that ERG is essentially normal and EOG shows unsteadiness of fixation in amblyopia.

EVALUATION AND DIAGNOSIS

Diagnosis of amblyopia is made by a reduced best corrected visual acuity that cannot be entirely explained on the basis of physical ocular abnormalities. Clinical evaluation of a suspected case of amblyopia should include the following:

1. Evaluation of visual acuity.
2. Neutral density filter test.
3. Test for crowding phenomenon.
4. Thorough ocular examination including fundus examination.
5. Refraction.
6. Evaluation for central versus eccentric fixation.
7. Tests for other sensory anomalies.

1. Evaluation for visual acuity. As mentioned above, clinical evaluation of visual acuity is most important for the diagnosis of amblyopia. Generally speaking, a difference of two lines between the best corrected visual acuity of the two eyes (e.g. OD 6/6, OS 6/12 or OD 6/5, OS 6/9) is considered diagnostic for amblyopia. For practical purposes, particularly after amblyopia treatment has started, any acuity difference is considered amblyopia.

Severity of amblyopia. In the "Amblyopia treatment study (ATS) group trials, amblyopia has been graded as below:

- *Mild to moderate* amblyopia is defined as visual acuity in the amblyopic eye of 20/80 or betta.
- *Severe amblyopia* is defined as visual acuity in the amblyopic eye of 20/100 to 20/400.

Methods employed to evaluate visual acuity depend upon the age of the patient and have been described in detail on page 48. However, for a ready reference, important points for different age groups are mentioned as follows.

Methods for evaluating visual potential in infants and very young children (up to 2½ years of age). Infancy and early childhood is probably the most important age to be bothered, since it is the most sensitive period to develop amblyopia. At the same time, testing of vision during this period is also not so easy. However, untiring efforts should be made to detect unequality of vision in two eyes. Certain useful methods are as follows:

Fixation behaviour test. Fixation behaviour test is a reliable and useful test in infancy to obtain a rough estimate of visual acuity. Each eye is covered alternately and behaviour of the infant is noticed. If vision is equal or nearly equal in both eyes, an infant or very young child will not object to having either eye covered. However, if the visual acuity is reduced in one eye, the child will show objection (in the form of a cry or pushing the occluder away) when the normal eye is covered. In such cases, one should suspect any ocular disease, high refractive error or amblyopia.

A rough estimate of visual acuity can be made by testing with brightly coloured toys of varying size while occluding one eye. It is noticed whether the child can fix and follow the toy.

Binocular fixation pattern (BFP). The binocular fixation pattern, indicating strength of preference for one eye or the other under binocular viewing conditions, is generally relied upon for estimating the relative level of vision in two eyes for very young children with strabismus. It is important to note that, when the infant's binocular fixation pattern is tested, an accommodative target such as small toy should be used. A child with extremely unequal vision will show great preference for the good eye. A child with nearly equal vision will have only mild preference for one eye. Five grades of binocular fixation pattern described while making the patient fix with the deviated eye (Table 8.2).

Binocular fixation pattern test is quite sensitive for detecting amblyopia but is sometimes false positive (showing a strong preference, when vision is equal or nearly equal in the two eyes), particularly with small-angle strabismic deviations.

Table 8.2 *Grading of binocular fixation pattern in strabismic patients*

Grade	Description of response
Grade 0	: Spontaneous alternation (no preference for one eye).
Grade 1	: Holds fixation through blink (simply prefers one eye but can use the other eye with nearly equal frequency).
Grade 2	: Holds fixation until blink, i.e. habitually fixing eye resumes fixation with the next blink (moderate fixation preference).
Grade 3	: Holds fixation for 1–2 seconds but switches before blinks (strong fixation preference but the other is used briefly for fixation.)
Grade 4	: Immediately switches fixation on removal of cover from non-deviating eye (strong fixation pattern, and patient uses only one eye for fixation.)

Prism-induced tropia test. Prisms can be used in a variety of ways to induce a tropia, thus allowing the binocular fixation pattern to be assessed in children with small angle strabismus:

- *25 dioptre base-in prism test (Cassin, 1982).* A 25D base-in prism is introduced over one eye and the child's eye preference is noticed. The prism is then placed over the other eye and preference is noted. This prism induces a large esotropia that cannot be overcome by most children and results in diplopia. Therefore, a child with equal vision will ordinarily use the eye without the prism to fixate regardless of which eye is viewing through the prism. If a child shows preference for one eye to fixate through the prism, the nonpreferred eye is considered amblyopic.
- *Vertical prism test (induced tropia test).* Ten to fifteen dioptre vertical prism test has also been recommended to assess eye fixation preference by producing tropia with diplopia, similar to 25D base-in prism test.

Note that the vertical prism test rectifies the high rate of misdiagnosis of amblyopia by standard fixation preference testing in patients with small-angle strabismus and monofixation syndrome. This is because the vertical prism breaks up the peripheral fusion and central scotoma complex, thus allowing the patient to fixate with either eye.

CSM method of rating monocular fixation. CSM method has been used to describe the fixation pattern of a too young patient for visual acuity measurement by some workers after examination with a handlight as follows:

- **C:** Stands for *'central'* which refers to the fact that angle kappa appeared equal in direction and magnitude.
- **S:** Stands for *'steady'* which means that fixation is not aimless or wandering as in amblyopia and also that nystagmus is absent.
- **M:** Stands for *'maintained'*, meaning thereby that there is no shift on the cover test, i.e. a manifest squint is not present.

It has been reported that rating of monocular fixation pattern as *central, steady* and *maintained* provides limited information. An eye with extremely poor visual acuity may also have central, steady and maintained fixation. Therefore, use of CSM should be avoided, particularly, if it replaces a visual acuity notation. Similarly the 'maintained' is no alternative to cover and cover-uncover test to detect manifest deviation.

Preferential looking test, optokinetic nystagmus and visually evoked potential. These tests are also used to measure visual acuity in infants and very young children (for details *see* page 40).

Methods of estimating visual acuity in preschool children (2½ to 4 years). Commonly employed tests are listed below (for details *see* page 45):
- Marble game test
- Hand chart test
- Illiterate E-game test
- Allen's preschool vision test
- Sheridan Gardiner test
- Stycar matching test

Methods of estimating visual acuity in school children and adults (age 5 and older). Most commonly used tests are as follows (for details *see* page 48):
- Snellen's test types
- E-chart for illiterate
- Landolt's broken-C chart

2. Neutral density filter test. Whenever possible, it is imperative to illucidate this important characteristic of amblyopic eye—that the amblyopic eye sees better under mesopic conditions (between scotopic and photopic condition). This can be tested with neutral density filter test. For details *see* page 184.

3. Test for crowding phenomenon should be performed to establish the separation difficulties—another important feature— exhibited by amblyopic eyes. For the detail *see* page 184.

4. Thorough ocular examination including fundus examination. A thorough ocular examination including a detailed fundus examination is very important to rule out any cause, other than amblyopia, of reduced visual acuity.

5. Refraction. The importance of a meticulous refraction cannot be overemphasized in the clinical evaluation of squint and amblyopia (*see* page 102).

6. Evaluation for central versus eccentric fixation. About one-half of all amblyopic eyes are associated with eccentric fixation. The fixation pattern can be evaluated by following methods:

i. *Angle kappa method.* An idea about eccentric fixation can be made by comparing the angle kappa in each eye. Though it is commonly used but comparatively less accurate method of detecting eccentric fixation. Angle kappa can be estimated by following methods:

- *Hand light method.* After occluding the non-fixing eye, patient is made to fix a hand light held directly below the examiner's eye to avoid an inaccuracy due to parallax. The location of corneal reflex is noted. The same procedure is repeated on the other eye. The angle is positive, when the corneal reflex is displaced nasally and negative, when it is displaced temporally (Fig. 8.12). A positive angle kappa of up to 5° is physiologic in emmetropic eyes.

  – *In central fixation,* the corneal reflex is located in a similar position in each eye.
  – *In eccentric fixation,* a significant difference in the location of corneal reflex in fixing and nonfixing eye will be noted.

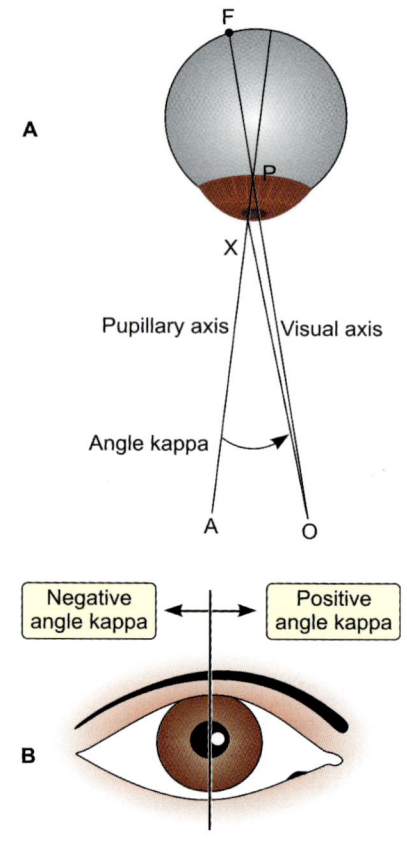

Fig. 8.12 *(A) Angle kappa (OPA) is formed between the visual axis (OF) and central pupillary line (AP). However, clinically angle kappa (OXA) is measured at a point on the cornea (X) that lies in the central pupillary line. (B) Angle kappa is labelled positive when the corneal light is displaced nasally and negative when it is displaced temporally.*

It is not an accurate method. Small degree of eccentric fixation is often missed. However, it is the only available method of testing eccentricity in infants.

- *Arc perimeter method.* In this technique, after occluding one eye, patient is asked to fix a centre mark on the perimeter, and a very fine light is moved along the perimeter arc until the light reflex is centred on the cornea. Location of light on the perimeter arc tells the angle kappa in degrees.
- *Major amblyoscope method.* Angle kappa is measured using special slides with synoptophore (*see* page 138).

ii. *Visuscope method.* In most clinical practice, visuscope or its ophthalmoscopic alternative is the most commonly employed method for testing eccentric fixation (*see* page 140). However, this technique requires patient's cooperation and thus can be used in patients above 4–5 years of age.

iii. *Haidinger's brushes method.* Patient is made to perceive the entoptic pattern of the Haidinger brushes and then asked to touch its centre with a pointer. In the presence of central fixation, patient will easily do so. However, if fixation is eccentric, a gross error will be made and patient will be unable, despite repeated attempts to correct the error. Being cumbersome, this method is not used routinely.

iv. *Maxwell's spot method.* Maxwell spot is a round, dark, purplish spot of about 3 arc degrees in diameter. It is perceived entoptically, when the eye is exposed to a homogenous blue or purple field. In central fixation, this spot is centred over the fixation target. In eccentric fixation, the Maxwell spot is displaced to the side of fixation target by an angular amount equivalent to the degree of eccentricity. Like Haidinger's brushes method, this is also sparingly used in common clinical practice.

7. **Tests for other sensory anomalies.** Amblyopia may be associated with ARC. Therefore, the tests employed for suppression (*see* page 171) and ARC (*see* page 129) may also be required for a thorough clinical evaluation of amblyopia.

PREVENTION AND EARLY DETECTION OF AMBLYOPIA

Early detection as well as early intervention is most essential for the effective treatment of amblyopia. The best way for prevention and early diagnosis of amblyopia is adoption of some screening programme.

Vision screening examinations should start at birth and continue as part of routine check ups by primary care physicians.

- *Acronym I-ARM* (Inspection—Acuity, Red reflex, and Motility) can be a helpful reminder of the essential parts of a paediatric screening examination. Table 8.3 summarizes the I-ARM screening eye examination for neonates, babies, and children.
- *Most important test for the newborn* is the red reflex test. If an abnormal red reflex is present, then an immediate referral to an ophthalmologist is required.
- *Infant screening examination* takes less than a minute, but this brief examination is quite powerful. If performed properly, it can detect the vast majority of eye pathologies.

Children with risk factor for amblyopia should have a comprehensive ophthalmic examination. Some risk factors include:

- Family history of amblyopia or strabismus
- Childhood cataract or glaucoma
- Premature birth of lens than 30 weeks gestation and/or less than 1500 gm weight

Brückner reflex test

The red reflex test is the single best vision screening exam for infants and young children. It is best performed using the Brückner modification, which is simply a simultaneous bilateral red reflex. Use the direct ophthalmoscope and view the patient's eyes at a distance of approximately 2 feet from the patient. Use a broad beam so that both eyes are illuminated at the same time. Dim the room lights and have the child look directly into the ophthalmoscope light.

Table 8.3 *Screening eye examination: I-ARM*

Step	Neonate (Birth–2 months)	Babies (3 months–2 years)	Children (3 years and older)
Inspection	Symmetry face and eyes	Face turn or head tilt	Face turn or head tilt.
Acuity	Poor fixation, pupillary response	Good fixation and smooth pursuit	Visual acuity: Allen cards, E-game,
Red reflex	Red reflex test	Binocular red reflex (Brückner)	Bilateral red reflex test (Brückner)
Motility	Gross alignment (70% small exotropia but esotropia probably abnormal)	Good alignment, light reflex and Brückner (esotropia is abnormal after 2 months of age).	Good alignment, light reflex and Brückner (any misalignment misalignment is abnormal)

Start with the ophthalmoscope on low illumination then slowly increase the illumination until a red reflex is seen. The examiner will observe a red reflex that fills the pupil and a small (approximately 1 mm) white light reflex that appears to reflect off the cornea . The white light reflex is actually a reflex coming from just behind the pupil and is called the "corneal light reflex" or the "Hirschberg reflex." Thus, the Brückner test gives both a red reflex and the corneal light reflex simultaneously. Blockage of the retinal image or large retinal pathology will result in an abnormal red reflex.

- *Cataract* can either block the red reflex or reflect light to give a white reflex.
- *Retinoblastoma* has a yellowish-white colour and will produce a yellow reflex.
- *Anisometropia* (difference in refractive error) will result in an unequal red reflex.
- *Strabismus* will cause a brighter red reflex in the deviated eye, and the corneal light reflex will be decentered.

Note. The key sign of a normal exam is symmetry.

TREATMENT OF AMBLYOPIA

Goal of amblyopia treatment is to maximise and potentially normalise visual acuity.

Strategies to treat amblyopia include:
- Elimination of the cause of visual deprivation and provision of clear retinal image in the amblyopic eye,
- Correction of ocular dominance
- Near visual activity, and
- Perceptual training.

I. ELIMINATION OF THE CAUSE OF VISUAL DEPRIVATION AND PROVISION OF CLEAR RETINAL IMAGE

1. Media clearance

Media clearance, whenever required, is the first step of amblyopia management.

Childhood cataract, when present should be operated as early as possible with appropriate aphakic correction depending upon the circumstances. Correction of amblyopia in congenital cataract is a challenge full of frustration. Important guidelines for treatment of childhood cataract are as follows:

- Significant congenital cataract should be removed during the first 2–3 months of life.
- In symmetric bilateral cases, the interval between operations on the first and second eyes should not be more than 1–2 weeks.
- Acutely developing severe traumatic cataracts in children under 8–10 years of age should be removed within a few weeks of injury, if possible.
- Refractive correction for aphakia following cataract surgery in childhood must be provided promptly with no further delay.

Severe congenital ptosis should be corrected at the earliest.

Corneal opacity should be treated by penetrating keratoplasty.

2. Correction of refractive error and spectacle adaptation

Refractive error, if any, should be fully corrected as determined with cycloplegic refraction before starting the amblyopia therapy.

Spectacle adoption for 3 to 4 weeks should be tried in anisometropic amblyopia before starting occlusion therapy. Refractive correction alone may improve vision in many cases.

II. CORRECTION OF OCULAR DOMINANCE

Correction of ocular dominance is done by stimulating the amblyopic eye with the use of following modalities alone or in combinations:
- Occlusion therapy
- Penalization
- Active stimulation
- Pleoptics
- Pharmacological manipulation

1. Occlusion therapy

Occlusion of sound eye is the most powerful means of treating amblyopia by forcing the patient to use amblyopic eye. Occlusion therapy has been the mainstay of treatment since 18th century.

Methods of occlusion

Occlusion can be accomplished by an adhesive patch on skin, gauze pad and tape, use of Doynes rubber occluder which can be stuck to spectacle lens, opaque contact lense, adhesive tape on glasses or any method that excludes the use of occluded eye (Fig. 8.13). *Adhesive skin patch is the best method*. However, problem may arise in children with sensitive skin. If application of tincture of benzoin before the patch is applied on the skin also does not help, then other methods may be tried as a substitute for a patch.

Programmable electronic glasses

The lenses are liquid crystal display (LCD), they can also be programmed to turn opaque, occluding vision in the left or right eye for different time intervals, acting like a digital patch that flickers on and off. Amblyz™ occlusion glasses were used for 4 hours daily in a study, where the lens over the eye with better vision switched from clear to opaque every 30 seconds (presented at AAO but not published).

Direct versus inverse occlusion

Direct occlusion refers to occlusion of the sound eye and *inverse or indirect occlusion* refers to occlusion of the amblyopic eye.

Previously, many workers recommended that in the presence of eccentric fixation, first one should occlude the amblyopic eye for some time, so that the eccentric fixation becomes less fixed. However, after long observations, now only direct occlusion is recommended even in the presence of eccentric fixation as discussed above.

Full-time versus intermittent (part-time) occlusion

Full-time occlusion involves placing the occluder over the eye as soon as the child gets up in the morning and removing only after the child goes to bed at night. Earlier, constant and total occlusion was considered the choice for initial treatment of amblyopia. Standard teaching has been that children need to be observed at intervals of 1 week per year of age, if undergoing full-time occlusion to avoid occlusion amblyopia in the sound eye. A simplified schedule for initial treatment of amblyopia previously recommended with a combination of full-time direct and inverse occlusion is shown in Table 8.4.

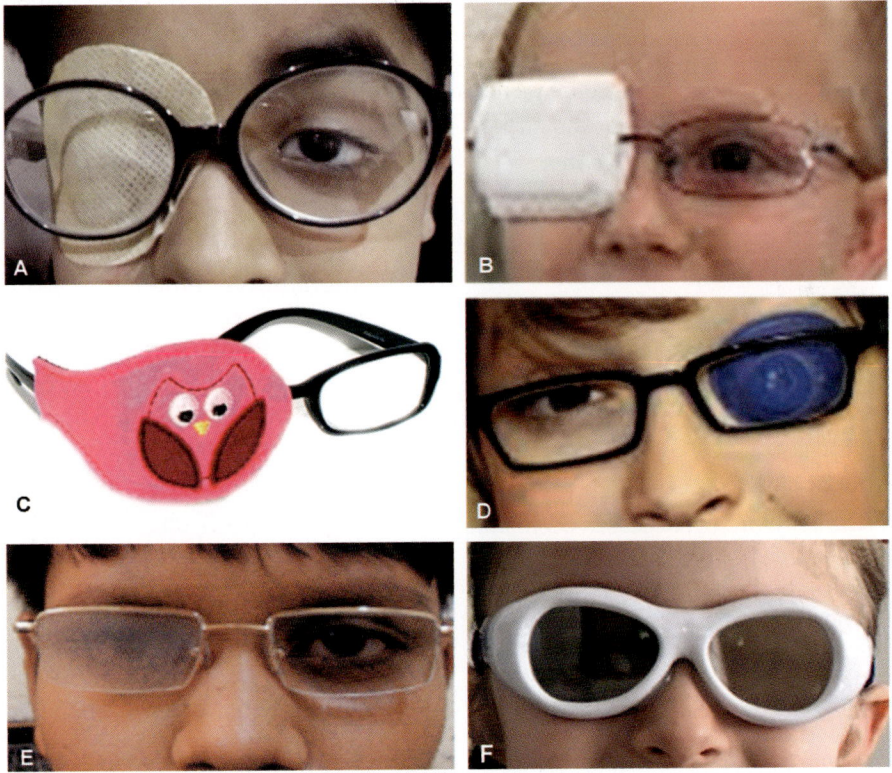

Fig. 8.13 *Methods of occlusion:* A, *Elastoplast orthoptic patch;* B, *Slip on nose pad;* C, *Spectacle mount orthoptic eye patch;* D, *Doyne's rubber occluder;* E, *Ground glass occluder, and* F, *Smart glasses for occlusion therapy.*

Table 8.4 *A simplified schedule for initial occlusion therapy for amblyopia*			
Age of the patient (in yrs.)	*Period of occlusion (days)*		*Follow-up after every*
	Direct :	*Inverse*	
Up to 2	2 :	1	15 days
3	3 :	1	15 days
4	4 :	1	1 month
5	5 :	1	1 month
6 and older	6 :	1	1 month

Part-time (intermittent) occlusion involves use of the occluder for a short time each day. Amblyopia treatment studies (ATS) have demonstrated:

- *In children aged 3–7 years with severe amblyopia* (visual acuity between 20/100 and 20/400), full-time patching produced a similar effect to that of 6 hours of patching per day.
- *In children aged 3–7 years with moderate amblyopia* (visual acuity better than 20/100), 2 hours of daily patching produced an improvement in visual acuity similar to that of 6 hours. In this study, patching was prescribed in combination with 1 hour of near visual activities.
- *In children aged from 7 years to younger than 13 years,* prescribing 2–6 hours a day of patching can improve visual acuity, even if the amblyopia has been previously treated.
- *In patients aged from 13 years to younger than 18 years,* prescribing 2–6 hours a day of patching might improve visual acuity, when amblyopia has not been previously treated; however, this is likely to be of little benefit, if amblyopia was previously treated with patching. Long-term results from these studies are still pending.

How to go about occlusion

Compliance is the keyword of success in occlusion therapy and should be ensured by motivating the child and parents. The initial phase is the uphill route; once the near vision and then the distance vision start improving, the task is easier.

How long to continue occlusion is decided as below:

- *In patients with improvement in vision,* assessed at monthly follow-up visits, the occlusion should be continued till the amblyopic eye has not only developed equal vision but also equal preference of fixation compared to the normal eye. On an average, it may take 3–6 months, depending upon the age of the patient and initial level of vision. The younger the patient the better is improvement in the visual acuity, when the occlusion is started, and the shorter is the duration of occlusion required.
- *In patients with no improvement with occlusion* on three consecutive monthly follow-up visits, further occlusion is unlikely to be fruitful. However, it is essential to once again rule out any organic disease and carefully recheck the refraction. Incomplete response to occlusion tends to be associated with anisohypermetropia and anisoastigmatism.

Maintenance occulsion treatment is done as below:

- Once the vision has been equalized, the maintenance occlusion should be continued till the amblyogenic age, i.e. up to at least 9 years of age and sometimes even till the child has reached early teens.
- Maintenance occlusion is accomplished by a part-time occlusion for 2–3 hours in a day with active vision exercises at home.

2. Penalization

Principle. The word penalization literally means to punish or to inhibit. The principle is to force the amblyopic eye to a greater use for distance, near or both by penalizing the sound eye for distance, near or both with the help of glasses and a cycloplegic drug.

Prerequisite to penalization is that the eyes should be straight and hence is best used in anisometropic amblyopia without deviation or with deviation after it has been corrected or surgically with prisms.

Indications. In the past, penalization therapy was reserved for children who would not wear a patch or in whom compliance was an issue. The amblyopia treatment studies, however, have demonstrated that atropine penalization in patients with moderate amblyopia (defined by the study as visual acuity better than 20/100) is as effective as patching. The amblyopia treatment studies were performed in children aged 3–7 years. Further, penalization may also be used for maintaining vision obtained through previous occlusion therapy.

Methods. Penalization can be done by two methods are given as follows.

i. Atropine penalization, and

ii. Optical penalization.

Note. Atropine penalization is a stronger method.

i. *Atropine penalization of non-amblyopic eye*

a. *Near penalization.* It is most commonly used. For near penalization, the fixing eye is atropinized and fully corrected for distance vision, while amblyopic eye is overcorrected with +2.0 to +3.0D. This forces the amblyopic eye to be used in near vision and stimulates alteration of two eyes for near and distance fixation.

Alternately, sound eye is atropinized and 1% pilocarpine is used in amblyopic eye. Pilocarpine gives pinhole effect due to constriction of pupil and improves near fixation due to facilitation of accommodation.

b. *Distance penalization.* Fixing eye is atropinized and overcorrected by +3.0D lens while the amblyopic eye is fully corrected. In this way, sound eye is penalized for distance and is used for near only, while amblyopic eye is used for distance.

c. *Total penalization.* Fixing eye is atropinized and undercorrected by 4.0 to 5.0D, while amblyopic eye is fully corrected. This prevents the fixing eye being used for near as well as distance.

ii. *Optical penalization*

Optical penalization is based on over-plussing (prescribing more plus sphere than needed) the sound eye to force fixation to the amblyopic eye for distance targets; the patient will usually use the sound eye for near targets. Optical penalization works well for mild amblyopia; however, some children will look over the tops of their glasses to use their sound eye.

3. Active stimulation therapy

Active stimulation therapy using CAM vision stimulator has been used in the past.

The word CAM stands for Cambridge (England), where this vision stimulator device was first used in 1978.

Method. In this technique, after occluding the sound eye, amblyopic eye is stimulated for 7 minutes by slowly rotating high contrast square wave grating of different spatial frequencies. The treatment is carried out once in a week for 3 to 4 weeks. The sound eye remains open between the weekly treatment sessions—an advantage over the conventional occlusion therapy.

Principle on which this treatment is based is the assumption that rotating grating provides specific stimulation for cortical neurons. However, equally good results are reported using grey discs instead of grating. Therefore, it may well be assumed that the combination of occlusion and near work requiring visual concentration is responsible for the improvement.

Present status of CAM vision stimulator. Though initial workers reported good results but subsequent workers reported that this technique is not as effective as conventional occlusion therapy. So it has failed to replace the time tested conventional occlusion therapy for the treatment of amblyopia. However, some workers believe that this method can be used as supplementary to occlusion therapy in co-operative patients with supportive parents who can carry out the treatment at home.

4. Pleoptics

The word pleoptics is derived from a Greek word meaning full vision. This technique generated a lot of excitement during 1950s and

1960s. But nowadays it is only of historical interest.

- Pleoptics was used for active stimulation of the fovea to overcome eccentric fixation and improves the visual acuity.
- In this technique, the peripheral retina including the eccentrically fixing area around the fovea is dazzled with an intense light while protecting foveal area.
- Supposedly, after the light source is turned off, the fovea functions better because the surrounding retinal area is in a state of hypofunction.
- This can be followed by direct stimulation of fovea as by pleoptophore (Bangerter's method) or indirectly by producing after-image (Cupper's method).
- The excitement over this technique abated, when it became obvious that the technique is complex and requires an absolute co-operation of the patient, his/her intelligence to appreciate after-images (which is possible in older children) and daily sittings for a longer period of time (with its own socio-economic problems) are required.
- Since occlusion of the dominant eye is a very successful simple and inexpensive method of treating eccentric fixation, so most practitioners have abundoned use of pleoptic methods.

5. Pharmacological manipulation

Role of levodopa. Studies indicate that plasticity of visual system during the sensitive period is dependent on input from non-adrenergic neurons and thus can be subjected to pharmacological manipulation. This aspect has been tried with the use of *levodopa* as a pharmacologic manipulator. Levodopa/carbidopa has been traditionally used to treat Parkinson's disease. Levodopa is a precursor for the catecholamine dopamine, a neurotransmitter/neuromodulator known to influence receptive fields. Levodopa/carbidopa has been studied as an adjunct to patching for the treatment of amblyopia. However, the role of levodopa remains controversial, as the visual acuity improvement has been relatively small, not clearly better than with patching alone and

there are questions regarding long-term stability of vision.

Role of Citicholine. See page 405

Role of omega fatty acid is also reported in development of vision and cognitive development.

III. ACTIVE THERAPY (NEAR VISUAL ACTIVITIES)

Active thrapy, in the form of near visual activities, using amblyopic eye has been suggested as an important supplement to occlusion therapy based on the assumption that these activities stimulate the visual system and thus causes easy recovery.

Active vision exercises by the amblyopic eye during occlusion therapy, which may enhance the success of occlusion include:

- *Simple tasks* like dotting the o's and encircling the e's in the newsprint, joining dots to make drawing, tracing, colouring threading beads, watching television, reading comics and story books may be quite useful and enchance the recovery.
- *Computer games,* especially designed for active vision exercises, are beging considered a very useful adjunct with occlusion therapy. The television, video games and mobile games for near vision activity are easily available and have become very popular with the children.

IV. ROLE OF PERCEPTUAL LEARNING IN AMBLYOPIA TREATMENT

Gibson (1963) defined perceptual learning as "Any relatively permanent and consistent change in the perception of stimulus array following practice or experience with this array...."

Over the last 15 years, number of studies suggest that 'perceptual learning (PL) may provide an important new method for treating amblyopia. Perceptual learning is reported to operate via a reduction of internal neural noise and/or through more efficient use of stimulus information by returning the weighting of the information. ***Perceptual learning employes*** repeatedly practicing a visual discrimination task, e.g:

- Positional acuity,
- Contrast sensitivity,
- Stereoacuity, etc.

Recommended period for preceptual learning is 2 hrs/day, 5 days/week, for a period of 9 months. *Role of preceptual learning* is still controversial, but utility is reported in adult amblyops.

V. BINOCULAR APPROACH FOR AMBLYOPIA TREATMENT

Recently, amblyopia is being considered a binocular problem caused by active suppression that's converts structurally intact binocular system into a functionally monocular system. So, treating unilateral amblyopia with a binocular approach using dichoptic stimuli is under active consideration. The dichoptic treatment presents a stimulus to each eye separately and the brain is forced to integrate the images into a single perception. In these treatment modalities; under binocular conditions, the signal strength coming into the patient's good eye is reduced enough so that it cannot suppress the amblyopic eye. The result is binocular perception in a patient with otherwise deep suppression of the amblyopic eye. Over time, the viewing conditions are changed and the image seen by the good eye is suppressed less until both eyes see approximately the same image. There are many popular softwares that are developing now-a-days promoting binocular vision therapy with 3D gaming and at the same time stimulating perceptual learning. These are believed to treat amblyopia not only in children but also in adults.

Examples of dichoptic stimuli are:
- Hess et al have developed antisupprression therapy as dichoptic stimuli using a 'Faling Blocks game' on an iPad.
- Li et al treated amblyopia with dichoptic stimuli using red-green glasses with reduced contrast for the non-amblyopic eye.

VI. ROLE OF OTHER MODALITIES IN AMBLYOPIA TREATMENT

Acupuncture in amblyopia

Acupuncture is a potentially useful complementary treatment modality that may provide sustainable adjunctive effect to refractive correction for anisometropic amblyopia in young children. Although the treatment effect of acupuncture appears promising, the mechanism underlying its success as a treatment for amblyopia remains unclear. Acupuncture at vision-related acupoints may modulate the activity of the visual cortex. Moreover, acupuncture has been shown to be effective in increasing blood flow to the cerebral and ocular vasculatures (including the choroid), stimulating the expression of retinal nerve growth factors and leading to metabolic changes in the central nervous system.

Transcranial magnetic brain stimulation in amblyopia

Transcranial magnetic stimulation (TMS) is a non-invasive method for stimulating parts of the brain by use of weak electric current that are induced into the tissue by use of rapidly changing magnetic currents. TMS produces effects that last slightly longer than the actual time of stimulation.

AMBLYOPIA TREATMENT STUDY REPORTS

Reports of various 'amblyopia treatment studies (ATS)' carried out under the 'Paediatric Eye Disease Investigation Group (PEDIG)' are summarised in Table 8.5.

PROBLEMS IN AMBLYOPIA TREATMENT

1. Problems in applying the occluder

Though occluding the sound eye may appear to be a simple procedure, and in many cases it is nevertheless, in the practical application of this simple treatment, several problems may arise. Some of the important difficulties encountered during this treatment are discussed as follows.

Occluder attached to spectacle lens is easy to wear but usually ineffective, since children are able to look over, around and under the patch. Further, most children will simply take their glasses off, when unobserved, and for this reason, most workers rarely use this method of occlusion.

Adhesive patch applied directly over the skin (Fig. 8.13) is the best method for a total and full-time occlusion. However, problems of skin reactions may arise in some children. Following measures have been recommended:

Table 8.5 *Summary of amblyopia treatment study reports*

Study	Aim	Age	No. of patients	Type of study	Follow up	Results
ATS 1	Occlusion versus pharmacologic therapy for moderate amblyopia to compare atropine and patching for moderate amblyopia	3–<7 yr	419	Randomised comparative trial	2 year	Improvement was initially faster in the patching group, but after 6 months the difference in visual acuity between treatment groups was insignificant; 3.16 lines (patching group) vs 2.84 lines (atropine group). Visual acuity >20/30 and/or improved by ≥3 lines in 79% of occlusion group and 74% of atropine group
ATS1-Ext	Atropine vs patching for treatment of moderate amblyopia: follow-up at 15 years of age of a randomized clinical trial	3–<7yr	188	Randomised comparative trial	15 years of age	At 15 years of age, most children treated for moderate amblyopia when younger than 7 years have good visual acuity, although mild residual amblyopia is common. The outcome is similar regardless of initial treatment with atropine or patching.
ATS 2A	A randomized trial comparing part-time versus minimal-time patching for moderate amblyopia	3–7yr	175	Randomised comparative trial	4 months	6 hrs of patching equally effective as full-time patching. 86% patients in the 6-hour group and 82% patients in the full-time group had improved by 3 lines from baseline.
ATS 2B	A randomized trial comparing part-time versus full-time patching for severe amblyopia	3–7yr	189	Randomised comparative trial	4 months	6 hrs of patching as effective as 2 hrs of patching. At 4 months, no difference in amblyopic eye acuity between groups
ATS 2C	An observational study on recurrence of amblyopia after disconti nuation of treatment	3–7 yr	156	Observational	52 weeks	Recurrence occurred in 35 (24%) of 145 cases and was similar in patients who stopped patching (25%) and in patients who stopped atropine (21%). In patients treated with moderately intense patching (6 to 8 hours per day), recurrence was more common (11 of 26, 42%) when treatment was not reduced prior to cessation than when treatment was reduced to 2 hours per day prior to cessation. Approximately one-fourth of successfully-treated amblyopic children experience a recurrence within the first year off treatment.

(Contd...)

Table 8.5 Summary of amblyopia treatment study reports (Contd...)

Study	Aim	Age	No. of patients	Type of study	Follow up	Results
ATS 3	To evaluate the effectiveness of optical correction alone *vs* 2–6 hr/day of patching combined with near visual activities plus atropine	7–13 yr	507	Observational phase and randomised trial phase	6 months	In the 7 to <13-year-old, 53% of the treatment group were responders compared with 25% of the optical correction group (P<0.001). In the 13 to <18-year-old, the responder rates were 25% and 23% respectively overall (adjusted P = 0.22), but 47% and 20% respectively among patients not previously treated with patching and/or atropine for amblyopia. For patients 7 to <13 years old, prescribing 2 to 6 hours per day of patching with near activities and atropine can improve visual acuity even if the amblyopia has been previously treated. For patients 13 to <18-year-old, prescribing patching 2 to 6 hours per day with near activities may improve visual acuity when amblyopia has not been previously treated but appears to be of little benefit if amblyopia was previously treated sheet with patching.
ATS 4	A randomized trial comparing daily atropine versus weekend atropine for moderate amblyopia	3–7 yr	168	Randomised comparative trial	4 months	Weekend atropine provides an improvement similar to that provided by daily atropine in moderate amblyopia.
ATS 5A	Prospective non-comparative trial to evaluate 2 hours of daily patching for amblyopia (eye glass only phase study)	3–7 yr	84	Prospective non-comparative trial	Up to 30 weeks	Amblyopia improved in 77% by optical correction and resolved in 27%.
ATS 5B	Randomized trial to evaluate 2 hours daily patching for amblyopia (randomization phase)	3–7 yr	180	Randomised trial	5 weeks	Refractive correction alone improves visual acuity in many cases and results in resolution of amblyopia in at least one-third of 3 to <7-year-old children with untreated anisometropic amblyopia. Following a period of treatment with spectacles, two hours of daily patching combined with one hour of near visual activities modestly improves moderate to severe amblyopia in children 3 to 7-year-old.

(Contd...)

Table 8.5 Summary of amblyopia treatment study reports (Contd...)

Study	Aim	Age	No. of patients	Type of study	Follow up	Results
ATS 6	A randomized trial of near versus distance activities while patching for amblyopia in children 3 to <7-year-old	3–7 yr	425	Randomised comparative trial	17 weeks	No difference in visual acuity improvement between children performing near activities and distance activities during patching.
ATS 7	Bilateral refractive amblyopia treatment study: Response to treatment of previously untreated presumed bilateral refractive amblyopia	3–11 yr	113	Randomised comparative trial	1 year	Bilateral refractive amblyopia improves with spectacle correction. Binocular visual acuity of 20/25 or better was achieved by 73%
ATS 8	To compare weekend atropine augmented by a plano lens with weekend atropine alone for moderate amblyopia.	3–7 yr	180	Randomised comparative trial	18 weeks	Augmentation of weekend atropine with a plano lens does not substantially improve amblyopic eye acuity
ATS 9	To compare patching with atropine eyedrops in the treatment of moderate amblyopia	7–12 yr	193	Randomised comparative trial	17 weeks	Atropine and patching achieve similar results among older children with unilateral amblyopia.
ATS 10	Randomized trial comparing bangerter filters vs part time occlusion for the treatment of moderate amblyopia	3–10 yr	186	Randomised comparative trial	24 weeks	Bangerter filters and patching was less than half a line, and there was lower burden of treatment on the child and family, Bangerter filter treatment is a reasonable option to consider for initial treatment of moderate amblyopia
ATS 11	Randomized trial to evaluate combined patching and atropine for residual amblyopia	3–10 yr	55	Randomised trial	10 weeks	Amblyopic eye VA improved similarly in both groups suggestive of no additional benefit of combined treatment in residual amblyopia

(Contd...)

Table 8.5 Summary of amblyopia treatment study reports (Contd...)

Study	Aim	Age	No. of patients	Type of study	Follow up	Results
ATS 12	A randomized trial comparing patching with active vision therapy to patching with control vision therapy as treatment for amblyopia in children 7 to <13 year old; to determine the feasibility of conducting a full-scale randomized clinical trial	7–<13 yr	19	Randomised trial	17 weeks	16-week treatment trial of vision therapy was feasible with respect to maintaining protocol adherence; however, recruitment under the proposed eligibility criteria, necessitated by the standardized approach to vision therapy, was not successfull
ATS 13	Nonrandomized prospective trial of glasses alone for strabismic and strabismic-anisometropic amblyopia	3–7 yr	146	Non randomised prospective trial	28 weeks	Treatment effect was greater for strabismic amblyopia than for combined mechanism amblyopia
ATS 14	A Pilot Study of Levodopa dosage as treatment for residual amblyopia	8–18 yr	33	Randomised trial	10 weeks	The results suggested that levodopa/carbidopa therapy for residual amblyopia in older children and teenagers is well tolerated and may improve visual acuity. There was a suggestion of partial regression of the improvement in visual acuity after treatment was discontinued.
ATS 15	Randomized trial of increasing patching for amblyopia	3–8 yr	169	Randomised trial	12 weeks	More improvement in VA after 10 weeks compared with continuing 2 hours daily.
ATS 16	Augmenting atropine treatment for amblyopia, the effectiveness of adding a plano lens (a lens without any prescription) to weekend atropine treatment after a patient's visual acuity has stabilized but amblyopia is still present.	3–8 yr			-	Not published

(Contd...)

Table 8.5 *Summary of amblyopia treatment study reports (Contd...)*

Study	Aim	Age	No. of patients	Type of study	Follow up	Results
ATS 17	Compare the efficacy and safety of oral levodopa and patching versus oral placebo and patching at 18 weeks, after 16 weeks of treatment followed by a two-week taper of oral medication.	7–13 yr	139	Randomised trial	18 weeks	For children 7 to 12 years of age with residual amblyopia after patching therapy, oral levodopa while continuing to patch 2 hours daily does not produce a clinically or statistically meaningful improvement in VA compared with placebo and patching.
ATS 18	Compare the effectiveness of 1 hour/day of binocular game play 7 days per week with 2 hours/day patching 7 days per week	5–<12 years	385	Non-inferiority randomised trial	16 weeks	In children aged 5 to younger than 13 years, amblyopic-eye VA improved with binocular game play and with patching, particularly in younger children (age 5 to <7 years) without prior amblyopia treatment. Although the primary noninferiority analysis was indeterminate, a post hoc analysis suggested that VA improvement with this particular binocular iPad treatment was not as good as with 2 hours of prescribed daily patching.
ATS 20	To compare the efficacy of 1 hour/day of binocular game play 5 days per week plus spectacle correction only, for treatment of amblyopia	4–13 years				Not published

- Tincture benzoins may be applied to the skin before applying the patch. This forms a protective layer over the skin and also increases adhesiveness of the patch so that child is less likely to remove it.
- Opticlude patch is claimed to be hypo-allergenic and can be replaced for ordinary sticking patch.
- If a skin problem does develop, the patch should be left on the eye until it falls off rather than removing it every night, since repeated removal of the patch aggravates the skin irritation.

Occluding soft contact lenses have been recommended where the above two methods prove to be frustrating because of one or the other reason. However, soft contact lenses have their inherent problem of difficulty in application and complications associated with soft contact lens use.

2. Problem of parental co-operation

A full co-operation of the parents is essential in keeping the sound eye of the child occluded. Many parents fail to co-operate for one or the other reason—may be their inability to devote time for their child or may be a lack of under-standing. Therefore, it is the duty of treating person to hammer on the parents' mind the importance of patching for the sake of their child, so much so, that even the parents should be warned that they will be held responsible for a permanent loss of vision of their child. Instilling a feeling of guilt in the parents is not wrong keeping in view the results of rightly and timely performed occlusion therapy.

3. Complications of occlusion

Two complications may accompany occlusion—occlusion amblyopia and occlusion esotropia.

i. *Occlusion amblyopia.* In very young child-ren, occlusion amblyopia in the sound eye may occur in as short a time as 2 to 3 weeks. Not only amblyopia but also eccentric fixation may develop in the previously normal eye when it is constantly occluded. It is, therefore, essential that visual acuity of the sound eye should be carefully monitored during occlusion therapy. If occlusion amblyopia does occur, it usually can be eliminated in about the same time it took to develop by changing the occlusion to the other eye.

Now, it has been established that chances of developing amblyopia in sound eye are more with the penalization technique than with total occlusion. It is because the blurred diffuse stimulus (a white noise type of stimulus) produced by penalization is more amblyogenic than the total occlusion.

ii. *Occlusion esotropia.* Sometimes, in anisome-tropic amblyopia, when no deviation exists and bifoveal single vision is present, constant occlusion may so disrupt binocular vision that an esotropia results. The parents should be warned of this possibility, but it should be explained that the risk is worthwhile in the interest of good visual acuity. The use of intermittent occlusion or partially transparent occlusion (which allows binocular fixation) is preferable to total occlusion as a precaution against the development of this complication. If a deviation does develop, it may not spon-taneously disappear once occlusion is discontinued.

4. Recurrence of amblyopia

Once amblyopia has been corrected, chances of recurrence are always there until child is visually mature (10 years of age). Therefore, a careful monitoring every month up to the age of 1 year, every 2 months up to the age of 2 years and then every 4–6 months up to the age of visual maturity is required. Not only this, a mainte-nance occlusion therapy (*see* page 192) should also be carried out.

PROGNOSIS

Prognosis of amblyopia therapy depends upon the age of patient, type of amblyopia and type of treatment as below:
- Younger the child better the prognosis.
- Amblyopia due to deprivation (e.g. due to congenital cataract) carries the poorest prognosis.
- Strabismic amblyopia has the best prognosis.
- Anisometropic amblyopia has a prognosis intermediate betwen strabismic amblyopia and deprivation amblyopia.

- Presence of eccentric fixation worsens the prognosis.
- Amblyopia with unilateral high hypermetropia has a poorer prognosis than the amblyopia with unilateral high myopia.
- Prognosis is better, when treated with total and full time occlusion than when treated with penalization or other methods.

ABNORMAL RETINAL CORRESPONDENCE

GENERAL CONSIDERATIONS

As we know, in a state of normal single binocular vision, there exists a precise physiological relationship between the corresponding points of the two retinae. And that the foveae of two eyes act as principal corresponding points and have the same visual direction. This adjustment is called normal retinal correspondence (NRC). When squint develops, patient may experience either diplopia or confusion. To avoid these, sometimes (especially in children with small degree of esotropia), there occurs an active cortical adjustment in the directional values of the two retinae. In this state, fovea of the normal eye and an extrafoveal point on the retina of the squinting eye acquire a common visual direction (i.e. become corresponding points). This condition is called abnormal retinal correspondence and the child gets a crude type of binocular vision. Thus, abnormal retinal correspondence (ARC) is a binocular sensory defence mechanism against peripheral diplopia and peripheral confusion. It is important to note that ARC is entirely a binocular phenomenon, i.e. when the eyes are used monocularly, there is no change in visual direction of any retinal element. While eccentric fixation is a monocular phenomenon in which patient takes fixation with an extrafoveal point. If the fixating eye of a patient with ARC is covered, he/she will turn the deviating eye to fixate either with his/her fovea (if he/she has central fixation) or with a peripheral area (if he has eccentric fixation). Only in a minority of patients are ARC and eccentric fixation related in such a manner that the point of anomaly during binocular single vision is also the point of eccentric fixation during monocular vision.

From the above description, an impression is created as if ARC is a new point-to-point correspondence between the two eyes leading to something like normal fusion, stereopsis, etc. However, in fact, this is not the case, rather the ARC is a fragile, variable form of binocular co-operation depending very much on the momentary conditions of binocular vision. Further, ARC does not replace NRC. In fact NRC appears to be suspended since on some tests it can be demonstrated that NRC co-exists with ARC.

Harmonious versus unharmonious ARC

Before exactly defining harmonious and unharmonious ARC, we should revise the definitions of objective and subjective angles of deviation and that of angle of anomaly.

- **Objective angle of deviation** is the amount of deviation measured, when no shift of the eyes is observed by the examiner on the prism and alternate cover test. When measured on synoptophore, it is the position of the instrument's arm when no shift occurs as the lights in the tubes are alternately turned off and on.

- **Subjective angle of deviation** when measured with the synoptophore, is denoted by the position of the instrument's arms at which the patient can superimpose the images of dissimilar test objects.

- **Angle of anomaly** refers to the difference between the objective angle of deviation and subjective angle of deviation. In NRC, the objective and the subjective angles of deviation are equal and so the angle of anomaly is zero. In ARC, the subjective angle is always less than the objective angle and so the angle of anomaly is more than zero. Depending upon the value of angle of anomaly, the ARC is of two types as follows:

1. Harmonious ARC is present, when the angle of anomaly equals the objective angle of squint. In other words, in harmonious ARC, subjective angle of deviation is zero indicating total compensation for the deviation.

2. Unharmonious ARC is present, when the angle of anomaly is less than the objective angle of deviation. In other words, in unharmonious ARC, the subjective angle of deviation is between zero and the objective angle, indicating thereby that the ocular deviation has not been fully compensated. In fact, unharmonious ARC is presently considered an artifact of the more dissociating testing conditions; since a more physiological test (e.g. Bagolini's test) reveals harmonious ARC and a more dissociating test (e.g. synoptophore or red-green glasses) may reveal unharmonious ARC in the same patient.

DEVELOPMENT OF ARC

Factors affecting development of ARC

ARC is a sensory adaptation that is brought about by an inherent desire for some form of binocular vision and to avoid diplopia and confusion that would otherwise take place. However, ARC does not develop in each and every case with strabismus. The factors that have been reported to favour and unfavour the development of ARC are as follows:

1. *Age of onset of squint.* ARC develops only in visually immature children who have acquired binocular single vision. Therefore, chances of ARC development are more, if the squint occurs between 1 and 6 years of age. Therefore, patients in whom binocular single vision is not developed due to presence of early infantile esotropia do not develop ARC. On the other hand, visually mature patients (beyond 6–7 years of age) who acquire strabismus are also incapable of developing ARC. In other words, in young children (below 6–7 years), with binocular single vision, the instability of the binocular reflexes leads to replacement of normal reflex development by abnormal binocular reflexes.

2. *Patient profile.* ARC develops more frequently in patients where binocular single vision has previously existed and the patient has a high degree of general adaptability and intelligence.

3. *Type and amount of strabismus*

- ARC develops more commonly in esotropes than in exotropes and is less common with vertical deviations.
- ARC develops more commonly in patients with uniocular squint than in patients with alternating squint.

- Patients with constant angle of squint are more likely to develop ARC as compared to those with variable angle of squint.
- ARC seems to develop more frequently, when the angle of esotropia is between 10D and 20D. This is because of the fact that the retinal area of the squinting eye, which receives the same stimulation as the fovea of the fixing eye, is close to the fovea and possesses good visual acuity, thus the false image is not only close to the true one but is also relatively clear and the resultant diplopia is troublesome, and in order to overcome this, ARC develops more rapidly.

Natural course of development of ARC

- During natural course of development of ARC, the angle of anomaly gradually increases until it equals the amount of objective deviation and the ARC becomes harmonious.
- During development of ARC, the NRC is not immediately and rarely totally suppressed. NRC and ARC may both coexist in some patients, especially in those with intermittent exotropia. Such patients may show NRC while fusing and ARC while tropic.
- The actual development of ARC appears to occur slowly. But once established the shift from ARC to NRC and back again can occur very rapidly.

ARC AND SUPPRESSION

Both ARC and suppression are the sensory adaptations to prevent diplopia and confusion. They may occur alone or may coexist in the same patient. Following observations have been made about occurrence of ARC and suppression:

1. In patients with large deviations suppression is the rule without associated ARC.
2. In patients with low degrees of strabismus (30D or less), ARC and/or suppression may develop.
3. The presence of suppression does not prevent the development of ARC. Rather some studies quote that suppression is a prerequisite for establishment of ARC.
4. Co-existence of ARC and suppression can be demonstrated, when Bagolini's striated glasses are used to test an esotropic patient.

As shown in Fig. 8.14, when the foveola of the non-deviating eye is aligned with an extrafoveal point in the deviating eye (Fig. 8.14B), the streak seen by the deviating eye has a gap in it (Fig. 8.14C). This gap corresponds to a suppression scotoma in the deviating eye. Since the patient sees the diagonal streaks as a cross and the streak seen by the deviating eye is in line with the fixation light, this indicates that in the periphery, ARC coexists with the central scotoma (Fig. 8.14).

5. Suppression and ARC when co-exist, are complementary mechanisms, since the extrafoveolar suppression in the deviating eye protects against central diplopia, while ARC eliminates peripheral diplopia and peripheral visual confusion.

QUALITY OF BINOCULAR VISION IN ARC

Simultaneous perception of images in the two eyes occurs in ARC due to correspondence of fovea of one eye with some extrafoveal area of the other eye.

Fusion in ARC. Possibly, restoration of some form of motor fusion occurs with the development of ARC. Since ARC provides a low-quality type of peripheral fusion, the occurrence of fusional movements might be expected in ARC. However, when a change in the strabismic angle occurs, patients with ARC should be expected to change the angle of anomaly to avoid peripheral diplopia. Peripheral fusion is thereby achieved without a fusional movement. Thus, the fusional movements, if they do occur in ARC, are probably limited. Further, some workers believe that the fusional movements noted in ARC may not be true fusional movements and instead might be the manifestations of covariations of the angle of anomaly. The covariation of angle of anomaly with the angle of deviation is believed to be possible because of a point-to-area relationship in ARC. Point-to-area relationship means that numerous retinal elements in the deviating eye can apparently be coupled with a single retinal element in the non-deviating eye.

Stereopsis and ARC. It has been concluded that ARC and stereopsis do not coexist. The absence of stereopsis is indicative of the low quality of ARC peripheral fusion.

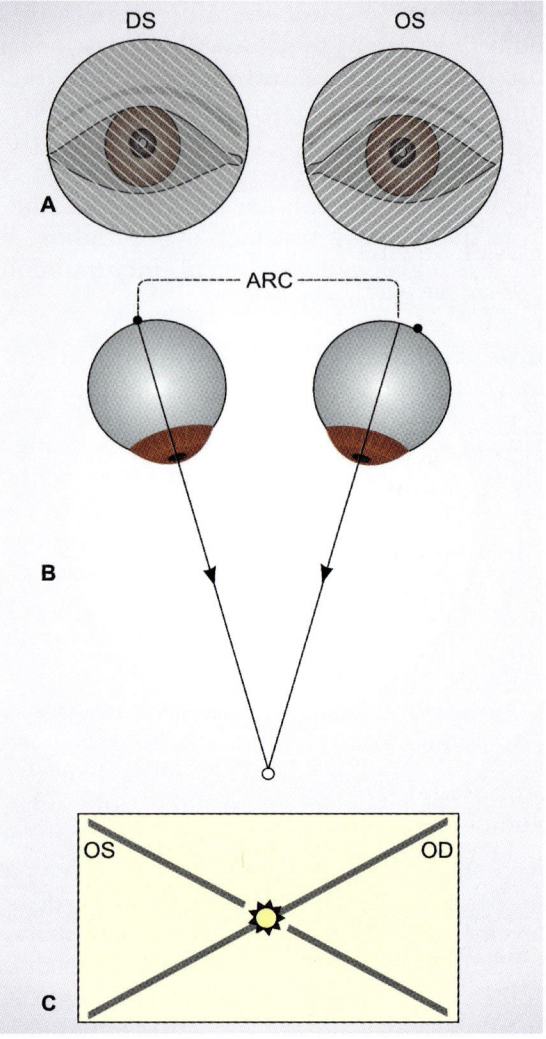

Fig. 8.14 *Bagolini's striated glass test depicting co-existence of suppression and ARC (for explanation, see text).*

It is important to remember that:
- Normal stereopsis (40 seconds or better), indicates bifixation, i.e. perfect central and peripheral fusion.
- Gross stereopsis (67–3000 seconds of arc), indicates monofixation, i.e. peripheral fusion without central fusion.
- Stereopsis is absent in peripheral fusion with arc. However, it has been reported that a gross stereopsis (usually less than 120 minutes of ARC), is a common finding in patients with ARC and small angle esotropia or microtropia which may occasionally even be demonstrable with random dot stereograms.

CLINICAL PHENOMENA ASSOCIATED WITH ARC

Paradoxical diplopia

Paradoxical diplopia is the one which is not expected in a particular type of deviation. Obviously, it occurs because of abnormal projection. In ARC, paradoxical diplopia occurs under following circumstances:

1. It can be elicited in patients with ARC, when both foveas are simultaneously stimulated with major amblyoscope. It can also be elicited with after-image test (*see* page 132 and Fig 6.33).

2. Paradoxical diplopia can also be perceived by a patient in which ARC continues after surgical correction of deviation. Though, in clinical practice, paradoxical diplopia is a fleeting phenomenon limited to the immediate postoperative period, which usually disappears after a few days or weeks of surgery. However, rarely it can persist long and may make the patient's life miserable.

Monocular diplopia

Monocular diplopia is a condition which sometimes occurs in patients with ARC, when an object stimulating a retinal area is projected in two different visual directions, i.e. the normal one and the abnormal one. Under binocular viewing, the patient may have binocular triplopia. In rare cases, binocular triplopia occurs spontaneously, but just like paradoxical diplopia, binocular triplopia can frequently be provoked instrumentally, e.g. by appropriate stimulation with synoptophore.

Postoperative changes in correspondence

Now most of the workers believe that in ARC there occurs point-to-area correspondence, i.e. numerous retinal elements in the deviating eye can apparently be coupled with a single retinal element in the deviating eye. Thus, with the change in the angle of deviating eye, the retinal point of the non-deviating eye starts corresponding with some other retinal point of the deviating eye. Thus, the angle of anomaly may adapt to considerable variations in the angle of strabismus. Disappearance of ARC after surgical correction of strabismus has been explained on the same basis. Following three stages have been postulated for the occurrence of changes in ARC after surgical correction of strabismus:

1. *Stage of ARC* (continues for some time).

2. *Stage of rivalry between normal and anomalous correspondence* (sometimes patient may complain of monocular diplopia during this stage).

3. *Stage of normal correspondence* (develops in favourable cases). It has also been reported that all patients may not develop NRC after surgical correction of strabismus.

Factors which influence the postoperative changes in correspondence are as follows:

- Age of the patient at the time of operation.
- Depth of ARC.
- Use of the eyes made by the patient.
- Individual adaptability.

TESTS FOR ARC

See page 129.

MANAGEMENT OF ARC

The important points to be noted are:

- *Great emphasis used to be laid on the treatment of ARC in the past before the surgical treatment of strabismus.* However, according to the current views, orthoptic treatment for ARC in patients with strabismus is not required.

- *Treatment modalities used for ARC in the past* (now of historical interest only) included: Occlusion therapy, prismatic overcorrection of the ocular deviation and use of major amblyoscope for retinal stimulation (retinal massage).

- Presently, it is believed that the *most effective treatment for terminating ARC*, is surgical realignment of the eyes.

- A small-angle, cosmetically inconspicuous residual strabismus with ARC is now considered an *acceptable or even desirable end stage of therapy in infantile esotropia.*

MOTOR ADAPTATIONS

As discussed above, suppression and ARC are the sensory adaptations which help the strabismus patients to deal with annoying diplopia and/or confusion. These mechanisms are available only to the visually immature children who acquire strabismus after developing singular binocular vision. The older, visually mature patients, have no capacity to develop sensory adaptations. However, these patients may deal with the confusion and/or diplopia by developing motor adaptations, which include:

- Control of ocular deviation by an alteration in tone of extraocular muscle,
- Compensatory head posture,
- Blind spot syndrome, and
- Blind spot mechanism.

CONTROL OF OCULAR DEVIATION BY AN ALTERATION OF TONE OF THE EXTRAOCULAR MUSCLES

Occasionally, a small degree of ocular deviation may be controlled by an alteration of tone of extraocular muscles, which may be of the nature of an active contraction or an active relaxation. The alterations in the extraocular muscles are induced by the compelling influence of the fusion reflexes so that there is a disappearance of the squint and a consequent absence of any diplopia or confusion. In this way, a manifest deviation is converted into a latent one. The success of such an adaptation, however, may be frustrated to some extent by an inadequacy of the fusional reserves, so that the deviation is controlled only at the expense of significant discomfort. However, sometimes this adaptation permits a satisfactory degree of functional control.

COMPENSATORY HEAD POSTURE

Compensatory head posture is a common motor adaptation used by visually mature patients to deal with the diplopia and/or confusion. It occurs under following circumstances:

1. Paralytic strabismus is a particularly common situation in which compensatory head posture is used to achieve fusion of the images seen by the two eyes. For details *see* page 289.

2. A- and V-pattern strabismus may also be associated with an abnormal head posture.

- *Chin is depressed* in A-pattern exotropia and V-pattern esotropia.

- *Chin is elevated* in A-pattern esotropia and V-pattern exotropia.

3. Nystagmus patients may place their head in such a way that the eyes are positioned in the null zone, thereby improving binocular visual acuity.

BLIND SPOT SYNDROME

The blind spot syndrome is a motor adaptation to cope up with the diplopia and/or confusion in patients with esotropia. It occurs, when the esotropia is of small to moderate degree with annoying diplopia and without sufficient divergence to regain foveal fixation. In this condition, a motor response tends to move the eye further to the esotropic side, projecting the image seen by the deviating eye on to the blind spot (optic disc) (Fig. 8.15).

Characteristics of blind spot syndrome
- Esotropia of 12° to 18° (25$^\Delta$ to 35$^\Delta$).
- Good visual acuity in each eye.
- Normal retinal correspondence (NRC).
- No suppression other than the fovea of the deviated eye.
- Normal fusional vergences.
- Diplopia is elicited, when the deviation is prismatically reduced.
- Occasional diplopia and/or confusion in casual seeing. Transitory diplopia is most

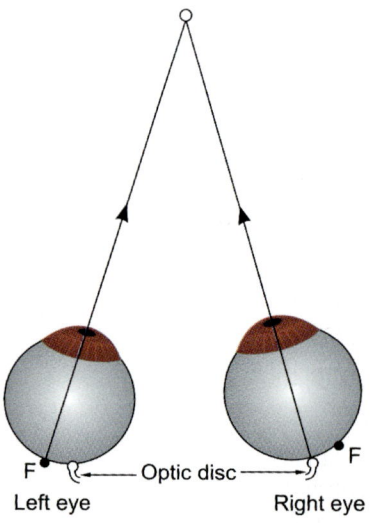

Fig. 8.15 *Blind spot syndrome or mechanism. Note, image in the right esotropic eye is formed on the optic disc.*

commonly noted, when approaching car lights are seen at night.
- Good fusion potentialities demonstrated on haploscopic devices.

BLIND SPOT MECHANISM

The blind spot mechanism is a coincidental type of esotropia in which the image of the fixated object falls on the blind spot (optic disc) of the deviated eye (Fig. 8.15).

Characteristics of blind spot mechanism
- Amblyopia of the non-dominant eye
- Abnormal retinal correspondence
- Deep suppression
- ARC and suppression may coexist

Presence of the above abnormal sensory findings makes the differential diagnosis between the blind spot syndrome and blind spot mechanism.

PSYCHOLOGICAL ADAPTATION

IGNORING

Ignoring is a psychological adaptation which is learnt by some visually mature patients to deal with the annoying diplopia. It probably falls somewhere between conscious and unconscious thought. All patients cannot learn to ignore diplopia. Further, it has also been reported that the patients with excellent acuity in each eye may be able to ignore the weaker image while the patients with poor vision cannot. How this occurs is not known exactly. Perhaps the individual's psychologic factors play an important role in the development of rare phenomenon of ignoring.

BIBLIOGRAPHY

1. Arden, GB, and Wooding, SL. Pattern ERG in amblyopia Invest Ophthalmol Vis. Sci. 26:88, 1985.
2. Assaf AA. The sensitive period: transfer of fixation after occlusion for strabismic amblyopia. Br J Ophthalmol 66:64, 1982.
3. Bagolini B. Presentazione di una sbarra di filtri a densita scalare assorbenti i raggi luminosi Boll Ocul 36:638, 1957.
4. Bagolini, B: Anomalous correspondence: definition and diagnostic methods. Doc Ophthalmol 23:346, 1967.
5. Bagolini, B: I Sensorial anomalies in strabismus (suppression, anomalous correspondence amblyopia). Doc Ophthalmol 41:1, 1976.
6. Bagolini, B: 11. Sensorio-motorial anomalies in strabismus (anomalous movements). Doc Ophthalmol 41:23, 1976.
7. Baker, FH, Grigg, P and Noorden, GK von: Effects of visual deprivation and strabismus on the response of neurons in the visual cortex of the monkey, including studies on the striate prestriate cortex in the normal animal. Brian Res. 66: 185, 1974.
8. Bielschowsky A: Lectures on motor anomalies, V Development and causes of strabismus. Am J Ophthalmol. 22:38, 1939.
9. Boeder, P: Anomalous retinal correspondence refuted. Am J Ophthalmol 58:366, 1964.
10. Bradley, A, and Freeman, RD: Is reduced vernier acuity in amblyopia due to position, contrast, or fixation deficits. Vision Res. 25:55, 1985.
11. Burian, HM: Sensorial retinal relationship in concomitant strabismus. Trans Am Ophthalmol Soc. 81: 373, 1945.
12. Burian, HM: Normal and anomalous correspondence. In Allen, JH, editor: Strabismus ophthalmic symposium I, St. Louis, 1950, Mosby-Year Book, Inc., p130.
13. Burian, HM: Anomalous retinal correspondence: Its essence and its significance in diagnosis and treatment. Am J Ophthalmol 34:237, 1951.
14. Burian, HM: Adaptive mechanisms. Trans Am Acad Ophthalmol Otolaryngol 57:131, 1953.
15. Burian, HM: Thoughts on the nature of amblyopia exanopsia. Am Orthopt J 6:5, 1956.
16. Burian, HM: The behavior of the amblyopic eye under reduced illumination and the theory of functional amblyopia. Doc Ophthalmol 23: 189, 1967.
17. Burian, HM, and Cortimiglia, RA: Visual acuity and fixation pattern in patients with strabismic amblyopia. Am Orthopt J 12:169, 1962.
18. Cantolino SJ: and Noorden. GK von: Heredity in microtropia. Arch Ophthalmol 81:753, 1969.
19. Capobianco, NM: The subjective measurement of the near point of convergence and its significance in the diagnosis of convergence insufficiency. Am Orthopt J 2:40, 1952.
20. Chavasse, BF: Worth's squint or the binocular reflexes and the treatment of strabismus, Philadelphia, 1939 P Blakiston's Son & Co. Inc.

21. Crawford MLJ, visual deprivation syndrome. Ophthalmology (Rochestter 85: 465, 1978.

22. Firth, AY: Pupillary responses in amblyopia. Br J Ophthalmol 74:676, 1990.

23. Garey L, Blakemore C: Monocular deprivation: Morphological effects on different classes of neurons in the lateral geniculate nucleus. Science 195:414, 1977.

24. Grunwald MJ, Parks MM: Amblyopia. In Tasman W, Jaeger EA (eds): Duane's clinical Ophthalmology, Philadephia, JB Lippincott 1990, VPI Ch. 101 pp 1-22.

25. Hielschowsky, A: Application of the afterimage test in the investigation of squint. Am J Ophthalmol 20:408, 1937.

26. Hubel, DN, and Wiesel, TN: Receptive fields, binocular interaction and functional architecture in the cat's visual cortex. J Physiol (Lond.) 160:106, 1962

27. Hubel, DH, and Wiesel,TN: Receptive fields of single neurons in the cat's striate cortex. J Physiol 148:574, 1959

28. Hubel, DH, and Wiesel, TN: Stereoscopic vision in macaque monkey, cells sensitive to binocular depth in area 18 of the macaque monkey cortex. Nature 225:41, 1970

29. Jampolsky, A: Characteristics of suppression in strabismus. Arch Ophthalmol 54:683. 1955.

30. Jampolsky, A: The prism test for strabismus screening. J Pediatr Ophthalmol 1:30, 1964.

31. Noorden, GK von: Pathogenesis of eccentric fixation. Doc Ophthalmol. 23:263, 1967.

32. Noorden, GK von: The etiology and pathogenesis of fixation anomalies in strabismus. Trans. Am. Ophthalmol. Soc. 67:698, 1969.

33. Noorden, GK von: Histological studies of the visual system in monkeys with experimental amblyopia Invest Ophthalmol 12:727, 1973.

34. Noorden, GK von: Mechanisms of amblyopia. Doc Ophthalmol 34:93, 1977.

35. Noorden, GK von: Infantile esotropia: a continuing riddle (Scobee Lecture). Am Orthopt. J 34:52, 1984.

36. Noorden, GK von: Idiopathic amblyopia. Am J Ophthalmol 100:214, 1985.

37. Noorden, GK von: Amblyopia: a multidisciplinary approach (Proctor Lecture). Invest. Ophthalmol. Vis, Sci. 26:1704, 1985.

38. Noorden, GK von, and Crawford, MLI: Morphological and Physiological changes in the monkey visual system after short-term lid suture. Invest Ophthalmol Vis. Sci. 17:762, 1978.

39. Noorden, GK von, and Maumenee, AE: Clinical observations on stimulus deprivation amblyopia (amblyopia exanopsia). Am J Ophthalmol 65: 220, 1968.

40. Noorden, GK von, and Middleditch PR: Histology of the monkey lateral geniculate nucleus after unilateral lid closure and experimental strabismus: further observations. Invest Ophthalmol 14:674, 1975.

HETEROPHORIA

DEFINITION

Heterophoria, also known as *'latent strabismus'*, is a condition wherein the tendency of the eyes to deviate is kept latent by the fusion reflex. However, when the fusion is interrupted, for example, by occluding one eye, the visual axis of the occluded eye deviates from its position and if the occluder is removed, the fusion reflex will turn the eye back into the orthoposition. While, *orthophoria* is a condition of perfect alignment of the two eyes which is maintained even after the removal of influence of fusion. However, orthophoria is just a theoretical ideal. Practically, a small amount of heterophoria is of universal occurrence and is known as *'physiological heterophoria'*. The incidence of distance heterophoria in primary position has been reported to be as high as 80% and that for near phorias close to 100%. When tested in different directions of gaze, almost everyone is found to have small degree of heterophoria.

ETIOLOGY

In general, the factors which play role in the etiology of heterophoria are the same as for heterotropia. For details *see* page 97.

TYPES OF HETEROPHORIA

Depending upon the direction of deviation, heterophoria may be:
- Esophoria
- Exophoria
- Hyperphoria, and
- Cyclophoria.

ESOPHORIA

In this condition, when fusion is interrupted, the non-fixating eye becomes convergent, i.e. deviates nasally. Esophoria is less frequent than exophoria. Only about 33% of all patients with a distance phoria are esophoric. Near esophorias occur even less frequently.

Clinical types

Esophoria may be:

1. *Convergence excess type*. Esophoria is greater on near fixation than on distant fixation.

2. *Divergence weakness type*. Esophoria is greater on distant fixation than on near fixation.

3. *Non-specific type*. Esophoria which does not vary significantly in degree for any distance.

Etiological types

The etiological factors have been discussed in general etiology of heterophoria. Common etiological types of esophoria are as follows:

1. *Accommodative esophoria*. It may be associated with:

a. *Uncorrected high hypermetropia.* In this condition, excessive use of accommodation in a bid to clear the blurred retinal image is associated with increased accommodative convergence. It may result in esophoria for distance and near in proportion to the accommodation used and the patient's fusional divergence.

b. *High AC/A ratio* may be associated with esophoria. Effect of AC/A ratio on basic esophoria is depicted in Table 9.1.

Table 9.1 *Effect of AC/A ratio on basic esophoria*	
AC/A ratio	Esophoria
Normal	E^1 slightly smaller than E
High	E^1 almost equal or greater than E
Low	E^1 smaller than E

2. *Tonic esophoria*. Most of the non-accommodative esophorias are due to increased tonic convergence which may be due to either overactivity or insufficient inhibition of the involved centres of the central nervous system.

3. *Esophoria due to other causes* includes those due to anatomical and innervational factors.

EXOPHORIA

In this condition, the non-fixating eye becomes divergent on dissociation, i.e. when fusion is interrupted. However, under condition of bifoveal single vision, the deviation is corrected by the fusional convergence. Exophoria is the commonest variety of heterophoria. It constitutes about 60% of all cases of heterophoria for distance and about 80% of all cases of heterophoria for near.

Types

Exophoria may be of following types:

1. *Convergence weakness type*. Exophoria is greater on near fixation than on distant fixation. In this condition, symptoms primarily occur during close work. Such patients frequently complain that during reading letters run together. The blurring is due to accommodation and occurs when fusional convergence becomes insufficient to cope up with the deviation, e.g. during prolonged close work.

2. *Divergence excess type*. Exophoria is greater on distant fixation than on near fixation. In such patients, asthenopic symptoms occur during activities connected with distant vision.

3. *Non-specific type*. This type of exophoria does not vary significantly in degree for any distance.

Relation of near exophoria to distance exophoria

The basic deviation in exophoria is measured while the patient fixates a distant target using his/her full optical correction and near exophoria is measured, when patient fixates a target at 33 cm. The patient's AC/A ratio influences the magnitude of near phoria (X') in relation to distance phoria (X) as depicted in Table 9.2.

Table 9.2 *Effect of AC/A ratio on near vs distance exophoria*	
AC/A ratio	Exophoria
Normal	X^1 slightly greater than X
High	X^1 almost same or smaller than X
Low	X^1 greater than X

HYPERPHORIA

It is a vertical deviation occurring on dissociation in which one eye rotates upwards or the other downwards depending upon the fixation. In orthoptic practice, the term hypophoria is avoided and it has become customary to use the term right or left hyperphoria depending upon the eye which remains up as compared to the other. For example, in a right hyperphoria, the right eye rotates upwards, when it is not fixating and when the right eye is fixating, the left eye rotates downwards, and reverse to it occurs in left hyperphoria.

The incidence of hyperphoria has been reported to be about 30%. Frequently, hyperphoria is combined with horizontal phorias. Since vertical fusional vergences are of small amplitude, asthenopic symptoms are more marked in hyperphorias than the horizontal phorias. For the same reason, even the minor prismatic action of glasses (due to vertical decentring) may be difficult to compensate.

A hyperphoria may be comitant or incomitant. Paresis of an extraocular muscle and anatomic anomalies of muscles and tendons and/or their insertions constitute the major causes of hyperphoria. Since, more frequently, hyperphoria is incomitant, measurements should be taken: (a) with either eye being the fixating eye, (b) in the cardinal positions, and (c) in the reading position. The latter is obviously more important since a special therapeutic solution has to be found, if the patient's deviation in the reading position differs from that in the primary position.

CYCLOPHORIA

It is the tendency of the either eye to wheel rotate around the anteroposterior axis on dissociation. When the 12 O'clock meridian of cornea rotates nasally, it is called *incyclophoria* and when it rotates temporally, it is called *excyclophoria*. Excyclophoria is of more frequent occurrence than the incyclophoria. In general, cyclophorias of clinical significance are of rare occurrence and are frequently associated with vertical deviation. Asthenopic symptoms are most marked with cyclophorias.

■ SYMPTOMS OF HETEROPHORIA

Symptoms that may be caused by phorias are of a very non-specific nature and they may also occur for other reasons. In general, the term *asthenopia* is used to denote the symptom complex produced by heterophoria. As already mentioned, asthenopia is most marked with cyclophoria followed by hyperphoria. Small degrees of esophoria and exophoria produce little or no symptoms.

Depending upon the symptoms, heterophoria can be divided into compensated and decompensated.

Compensated heterophoria. It is associated with no subjective symptoms. Compensation of the phoria depends upon the reserve neuro-muscular power to overcome the muscular imbalance and individual's desire for maintenance of binocular vision.

Decompensated heterophoria. It is associated with multiple symptoms which may be grouped as under:

1. *Symptoms of muscular fatigue.* These result due to continuous use of the reserve neuro-muscular power and are usually more marked after the day's work. These include:

- *Headache and eye ache* after prolonged use of eyes, which is relieved when the eyes are closed for a while.
- *Difficulty in changing the focus* from near to distant objects of fixation or vice versa.
- *Photophobia, itching* and *burning* may also be experienced by some patients. Photophobia due to muscular fatigue is not relieved by using dark goggles, but is relieved by closing one eye.

2. *Symptoms due to failure to maintain binocular vision.* These include:

- *Blurring or crowding* of words while reading.
- *Intermittent diplopia* due to temporary manifest deviation under conditions of fatigue.
- *Intermittent squint* (without diplopia) may occur in patients who involuntarily learn to suppress. It is usually noticed by the patient's close relations or friends.

3. *Symptoms of defective postural sensations* cause problems in judging distances and positions, especially of the moving objects. This difficulty may be experienced particularly by cricketers, tennis players and pilots during landing.

■ EXAMINATION (EVALUATION) OF A CASE OF HETEROPHORIA

It should include the following tests:

1. *Testing of visual acuity and refraction.* It is of prime importance in management of heterophoria.

2. *Testing for ocular movements.* Uniocular as well as binocular movements should be tested meticulously (*see* page 113).

3. *Cover-uncover test.* It is quite useful in detecting the presence of a heterophoria. When using an occluder to dissociate the eyes, the fusion reflex innervation does not immediately close completely covering one eye, although all

fusional stimuli are excluded by the cover. Therefore, the cover should be kept in front of the eye for a few moments before proceeding with the test.

4. Measurement of heterophoria. A heterophoria should be measured for both distance and near. To obtain the basic measurement of a heterophoria, the patient should fixate a distant target and should not accommodate. It is necessary, therefore, that he/she wears full optical distance correction. It should also be kept in mind that lenses that are decentred before the eye have a prismatic effect and that this may obscure the true situation because the patient has to overcome such an effect during binocular vision through fusional vergence. Thus a phoria may be simulated or depending on the direction of prismatic displacement, an existing phoria may be exaggerated or minimized, if lenses of sufficient power are decentred to a significant degree during the phoria test.

The near phoria should be measured at a fixation distance of about 33 cm using a target which requires accommodation rather than a flashlight. In presbyopes, the near phoria should be determined while they fixate through their reading glasses.

Commonly employed tests to measure the heterophoria are as follows:

Objective tests: Prism and cover test (page 105)

Subjective tests include:

- Maddox rod test (page 109)
- Maddox wing test (page 111)
- Double prism test (page 113)

5. Measurement of convergence, accommodation and AC/A ratio. A knowledge about these parameters is quite useful in the management of heterophoria.

6. Measurement of fusional reserve. It is essential to examine the patient's fusional vergence amplitude to form a meaningful opinion of the significance of his/her phoria. During this examination, an excessive demand is placed on the vergence mechanism. This may induce a transient phoria in some patients. *Therefore, in clinical practice, the phoria should be measured first and the vergence amplitude determined afterward.*

The power of the fusional vergence that opposes and overcomes the phoria during bifoveal vision is very important in planning the treatment of phoria. The fusional vergence available in excess of the amount necessary to overcome the phoria and to bring the eyes into orthoposition is called the *fusional reserve* or the *relative vergence.* Though there does not exist any relationship between the amount of fusional reserve and degree of phoria producing symptoms, but, in general, bifoveal vision is comfortable, when the fusional reserve is twice as large as the phoria.

7. Assessment of state of binocular vision. It is also helpful in planning the management of a heterophoria. For details of the various tests, *see* page 83.

TREATMENT OF HETEROPHORIA

INDICATIONS OF TREATMENT

- *In adults,* treatment is indicated only if the patient is suffering from symptoms. Sometimes it is difficult to decide whether or not the asthenopic symptoms are due to the phoria. In such cases, occlusion may be used to diagnose. If this relieves the symptoms, it is very likely that the phoria is the cause.
- *In children,* however, treatment is indicated, if the phoria is showing a tendency to decompensate into a manifest deviation, whether symptoms are present or not.

CHOICE OF TREATMENT

The treatment modalities employed in heterophoria includes, glasses, miotics, orthoptic exercises, prismotherapy and surgery. The choice of a particular modality in a given patient depends upon different factors, some of which are as follows:

1. *Age and cooperation* of the patient, e.g. in a small child, miotics may be used to facilitate accommodation.

2. *Etiology of heterophoria*

- If a phoria is entirely or partly caused by a refractive error, glasses will eliminate or improve the condition.
- When a phoria is due to abnormal AC/A ratio, orthoptic exercises to increase the fusional amplitudes are the method of choice.

- Surgery is indicated in phorias of anatomic or paretic origin for which other treatment methods cannot be successful.

3. *Size and type of heterophoria*

- When the heterophoria is too large to be controlled easily with other methods, surgery will be necessary.
- When vertical phorias are associated with horizontal phorias, an attempt should be made to eliminate the vertical deviation first, since in a number of instances, this will enable the patient to control the horizontal phorias with much less effort.

4. *The speed of recovery to binocular single vision on cover test.* Symptomatic phorias with very slow recovery require surgical treatment more often than those with a quick recovery.

TREATMENT MODALITIES

1. Optical correction

In all cases, a meticulous refraction should be performed and correct glasses prescribed. Optical correction may eliminate the underlying cause of the phoria in some patients. General guidelines for prescribing glasses are as follows:

- Astigmatic errors and spherical differences between the two eyes should be eliminated completely.
- In *exophoria*, both eyes may be undercorrected by an equal amount of spherical plus power. This forces the patient to accommodate constantly and accordingly induces accommodative convergence. However, it should be kept in mind that constant accommodation itself may lead to eye strain.
- In *esophoria*, the patient should receive as much spherical plus correction as is compatible with his/her best visual acuity. Bifocal glasses decrease or eliminate the need for accommodation during near vision and thus may be useful in patients having esophoria of convergence excess type. Bifocals should be used as a temporary aid to orthoptic treatment aiming to reduce the bifocal segment as soon as possible.
- In *hyperphoria*, if feasible, the lenses of the patient's optical correction may be decentred

to achieve a prismatic effect thus relieving the stress on patient's vertical vergence control.

- In *cyclophoria*, the best efforts should be made to correct the astigmatic refractive error, when associated.

2. Orthoptic treatment

Aim of orthoptic treatment of heterophoria is to improve fusional reserves so that the bifoveal single vision can be maintained without efforts.

Orthoptic treatment also known as 'vision therapy' includes:

A. *Conventional or non-computerised excercise for:*
- In-office vision therapy, and
- Home vision therapy

B. *Computerised orthoptic excercises for:*
- In-office vision therapy, and
- Home vision therapy

Note: Conventional, i.e. non-computerised excercises are described here. For computerised exercises *see* page 146.

Orthoptic exercises for esophoria

In general, the orthoptic treatment of esophoria is aimed at improving the amplitude of fusional divergence (relative negative convergence). This can be accomplished by the following exercises:

a. *Divergence exercises with prisms.* Prisms of increasing strength are placed base-in before one eye while he/she is fixating an object at any distance (preferably at a distance where the esophoria is maximum). Patient is trained to maintain a single vision by relaxing the convergence.

Loose prisms, a prism bar or rotatory (Risley) prisms may be used for this purpose. A prism bar should be preferred. Prism exercises are performed for a few minutes at each weekly visit.

b. *Divergence exercises on synoptophore.* These exercises are performed on synoptophore using stereopsis slides, because they provide the strongest stimulus to fusion. After fusing the two pictures, patient is trained to maintain a single vision (by relaxing convergence) while the instrument tubes are diverged. These exercises should be performed for about 5 minutes at each weekly visit.

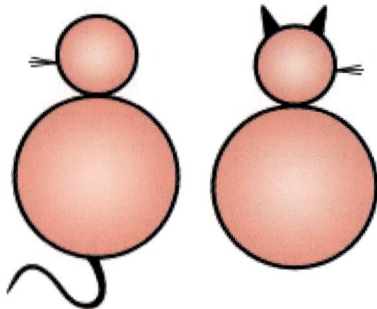

Fig. 9.1 *Stereogram card.*

c. *Physiologic diplopia exercises using stereograms in the crossed position.* To perform this exercise, patient is first trained to appreciate crossed physiological diplopia with a flash light or pencil. Once the patient is trained, the exercise is performed as below:

While the patient is fixating a distant object, the stereogram card (Fig. 9.1) is held about 25 cm in front of his/her eyes. Patient will perceive four pictures (because of crossed physiological diplopia). He/she is trained to adjust its position until the two central pictures are fused and patient perceives three pictures (Fig. 9.2). Patient is trained to maintain the joined pictures and to see it clearly. While doing so, patient is converging for the distant target but accommodating for near (distance of the card) and thus relatively relaxing his/her convergence.

Once the patient is trained to perform this exercise, he/she can practice at home for a few minutes several times a day.

d. *Exercises using diploscope.* For details *see* page 141.

e. *Exercises using Remy separator.* For details *see* page 143.

f. *Reading bar exercises.* For details *see* page 143.

Orthoptic exercises for esophoria should be carried out weekly in the clinic and should be supported by home exercises as discussed above. It is important to ensure that constant efforts to relax convergence have not resulted in an inability to obtain a normal near point of convergence. This should be checked at regular intervals.

It is more difficult to improve relative negative convergence than relative positive convergence. Therefore, esophorias respond less well to orthoptic treatment alone.

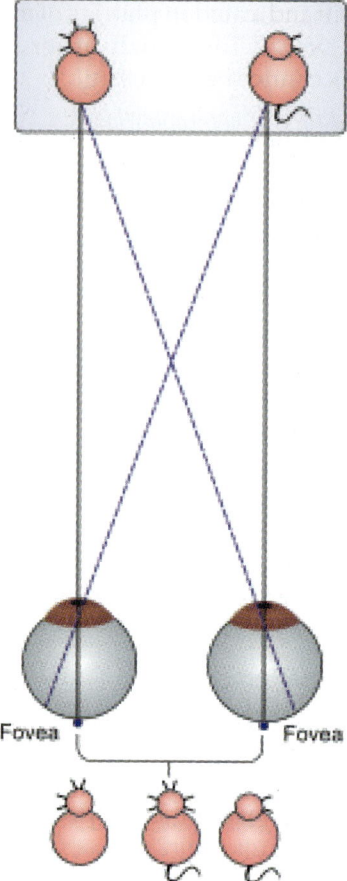

Fig. 9.2 *Physiologic diplopia excercises using stereogram in the crossed position.*

Orthoptic exercises for exophoria

The aim is to improve the fusional convergence (relative positive convergence). This can be accomplished by the following:

a. *Convergence exercise with prisms.* It is similar to that described for esophoria, except that in it, prisms are placed base-out in front of the eyes. While the patient is performing this exercise, the orthoptist should watch the patient's eyes to make certain that he/she is converging and has not diverged and suppressed.

b. *Convergence exercise using synoptophore.* It is performed as described for esophoria, except that in it, the instrument arms are slowly converged, beginning at an angle at which patient can fuse the picture.

c. *Physiologic diplopia exercise using stereogram in the uncrossed position.* To perform this exercise, the stereogram card is held at arm's length in front of the patient and a pencil (fixation point) is placed midway between his/her eyes and the card. When he/she looks at the pencil, he/she will notice diplopia (uncrossed) of the card and will see four instead of two pictures. Patient is trained to adjust the position of the pencil in such a way that the two central pictures are joined into one so that now he/she sees three pictures (Fig. 9.3). The patient is trained to see the fused central picture clearly. In doing so, he/she is converging for the fixation object and accommodating for the distance of the card, i.e. he/she is converging relatively more than he/she is accommodating. Patient can practise this exercise at home for a few minutes several times a day.

d. Convergence exercise using diploscope. *See page 141.*

e. Exercises for improving near point of convergence. These are as follows:

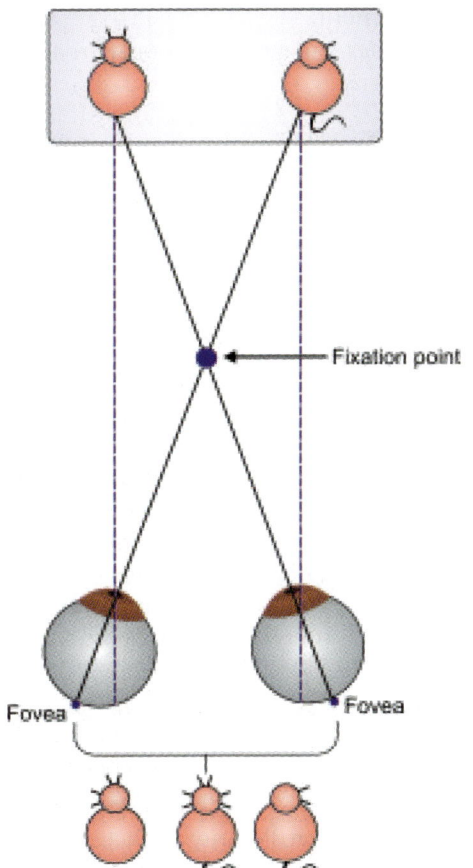

Fixation point

Fovea   Fovea

Fig. 9.3 *Physiologic diplopia excercises using stereogram in the uncrossed position.*

i. *Advancement exercise.* It is a good convergence exercise which can be done at near. In it, patient is asked to hold a target (preferably a small detailed picture or fine print) away from his/her nose where fusion is possible. He/She is asked to slowly advance the target towards his/her nose until diplopia is appreciated. At this point, he/she is asked to stop and try to converge more and, thus to unite the two images again. If he/she cannot do this, he/she should move the target back to a small distance to get single vision and then try to bring it closer again. This should be repeated until the patient can converge to his/her nose or at least reasonably close to it.

ii. *Jump convergence exercise.* Jump convergence is more elaborate and more effective form of the 'picture-to-nose' convergence exercise. It trains the patient to achieve bifoveal single vision following a sudden change in the convergence requirement. This is usually possible only after convergence has been improved to some extent by other exercises and therefore, is not used before the fourth week of convergence training, depending upon the progress. This exercise may be carried out by any of the following methods:

- The simplest way of doing this exercise is to have two fixation targets, one fixed target at a distance of about 6 metres and other movable target held about 33 cm in front of the eyes. The patient is asked to change his/her fixation repeatedly between the distance and near targets. Subsequently, the near target is brought closer to the eyes until he/she can eventually change from distant fixation to fixation at 5 cm while keeping one image of the near object, even though it may be very blurred.

- Another way of performing jump convergence exercise is the use of prism. Patient is asked to fixate an object and a 10D prism is placed base-out in front of one eye. Patient is instructed to try to maintain single vision. In doing so, he/she has to converge his/her eyes. The prism is then removed and convergence is relaxed for a few seconds. This is repeated several times with prisms of increasing strength until eventually the patient can converge to overcome a 40D prism.

- Jump convergence exercise can also be performed with synoptophore. Patient is asked to join the two pictures from stereopsis slides. He/she is then asked to look up on a distant target, while the orthoptist moves the tubes of instrument into slightly more convergent position. Patient is then asked to look back at the pictures. Patient will have to converge to obtain single vision. This is repeated several times, converging the instrument tubes more each time, until the patient can converge to overcome an angle of 60D.

3. Role of miotic drugs in the treatment of heterophoria

Miotic drugs are the treatment of choice in near esophoria due to a high AC/A ratio. Miotics facilitate accommodation, so that less than normal innervation is necessary to obtain a given accommodative response and consequently there occurs less accommodative convergence. Therefore, miotics are useful aid to orthoptic treatment in convergence excess type of decompensating esophorias, if orthoptic treatment alone is insufficient to relieve the symptoms.

Miotics do not affect the distance deviation, for distance vision, no accommodation is necessary, if full correction is provided by glasses. However, if for some reasons, full optical correction has not been provided, the distance esophoria will also show a decrease.

Usually, phospholine iodide 0.06%, or 0.125% is used once daily.

4. Role of prisms

- Prisms may be used as a training device for orthoptic exercises as discussed above. They may also be incorporated as a permanent correction in the patient's glasses, or they may be clipped on by the patient for specific purposes only.
- Role of prisms as a permanent correction in horizontal phorias is debatable. They should be considered only after other measures have failed to relieve the symptoms. For exophoria, base-in prisms and for esophoria base-out prisms are incorporated into the glasses.
- Primarily, prisms are prescribed as a permanent correction in the treatment of comitant vertical phorias. A vertical prismatic correction of 10D is the maximum amount that

can be tolerated. There is no fixed rule as to the amount of prism correction to be given in a particular patient. However, in practice, prism is prescribed with apex towards the phoria to correct only half or at the most two-thirds of total heterophorias.

5. Surgical treatment of heterophoria

Indications

- *Horizontal phorias.* Surgery becomes necessary only when symptoms cannot be relieved by other methods. This is most frequently true, when the basic deviation is too large to be controlled despite good fusional vergence. An operation is also indicated in phorias of anatomic or paretic origin for which other treatment methods cannot be successful.
- *Vertical phorias.* In many hyperphorias, especially those of paretic origin and those too large to be corrected by prisms, surgery is the best treatment.
- *Cyclophorias.* Surgery is the only treatment of cyclophorias.

Amount of surgery

It is an erroneous attitude to think that lesser amount of surgery is required in heterophorias in comparison to heterotropias. In fact, the amount of surgery must be aimed at the basic deviation and the goal to align the eyes, regardless of whether it is a latent, intermittent or manifest deviation. However, a conservative approach has been recommended when considering surgery in patients beyond 50 years of age.

BIBLIOGRAPHY

1. Crone RA: A new theory about heterophoria. Ophthalmologica 1971;162:199.
2. Flynn JT, Grundmann S, Mashikian M: Binocular suppression of scotoma: its role in phorias and intermittent tropias. Am Orthopt J 1970;20:54.
3. Jampolsky A, Flom B, Fried A: Fixation disparity in relation to heterophoria. Am J Ophthalmol 1957;43:97.
4. Palmer EA, Noorden GK von: The relationship between fixation disparity and heterophoria. Am J Ophthalmol 1978;86:172.
5. Scobee RG: The oculorotary muscles, 2nd ed., St. Louis. 1952, Mosby-Year Book, Inc.

Chapter
10
Concomitant Esotropias and Exotropias

Chapter Outline

CONCOMITANT ESOTROPIAS

- Definition
- Classification
- Infantile esotropia
- Accommodative esotropias
- Refractive
- Nonrefractive
- Hypoaccommodative
- Partial accommodative
- Acquired non-accommodative esotropias
- Sensory esotropia
- Consecutive esotropia

CONCOMITANT EXOTROPIAS

- Congenital (infantile) exotropia
- Primary exotropia
- Etiology
- Classification
- Intermittent exotropia
- Constant exotropia
- Sensory exotropia
- Consecutive exotropia

CONCOMITANT ESOTROPIAS

DEFINITION

Concomitant esotropia is the term used to describe any manifest convergent deviation of the visual axes in which the amount of deviation in the squinting eye remains constant (unaltered) in all the directions of gaze and there is no associated limitation of ocular movements.

In general, development of an esodeviation has got three stages:

1. *Stage of latent esodeviation.* In this stage, the esodeviation is kept latent by the control of fusional divergence reserve. It is also called the stage of *esophoria.* It has been described in detail on page 209.

2. *Stage of intermittent esodeviation.* In this stage, the fusional divergence reserves which usually keep the deviation latent, become inadequate intermittently resulting in intermittent manifest esodeviation (*intermittent esotropia).*

3. *Stage of constant esodeviation.* When the fusional divergence amplitude becomes inadequate to maintain the latency of deviation, a permanent manifest esodeviation, i.e. *constant esotropia* occurs. Constant esotropia may be unilateral esotropia or alternating esotropia.

Note. Since the fusional divergence mechanism is much weaker (amplitude 4 to 6 PD) than fusional convergence (amplitude >30 PD), the esodeviations usually become constant with poor stereoacuity. While in contrast, exodeviations tend to remain intermittent with good stereoacuity for a longer period.

CLASSIFICATION

Concomitant esodeviations can be classified into following clinico-etiological groups:

1. *Infantile (congenital) estropia.* It is a large angel estropia that is constantly mainfest and occurs during first few months of life.

2. *Accommodative esotropia.* The deviation increases, when accommodation is exerted. It may be:

i. Refractive accommodative esotropia

ii. Non-refractive accommodative esotropia

  – Hyperaccommodative (high AC/A ratio)

iii. Hypoaccommodative (weak accommodation)

iv. Mixed or partially accommodative esotropia.

3. Acquired non-accommodative esotropia. The acquired esotropia, in which deviations not affected by the state of accommodation, includes:

i. Essential acquired or late onset non-accommodative esotropia, which can be:
- Basic esotropia
- Convergence excess esotropia
- Divergence insufficiency esotropia

ii. Acute concomitant esotropia

iii. Microtropia

iv. Nystagmus blockage syndrome

v. Cyclic esotropia

vi. Divergence pareses

vii. Stress-induced esotropia

viii. Esotropia in myopia

ix. Esotropia due to spasm of near reflex.

4. Sensory esotropia. It results from a poor vision in one eye.

5. Consecutive esotropia. It results following surgical over correction of exotropia.

Unilateral versus alternating esotropia

Primary constant esotropia of any type may be either unilateral or alternating depending upon the type of fixation. Some of the important points worth mentioning about each type are given below.

Unilateral esotropia

- It occurs more frequently than alternating esotropia.
- In it, one eye is habitually preferred for fixation and the other eye is always deviated.
- If an anisometropia exists, almost invariably the eye with the lesser spherical or astigmatic error will be fixating eye.
- In patients with small angle esotropia (up to about 15Δ), harmonious anomalous retinal correspondence and moderate degree of amblyopia are found more frequently than in those with larger deviations, in whom

profound amblyopia and normal retinal correspondence prevail.

Alternating esotropia

- In alternating esotropia, either eye is used alternately for fixation while the other one assumes the deviated position.
- The patients frequently use crossfixation, especially when the angle of deviation is large.
- Visual acuity is almost equal in both eyes.
- Sensory adaptations in alternating esotropia are such that while one eye fixates, the deviating eye is either suppressed or participates through anomalous retinal correspondence (ARC) in binocular vision. Incidence of ARC is high and is found with greater frequency in patients with small angle deviations than in those with large angles in whom NRC prevails.
- Since either eye is used for fixation part of the time, there is no amblyopia.

■ INFANTILE ESOTROPIA

Infantile esotropia (old name—congenital esotropia) is a distinct clinical form of esotropia which usually presents at 1–2 months of age. However, it may be detected shortly after birth or any time within the first 6 months of life. Previously, it was known as 'congenital esotropia'.

ETIOLOGY

The exact etiology of infantile esotropia is obscure. Following factors have been implicated:

1. Innervational disturbance in the form of an imbalance between tonic convergence and divergence is being considered the probable cause rather than the anatomic cause. This view has been derived from the observation that many a time, the eyes of such a patient become straight or even divergent under anaesthesia.

2. Role of accommodation. It has also been reported that an accommodative element may be responsible partially or wholly in some cases of infantile esotropia. Further, in some cases, an accommodative element may be superadded over the basic deviation at the age of 2–3 years.

3. *General and environmental factors* include low birth weight, prematurity, perinatal hypoxia, maternal-smoking, drugs and alcohol abuse.

CLINICAL FEATURES

1. *Time of onset.* In most of the cases, squint manifests within first 6 months of birth in an otherwise normal infant.

2. *Angle of deviation.* Most patients with infantile esotropia (Fig. 10.1) have a large angle

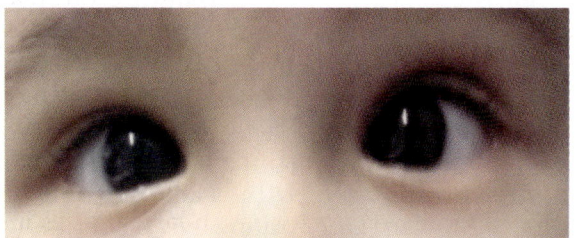

Fig. 10.1 *A child with infantile esotropia.*

of deviation for both distance and near fixation. In half of the patients, the deviation measures 30° or more. The angle of deviation is usually stable except in a few cases having an accommodative element in the etiology.

3. *Fixation pattern.* Usually an alternate fixation occurs in primary gaze and crossed fixation in lateral gaze, i.e. the infant fixates the objects in the left field with right eye and the objects in the right field with the left eye (Fig. 10.2).

4. *Apparant limitation of abduction.* The cross-fixation makes the abduction of either eye unnecessary and thus on initial examination, the impression of bilateral sixth nerve palsy may be given. However, following examination techniques may help in demonstrating the presence of abduction:

a. *Doll's head phenomenon test.* This is simple, easy and best method of demonstrating presence of abduction in an infant. In this technique, the examiner grasps the top of the infant's head and quickly turns it in horizontal direction. During this manoeuvre, an observation for the occurrence of abduction is made in the eye opposite to head turn, i.e. when head is suddenly turned towards the right, the observation should be made in left eye and vice versa.

b. *Rotating the child for demonstrating abduction.* In this technique, the examiner holds the infant in his hands and rotates him completely first in one direction and then the other. While rotating towards his right the examiner should look for a quick abductive movement in the infant's right eye and vice versa (Fig. 10.3).

c. *Alternate patching.* If the above described two techniques fail to demonstrate abduction, then an alternate patching of the either eye should be done for several hours. If there is no lateral rectus palsy in the unpatched eye, the ability to abduct will become apparent (Fig. 10.4).

5. *Visual acuity* is normal and equal in both eyes of patients who freely alternate fixation. If, however, one eye is preferred, amblyopia will develop in the other eye.

6. *Refractive errors.* The refractive errors are not prominent, but are consistent with the patient's age group.

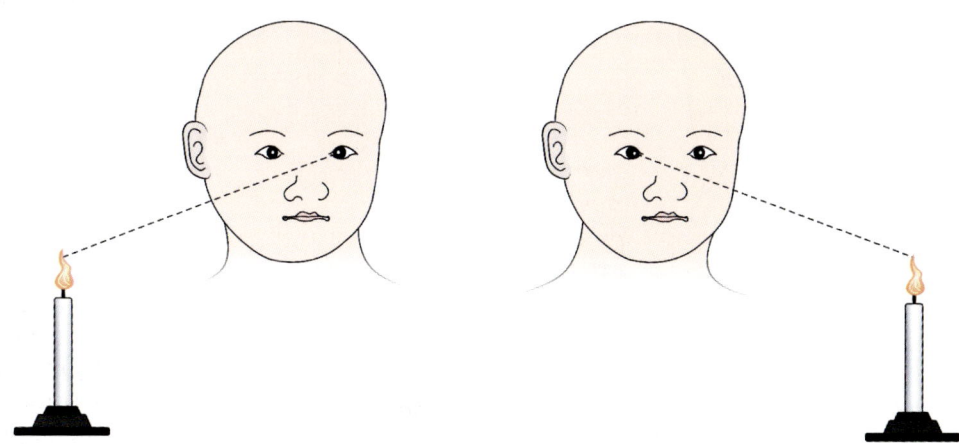

Fig. 10.2 *Diagrammatic depiction of crossfixation in a patient with infantile esotropia.*

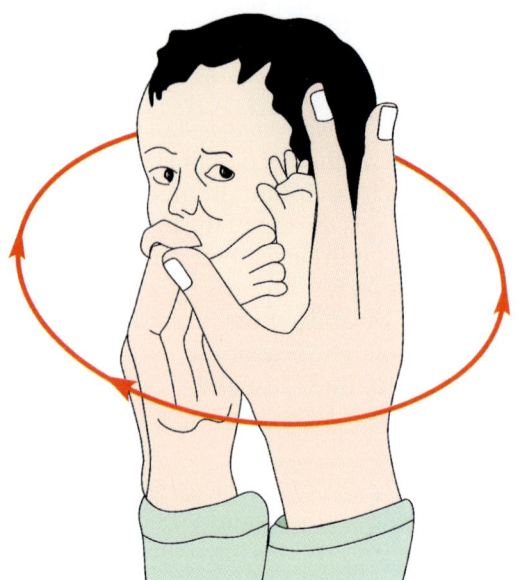

Fig. 10.3 *Rotation of an infant to determine lateral rectus palsy (for explanation see text).*

Associations

Infantile esotropia is frequently associated with other ocular abnormalities. Under such circumstances, the condition is labelled as *infantile esotropia syndrome.* Components other than esotropia of this syndrome are as follows:

1. *Inferior oblique overaction.* A marked degree of overaction of one or both inferior oblique muscles may be seen in about 50–60% of patients above one year of age. Before this age, it is rarely seen suggesting that probably it represents an evolutionary stage in the development of infantile esotropia syndrome.

2. *Dissociated vertical deviation (DVD).* It is an important component of the syndrome, seen in about 70 to 90% of cases. For details of DVD, *see* page 264.

3. *Latent nystagmus.* A jerk type of latent nystagmus having a decreasing exponential slow phase is another component of the syndrome seen in about 33% cases. The nystagmus occurs in both eyes, on occluding one eye, with the fast component directed towards the fixating (uncovered) eye. In patients having alternate squint, nystagmus may occur while both eyes are open, with a fast component directed towards the fixating eye. Under these circumstances, it might be confused with the true congenital nystagmus and thus electro-oculography may be indicated for differentiation.

4. *Lack of bifixation.* Inherent lack of capacity for bifixation is another component of the syndrome. Therefore, many patients with infantile esotropia syndrome, even after full surgical correction performed in time, do not achieve normal stereopsis. This is one of the causes of *monofixation syndrome* which has been described on page 235.

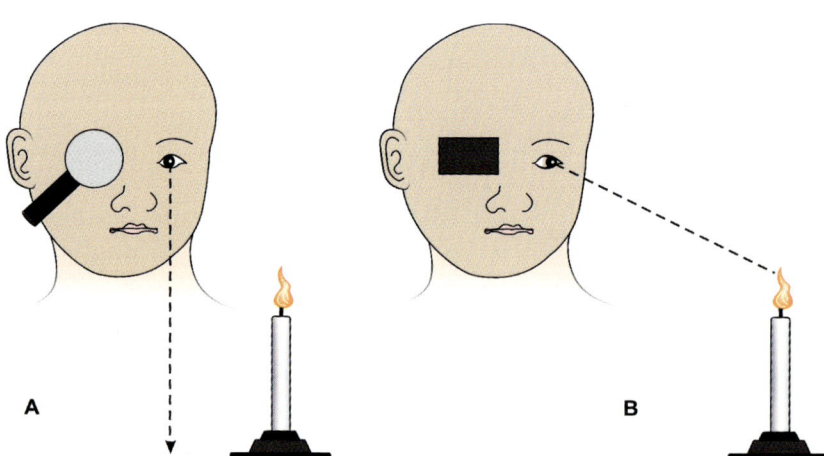

A   **B**

Fig. 10.4 *Patch test to detect ability of abduction in an infant: A, momentary occlusion of the fixing eye may not suffice to force the fellow eye to take up fixation; B, patching for several hours may be required to detect abduction ability in the originally non-fixing eyes.*

MANAGEMENT

Management of a case of infantile esotropia can be considered under following heads:
- Clinical evaluation and differential diagnosis
- Non-surgical treatment
- Surgical treatment
- Surgical results and post-surgical treatment

A. Clinical evaluation and differential diagnosis

The essential infantile esotropia usually manifests between birth and 6 months of age and thus needs to be differentiated from following conditions:

1. *Pseudoesotropia* or aparant esotropia may occur in infants due to following associations:
- Prominent epicanthal folds (Fig. 5.3)
- Small interpupillary distance
- Negative angle kappa, and
- Excessively broad nasal bridge

2. *Infantile accommodative esotropia.* Though accommodative esotropia usually occurs between 2 and 3 years of age but can occur in infants as young on 2 months of age and is often diagnosed as infantile esotropia. The key features which help to differentiate infantile accommodative esotropia from infantile (congenital) esotropia are:
- Presence of straight eyes for the first 2–3 months of life,
- Variable angle of strabismus, and
- Hypermetropia >2D.

3. *Sensory esotropia* may occur rarely in infants with early onset retinoblastoma and other disorders of optic nerve and retina.

4. *Ciancia syndrome,* though a variant of infantile esotropia, is a distinct clinical entity characterized by following features:
- *Large angle esotropia* (>60 PD) with cross-fixation and both eyes appear to be stuck in towards the nose.
- *Face turn* towards fixing eye.
- *Limited abduction* bilaterally with good abduction saccades.
- *Jerk-end-point nystagmus* on attempted abduction with minimal or no nystagmus on adduction.

- *Tight medial rectus muscle* revealed on forced duction test.
- *Vision* is most comfortable with the eye in adduction leading to face turn towards the fixing eye.

5. *Congenital fibrosis syndrome,* also known as *strabismus fixus* (*see* page 350) may present as large angle congenital esotropia with severe limitation of abduction of one or both eyes. This is a congenital restrictive strabismus, often inherited as an autosomal dominant trait.

6. *Congenital sixth nerve palsy* unilateral or bilateral also needs to be differentiated from infantile esotropia.

Clinical work-up which may help in arising at the diagnosis should include:

1. *Examination of anterior segment* to rule out corneal pathology and congenital/developmental cataract.

2. *Estimation of visual acuity* in an infant can be made by OKN, PVT or VEP as described on page 40.

3. *Examination of fundus and media* is quite useful in diagnosing retinoblastoma and other abnormalities responsible for sensory squint.

4. *Refraction under atropine cycloplegia* helps in discovering refractive accommodative esotropia due to high hypermetropia. In essential infantile esotropia, cycloplegic refraction characteristically reveals only 1–2 D of hyperopia. Repeat refractions are important because an accommodative component is sometimes discovered on follow-up in patients with infantile esotropia.

5. *Measurement of AC/A ratio.* The lens gradient method (*see* page 119) can be used to know the approximate AC/A ratio.

6. *Measurement of deviation.* Usually, an approximate idea is made by observation for *distance deviation*, since it is not possible to get cooperation from the infant for a distance fixation. However, attempts may be made to measure the near deviation with the help of Krimsky test (described on page 107).

7. *Differentiation from simulated bilateral sixth nerve paralysis* can be made by Doll's head phenomenon test, i.e. rotating the child to demonstrate abduction or by alternate patching test as described earlier (Fig. 10.2).

Note. Most of the times, the above examinations and the typical clinical features are helpful in establishing the diagnosis of essential infantile esotropia. *Once diagnosed, treatment of choice for infantile esotropia is surgical alignment of the eyes.* However, some non-surgical treatments may be needed before the surgery is performed.

B. Non-surgical treatment

Non-surgical measures needed before the surgery is undertaken include the following:
1. *Correction of refractive error.* Usually correction of physiologic hypermetropia of 2D to 3D has little effect on the deviation. However, it has been advocated that when hypermetropia is more than +1.5D, glasses should be prescribed and child should be reassessed after 6 weeks. This time it may be possible to determine the AC/A ratio accurately, because accommodation will now be controlled by the patient's glasses. *Miotics* may be tried as an alternative to spectacles in unco-operative infants.
2. *Treatment of amblyopia.* Amblyopia, when present, should always be treated rigorously before rather than after the surgery. For treatment of amblyopia, *see* page 190. Failure to treat amblyopia will compromise a stable surgical alignment of the eyes.

C. Surgical treatment

Time of surgery

It has been and still continues to be a controversial and debatable question. However, experienced strabismologists have recommended that before surgery is performed for infantile esotropia, following *prerequists* should be ascertained:
- *Deviation* should be constant and stable.
- *Fixation* should be alternating or only a mild fixation preference should be present.
- *Accommodative element* should be absent.
- *Sensory esotropia* should have been ruled out.
- *Amblyopia* should have been treated.
- *Associated vertical deviation or A/V patterns* should be revealed.

The above information can be obtained between the age of 6 months and 2 years depending upon the cooperation of the child as well as patience and understanding of the examiner.

- In general, it has been reported that the sooner the child can be operated after fulfilling the above criteria, the better it is.
- *Peripheral fusion* (monofixation syndrome) is achieved in most cases (80%), if the surgery is done by the age of 2 years and in some patients if it is done by the age of 4 years (20%).
- *After the age of 4 years*, a functional cure in the form of peripheral fusion is unlikely.

Choice of surgery

- *Bimedial recessions* are preferred over the unilateral recess-resect procedure in the absence of amblyopia. However, by and large, it is surgeon's perference.
- It has recently been recognized that a maximum of 8 mm of medial rectus recession may be performed without crippling its function as against the traditionally suggested upper limit of 5.5 mm.
- *Unilateral recess-resect* operation on the non-dominant eye may be performed in patients who have failed to respond to amblyopia treatment.
- *Amount of muscle surgery* to be performed for horizontal deviation depends upon the angle of squint, age of the patient, duration of squint, visual status and the surgeon's previous experience. However, the figures given in Table 10.1 can serve as a rough guideline for the beginners. From the Table 10.1, it is clear that now the surgeon has an alternative to three and four muscles surgery for a large angle esotropia.

Table 10.1 *Rough guidelines for amount of surgery in infantile esotropia*

Deviation in prism dioptres	Monocular surgery in mm		Binocular surgery in mm
	Recession of MR	Resection of LR	Bilateral MR recession
15	3.0	4.0	3.0
20	3.5	5.0	3.5
25	4.0	5.0	4.0
30	4.5	6.0	4.5
35	5.0	7.0	5.0
40	5.5	7.0	5.5
50	6.0	8.0	6.0
60	6.5	9.0	6.5
70	7.0	10.0	7.0

- *Recession of both inferior oblique muscles*, if indicated, should be performed along with the horizontal muscle surgery.
- *Surgical treatment of DVD*, if associated with infantile esotropia, may be postponed for a later date.

D. Surgical results and post-surgical treatment

Post-surgical treatment will depend upon the outcome of surgery. Von Noorden has graded the surgical results of infantile esotropia as follows:

1. Subnormal binocular vision. It is the best possible therapeutic result that can be expected following surgery for infantile esotropia. It is usually achieved, if surgery is performed before 2 years of age. It is characterized by:

- Orthophoria or asymptomatic heterophoria; alignment is stable.
- Normal visual acuity in both eyes.
- Peripheral fusion develops, which allows a low grade of stereopsis from 67 to 3000 seconds of arc as well as normal fusional vergence amplitudes.
- Normal retinal correspondence.
- Foveal suppression in one eye in binocular vision.

Post-surgical treatment. Such patients do not require further treatment, regular follow-up is required for:

- Correction of refractive error,
- Maintenance amblyopia therapy, and
- Late development of under or overcorrection.

2. Microtropia. Postoperative microtropia (deviation less than 10^Δ) is the *desirable* treatment result. It is characterized by:

- Inconspicuous shift or no shift on cover test. Alignment is usually stable and thus no further treatment except amblyopia prevention is required.
- Mild amblyopia is common.
- Peripheral fusion usually develops, which may allow a low grade stereopsis and normal fusional vergence amplitudes.

3. Small-angle residual esotropia or small-angle exotropia due to overcorrection is considered an acceptable treatment result. It is characterized by:

- Small-angle esotropia or exotropia (less than 15^Δ) which is cosmetically acceptable. There is less stability of angle.
- About 80% patients have anomalous retinal correspondence.
- Stereopsis is of low grade or absent.

Treatment. No further treatment is required except amblyopia prevention.

4. Large-angle residual esotropia (undercorrection) is an unacceptable treatment result. Its features are:

- Large-angle esotropia (more than 20D) is usually cosmetically unacceptable and needs repeat surgery.
- Suppression amblyopia is of frequent occurrence.
- Stereopsis is absent.

Post-surgical treatment: Resurgery may be required for large residual esotropia and should be done within 3 months of origin surgery. Prism adaptation test may be preformed before surgery to identify patients with binocular potential and to uncover the maximum underlying deviation prior to any further surgery.

Choice of surgery

- Bilateral LR resection may be performed, if the primary surgery was bilateral MR recession.
- When the primary surgery was LR resection and MR recession, then the similar surgery should be performed in the other eye.

5. Large-angle consecutive exotropia (over-correction) should be managed as below:

i. *Children below 2 years of age* having fusion potential with consecutive exotropia of more than 15 PD, surgery should be taken up early to give the child a chance of developing peripheral fusion. *Principle:* Copper's dictum, i.e. a decision about type of surgery should be based on thorough reassessment as a new case of exotropia.

Surgical options include

- *LR recession with advancement* of the previously recessed MR is an effective treatment.
- *Bilateral LR recession* is another equally effective option.
- *LR recession + MR resection* of the other eye may also be considered.

Note

- The diagnostic value of preoperative prismatic correction of the deviation is very limited.
- Exotropia drift is common after consecutive exotropia surgery.
- Therefore, a suitable ocular alignment immediately after surgery for consecutive exotropia is a small-angle esotropia of 5–10 PD.

ii. *In patients above 8 years of age,* i.e. visually mature group with bifoveal fusion, wait for 6 to 8 weeks and perform surgery, if deviation is more than 20 PD. If adduction is near normal, the decision of whether or not to perform more surgery should be based purely on the desire for improved cosmesis.

◼ ACCOMMODATIVE ESOTROPIAS

Accommodative esotropia refers to esotropia which is caused by over convergence in response to accommodation. Therefore, the convergent deviation of the eyes varies in degree according to the amount of accommodation exerted.

Characteristics. All accommodative esodeviations are acquired and have the following characteristics in general:

- *Onset age* is usually between 2 and 3 years. Most cases occur between 6 months and 7 years of age. However, rarely it may occur as early as 3–4 months of age (infantile accommodative esotropia).
- Esodeviations is usually intermittent at onset becoming constant with passage of time.
- Often hereditary.
- *Precipitated* sometimes by trauma or illness.
- *Amblyopia* is frequently associated.

Types

Depending upon the mechanism of occurrence, accommodative esotropia is of following types:

1. Refractive accommodative esotropia (high hyperopia with normal AC/A ratio)
2. Non-refractive accommodative esotropia (high AC/A ratio)
3. Hypoaccommodative esotropia
4. Mixed or partially accommodative esotropia

REFRACTIVE ACCOMMODATIVE ESOTROPIA

Definition

Refractive accommodative esotropia refers to that type of esotropia which:

- Varies in degree depending on the amount of accommodation exerted,
- Is caused by hypermetropia, and
- Wearing of spectacles (to correct the hypermetropia) eliminates the esotropia in all fixation distances and in all gaze positions.

Etiopathogenesis

All children with uncorrected hypermetropia do not develop accommodative esotropia. This implies that in addition to hypermetropia, there are some other factors also which play an important role in the occurrence of accommodative esotropia.

Factors implicated are:

- Uncorrected hypermetropia,
- Fusional divergence amplitude,
- AC/A ratio, and
- Child's personality

Course of events, depending upon the interplay of above factors as described by von Noorden and Helveston (Fig. 10.5), is as follows:

1. It is unequivocal that the uncorrected hypermetropia causes a *retinal image blur.* Thus the patients with hypermetropia must accommodate to clear the retinal image at distance. Whether the child will accommodate to clear the image or not depends less on the degree of hypermetropia than on the child's personality. It has been reported that the more relaxed and easy going children may not accommodate and thus remain orthotropic (because they prefer blurred vision over the constant effort to accommodate excessively). However, these patients may develop *bilateral ametropic amblyopia* with or without accommodative deficiency (Fig. 10.5A).

2. Many patients with uncorrected hypermetropia (especially fastidious and exacting children) will accommodate to clear the retinal image blur. Because of the near synkinesis, the accommodation in turn will cause *excessive accommodative convergence.* The final outcome of

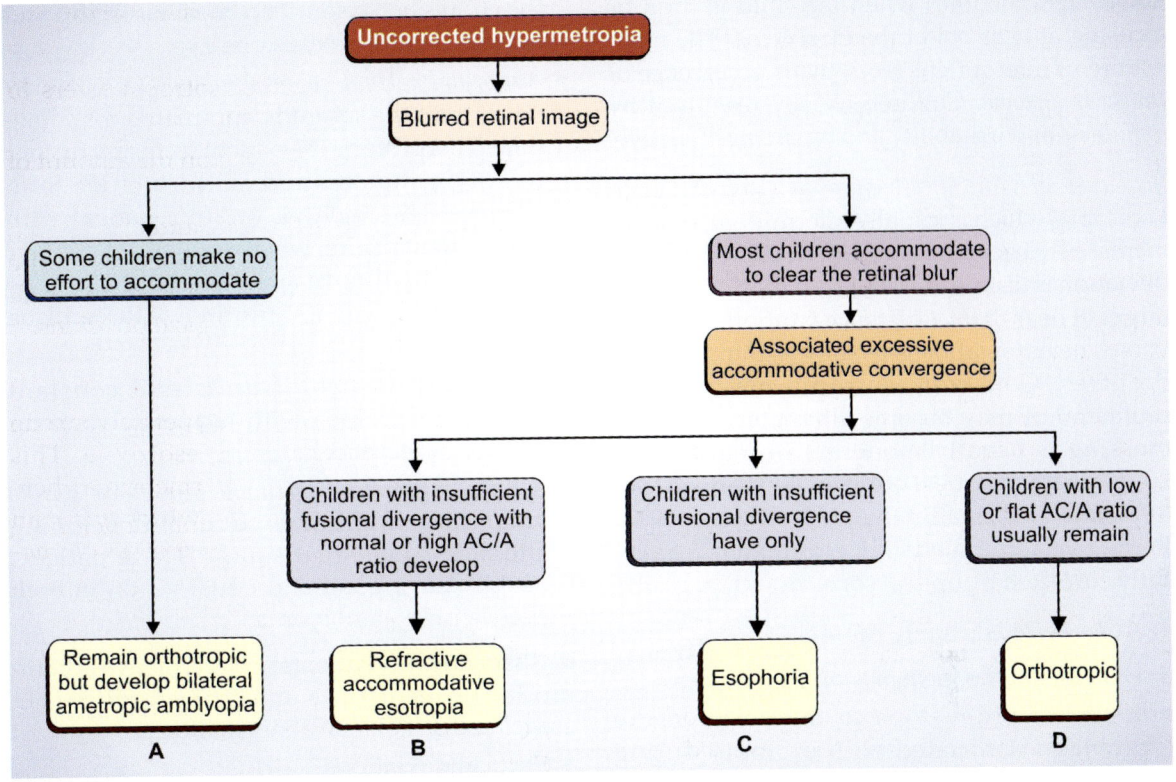

Fig. 10.5 *Course of events in patients with uncorrected high hypermetropia.*

this excessive use of accommodative convergence, depending upon the fusional divergence amplitude of the patient, may be any of the three:

i. *Refractive accommodative esotropia* will develop in children with insufficient fusional divergence to handle the excessive accommodative convergence and a normal AC/A ratio (Fig. 10.5B).

ii. *Intermittent esotropia and esophoria.* Esophoria will develop in children with sufficient fusional divergence amplitude to handle the excessive accommodative convergence and thus have straight eyes under binocular vision (Fig. 10.5C). However, at times patient's fusional reserve may be depleted resulting in *intermittent esotropia. Factors affecting fusional reserve* are:

• Any severe illness
• Emotional stress
• Fatigue, etc.

iii. *Orthotropia* will be there in children with low or flat AC/A ratio who may not become esotropic inspite of uncorrected hypermetropia, since the

convergence induced by excessive accommodation is normal or even subnormal (Fig. 10.5D).

Clinical characteristics

1. *Time of onset.* Most of the times, the accommodative esotropia manifests between the age of 2 and 3 years. However, in rare circum-stances, it may develop anytime between birth to 7 years of age.

2. *Hypermetropia.* Children developing refractive accommodative esotropia usually have hypermetropia ranging between 2 and 6 dioptres with a mean of 4.75 dioptres.

3. *Ocular deviation.* Development of accommodative esotropia usually passes through stages of esophoria and intermittent esotropia. However, in a child features of these stages may not be noticed every time and constant esotropia may be the first complaint by the parents.

Features during stage of intermittent esotropia. Parents often give a history that the eyes are straight, however, sometimes when the child is tired or focusing at near object the eyes cross. The main feature of intermittent esotropia is occurrence of *transient diplopia*. Children usually react to it by *fretfulness* and irritability and by *closing of one* eye.

Features of constant esotropia (Fig. 10.6A). Esotropia, which is initially intermittent, quickly increases to become a constant deviation. Ocular deviation is usually variable and may be slightly larger at near than at distance fixation. Distance versus near deviation is usually within 10 prism dioptres. Constant esotropia may remain unilateral or may become alternate. Degree of crossing is usually moderate in magnitude, 20–40 prism dioptres, but may be more or less. Typically, it is smaller than infantile esotropia. Refractive accommodative esotropia is usually fully corrected by optical correction (Fig. 10.6B).

4. AC/A ratio is usually normal.

5. Development of sensory adaptations.

- *Suppression* develops to take care of the problems associated with diplopia during stage of intermittent squint. It usually develops within a week of the onset of squint and then the child's behaviour becomes less fretful and he/she no more closes one eye.

- *Abnormal retinal correspondence (ARC)* may develop, if the squint is not treated for a long time. This protects the patient from any further sensory symptoms and allows a crude form of binocular single vision. In a patient with intermittent squint, when the eyes are straight normal retinal correspondence (NRC) will be present and when squinting, ARC will be present.

- *Amblyopia* ensues, if unilateral constant esotropia develops with moderately strong fixation preference.

- *Alternate fixation with no binocular single vision* occurs in some patients developing alternate convergent squint. These patients usually have good and equal vision in both eyes, with no amblyopia.

6. Associations. Patients with refractive accommodative esotropia may have following associated strabismic abnormalities:

- Vertical deviations
- A–V pattern

Clinical evaluation and diagnosis

Accommodative esotropia usually develops at the age of 2–3 years and needs to be differentiated from sensory esotropia. Rarely, it may develop early and must be differentiated from essential infantile esotropia. Each case needs a detailed work-up as described on page 100, but the key features which need a special mention are as follows:

1. Measurement of deviation for far and near and in all cardinal positions of gaze is important.

2. Cycloplegic refraction is the most important investigation in the evaluation of a case of squint with a special reference to refractive accommodative esotropia. It is preferred to use 1% atropine eye ointment, three times a day for three consecutive days to achieve cycloplegia. Use of atropine not only allows a complete cycloplegia, but also provides a brief period of relaxed accommodation during which child starts tolerating the glasses. Further, incidence of systemic complications is much less with the use of atropine eye

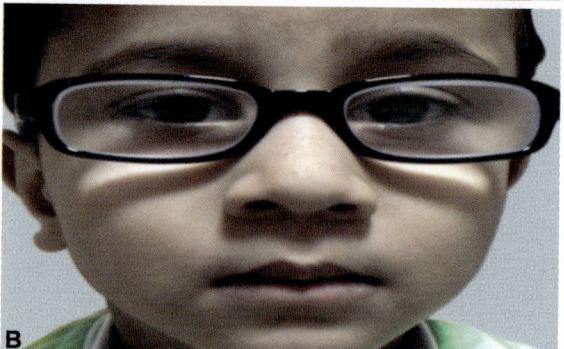

Fig. 10.6 *A patient with accommodative esotropia* (A), *corrected with glasses* (B).

ointment than with the eyedrops. However, recently some clinicians contest that 1% cyclopentolate is good enough for the cycloplegia.

3. *Measurement of fusional divergence amplitude* is also an important parameter in such cases, since it plays an important role in the development of refractive accommodative esotropia (see etiology). Normal fusional divergence amplitude at distance is 4–6$^\Delta$ and at near it is 8–12$^\Delta$.

4. *Examination of fundus and ocular media* is quite useful in diagnosing retinoblastomas and other abnormalities responsible for sensory squint. Fundus examination should be performed along with the cycloplegic refraction.

Treatment

1. Optical correction

- *A full optical correction* usually eliminates the refractive accommodative esotropia (Fig. 10.6) and converts it into a phoria. However, it may take several weeks before the glasses become fully effective.
- *Role of atropinization.* A child who has never worn glasses and has been accommodating for years may not accept glasses immediately. Such children require atropinization for a period of a few weeks to relax their accommodation before the glasses are tolerated.
- *Importance of full time wear of spectacle correction must be emphasized to the parents.* A common cause of treatment failures or partial responses to anti-accommodative management is inconsistent spectacle wear.

Method of prescribing optical correction and follow-up

The follow-up regime varies slightly from age to age, as follows:

i. *From birth to 6 months.* An infant below 6 months (with a definite intermittent or constant esotropia) usually has non-accommo-dative infantile esotropia. However, all such infants having hypermetropia of +2.0 dioptres or more should be given glasses. The prescription should include full retinoscopic findings plus an additional +1.5D. The additional plus will provide clear vision up to 66 cm which is the usual limit of the young infant's world.

These infants should be seen every 2–3 weeks until it is certain that the glasses have controlled the deviation. If the esotropia persists, retinoscopy should be repeated and if additional hypermetropia is discovered, the glasses should be changed. However, if no change in retinoscopy is observed, the diagnosis should be changed to infantile type.

ii. *From 6 months to 6 years.* Esotropic children of this age group having hypermetropia of more than +1.5D should be prescribed full retinoscopic finding without any additional plus lens and should be followed every month till their deviation is stabilized. Once a patient is stabilized under 1 year of age, retinoscopy should be repeated at least every 3 months. For the children between 1 and 5 years of age, retinoscopy should be repeated every 6 months.

iii. *Above 6 years of age.* In children above 6 years of age, the optical prescription should include the minimum power lens that should provide both binocular single vision with esophoria and maximum visual acuity. At this stage, to obtain esophoria rather than orthophoria is useful since with the former fusional divergence, amplitude continues to be exercised. These patients should be followed every 6 months for 2 years and then every year.

Note. When, after full hypermetropic correction for 4 to 8 weeks, the residual esotropia is greater than 15 PD, the diganosis should be revised as below:

- *Partial accommodative esotropia* is labelled, when residual esotropia is for both distance and near. In such cases, surgery is indicated (*see* page 232).
- *High AC/A ratio* should be considered, when eyes are aligned for distance and residual esotropia is present for near. Such patients need bifocals (*see* page 230).

2. Role of miotics

Though some people have recommended use of topical miotics, but it is best to avoid their use in refractive accommodative esotropia. However, in extremely uncooperative and hyperexcited children, miotics may be prescribed as a short-term alternative to spectacles.

3. Amblyopia therapy

It is indicated, when a child is brought late with a constant unilateral accommodative esotropia with amblyopia. For details of amblyopia, *see* page 190. However, in general, full hypermetropic correction and occlusion therapy may improve the vision.

4. Orthoptic treatment

Once the occlusion therapy improves visual acuity, the orthoptic treatment aims at overcoming the suppression and improving the negative fusional convergence. Before starting orthoptic treatment, it should be ensured that:

a. Child has worn glasses for several weeks;
b. Amblyopia, if any, has been treated; and
c. Child is cooperative enough for exercises.

- *Antisuppression exercises.* For details, *see* page 174.
- *Exercises to improve negative fusional convergence (fusional divergence)* include divergence exercises with prisms, exercises with synoptophore, physiological diplopia exercises using stereogram in the crossed position, exercises using diploscope, exercises using Remy separator and bar reading exercises. For details, *see* page 143.

Antisuppression and fusional divergence exercises combined with the full hypermetropic correction may be successful in maintaining single binocular vision.

5. Role of surgery

- As a general principle, surgery for refractive accommodative esotropia should not be recommended, since it causes more harm than any benefit. Therefore, it would be an error of commission to surgically correct accommodative esotropia.
- Patients, who have an associated vertical deviation of A–V-pattern, will require surgery for these strabismic abnormalities in addition to the proper refractive correction for their accommodative esotropia.
- In the rare event of deteriorations despite a satisfactory initial response to optical correction for the hypermetropia, a recession of both medial rectus muscles will restore fusion.

Course of untreated accommodative esotropia

If anti-accommodative therapy is delayed for several weeks to months:

- Some or all of the esodeviations will not respond fully to appropriate anti-accommodative therapy.
- When hypermetropia is greater than 5.0D, there is a major risk of bilateral ametropic amblyopia.

NON-REFRACTIVE ACCOMMODATIVE ESOTROPIA (ESOTROPIA WITH HIGH AC/A RATIO)

Definition

It refers to that type of accommodative esotropia which is caused by a high AC/A ratio and thus the esotropia is significantly greater at near than distance fixation. It is unrelated to refractive error and the near point of accommodation is normal for the age of the patient.

Etiopathogenesis

High AC/A ratio. The principal factor in the etiopathogenesis of non-refractive accommodative esotropia is occurrence of an excessive amount of accommodative convergence associated with a normal amount of accommodation (i.e. high AC/A ratio).

Amplitude of fusional divergence modifies the deviation as follows:

- *Esophoria for near will occur*, when the fusional divergence is sufficient to cope up with the increased convergence at near fixation.
- *Esophoria for distance and esotropia for near will occur*, when the fusional divergence is able to cope up with the convergence exerted during distance fixation but is insufficient to cope up with the excessive convergence at near fixation.
- *Esotropia greater at near than at distance fixation occurs*, when the fusional divergence is insufficient to counter the convergence exerted even for distance fixation.

Clinical characteristics

1. Time of onset. Like the refractive accommodative esotropia (RAE), the peak age of onset of non-refractive accommodative esotropia (NRAE) is also 2–3 years, but may occur anytime between 6 months to 7 years of age.

2. *Ocular deviation.* Like the RAE, to begin with, deviation in NRAE is also small and intermittent. However, unlike RAE (where distance and near esotropias are approximately equal), in NRAE, the near esotropia is typically much greater than the distance esodeviation. In fact, there is little or no deviation for distance in NRAE.

Near-distance disparity, depending on the degree, can be classified as below:
- *Grade I:* 10–19 PD more deviation for near,
- *Grade II:* 20–29 PD more deviation for near, and
- *Grade III:* ≥30 PD more deviation for near.

3. *AC/A ratio.* It is characteristically high.

4. *Development of sensory adaptations*

- *Suppression.* During periods of manifest deviation (near fixation), the patient soon learns to suppress to avoid problem of diplopia. Before the development of suppression, child may be irritable, fretful and may close one eye.
- *Abnormal retinal correspondence.* Development of suppression is soon followed by development of abnormal retinal correspondence (ARC). Thus, in such patients, retinal correspondence is normal (NRC) for distance fixation and abnormal (ARC) for near fixation.
- *Amblyopia.* Like RAE, development of amblyopia is a particular danger in patients with high AC/A ratio esotropia. A proper optical correction with regular follow-up is must to avoid the amblyopia.

5. *Associations.* Like RAE, patients with NRAE may also have following strabismic abnormalities:
- Vertical deviations
- A–V-pattern

Clinical evaluation and diagnosis

Each case of strabismus needs a complete work up (*see* page 100). The most important aspects of strabismic work for non-refractive accommodative esotropia which need special mention are as below:

1. *Measurement of deviation.* It should be performed for far and near by prism and alternate cover test. While measuring deviation for near fixation, special care should be taken to ensure that child is fully accommodating. This can be achieved with the use of a fixation target that requires full accommodation to identify small details.

2. *Cycloplegic refraction.* Cycloplegic refraction should be carried out in each case. Non-refractive accommodative esotropia may occur in emmetropia, hypermetropia or even myopes. However, moderate degree of hypermetropia is a more frequent association.

3. *Measurement of AC/A ratio.* It can be performed with lens gradient method or heterophoria method, former being more reliable. Normal AC/A ratio is 3 to 4 : 1 (For details, *see* page 119).

4. *Measurement of fusional divergence amplitude.* It is also an important factor. Its role has been discussed in etiopathogenesis. For details, *see* page 116.

5. *Examination of fundus and ocular media* is quite useful in differentiating from sensory deviation. Fundus examination should be performed along with cycloplegic refraction.

Diagnosis of NRAE is usually based on following observations:

- *Near esotropia is typically much greater* than the distance esotropia with the refractive error fully corrected.
- *Establishment of high AC/A ratio* by lens gradient method in the presence of a normal near point of accommodation.
- Special care and caution is needed in not to confuse a V-pattern esotropia with NRAE due to high AC/A ratio. In V esotropia, the deviation increases characteristically in down gaze at either distance or near fixation. While in esotropia due to high AC/A ratio, deviation increases at near fixation irrespective of the position of the eyes.

Treatment

1. Amblyopia therapy. Before treatment is begun, any amblyopia should be eliminated or improved.

2. Bifocal glasses. Since near deviation is the primary obstacle to normal binocular vision, a bifocal add of about +3.0 D over the full cycloplegic refraction with simultaneous orthoptic exercises is extremley useful in the treatment of non-refractive accommodative esotropia.

Prerequisites for use of bifocals
- Non-refractive accommodative esotropia usually occurs at 1½ to 2½ years of age. However, sometimes it may occur even in an infant. Bifocals need not be prescirbed in cases below 6 months of age. As a general principle, all infants below 6 months with definite esotropia (intermittent or constant) should be prescribed the full retinoscopic finding plus an addition of +1.5D as a single vision glasses. Bifocals are not required below 6 months because visual acuity of such infants is usually limited to 66 cm. These infants should be followed up as described for refractive accommodative esotropia (*see* page 227).
- Above 6 months of age, a focal add of +3.0D should be given.
- Bifocals should be prescribed only in patients with marked esotropia for near and ortho-tropia or minimal esotropia for distance with full cycloplegic refraction worn for at least 4–8 weeks.
- Bifocals should be continued in patients whose near esotropia is fully corrected with their use.
- Bifocals should not be prescribed in the presence of amblyopia. Rather amblyopia should be treated first.

Prescription of bifocals
Usually about +3.0D add is required in bifocal glasses to correct the non-refractive accommodative esotropia. However, the exact power of bifocal add is determined by hit and trial method. To begin with, +1D is added to the distance correction in the trial frame and then the power is increased in steps of +0.5D up to a maximum of +3.0D till all the near esotropia is corrected.

The success of bifocal therapy depends largely on the *proper bifocal segment*. Executive type of bifocals in which the separation line between the distance and near segments is properly located so that it bisects the pupil or touches its lower border, when the child looks straight ahead (Fig. 10.7) should be preferred.

Follow-up examination should be done every 3 months up to one year of age, every 6 months up to 2 years of age and thereafter every year.

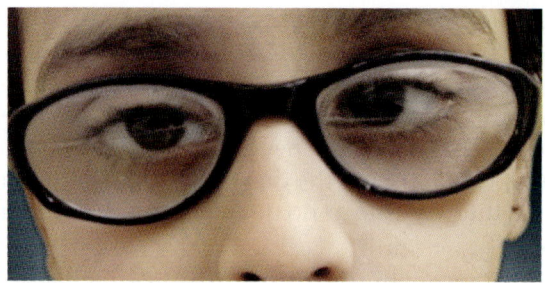

Fig. 10.7 *Use of executive type of bifocal glasses in a patient with high AC/A ratio.*

At each follow-up visit, retinoscopy should be performed and new glasses should be prescribed, if there is difference of 1D or more.

Wearing of bifocals
If, with the use of bifocals, bifoveal single vision can be maintained at near, the fusion reflex may gain in stability. Under these circumstances, the bifocals should be continued up to 5 years of age, after which the bifocals may be reduced step by step in decrements of +0.75 to +1D. The aim is to maintain the patient's fusion while leaving him/her esophoric at near so that patient excercises divergence amplitude continuously. Preferably, the patient should be completely weaned from the bifocal segment by 10 years of age.

During the weaning period, the antisupp-ression exercises and exercises to increase fusional divergence amplitudes may be helpful for maintaining fusion.

Some patients may become dependent on bifocals and weaning may not be possible even in early teens. Under these circumstances, a Faden or bilateral MR recession may be preferred to remove the near add. However, spectacles without near add still may be required.

3. Miotics
Mechanism of action. Miotics facilitate accommo-dation and thus reduce the accommodative convergence. Because of this action, miotics are quite useful in patients with non-refractive accommodative esotropia due to high AC/A ratio.

Suitable cases. Presently bifocals are preferred over miotics in general, but some physicians do prefer use of miotics. Perhaps following are the guidelines for suitable cases for use of miotics:

- Patients of younger age group than bifocals.
- When the child is unlikely to wear glasses for the entire day.
- Probably, the best and most appropriate use of miotics is to assist in withdrawing bifocals.
- May be used for residual deviations post-operatively.
- Miotics should not be used unless some degree of binocularity can be achieved. A slight reduction in the angle of esotropia is of no benefit to the patient with respect to restoring normal binocular function.

Preparation and dosage schedule for miotics is as below:

- Two most commonly used miotics are phospholine iodide (0.06%, 0.125%) solution and disopropyl fluorophosphate (DFP 0.025% ointment).
- To begin with, higher strength of phospholine iodide may be used. Where, with the help of miotics, bifoveal single vision can be achieved for near, continue the drug for several weeks. Gradually discontinue, reducing strength of the phospholine iodide.
- It is unequivocal to say that a hypermetropic patient must wear the full distance correction during treatment with miotics so that the need for accommodation during near vision is minimum. Any significant astigmatism should also be corrected since clear images promote better vision.
- While using miotics, patient should be reviewed at fortnightly intervals and checked for the side effects.

Complications of miotics include

i. *Anaesthetic risk.* Inadvertent use of depolarizing muscle relaxant such as succinylcholine, during general anaesthesia, may result in life-threatening apnoea. Therefore, anaesthetist must be informed about the use of these medicines.

ii. *Systemic complications* such as headache, stomach cramps, hallucinations, nausea, vomiting and diarrhoea have been reported with the use of topical anticholinestrase agents, but are rare.

iii. *Ocular side effects* include pain on instillation, iris cyst formation, spasm of accommodation, anterior subcapsular cataract and rarely retinal detachment. Iris cyst formation is not uncommon, but immediate cessation of miotic treatment will lead to the spontaneous disappearance of the cysts.

4. Orthoptic exercises

Orthoptic exercises rarely achieve results alone. These should be best combined with bifocal glasses and/or miotics. Orthoptic exercises require good co-operation from the patient. Some exercises are only suitable for older children. So, in practice, it is often impossible to carry out orthoptic treatment satisfactorily.

The aim of orthoptic treatment is to overcome suppression and to improve negative fusional convergence, i.e. fusional divergence (*see* pages 174 and 213).

These orthoptic exercises have been described in the section of refractive accommodative esotropia (*see* page 228).

5. Surgery

Surgery is indicated in patients with large angle of squint in which deviation cannot be corrected by above described measures.

Generally, these patients respond well to bilateral medial rectus recessions. Occasionally, recession may have to be combined with bilateral Faden operation on medial recti. The amount of surgery should always be based on the near deviation.

HYPOACCOMMODATIVE ESOTROPIA

Hypoaccommodative esotropia is the term coined by Costenbader for the accommodative esotropia which is associated with weakness of accommodation. Costenbader hypothesized that to overcome accommodation, there is an increased accommodative effort which in turn results in increased convergence resulting in near esotropia.

Clinical characteristics

Hypoaccommodative esotropia is characterized by following features:

- *Esotropia is large* for near fixation and small for distance fixation.
- *Esotropia is not related* to uncorrected hypermetropia.
- *AC/A ratio* is not high.
- *Near point of accommodation* (NPA) is definitely remote, i.e. there is weakness of accommodation.

Treatment

1. *Bifocal glasses.* A near add of plus lenses to compensate for the weak accommodation may be useful.

2. *Orthoptic exercises* to improve accommodation.

PARTIALLY ACCOMMODATIVE ESOTROPIA

Definition

Partially accommodative or mixed esotropia is the term used to describe an esotropia which is partly due to some accommodative factors (hypermetropia, or high AC/A ratio) and partly due to some non-accommodative factors.

Clinical types

In clinical practice, two types of partially accommodative esotropia are described:

1. *Infantile esotropia with superadded accommodative esotropia.* In this clinical situation, child first develops typical infantile esotropia before 6 months of age which is non-accommodative (for details *see* page 218). This is superadded by accommodative esotropia, usually, by the age of 2–3 years, often accompanied by a larger hypermetropia than was first measured.

2. *Decompensated accommodative esotropia with superadded non-accommodative esotropia.* In this clinical situation, the accommodative esotropia is well corrected with glasses or bifocal lenses. But, after some period of initial alignment of the eyes, the esotropia again develops due to some superadded non-accommodative factors. It has been postulated that in decompensated accommodative esotropia, either increased convergence tone or mechanical factors such as hypertrophy or contracture of the medial rectus muscles, conjunctiva or Tenon's capsule may play a role.

Note: Partially accommodative esotropia is usually constant and, therefore, typically associated with suppression, ARC and amblyopia.

Treatment

1. *Correction of accommodative part of esotropia* should be carried out first.

2. *Amblyopia* is usually associated and should be treated (as described on page 190) before the surgery is undertaken.

3. *Surgery.* It is important to note that only non-accommodative part of the squint needs to be corrected surgically.

- *Measurement* should, therefore, be taken with full optical correction for near and distance; and the amount of surgery should be based on the amount of residual esotropia measured at distance with full correction.

- *Parents* should also be explained that even after the surgery, the child will require glasses to correct the esotropia.

- *Bilateral medial rectus recession* should be preferred. However, in the presence of uncorrected amblyopia, parents may insist for surgery on the affected eye only.

- *In the presence of high AC/A ratio,* it has been observed that a slightly larger recession is required. For example, if ordinarily bilateral medial rectus recession of 3 mm is required to correct an esotropia of 18D at distance, this should be increased to bilateral 3.5 mm recession. Bilateral Faden operation on the medial recti may also be required.

- *To prevent undercorrection* in patients with the so-called decompensated, deteriorated, residual or non-accommodative portion of the mixed mechanism squint, following measures have been recommended:

  - *Surgery after prism adaptation.* Patient is given full hyperopic correction as usual with added press-on prism to neutralize any residual esodeviation. The patient wears the glasses with press-on prism for 1 or 2 weeks and is then re-examined. If the esodeviation increases with the prism, new prisms are prescribed to neutralize the deviation. In some patients, the esodeviation will increase as the patient 'eats-up' the prism. Surgery is planned for the full prism-adapted deviation.

  - *Enhanced or augmented surgery* has been advocated by some workers as an alternative to surgery with prism adaptation.

Note. Various formulas are used to augment standard surgery. A simple and effective method to determine the target angle is by averaging the near deviation without correction (largest deviation) and the distance deviation with correction (smallest deviation).

INFANTILE ACCOMMODATIVE ESOTROPIA

Infantile accommodative esotropia is the term used for rare cases of accommodative esotropia occurring at 3 to 4 months of age.

Differential diagnosis from essential infantile esotropia can be made by:
- Presence of straight eyes for the first 2 to 3 months,
- Variable angle of deviation at the onset, and
- Presence of hypermetropia >2D.

Treatment consists of:
- *Full hypermetropic correction* should be done immediately after cycloplegic refraction.
- *Amblyopia* should be treated, when present.
- *Surgery* is indicated when spectacles correction cannot allign the eyes to within 10 PD (see partially accommodative esotropia).

ACQUIRED NON-ACCOMMODATIVE ESOTROPIAS

This group includes all the acquired esodeviations in which the amount of deviation is not affected by the state of accommodation. These include the following clinical entities:
- Essential acquired or late onset esotropia
- Acute concomitant esotropia
- Microtropia
- Nystagmus blockage syndrome
- Cyclic esotropia
- Divergence paresis
- Stress-induced esotropia
- Esotropia in myopia
- Esotropia due to spasm of near reflex

ESSENTIAL ACQUIRED ESOTROPIA OR LATE ONSET ESOTROPIA

In general, all forms of non-accommodative esodeviations other than essential infantile esotropia may be labelled as 'acquired non-accommodative esotropias'. However, in strabismic practice, the term acquired non-accommodative esotropia or the late onset non-accommodative esotropia or essential acquired esotropia by common use has come to mean a non-accommodative esotropia that occurs during the first few years of life and that cannot be grouped with other forms of esotropia. It includes following clinical types:

- Basic esotropia
- Non-accommodative convergence excess esotropia
- Divergence insufficiency esotropia

Basic esotropia

Clinical features

1. *Onset* is in childhood (early a few years of life) but decidedly after 6 months of age.

2. *Deviation* is usually equal at distance and near. At the onset, the angle of deviation is smaller than essential infantile esotropia but the angle may increase to 30^Δ to 70^Δ.

3. *Accommodative factor* is characteristically absent.

4. *Refractive error* is insignificant.

5. *AC/A ratio* is normal.

Etiopathogenesis

In view of the above clinical features, Costenbader postulated that this deviation is due to *excessive convergence* tonus and so suggested the term 'acquired tonic esotropia' for basic esotropia.

Clinical work-up

- It should be on the general lines for work up of any squint patient.
- A special word of caution has been conveyed by many reports in the literature to rule out any possibility of an underlying lesion of malformation in the central nervous system in all patients with 'acquired non-accommodative esotropia'.

Treatment

1. *Amblyopia,* when present, should be treated first of all (see page 150).

2. *Surgery* is the ultimate treatment for basic esotropia. It should be performed as early as possible after the amblyopia therapy. Results, in terms of binocular visual potential, are better than the infantile esotropia.

Non-accommodative convergence excess esotropia

Clinical features

It is characterized by following features:

1. *Onset* of deviation is usually between 2 and 5 years of age.

2. *Deviation* is characteristically large-angle esotropia for near with a small angle esotropia/esophoria or orthophoria at distance (similar to non-refractive accommodative esotropia). Near distance disparity is ≥15 PD.

3. *AC/A ratio* determined by lens gradient method is normal or even low and the use of bifocals has no effect on near deviation (unlike non-refractive accommodative esotropia due to high AC/A ratio). In view of the above, determining the AC/A ratio by heterophoria method (by comparing the near and distance deviation) is likely to miss such a condition and patient may be wrongly prescribed bifocals to which they will not respond.

4. *Near point of accommodation* is within normal limits. This observation differentiates the condition from the hypoaccommodative type of non-refractive accommodative esotropia.

5. *Refractive error.* Patients are usually hypermetropic or emmetropic.

Treatment

Surgical correction by bilateral medial rectus recession with Faden operation (suturing the muscle to the sclera 12 mm behind the muscle insertion) is the treatment of choice. von Noorden has reported that conventional recession procedure of bilateral medial rectus (4 to 5 mm) with or without Faden operation is usually ineffective. Therefore, a large recession between 5 and 8 mm should be planned.

Divergence insufficiency esotropia

Clinical features

- It is characterized by a greater deviation for distance than near. Near-distance disparity should be ≥15 PD.
- It is usually comitant; but the possibility of an underlying neurological lesion causing mild sixth nerve palsy should always be ruled out.

Treatment

Base-out prism may be tried to help the patient. However, often surgical treatment with bilateral rectus resection is required.

ACUTE CONCOMITANT ESOTROPIA

It refers to sudden onset of large-angle concomitant esotropia without any paralytic element. It is typically associated with diplopia. Voluntary closure of one eye may often be the only sign in preverbal infants. Following two forms of acute concomitant esotropia have been reported.

1. Acute strabismus after artificial interruption of fusion

- It has been reported to occur in patients with no previous history of squint, after interruption of fusion under following conditions:
  - Prolonged bandaging of one eye for any surgery or perforating injuries.
  - Occlusion of one eye for treatment of ambylopia without squint (e.g. anisometropic amblyopia).
  - Swelling of the lids following blunt trauma.
- It has been postulated that perhaps these patients have latent esodeviation and/or uncorrected hypermetropia which was fully controlled by the well-functioning fusion mechanism without any symptoms. However, the deviation becomes manifest after the fusion is disrupted and the compensatory mechanism is thus suspended following occlusion of one eye.

Treatment

- *Spontaneous improvement* occurs in some patients after the occlusion is removed.
- *Correction of underlying hypermetropia* may straighten the eyes in other patients.
- *Surgery* may be required to correct esotropia in a few patients.

2. Acute concomitant esotropia without preceding disruption of fusion

Etiopathogenesis

It has been postulated that perhaps such patients have an asymptomatic esophoria with only a slim reserve of fusional amplitude that maintains alignment of the eye over the years but that may become lost under the influence of physical or emotional strain.

Clinical features

- *Onset* is acute with diplopia.
- *Deviation* is relatively large.
- *Refractive error* is insignificant.

- *Disruption of fusion* is not the associated factor.
- *No signs* of paralysis of lateral rectus muscle.
- Good potential for binocular co-operation is there.

Treatment

Excellent functional results are obtained in such patients with surgical treatment.

MICROTROPIA

Depending upon the degree of deviation, Lange classified heterotropia as follows:

- Microtropia: 1°–5°
- Small angle esotropia: 5°–12°
- Large angle esotropia: >12°

Monofixation syndrome versus microtropia

The sine quo non of the monofixation syndrome is the absence of bifoveolar fusion with the presence of peripheral fusion. There are various causes of monofixation syndrome. Microtropia is the most common cause of monofixation syndrome (Park's syndrome). Thus, microtropia is a cause and not synonymous with mono-fixation syndrome as used previously in the strabismic literature.

An array of other terms have also been used to describe the microtropia. Some of these are: Fixation disparity, fusion disparity, mono-fixational esophoria, retinal slip, retinal flicker and minisquint.

Diagnostic features

Based on the fixation pattern, Lang has described three types of microtropia:

- *Type-I*—central fixation,
- *Type-II*—eccentric fixation without identity, and
- *Type-III*—eccenteric fixation, with identity, i.e. angle of anomaly is same as the eccentricity of fixation.

Features of microtropia as described by Lange and also adopted by von Noorden et al can be grouped as:

- Consistent findings, and
- Variable findings.

Consistent findings

1. *Amblyopia.* A microtropia should always be suspected in unilateral decrease of visual acuity (usually not worse than 6/18) for which no organic cause can be found in patients without apparent strabismus or a history of such and without significant refractive error or anisometropia. Amblyopia is not the cause but a result of microtropia.

2. *Abnormal retinal correspondence (ARC) as determined with:* (i) Bagolini's striated glasses (page 129) and (ii) Foveo-foveal test of Cupper (page 134).

3. *Relative scotoma on the fovea* or in the case of parafoveal fixation, the fixation point of the deviated eye. Tests for identifying a monocular scotoma in the binocular visual field include:

- Worth four-dot test (page 132)
- Binocular scotometry (page 185)
- 4^Δ base-out prism test (page 171)
- Bagolini striated glasses (page 129)
- A–O Vectographic Project-O-Chart slide (page 173).

4. *Normal or near normal peripheral fusion with amplitudes* is present in patients with microtropia despite the fact that such patients have 3°–5° central scotoma in one eye during binocular viewing and retinal image disparity of up to 10^Δ. This is possible because the Panum's fusional space is wide in the peripheral retina (up to 5°) as compared to central retina (only 20 minutes of arc). It has been reported that peripheral fusion begins at some point in the retina that is anywhere from 9° to 12° from the foveola.

5. *Defective stereoacuity.* Stereoacuity for near should at least be 3000 seconds of arc. A minimal requirement for gross stereopsis of distance is not necessary for diagnosis. However, about one-third patients with monofixation syndrome have a distance stereoacuity between 240 and 120 seconds of arc.

Variable findings

1. *Size of deviation* can measure up to 10^Δ horizontally and up to 3^Δ vertically.
2. *Fixation pattern* is non-foveal but may be foveal. Diagnosis of microtropia is difficult in patients with minute degrees of fixation anomalies.

3. *Anisometropia* may or may not be present. Identification of microtropia is more difficult in isometropic patients.

4. *Cover test* may be positive or negative. In patients with positive cover test, diagnosis is clearly established by a very small fixation movement (flick) of the deviated eye upon covering the fixating eye. When the cover test is negative (Fig. 10.8), special diagnostic procedures are required to differentiate a microtropia with identity from non-strabismic causes of decreased vision in one eye.

Treatment

1. *In young patients* who are visually immature (age 6 or under), full-time occlusion therapy should be done to treat amblyopia after full *refractive correction*. Even microtropia is reported to disappear following energetic occlusion therapy. In patients showing recurrence, part-time occlusion should be continued for a long time.

2. *Older children or adults* with microtropia need not be treated, since they have comfortable and nearly normal binocular vision with good peripheral fusional amplitude.

NYSTAGMUS BLOCKAGE SYNDROME

Definition and etiology

The term 'nystagmus blockage syndrome' has been suggested for the occurrence of esotropia in a child with congenital nystagmus. It has been reported that in a bid to dampen the nystagmus, there occurs adduction or excessive convergence which results in esotropia. Others believe that nystagmus is not the sole cause of esotropia. Such patients usually have a static angle infantile esotropia unrelated to nystagmus on which is superadded a dynamic angle due to convergence for dampening nystagmus.

Clinical features

1. *Esotropia.* Nystagmus blockage syndrome is characterized in its acute form by an esotropia

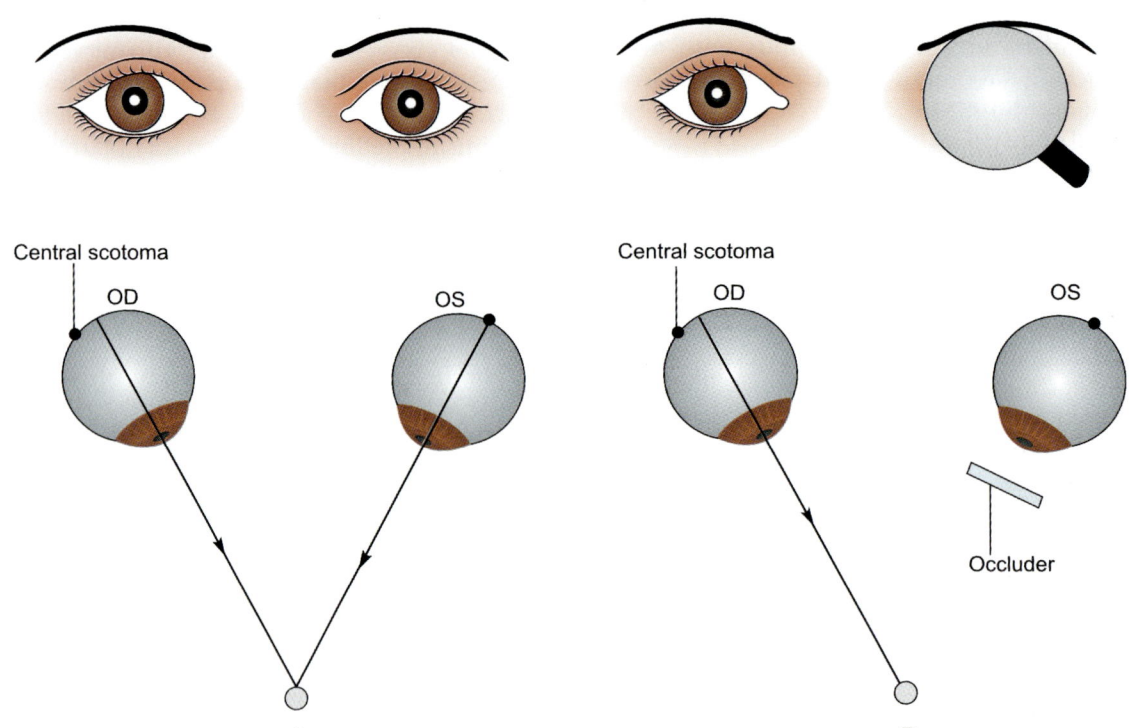

Fig. 10.8 Microtropia with identity: A, *Eyes appear straight and both eyes take up fixation; the right esotropic eye has parafoveal fixation due to central scotoma; B, on cover test, right eye continues to fixate with the same parafoveal point and thus there occurs no fixation movement.*

of early onset with a variable angle, changing from *orthotropia with manifest nystagmus* during periods of visual inattention to *esotropia without nystagmus* during visual attention. Eventually esotropia may become constant.

2. *Nystagmus* intensity is inversely proportional to the angle of deviation. Nystagmus appears as the fixing eye moves from adduction to abduction. This is an important distinguishing feature from infantile esotropia with associated latent nystagmus which lacks inverse relationship.

3. *Pseudoparalysis of both lateral recti* results due to maintaining the eyes in a position of convergence. It can be differentiated from a true paresis of lateral recti by means of the Doll's head manoeuvre (*see* page 219).

4. *Fixation* occurs with the adducting eye.

5. *Head turn* may exist towards the side of fixating eye. When one eye is covered, a face turn in the direction of the uncovered eye may be demonstrated. A periodic shifting of the head from side to side may be observed in the presence of alternate fixation.

6. *Visual acuity* is increased with adduction due to dampening of nystagmus. Therefore, best visual acuity is at near fixation.

Treatment

Treatment is surgical but unsatisfactory.

1. *In the presence of a face turn,* a recession of the medial rectus combined with Faden operation and a resection of the lateral rectus of the adducting eye should be performed. This procedure will relieve the face turn and also correct esotropia.

2. *In the absence of face turn,* a bilateral medial rectus recession with Faden operation should be preferred.

CYCLIC ESOTROPIA

It is rare but fascinating form of esotropia characterized by a strabismic and a non-strabismic phase of 24 hours each. This 48 hour cycle is encountered most commonly, but 72 hours and 96 hours cycles have also been reported in the literature.

Onset. Cyclic esotropia can be acquired at virtually any age but most frequently occurs between 2 and 6 years of age.

Cyclic nature of strabismus may last from 4 months to several years, after which the cycle breaks and esotropia becomes constant.

Clinical features

1. *During strabismic phase* (24 hours)
* *Deviation* is usually large, 40^Δ to 70^Δ, and is consistent on subsequent examinations.
* *Suppression* occurs in deviated eye, so usually there is no history of amblyopia.
* *Fusional amplitudes* are defective or absent.

2. *During non-strabismic phase* (next 24 hours)
* *Deviation.* There is no manifest deviation, however, esophoria may be present.
* *Fusion and stereopsis* are both normal.

Treatment

* *Surgery* in the form of either bilateral medial rectus recessions or recession of the medial rectus and resection of the lateral rectus constitutes the treatment.
* *Amount of muscle surgery* is based on the degree of deviation during strabismic phase.
* *No overcorrection* is seen on alternate days, as is expected.

DIVERGENCE PARESIS

It is a poorly understood condition characterized by comitant esodeviation present at distance fixation in patients having normal ductions and versions.

Etiology

1. *Idiopathic.* Etiology is not known in many cases. These cases are usually self-limiting.

2. *Neurological disorders* may be associated in some cases, so neurologic consultation is indicated for all such cases. A few reported causes include tabes, encephalitis, disseminated sclerosis, poliomyelitis, influenza, pontine tumour, increased intracranial pressure, trauma, and Arnold-Chiari syndrome.

Clinical features

1. *Diplopia.* There is history of sudden onset of uncrossed diplopia at distance fixation. When an object is brought near to the patient, the images become closer, and patient fuses them at 25–50 cm.

2. Deviation. Esotropia is usually more for distance with a near-distance disparity of ≥15 PD. The angle of esotropia remains unchanged or may decrease on lateroversion.

3. Abduction and versions are completely normal bilaterally.

4. Field of fixation is unrestricted.

Differential diagnosis

1. Sixth nerve palsy. The condition is differentiated from either unilateral or bilateral sixth nerve palsy by the fact that in diversence paresis, the deviation is equal in both right and left lateral gaze and that abduction is completely normal bilaterally.

2. Convergence spasm. Occasionally, divergence paralysis may be confused with convergence spasm, since in both the conditions patient presents with uncrossed diplopia at distance fixation. However, presence of unimpaired fusional divergence and decreased visual acuity for distance are diagnostic features of convergence spasm. Further, the esotropia will be more for near (≥15 PD) than distance.

Treatment

Note. Neuroimaging studies, as well as neurologic consultation are indicated to rule out possible neurologic disease.

1. Prismotherapy. Since in most of the cases, divergence paralysis is self-limiting and disappears within 5–6 months, so *base-out prisms* may provide adequate relief from diplopia. The minimum power that gives the patient comfortable single vision at distance fixation should be used and should be decreased periodically as the deviation improves.

2. Surgery. If the condition does not disappear within 6 months, resection of both lateral rectus muscles should be considered.

▮ SENSORY ESOTROPIA

DEFINITION

It refers to the esotropia which develops due to poor visual function in one eye in the childhood.

ETIOPATHOGENESIS

Sensory esotropia results from *monocular lesions* (from infancy to childhood) which either prevent the development of normal binocular vision or interfere with its maintenance. Examples of such lesions are: Congenital or acquired cataracts, paediatric aphakia, corneal opacities, anisometropia, optic atrophy, retinoblastoma, macular lesions, severe congenital ptosis and so on.

It has been reported that if the loss of vision in one eye occurs in the first few months of life, there may occur sensory esotropia or exotropia; and after that till childhood, usually there occurs sensory esotropia. Occurrence of poor vision in adulthood due to any reason tends to cause a sensory exotropia. However, Sidikaro and von Noorden have reported that up to 5 years of age, there are almost equal chances of getting sensory esotropia and sensory exotropia; and after 5 years definitely there are more chances of developing sensory exotropia.

Mechanism of sensory heterotropia. The exact mechanism of development of sensory heterotropia is not known; however, following views have been put forward:

1. Chavasse's theory. He reported that possibly strong tonic convergence during childhood and perhaps the diminishing tonic convergence with age contribute to the direction of sensory heterotropia.

2. Bielschowsky's theory. He explained the increased incidence of sensory exotropia with advancing age as a gradual change of topographic anatomic orbital factors in adolescence, favouring divergence rather than convergence. This explanation is difficult to reconcile with the observation by Mann that the orbital axes actually converge rather than diverge.

3. Worth's theory. Worth speculated that the direction of a sensory heterotropia is determined by the refractive error of the sound eye; that is, the blind eye will diverge, if the sound eye is myopic, and will converge, if the sound eye is hypermetropic. However, this view has not been supported by other workers. Sidikaro and von Noorden have reported an equal distribution of refractive errors in patients with sensory squint.

4. Spielmann's theory. He reported that there is a frequent association between monocular vision loss, esotropia and manifest latent nystagmus. He suggested that these signs together with optometeric asymmetry are manifestations of optokinetic immaturity occurring from lack of normal binocular inputs during early infancy.

From the above discussions, it is quite clear that still the mechanism of sensory esotropia is illusive.

CLINICAL FEATURES

1. *Monocular visual loss* due to any cause is always associated.

2. *Deviation.* Sensory esotropia is always comitant. However, limitation of abduction due to contracture of medial rectus or conjunctiva or both may occur in long-standing cases. Vertical deviation due to overaction of inferior oblique muscle is a frequent association.

3. *Amblyopia* may be superimposed over the originally caused organic visual loss.

TREATMENT

- *Surgical treatment is usually required* to improve cosmetic appearance, since visual loss is due to some intractable organic lesion. However, in all such cases, the refractive error and accommodational status of the straight eye needs to be evaluated before contemplating cosmetic surgery.
- *In children with sensory esotropia* due to un-corrected aphakia or traumatic cataract, functional results may be obtained sometimes. In these cases, cataract surgery, treatment of aphakia and occlusion therapy for amblyopia should be tried first, followed eventually by squint surgery.
- *Medial rectus recession with or without lateral rectus resection* depending upon the size of deviation. Should always be performed on the eye with poor vision. Inferior oblique weaken-ing should be performed for associated overaction of this muscle.
- *Patients should always be informed* that an esotropia may recur or a consecutive exotropia may develop years after.

CONSECUTIVE ESOTROPIA

Consecutive esotropia refers to occurrence of esotropia in an eye which was previously exotropic. It has been reported to occur under following two clinical situations:

1. *Surgical overcorrection of exotropia,* is the cause of consecutive esotropia in almost all the cases. Its management has been discussed in detail on page 248.

2. *Spontaneous consecutive esotropia,* i.e. change of exotropia into esotropia without any exogenous mechanical factor or an acquired paralysis of lateral rectus muscle is an extremely rare condition. Hardly any such case has been reported in the literature.

CONCOMITANT EXOTROPIAS

Concomitant exotropia is the term used to describe any manifest divergent deviation of the visual axes in which the amount of deviation in the squinting eye remains constant (unaltered) in all the positions of gaze and there is no associated limitation of ocular movements.

Concomitant exotropia may be divided into four types:
- Congenital (infantile) exotropia
- Primary exotropia
- Sensory exotropia
- Consecutive exotropia

CONGENITAL (INFANTILE) EXOTROPIA

Congenital (infantile) exotropia is an extremely rare condition.

Systemic associations. It is reported to occur in patient with:
- Craniofacial anomalies,
- Ocular albinism, and
- Cerebral palsy
- Prematurity

Characteristic features of congenital exotropia include:
- *Onset*, usually before 6 months of age
- *Large angle constant exodeviation* mostly more than 35 PD. Equal at distance and near
- *Fusion*, prospectives are poor
- *Amblyopia,* incidence is much higher than intermittent exotropia
- *Patterns.* V-pattern more common than A-patten
- *Associations* include dissociated vertical deviation (DVD), primary inferior oblique overaction (IOOA). Rarely superior oblique overaction (SOOA) is also reported.

Differential diagnosis. Congenital exotropia needs to be differentiated from variable small-angle exodeviation seen in 70% of normal newborn infants, which is a transient exodeviation and resolves by 2 to 4 months of age.

Treatment consists of:
- *Amblyopia therapy* to be started at the earliest.
- *Surgical treatment* in the form of bilateral lateral rectus recession should be performed after 6 months of age, usually before the age of 24 months.

▓ PRIMARY EXOTROPIA

Primary exodeviation is an idiopathic condition in which the deviation is the essential feature, in contrast to other types in which divergence occurs as a result of certain obstacles in the development or maintenance of binocular single vision or due to defective action of the extraocular muscles.

ETIOLOGY

Etiology of primary exotropia is speculative. Following factors have been implicated:

Predisposing factors

1. *Mechanical factors,* which have been implicated to predispose a person for development of exotropia include:
- Shape and axes of the orbit,
- Interpupillary distance,
- Size of the eyeball,
- Mechanical properties of the conjunctiva or Tenon's capsule and
- Extraocular muscle characteristics.

2. *Innervational factors* perhaps have been thought to play more important role than the mechanical factors in development of primary exotropia. Duane hypothesized that primary exotropias are caused by an innervational imbalance that upsets the reciprocal relationship between active convergence and divergence mechanism. He suggested that exodeviation is caused either by hypertonicity of divergence or convergence insufficiency or both.

Precipitating factors

Precipitating factors which cause decompensation of exophoria to intermittent exotropia include bright light, fatigue, ill health and day dreaming.

Stages of development of exodeviation

In general, development of an exodeviation has got three stages:

1. *Stage of latent exodeviation.* In this stage, exodeviation is kept latent by the control of fusional convergence reserve. It is also called as stage of exophoria. It has been described in detail on page 209.

2. *Stage of intermittent exotropia.* In this stage, the fusional convergence reserves which usually keep the deviation latent, become inadequate intermittently resulting in intermittent manifest exodeviation (intermittent exotropia).

3. *Stage of constant exodeviation.* When the fusional convergence amplitude becomes inadequate to maintain the latency of deviation, a permanent manifest exodeviation, i.e. constant exotropia occurs. Constant exotropia may be unilateral or alternating.

CLASSIFICATION

I. In terms of the state of fusion, the exodeviations can be classified into:
- Exophoria (*see* page 209),
- Intermittent exotropia, and
- Constant exotropia (unilateral or alternating)

II. Duane's classification. It is based on the assumption that divergence is an active process rather than relaxation of the convergence with a return of the eyes to parallelism or a divergence position by mechanical or elastic forces. In Duane's classification, the primary comitant exodeviations (which include exophoria, intermittent exotropia and constant exotropia) are further subdivided as follows:

1. *Basic exodeviation.* Exodeviation is equal at distance and at near, i.e. within 10PO of each other. It is thought to be associated with both divergence excess and convergence insufficiency. Therefore, it is also called mixed type exodeviation.

2. *Divergence excess type.* The exodeviation is at least 10^Δ greater at distance than at near even after performing the patch test.

Note: Most of the patients with true divergence excess type exotropia have high AC/A ratio, and such patients are prone to postoperative overcorrection, if the distance measurement is used as the target angle.

3. *Pseudodivergence excess type*. Apparently, the exodeviation appears to be greater at distance than at near (e.g. XT 25D at distance and 10D at near). However, with special tests such as the patch for 30 minutes, the pattern is shown to be basic type. (e.g. 25D at distance, 25D at near).

This occurs because patients with pseudo-divergence excess have increased tonic fusional convergence, which acts more at near. The prolonged monocular patching dissipates tonic fusional convergence, thereby disclosing the full latent deviation. Short period of monocular occlusion that occur with alternate cover test is not enough to break the tonic fusional convergence.

4. *Convergence insufficiency type*. The exo-deviation is at least 15^Δ greater at near than at distance.

These four varieties of primary exodeviation must not be considered as being in 'water-tight' compartments.

III. Phases of divergence excess type of exodeviation: Calhounz et al. have described four phases of divergence excess type of exodeviation (Table 10.2).

IV. Kushner's classification of intermittent exotropia is depicted in Table 10.3.

Table 10.2 *Phases of exodeviations and clinical presentations*

| Phase | Clinical presentation | | |
	Deviation at distance	Deviation at near	Other features
I	Exophoria	Orthophoria	Asymptomatic goes undetected
II	Intermittent exotropia	Orthophoria or exophoria	Symptomatic for distance (no suppression scotoma)
III	Exotropia	Exophoria or intermittent exotropia	Binocular vision for near, suppression, scotoma for distance
IV	Exotropia	Exotropia	No binocular single vision

INTERMITTENT EXOTROPIA

Intermittent exotropia occurs much more frequently than constant exotropia. It comprises between 70% and 90% of all exotropias.

As discussed earlier, intermittent exotropia is usually preceded by a stage of exophoria. In intermittent exotropia, the deviation becomes manifest intermittently when the fusional convergence fails to control the deviation.

Clinical features

1. *Time of onset*. The onset of intermittent exotropia is usually in early childhood. About 50% of the children develop intermittent exodeviation before 6 months of age and nearly

Table 10.3 *Kushner's classification of intermittent exotropia*	
Type	*Definition*
Basic	Distance and near measurements are equal
Tenacious proximal fusion	Distance measurement initially exceeds near, but the near measurement increases after 30–60 minutes of monocular occlusion
High AC/A ratio	Distance measurement exceeds near measurement, even after 60 minutes of monocular occlusion and a high AC/A ratio is present
Proximal convergence	Distance measurement exceeds near measurement, even after 60 minutes of monocular occlusion. AC/A ratio is normal
Low AC/A ration	Near measurement exceeds distance measurement. A low AC/A ratio is demonstrated
Fusional convergence insufficency	Near measurement exceeds distance measurement. Patient has poor fusional convergence amplitudes
Pseudoconvergence insufficiency	Near measurement exceeds distance measurement, but distance measurement increases with 60 minutes of monocular occlusion.

AC/A = Accommodative convergence/accommodation

70% develop within first two years of life. Some begin at birth or shortly thereafter. Only a few develop the exotropia after 5 years of age.

2. Sex distribution. Exodeviations are more common in females (70.0%) than males (30.0%). The exact reason for female preponderance is not known, possibly there might be some genetic factor.

3. Refractive errors. Earlier reports suggested that myopia was more common in exotropia. However, recent view is that distribution of refractive errors in exotropes resembles that in the orthotropes and that there is no role of underlying refractive errors in the etiology of primary exotropia.

4. Precipitating factors. The heterotropic phase of intermittent exotropia most commonly occurs under conditions of fatigue, ill-health, bright light, day dreaming, drowsiness or visual inattention.

5. Symptoms are as follows:

i. *Transient diplopia* may be experienced in the beginning. However, suppression and later anomalous retinal correspondence (ARC) develop quickly to protect the patient from diplopia.

ii. *Closing of one eye in bright light,* conventionaly referred to as *photophobia* is a conspicuous symptom of intermittent exotropia. The usual history is that child closes one eye in bright light. No convincing explanation is available in the literature for this phenomenon. Recent view is that, perhaps, the bright light adversely affects the amplitude of fusional convergence in patients who maintain a delicate balance between exophoria and intermittent exotropia, causing them to close one eye.

iii. *Asthenopic symptoms* may occur in the initial phases, when fusion begins to succumb and the eyes deviate momentarily from the ortho-position. Patient may experience eye strain, blurring, headache, difficulty with prolonged periods of reading and other asthenopic symptoms. However, soon the children become asymptomatic due to development of sensory adaptation. While adult patients with inter-mittent exotropia commonly have symptoms of decompensated exophoria.

iv. *Micropsia* is a comparatively less known symptom of intermittent exodeviation. It is explained to occur owing to use of accommo-dative convergence to control the exodeviation.

6. Deviation. At first, the deviation is typically manifest only at distance. With increasing age, the deviation progresses and there occurs an increase in the duration and frequency of the tropia phase. Ultimately, a manifest deviation appears at near also (Tables 10.2 and 10.3). *Factors that may influence progression are:*

• Decline in tonic convergence with increasing age,
• Gradual lessening of accommodative power,
• Development of suppression, and
• An increase in the divergence of the orbits with advancing age.

Associations

Intermittent exotropia may be associated with:
• A–V-pattern (common)
• Comitant verstical deviation
• Dissociated vertical deviation
• Incomitant vertical deviation

Sensory adaptations

• Suppression and anomalous retinal corres-pondence develop quickly to protect the patient from diplopia during exotropic phase.
• During non-strabismic phase, normal retinal correspondence is present.
• Deep amblyopia with eccentric fixation is a rare finding in exotropia.

Clinical evaluation

Detailed clinical evaluation should be carried out on the general lines (*see* page 100). However, the points which need special attention are mentioned here.

1. History should provide information about: Age of onset, change since onset, frequency of manifest phase and general health.

2. Visual acuity is usually good. If unequal, suspect: Anisometropia, microtropia or fundus pathology.

3. Cycloplegic refraction and fundus exami-nation should be carried out in each case.

4. Cover test should be performed to assess at 1/3 m, 6 m and far distance.

5. Measurement of deviation with prism bar cover test (PBCT) should be performed in all the cardinal positions of gaze at near and distance fixation to discover any associated A- or V-pattern and presence of lateral gaze incomitance (LGI, i.e. 20% reduction in the angle of squint in lateral gaze). Detection of LGI is important to prevent surgical overcorrection.

Measurement of squint should also be made at a far distance beyond 6 metres since many a time a larger angle of deviation may be detected.

6. *Measurement of stereopsis* should be made during the phoric phase. Both near and distance stereoacuity should be tested. A progressive decline in stereopsis is a clear indication to correct exotropia. Distance stereopsis deteriorates earlier than the near stereopsis.

7. *Occlusion test.* It is very important for the differentiation between true and simulated divergence excess type of exotropia. Thus in every child with intermittent exotropia at

distance only or with at least 15^Δ greater exotropia at distance than near the occlusion test must be performed. Preferably one eye should be patched for 24 hours. However, recently it has been reported that only brief period of occlusion (30 minutes to one hour) is sufficient. The detailed procedure of the occlusion test is as follows:

- First of all perform alternate cover test at distance and near to measure the angle of exotropia (Fig. 10.9A to C). Let us presume this step has revealed that exotropia is significantly greater (15^Δ or more) at distance than at near.
- Patch is placed over one eye for one hour to dissociate the eyes thoroughly (Fig. 10.9D).
- After one hour, the fellow eye is covered with an occluder and the patch is removed (Fig. 10.9E and F). It is very important to

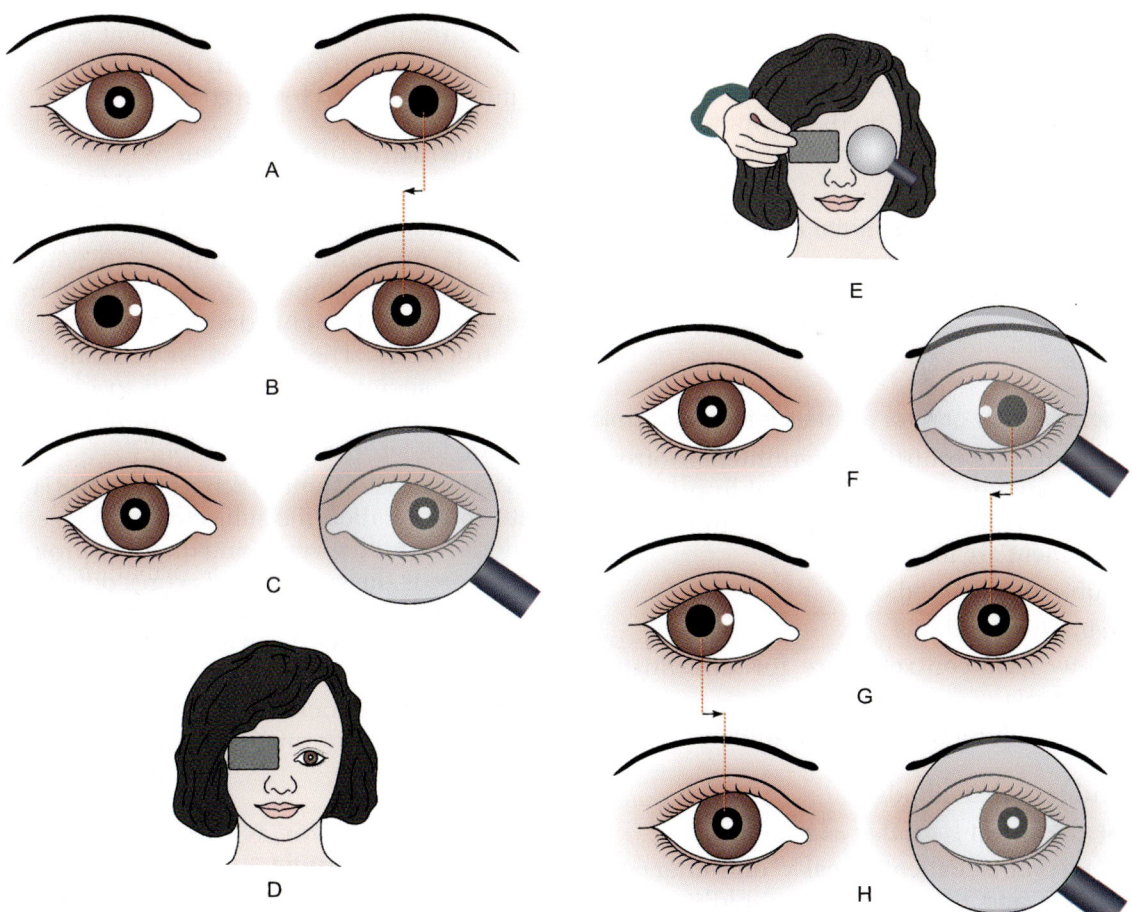

Fig. 10.9 *Patch test for simulated divergence excess type exotropia (for explanation, see text).*

prevent the patient from using both eyes simultan-eously even momentarily, since only a brief binocular exposure may be sufficient to decrease the near deviation by fusional convergence.

- Again alternate cover test is performed at near and deviation measured (Fig. 10.9 G and H). In patients with simulated divergence excess type exotropia, the angle of deviation for near will increase markedly and will become equal to the angle for distance (basic type); whereas with true divergence excess, the near deviation will remain unchanged, i.e. deviation for distance will be ≥15 PD more than the near.

8. +3.0D spherical lens test. In this test, measurement for near is performed with and without +3.0 DS lens in front of the exotropic eye using an accommodative target which must be seen clearly. This test is not an alternative to occlusion test in planning the surgical therapy (since, the occlusion test removes binocular fusional stimuli, whereas +3.0 DS lenses provide only an indication of AC/A ratio). The +3.0 DS lens test is useful in predicting how a patient may respond to plus lenses, if surgical over-correction results.

9. *Measurement of fusional amplitudes*
- *Convergence amplitudes* are usually normal at near and poor to good at distance.
- *Divergence amplitudes* may be excellent to poor.

Assessment of control of intermittent exotropia

Assessment of control of intermittent exotropia before any intervention is useful in predicting surgical outcome. Following methods of assessment are in vague:
- Subjective methods
- Objective methods
- Newcastle control score for intermittent exotropia
- Mayo scale for control in intermittent exotropia

I. Subjective methods

Office control is graded as below:
- *Good control*: Patient "breaks" only after cover testing and resumes fusion rapidly without need for a blink or refixation.

- *Fair control*: Patient blinks or refixates to control the deviation after disruption with cover testing.
- *Poor control*: Patient who breaks spontaneously without any form of fusion disruption.

Home control: At home, parents are told to keep a chart noting the control of deviation in terms of the percentage of waking hours the manifest deviation is noticed at home.

II. Objective methods

Distance stereoacuity testing is useful in noting the deterioration of fusion, that occurs early in this disorder. Normal distance stereoacuity indicates good control with little or no suppression. The Mentor BVat II BVS assesses distance stereoacuity using both contour circles and the 'Random dot E test' from 240 to 15 seconds of arc disparity.

Near stereoacuity: It does not correlate well with the degree of control in intermittent exotropia and that performance in this test is only minimally affected by surgery.

III. Newcastle scoring system

Since the clinic control does not take into account the duration of tropic phase and the fact that there is no standardization as to when to intervene, a novel method was put forth by H. Haggerty and Richardson, the Newcastle Control Score. The revised New Castle Score system seems to be useful in grading the severity of intermittent exotropia and as a criteria for surgical intervention.

The Newcastle Control Score (Table 10.4) takes into consideration the subjective and objective criteria to grade severity and quantify progress. The score is the sum total of scores obtained in home control and in the clinic for near and far. Total score can vary from 0–7 and patients with a score of 3 or more are considered to need surgical intervention. It is a consistent method of rating severity and enables one to easily monitor progress.

IV. Mayo scale for scoring of control in intermittent exotropia

Mayo scoring system (Table 10.5) is based solely on times observations. An average of three score

Table 10.4 *The Newcastle Control Score*

Newcastle control score

Score	Component
Home control	
0	Squint/monocular eye closure never noticed
1	Squint/monocular closure seen occasionally (<50% of time) for distance
2	Squint/monocular eye closure seen frequently (>50% of time) for distance
3	Squint/monocular closure seen for distance and near fixation
Clinic control near	
0	Manifest only after CT and resumes fusion without need for blink or refixation
1	Blink or refixate to control after CT
2	Manifest spontaneously or with any form of fusion disruption without recovery
Clinic control distance	
0	Manifest only after CT and resumes fusion without need for blink or refixation
1	Blink or refixate to control after CT
2	Manifest spontaneously or with any form of fusion disruption without recovery
	The score varies from 0–7: score of 3 or more significant

Table 10.5 *Mayo score for scoring control of intermittent exotropia*

Observation	Score	
	Near	Distance
• No exotropia, unless dissociated and recovers in <1 second (exophoria)	0	0
• No exotropia, unless dissociated and recovers in 1–5 seconds (exophoria)	1	1
• No exotropia, unless dissociated and recovers in >5 seconds (exophoria)	2	2
• Exotropia <50% of the examination before dissociation	3	3
• Exotropia > 50% of the examination before dissociation	4	4
• Constant exotropia	5	5

is taken to be more reliable. Score (0 to 5) is measured both at distance and near fixation. So a total score of 0–10 can be obtained.

Treatment

1. Optical treatment

- *Myopia*, when present, should be fully corrected.
- *Hypermetropia* up to +2.0 DS need not be corrected.
- *Over minus lenses* of 2 to 3D prescribed in emmetropes or over prescribed in myopes, is reported to correct x(T) in some children.

2. Prismotherapy

Some strabismologists recommend use of *base-in prisms* to enforce bifoveolar stimulation. They correct one-half to one-third of deviation by prisms in order to stimulate fusional covergence. While other strabismologists like von Noorden do not prefer to use prisms. However, prismotherapy may be useful in children where surgery is to be postponed for some period.

3. Orthoptic treatment

Most of the strabismologists agree that, there is not much role of preoperative orthoptics treatment in patients with exotropia. However, following measures may sometimes be useful. Aim is to make the patient aware of manifest deviation and to improve the patient's control over it.

i. *Antisuppression exercises.* An attempt should be made to eliminate suppression so that the patient experiences diplopia whenever the deviation becomes manifest. Suppression scotoma usually and initially is amenable to therapy by flashes and then the BSV should be maintained by antisuppression exercises such as bar reading, cheiroscope or on synoptophore. The methods of antisuppression treatment are described in Chapter 8 page 174.

ii. *Exercises to improve the patient's control of the deviation by strengthening the fusional vergences.* Improvement of fusional positive relative convergence is of particular value in patients with intermittent exotropia at near only. The methods described in the treatment of exophoria (page 214) may be used with the aim of ultimately obtaining a normal near point of convergence. Occasionally, a patient is unable to control the near exotropia with orthoptic treatment, in which case, surgery should be indicated. In such cases, postoperative treatment to improve the fusional vergences should be given.

Some people have questioned the effectivity of convergence exercises in controlling exodeviations. They cannot and do not affect the basic deviation but by improving the fusion control decrease the manifestation of an exodeviation, a tropia being converted into a phoria. The lack of effect is only due to poor case selection (cases having suppression may require anti-suppression exercises first) or improper method of exercising. Appreciation of physiological diplopia should be taught as the first step. Secondly, training should be done to increase both the phasic and tonic control, to improve the convergence sustenance. Just like any other physical exercises, the results last till the exercises are continued. Synoptophore exercises may be desirable to start with but are insufficient, if not supplemented by proper home exercises.

For home exercises, special cards or a line on a plain paper may be made use of or a properly done "pencil-pushups" may be done.

It should be noted that no convergence exercises should be done by patients with intermittent exotropia at distance only, in whom surgery is planned, for this may lead to postoperative overconvergence.

iii. *Occlusion therapy.* It has been reported that occlusion of preferred eye for 3 to 5 hours a day for a long period is useful in decreasing the angle of deviation. In one study, it has been reported that about 40% patients with intermittent exotropia become exophoric. The recommended schedule of occlusion is as follows:

Initially, the results are evaluated after 4 months of occlusion. If the angle of deviation is decreased, the occlusion should be continued and assessment made every 4 months until no further change occurs. In case, there is no improvement after initial occlusion for 4 months, it should be discontinued.

von Noorden reports that alternate occlusion for 3 months may be employed in lieu of surgery with useful results in patients with small-angle intermittent exotropia.

4. Surgical treatment

Indications for surgery

i. Surgery is advisable, when the exotropia occurs during more than 50% of waking hours, or causes asthenopic symptoms or when the deviation exceeds 20$^\Delta$.

ii. When the patient is exophoric most of the time and becomes exotropic only two or three times a day, surgery should be preceded by several months of observation, since the disease does not progress in all patients. However, surgery should be undertaken, if during observation patient shows one or several of the following signs and symptoms of progression:

- Gradual loss of fusional control as evidenced by increasing frequency of the manifest phase of squint.
- An increase in the size of basic deviation (more than 20$^\Delta$).
- Development of secondary convergence insufficiency with asthenopic symptoms.
- Development of suppression as indicated by absence of diplopia during manifest phase.
- Gradual deterioration of stereopsis (it is a frequently used argument for early surgical therapy).

Age for surgery

There are two schools of thought:

i. *Early surgery.* Knap and many other workers advocate early surgery. These workers state that, "surgery is dictated by the amount and frequency of the exodeviation, not by the patient's age. As long as the patient is 6 months or older, surgery can be performed." However, they do caution that in visually immature children a slight undercorrection should be attempted to prevent occurrence of mono-fixation syndrome from consecutive esotropia.

ii. *Delayed surgery.* Jampolsky and a few other workers recommend that surgery should be delayed in visually immature infants to avoid consecutive esotropia and occurrence of monofixation syndrome. It is advisable that to get good results, surgery may be delayed up to 4 years of age. Till then child should be kept under observation to watch: Visual acuity, convergences, and parent's observation of frequency of squint. Further, in the interim, binocular vision should be reinforced with prisms base-in or minus lenses. However, in case there is very rapid functional deterioration of fusional control in spite of prismotherapy and orthoptics, an early surgical therapy may be considered.

General guidelines

General guidelines adopted from the observation of various workers are as follows:

- In *true divergence excess* type of exotropia, a bilateral recession of lateral recti should be preferred.
- In *basic exotropia and simulated divergence excess type*, a unilateral lateral rectus recession and medial rectus resection should be preferred. However, Parks has shown that bilateral rectus recession works for these patients also.
- In *convergence insufficiency type of exotropia*, a bilateral medial rectus muscle resection may be preferred.
- In *the presence of lateral gaze inhibition* (i.e. 20% reduction in the amount of squint in right and left lateral gaze), there is danger of over-correction with the usual surgery especially so in visually immature patient. Therefore, in the presence of LGI, a bilateral lateral rectus recession should be avoided and also, the recession and resection done on the nonpreferred eye should each be 1 mm less.
- In *small children (visually immature patients)*, a slight undercorrection should be attempted to avoid hazards of consecutive esotropia.
- In *visually mature patients*, many strabismologists feel that the surgeon should aim at an overcorrection of 10^D to 20^D to ultimately produce more stable results. However, it has been observed that it is not possible to accomplish this goal other than by pure chance.
- *Single muscle surgery* is almost useless in exotropias, it has been reported in the literature.

Table 10.6 *Rough estimate of amount of surgery to be performed in patients with intermittent divergent squint of true divergence excess type*

Deviation in prism dioptres	Bilateral lateral rectus recession
15	4.0
20	5.0
25	5.5
30	6.0
35	6.5
40	7.0
50	8.0
60	9.5
70	8.0 + 8 mm MR resection in one eye
80	8.0 + 8 mm MR resection in both eyes

Table 10.7 *Rough estimate of amount of surgery to be performed in patients with intermittent exotropia of basic and simulated divergence excess type*

Deviation in prism dioptres	Binocular surgery in mm Bilateral LR recession	Uniocular surgery in mm LR recession	Uniocular surgery in mm MR resection
15	4.0	4.0	3.0
20	5.0	5.0	4.0
25	5.5	6.0	4.5
30	6.0	7.0	5.0
35	6.5	7.5	5.0
40	7.0	8.0	6.0
50	8.0	9.0	7.0
60	9.5	10.0	8.0
70	8.0 + 8.0 MR resection in one eye		
80	8.0 + 8.0 MR resection in both eyes		

Table 10.8 *Rough estimate of amount of surgery to be performed in patients with intermittent exotropia of convergence insufficiency type*

Deviation in prism dioptres	Bilateral medial rectus resection
15	3.0
20	3.5
25	4.5
30	5.5
35	6.0
40	6.5
50	7.5
60	8.0
70	8.0 LR recession of one eye + 8.0
80	8.0 LR recession of both eyes + 8.0

Amount of surgery

The actual amount of surgery performed will vary according to an individual surgeon's technique. However, guidelines given in Tables 10.6, 10.7 and 10.8 may be useful as rough estimate of amount of surgery to be performed.

Management of associations

1. *Pattern deviations*
   i. A-pattern exotropia (*see* page 285)
   ii. V-pattern exotropia (*see* page 285)

2. *Comitant vertical deviation* (*see* page 255)
3. *Dissociated vertical deviation* (DVD). Though very rare, but may be associated with exotropia (*see* page 264).

Surgical results and postoperative management

After squint surgery, the eyes may be in orthoposition, still exotropic (undercorrection) or consecutive esotropic (overcorrection). Depending upon the position of the eyes, the postoperative management will be as follows:

1. Orthoposition

Undoubtedly, it is ideal to get a permanent orthoposition, but there is always a tendency of the eyes to diverge postoperatively. Therefore, it is extremely important to *strengthen the positive fusional convergence* with orthoptic exercises in order to improve control of the newly acquired bifoveal single vision.

Orthoptic exercises required to strengthen the positive fusional convergence are the same as described for exophoria (page 214).

2. Consecutive esotropia (overcorrection)

A very large overcorrection with gross limitation of ocular motility noted on the very next day is possibly due to lost or slipped lateral rectus muscle. Under such circumstances, patient should undergo surgery again within 24 hours.

Small to moderate (10$^\Delta$ to 50$^\Delta$) overcorrection needs to be managed depending upon the age of the patient:

A. *In adults* (visually mature patients), as described earlier, an overcorrection of 10$^\Delta$ to 20$^\Delta$ is desirable to ultimately achieve stable results.
- If overcorrection is more than 20$^\Delta$ after at least six weeks of surgery, then following *non-surgical measures* should be tried during the wait and watch period of 6 months.

   – *Rerefraction* should be done and if hypermetropia is detected, it should be fully corrected.
   – *Bifocals or miotic therapy* may be prescribed, if near esotropia is more than the distance.
   – *Prismotherapy* in the form of Fresnel membrane prism that fully correct the deviation should be prescribed. The prism power should be adjusted monthly depending upon the latest examination results.
- *Re-surgery* is indicated in patients where overcorrection of more than 20$^\Delta$ continues even after the above described non-surgical therapy for a period of 6 months.

   It has been recommended that in planning second surgery, *Cooper's dictum* (i.e. the decision about choice and amount of surgery should be made as if the present patient is a fresh case of squint) should be followed.

B. *In small children* (i.e. visually immature patients), as stated earlier, the consecutive esotropia is associated with a greater danger of developing monofixation syndrome and suppression amblyopia. So these patients need a special care. Following measures should be taken *within 2 weeks* of the surgery.
- *Re-refraction* should be done and any hypermetropic error should be fully corrected.
- *Bifocals or miotics* should be prescribed, if the deviation is greater at near.
- *Occlusion therapy.* Initially, when there is no fixation preference, *alternate occlusion* should be done for a few weeks. If the child develops moderate fixation preference, *conventional occlusion* of the preferred eye should be used till either there occurs alternate fixation or only a mild fixation preference.
- *Prismotherapy* in the form of 'Press on' base-out Fresnel membrane prism should be started at this stage to maintain bifoveal fixation. The prism power should fully correct the deviation and be adjusted monthly depending upon the latest examination results.
- *Re-surgery* is indicated, if the child remains overcorrected by 15$^\Delta$ or more in spite of the above described non-surgical therapy.

   For a re-operation, the *Cooper's dictum* (as stated above) should be followed.

3. *Residual exotropia* (undercorrection)

i. *Small residual exotropia* (15^Δ to 18^Δ) should be managed by following non-surgical measures:

- *Optical correction.* Refraction should be done and if the patient is myopic, a full optical correction should be ordered.
- *Cycloplegics.* In hypermetropic or emmetropic patient, 1% cyclopentolate eyedrops may be instilled twice a day to stimulate accommodative convergence. Once the alignment of the eyes and fusion are achieved, the frequency of instillation should be reduced progressively, i.e. once a day, then on alternate day to every third day. The regime may be continued for several months till full alignment is achieved.
- *Orthoptic exercises* in the form of antisuppression exercises (page 174) and fusional convergence exercises (page 214) should be continued till the goal is achieved.
- *Prismotherapy* in the form of base-in prisms that equals the undercorrection may be useful in visually mature patients.

ii. *Large residual exotropia* (more than 15D to 18D) needs resurgery which can be performed within *6–8 weeks of primary procedure*. For a repeat surgery, the planning should be done as on a new case (Cooper's dictum). Depending upon the type of residual exotropia and primary procedure done, the secondary procedure can be planned as shown in Table 10.9.

Criteria for success of management

The criteria for classification of excellent and poor success in the management of exotropia are as described below.

Excellent success

- Phoria for distance and near in the primary position and reading position.
- Absolute convergence not less than 20 p.d. for distance and near.
- Relative convergence not less than 15 p.d. for distance and near.
- Unlimited near point of convergence (5 cm or closer).
- No suppression.
- Excellent awareness of diplopia during testing situation.
- Comfortable without asthenopic symptoms.

Table 10.9 *Plan of secondary surgical procedures in patients with large residual exotropia*

Type of residual exotropia	Primary procedure performed	Secondary procedure required
Basic exotropia (equal for near and distance)	Recess-resect operation	Recess-resect operation on the other eye.
	Bilateral lateral rectus recession	Ipsilateral medial rectus resection and lateral rectus marginal myotomy
Divergence excess type (greater at distance than near)	Bilateral lateral rectus recession	Further recession or myotomies of lateral recti.
Convergence insufficiency type (greater at near than distance)	Recess-resect procedure	Recession of the virgin lateral rectus and further recession or marginal myotomy of the already recessed lateral rectus muscle

Failure

- Tropia at any distance or intermittent at two of the four testing distances.
- Absolute convergence less than 10 p.d. for distance.
- Relative convergence less than 5 p.d. for distance and near.
- Near point of convergence less than 8 cm.
- Peripheral and foveal suppression.
- No awareness of diplopia.
- Asthenopic symptoms.

PRIMARY CONSTANT EXOTROPIA

Primary constant exotropia (Fig. 10.10) does not occur as frequently as intermittent exotropia, and both groups combinedly occur less frequently than esotropias (constant exotropia, aetiologically, may be primary, secondary, sensory and consecutive). The number of primary constant exotropias is small compared to the number of secondary forms.

Clinical features

1. *Time of onset*

Two types of primary constant exotropias have been described depending upon the time of onset:

1. *Primary constant, infantile exotropia.* It is an extremely rare condition with onset shortly after birth. It has been reported that this form of exotropia is more common in the African than in the white race. It has been described on page 239.

2. *Primary constant exotropia due to decompensated intermittent exotropia.* The primary constant exotropia almost invariably results from decompensated intermittent exotropia, and thus such patients usually do not possess a significant amount of amblyopia. It has been reported that in many patients intermittent exotropia may not decompensate for a long period. Therefore, it has been recommended that patients with intermittent exotropia need to be evaluated over a period of time to ascertain whether progression is taking place and surgery is warranted, particularly those in whom a constant deviation is present less than 50% of the time.

2. Fixation pattern

The patients with constant exotropia may fix alternately, fix with one eye only or show a mild, moderate or strong fixation preference. According to the fixation behaviour, constant exotropia may be classified as unilateral or alternating:

(a) Alternating exotropia

i. *Fixation.* In constant alternating exotropia, the patient uses each eye alternately for fixation (Fig. 10.10).

ii. *Visual acuity.* Usually, there is little or no difference between the visual acuity of the two eyes.

iii. *Deviation.* The angle of deviation is usually large and tends to be equal for distance and near fixation. The near deviation is determined by the effect of proximal and accommodative convergence. Very frequently there is a secondary vertical deviation, the deviating abducted eye being elevated.

iv. *Sensory adaptations.* In cases with acquired alternating exotropia, the patients had normal retinal correspondence and bifoveal fusion before the deviation became constant. If normal correspondence persists, there occurs complete suppression of the deviating eye. However, if ARC develops, both eyes co-operate in binocular vision. Sometimes a form of binocular vision is achieved whereby each half of the visual field is perceived by the homolateral eye while the information from the other half is

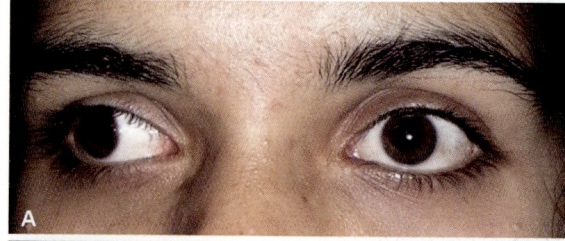
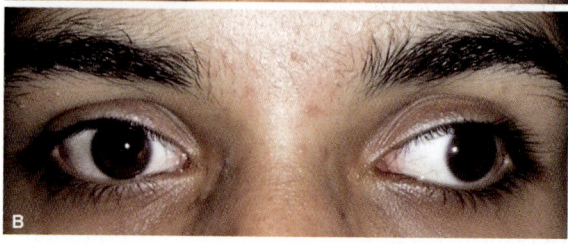

Fig. 10.10 *A patient with primary alternate divergent squint (ADS): A, Right exotropia while fixing with left eye; and B, left exotropia while fixing with right eye.*

suppressed. Thus the left eye would perceive the left half of the field but suppress the right half, while the right eye would see the right half and suppress the left. The fixation point and its vicinity, in this case, is seen by the fixating eye and is included in the suppression area of the deviating eye.

(b) Unilateral exotropia

i. *Fixation.* In constant unilateral exotropia, the same eye is used for fixation while the other is deviated. Fixation preference may be mild, moderate or strong:

- *In mild fixation preference,* one eye is preferred, but when it is covered, the other eye easily takes up fixation and maintains it even when the cover is removed from the first eye. Such patients usually do not have a significant amount of amblyopia.
- *In moderate fixation preference,* one eye is preferred and when it is covered, the other eye will take up fixation; but after the cover is removed from the first eye, the other eye will hold fixation only until the patient blinks or changes fixation.
- *In strong fixation preference,* one eye is preferred and when it is covered, the other eye will take up fixation, but only as long as the cover is left over the first eye.
- *In unilateral fixation,* only one eye is preferred and when it is covered, the other eye does not

take up fixation but makes irregular jerky movements, suggesting loss of central fixation and a deep amblyopia.

ii. *Deviation* is usually large. In patients with long-standing neglected deviations, anatomic changes may occur in the contracted muscles.

iii. *Sensory adaptations.* There is marked *suppression* in the deviating eye, but amblyopia is less severe than in esotropia. ARC may be present but is of little importance since suppression prevails. Since the majority of unilateral exotropias are acquired, most of the patients have had normal retinal correspondence previously.

Associations

Primary constant exotropia may be associated with:
- A- or V-pattern (Fig. 10.11) with or without oblique muscle by function
- Comitant vertical deviation muscle dept function
- Dissociated vertical deviation (DVD)

Clinical evaluation

The aim of clinical evaluation is to diagnose type of deviation and to assess potential for binocular single vision. The complete clinical evaluation should be carried out in each case of strabismus. Points pertinent to the evaluation of primary constant exotropia are similar to those described for the intermittent exotropia.

Treatment

The treatment of constant exotropia is almost always surgical. Orthoptic treatment is given both preoperatively and postoperatively, if fusion ability can be demonstrated. Any patient over 6 months of age can be taken for surgery. The type and amount of surgery to be performed is similar to that for intermittent exotropia.

SENSORY EXOTROPIA

Definition

It refers to unilateral exotropia that develops as a result of poor visual function in one eye.

Etiopathogenesis

Sensory exotropia results secondary to some sensory deficit such as anisometropia, unilateral cataract, unilateral aphakia, corneal opacity, optic atrophy, macular lesion and any other organic cause of unilateral loss of vision.

It has been reported that both infants and young adults with poor vision in one eye develop sensory exotropia and the older children tend to develop a sensory esotropia. The mechanisms and theories about development of sensory esotropia and exotropia have been described on page 238.

Clinical features

1. ***Monocular visual loss*** due to any cause is always associated.
2. ***Deviation*** is unilateral and constant and involves the eye with poor vision (Fig. 10.12).

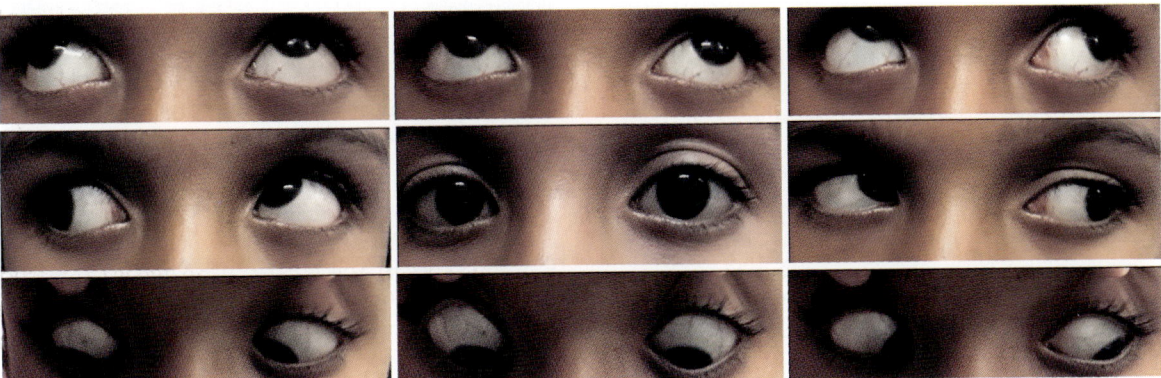

Fig. 10.11 *Nine gaze photographs of a patient with alternate divergent squint with V-pattern with inferior oblique over action (IOOA).*

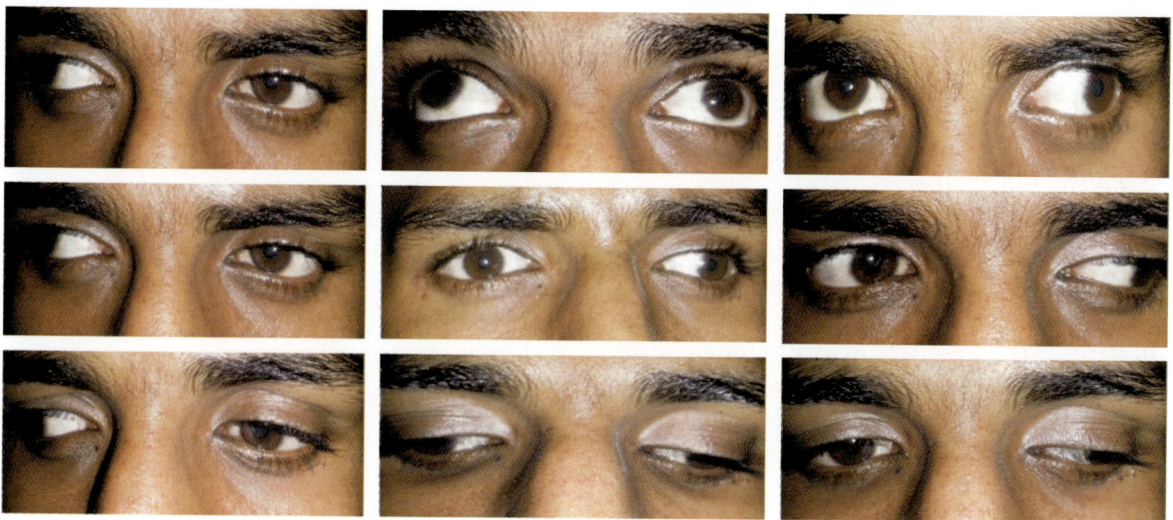

Fig. 10.12 *Nine gaze photographs of a patient with left sensory exotropia.*

Treatment

• *Cosmetic surgery* is the treatment for most sensory exotropias. However, some scope of functional recovery may be there in children with sensory exotropia due to anisometropia including unilateral aphakia.

• *Choice of surgery* for sensory exotropia is usually recess-resect operation on the same eye. In large exodeviation, one can recess lateral rectus up to 10 mm and can resect medial rectus also up to 10 mm. Though, it may result in limitation of horizontal movements in the operated eye.

• *Adjustable suture surgery* may be preferred in patients above 10–11 years of age with sensory exotropia.

CONSECUTIVE EXOTROPIA

Consecutive exotropia refers to occurrence of exotropia in an eye which was previously esotropic.

Clinical types

It has been reported to occur under following two clinical situations:

1. Surgical overcorrection of esotropia may result in consecutive exotropia (Fig. 10.13).

2. Spontaneous consecutive exotropia is change of esotropia into exotropia without exogenous mechanical factors or an acquired paralysis of

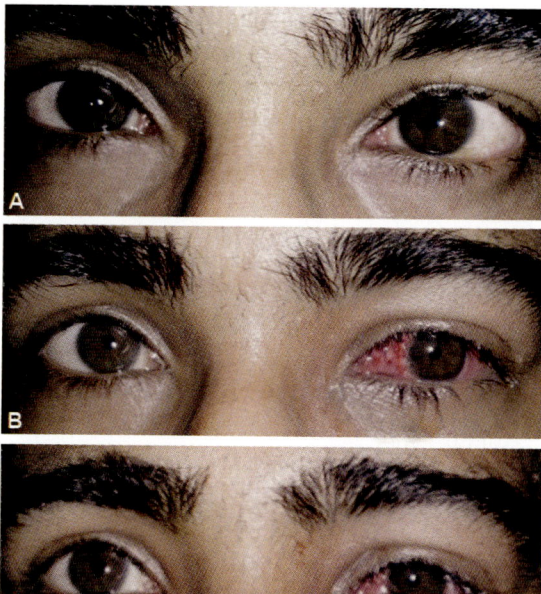

Fig. 10.13 *A patient with esotropia (A), who developed consecutive exotropia after surgery (B), which was surgically corrected to orthotropia (C).*

medial rectus muscle. Spontaneous consecutive exotropia is known to occur more commonly under following circumstances:

• Esotropia with poor vision in the deviating eye.

• Infantile esotropia associated with a high hypermetropia.

Treatment

1. Refractive error, if any, kind should be corrected.
2. Assess state of binocular sensory cooperation:
   i. *If normal retinal correspondence and bifoveal fusion can be demonstrated* (especially in patients with overcorrected esotropia):
      - Overcome suppression
      - Improve fusional convergence
      - Perform surgery
   ii. *If bifoveal fusion cannot be demonstrated*, assess cosmetic appearance:
      - If good, leave alone.
      - If poor, perform cosmetic surgery.

BIBLIOGRAPHY

1. Burian HM: Pathophysiology of exodeviations. In Manlev DR (ed): Symposium on Horizontal Ocular Deviations. St. Louis. Mosby, 1971. p 119
2. Burian HM, Noorden GK von: Binocular Vision and Ocular Motility. St. Louis, Mosby, 1974.
3. Burian HM: Exodeviations : Their classification, diagnosis and treatment. Am J Ophthalmol 62:1161, 1966.
4. Cooper El: Purposeful overcorrection in exotropia. In Arruga A(ed): International Strabismus Symposium (University of Geissen, 1966). Basel/New York, S Karger, 1968, p 311.
5. Costenbader FD: Roundtable discussion. In Allen JH (ed): Strabismic Ophthalmic Symposium II. St. Louis, Mosby, 1958, p 484.
6. Costenbader FD: Infantile esotropia. Trans Am Ophthalmol Soc. 59:397, 1961
7. Calhou JC, Nelson LB, Harley RD Atlas of Ped. Ophthal Surgery Philadelphia Saunders. 1987 pp 8-10.
8. Crone RA. Everhard-Halm Y: Cyclofusion. In Moore 5, Mein J (eds): Orthoptics: Past, Present, and Future. New York, Stratton Intercontinental, 1976, p 409.
9. Dell' Osso LF, Ellenberger CJr, Abel LA et al: The nystagmus blockage syndrome: Congenital nystagmus, manifest latent nystagmus or both? Invest Ophthalmol Vis Sci. 24: 1580-87, 1983.
10. Duane A: A new classification of the motor anomalies of the eye based upon physiological principles, together with their symptoms, diagnosis and treatment. Ann Ophthalmol Otolaryngol 5:969, 1896; 6:84, 247, 1897.
11. Helveston EM: Cyclic strabismus. Am Orthopt J 23: 48-51, 1973.
12. Havener WH: Ocular Pharmacology, St. Louis, Mosby, 1978.
13. Henson DB, Williams DE: Depth perception in strabismus. Br J Ophthalmol 64:349, 1980.
14. Hiles DA: Surgery for congenital esotropia. Int Ophthalmol Clin 16 (3) : 75, 1976.
15. Hoyt WF, Daroff RB: Supranuclear disorders of ocular control systems in man: Clinical, anatomical and physiological correlations. In Bach-y-rita P, Collins CC, Hyde JE(eds): The Control of Eye Movements New York. Academic Press, 1971, p 175.
16. Ing MR: Early surgical alignment for congenital esotropia. J Pediatr Ophthalmol Strabismus 20:11-18, 1983.
17. Jotterand VH, Isenberg SJ: Enhancing surgery for accommodative esotropia, Ophthalmic Surg 19:263-266, 1988.
18. Krzystkowa, K and Paja Kowa J, The sensorial state in divergent strabismus. In orthoptics, Proceeding of the second international orthoptics congress, Amsterdam, 1972, Excerpta media foundation, p 72.
19. Kushner BJ: Exotropic deviations: A functional classification and approach to treatment. Am Orthoptic J 38:81-93, 1988.
20. Manle DR: Classification of the exodeviations, in Manley DR (ed): Symposium on Horizontal Ocular Deviations. St. Louis. Mosby, 1971.p 128.
21. Nelson LB Bacal Da Burke MJ An alternative approach to the surgical management of exotropia : the unilateral lateral rectus recession. J.Ped. Ophthalmol strabismus 1992. 29 (6) 357–60.
22. Noorden GK von: Divergence excess and simulated divergence excess, diagnosis and surgical management, Ophthalmologica 26: 719, 1969.
23. Noorden GK von: Some aspects of exotropia, presented before meeting of the Wilmer Resident Association, John Hopkins Hospital, April 26, 1966.
24. Noorden GK von: The nystagmus compensation (blockage) syndrome. Am J Ophthalmol 82:283, 1976.
25. Noorden GK von: Indications of the posterior fixation operation in strabismus. Ophthalmology (Rochester) 85:512, 1979.
26. Parks MM: The monofixation syndrome. Trans Am Ophthalmol Soc 67:609. 1969.
27. Prism Adaptation Study Group: Efficacy of prism adaptation in the surgica management of

acquired esotropia. Arch Ophthalmol 108:1228-1256, 1993.

28. Reinecke RD: Accommodative esotropia. J Continuing Educ Ophthalmol 40:11,1978.

29. Rogers GL, Chazen S, Fellows R, et al: Strabismus surgery and its effect upon infant development in congenital esotropia. Ophthalmology 89:479-483, 1982.

30. Sanfilippo S. clahane AC The effectiveness of orthoptics alone in selected cases of exodeviations the immediate result and several years later Am Orthopt J. 1970: 20: 104-17.

31. Tychsen L, Lisberger SG: Maldevelopment of visual motion processing in humans who had strabismus with onset in infancy. J Neurosci 6:2495-2508, 1986.

32. Wright KW, Bruce-Lyle L: Augmented surgery for esotropia associated with high hypermetropia. J Pediatr Ophthalmol Strabismus 30:167-170, 1993.

Chapter
11
Vertical Strabismus and Cyclodeviations

VERTICAL STRABISMUS

CLASSIFICATION

A. *Depending upon constancy of deviation*
  1. Hyperphoria (H)
  2. Intermittent hypertropia (H [T])
  3. Hypertropia (HT)

B. *Depending upon the direction of deviation in the non-fixing eye*
  1. Hypertropia
  2. Hypotropia

C. *Depending upon comitance of deviation*
  I. *Comitant vertical deviation*
   1. Induced (refractive)
   2. End result of long-standing paralytic deviation
  II. *Incomitant vertical deviations*
   Depending upon the innervational etiology, the incomitant vertical deviations can be further subdivided into following types:
   1. Apparent oblique muscle dysfunction
   2. Paretic vertical deviations
   3. Restrictive vertical deviations

  III. *Dissociated vertical deviation (DVD)*
   - Monocular DVD
   - Bionocular or alternating DVD

COMITANT VERTICAL DEVIATIONS

The prevalence of comitant vertical deviations in general is not low. Vertical deviations may occur as isolated anomalies or in association with horizontal deviations.

Prevalence. Following observations have been made regarding prevalence of vertical deviations:
- Approximately, half of the patients with motility disorders have isolated vertical anomalies.
- Approximately, one-third of all patients with motility disorders have a combined horizontal and vertical deviation.
- An associated vertical deviation has been reported in 43% of all exotropias.

Types. Comitant vertical deviations include:
1. *Hypertropia.* In this condition, non-fixating eye is higher than the fixating eye.
2. *Hypotropia.* In this condition, non-fixating eye is lower than the fixing eye.

Etiology

Exact etiology is not known. Following factors have been blamed:

- *Correction of unequal refractive error* may induce comitant hyperdeviations.
- *Anomalous position of rest* caused by orbital or other anatomical anomalies or mechanical factors or abnormal innervation may be causative mechanism.
- *Convertion of incomitant paralytic hyperdeviation* to comitant with the passage of time (as secondary changes occur) is also common to find.

Clinical features

- Symptoms can be marked in hyperdeviations, even when the magnitude is low. Patients often present with frontal headache, diplopia, ocular discomfort or pain, due to overuse of fusional vergence.
- Hypertropias are more frequently intermittent than constant deviations.
- Suppression, amblyopia, or vertical anomalous retinal correspondence may occur.
- In deviation of lesser magnitude, the patient may obtain bifoveal fusion by tilting the head.
- Typically, patients with small comitant vertical deviations have a moderate to large horizontal strabismus (exotropia or esotropia) as well.
- Repeated measurements in the diagnostic positions of gaze in majority of patients may reveal a paretic component or a primary overaction of one or several cyclovertical muscles.

Note. Large primary comitant vertical deviations are rare. The primary vertical deviation must be differentiated from skew deviation, which is rather abrupt in onset, variable, and associated with symptoms caused by intracranial or labyrinthin disease.

Treatment

1. Orthoptics. Amblyopia, when present, should be treated. If a bifoveal fusion potential and normal correspondence can be demonstrated in patients in whom the deviation was acquired after a period of normal binocular vision, orthoptic treatment to eliminate suppression may be indicated prior to surgery. It is almost impossible to improve vertical fusional vergence through orthoptic training.

2. Prismotherapy. Comitant vertical deviations smaller than 10D can be corrected with prism. The prism power should be distributed equally before the two eyes with a base-down prism in front of the hypertropic eye and a base-up prism infront of hypotropic eye. The minimal prismatic power that provides comfortable single binocular vision should be prescribed.

3. Surgery. Following procedures are indicated:

- *A comitant vertical deviation up to 11D to 14D* associated with horizontal deviation can be eliminated by simply lowering the horizontal muscle insertion (by 5 to 8 mm) of the hypertropic eye or by raising the insertions of hypotropic eye; while performing the horizontal squint surgery.
- *For large vertical deviations (between 15D and 25D)*, a 3 to 4 mm recession of the appropriate vertical rectus muscle is recommended. For example, in a patient with right hypertropia of 25D, the right superior rectus and left inferior rectus should each be recessed by 4–5 mm.

INCOMITANT VERTICAL DEVIATIONS

CLASSIFICATION

Incomitant vertical deviations can be classified as below:

1. Apparent oblique muscle dysfunction

i. *Inferior oblique overaction (strabismus surso-adductorious)* is now termed as *over-elevation in adduction* (OEA). It can be:
   - Primary OEA, or
   - Secondarry OEA.

ii. *Inferior oblique underaction*, is now termed as *under-elevation in adduction* (UEA). It can be:
   - Primary UEA, or
   - Seconday UEA

iii. *Superior oblique overaction (strabismus deorsadductorious)* is now termed as *over-depression in adduction* (ODA). It can be:
   - Primary ODA, or
   - Seconday ODA.

iv. *Superior oblique underaction* is now termed as *under-depresson in adduction* (UDA). It can be:
- Primary UDA, or
- Secondary UDA.

2. *Paretic vertical deviations*
- Congenital unilateral superior oblique paresis.
- Non-congenital superior oblique paresis.
- Bilateral superior oblique paresis.
- Monocular elevation deficiency (MED), (old name: Double elevator palsy).
- Monocular depression deficiency (MDD); (old name: Double depressor palsy).
- Superior rectus paresis (isolated).
- Inferior rectus paresis (isolated).
- Skew deviation.
- Inferior oblique paresis

3. *Restrictive vertical deviations*
A. *Restrictive vertical deviations due to misdirected muscle force*, as seen in:

i. Congenital cranial dysinnervation disorders (CCDDs) primarily affecting vertical ocular motility.
  - Congenital fibrosis of extraocular muscles (CFEOMs)

ii. Iatrogenic displacement of inferior oblique muscle after its anteriorization.

B. *Restrictive vertical deviation due to mechanical restrictions* as seen in:

i. *Tight extraocular muscles,* e.g.
  - Congenital Brown's syndrome (new name restrictive hypotropia in adduction, i.e. RHA).
  - Hypotropia due to incarceration of inferior rectus in blow-out fracture of orbital floor.
  - Hypotropia due to inferior rectus thickening in thyroid ophthalmopathy.
  - Hypotropia in monocular elevation deficiency (MED) caused by fibrotic inferior rectus muscle.

ii. *Restrictive vertical deviation due to structural adhesions* (induced adhesive syndromes), e.g.:
  - Acquired Brown's syndrome due to scarring around the trochlea.

- Due to fat adherence as seen after retinal detachment surgery.
- Post-radiation orbital scarring.
- Due to conjunctival and Tenon's capsule scarring:
  - Postoperative
  - Post-traumatic
  - Post-chemical burns

iii. *Restrictive vertical deviation due to orbital mass lesions*, e.g. as in:

- Orbital tumours
- Glaucoma explant with large bleb causing mass effect.

Note. Incomitant vertical deviations caused by overaction of superior and inferior oblique muscles are discussed here.

Incomitant vertical deviations caused by weakness, paralysis or restriction of the cyclovertical muscles are discussed in Chapter 12.

■ APPARANT OBLIQUE MUSCLE DYSFUNCTION

INFERIOR OBLIQUE OVERACTION

Inferior oblique muscle overaction, also referred to as *strabismus sursoadductorious*, is now termed as *over-elevation in adduction* (OEA). It is characterized by an upshoot of the eye in adduction.

Etiology

1. *Primary overaction of the inferior oblique muscle* is etiologically not well understood. Perhaps it may be due to mechanical or innervational causes or a combination of the two. It may occur as an isolated phenomenon or in association with esotropia or exotropia-often of V-pattern.

2. *Secondary overaction of the inferior oblique muscle* is caused by paralysis or paresis of either its antagonist muscle (ipsilateral superior oblique muscle) or its yoke muscle (contralateral superior rectus muscle). Another cause of secondary overaction of the inferior oblique, unrelated to paralysis is non-parallelism of the plane of superior and inferior oblique muscles. (The term desagittalization has been suggested to describe this dysfunction.)

Clinical features

Clinical features of primary inferior oblique overaction (PIOO) versus secondary inferior oblique overaction (SIOO) are as follows:

1. Age of onset. PIOO usually occurs after one year of age, while SIOO can occur at any age. SIOO occurs either spontaneously or few weeks to months following paresis of the ipsilateral superior oblique muscle or contralateral superior rectus muscle.

2. Bilaterality. PIOO is frequently bilateral (72%) and often asymmetric while SIOO is occasionally bilateral.

3. Upshoot or over-elevation of the eye in adduction is the clinical characteristic of primary as well as secondary inferior oblique overaction. That is, with the eyes in lateral gaze and the abducting eye fixing, the adducted eye is over elevated. When the eyes are in lateral gaze and the adducting eye is made to fix, the abducted eye will be depressed and manifest a hypotropia on alternate cover testing. (c.f. DVD page 267). Clinically, the upshoot of the eye can be graded on a scale of +1 to +4 (page 115). In a +4 overaction, the cornea nearly disappears (Fig. 11.1).

4. Associated horizontal deviation in primary position. PIOO is commonly (but not universally) associated with some horizontal deviation such as infantile esotropia (72%), accommodative esotropia (34%) and intermittent exotropia (32%). The associated horizontal deviation is usually of V-pattern. It may be a part of infantile esotropia syndrome (page 218). In contradiction to it, SIOO is usually not associated with any form of concomitant deviation.

5. Associated vertical deviation in primary position is either absent or less than 5PD in PIOO. While a vertical deviation of 10–22PD is characteristic of SIOO, a vertical deviation of more than 22PD usually suggests a coexisting vertical rectus muscle weakness. Bilateral inferior oblique overaction produces a left hypertropia in right gaze, a right hypertropia in left gaze and little or no vertical deviation in primary position. Further, primary IOOA is commonly associated with DVD also.

6. Head tilt is typically present in patients with SIOO, when the onset is after 6 years of age, while it is usually absent in patients with PIOO. Distinguishing PIOOA from SIOOA is largely dependent on the head tilt test. If the head tilt test is negative this indicates a PIOOA, whereas a positive head tilt test (increasing hypertropia with tilt to the side of IOOA) indicates a superior oblique paresis or secondary inferior oblique overaction.

7. Associated excyclodeviation. Objective excyclodeviation, as evidenced by a disturbed relationship of the optic disc with foveola (normally the foveola is aligned approximately with the junction of the middle and lower third of disc), can be demonstrated both in patients

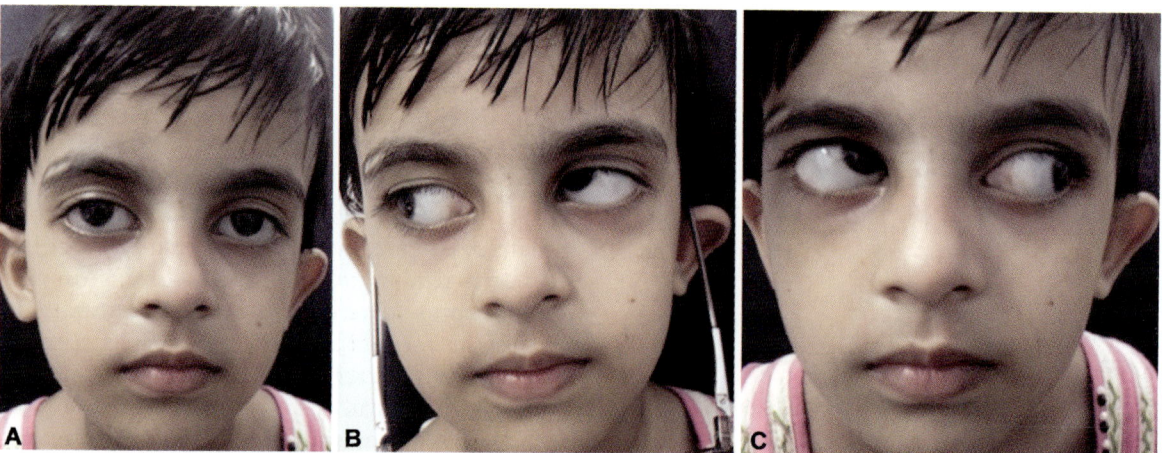

Fig. 11.1 *A patient with bilateral primary inferior oblique overaction.* A, *no vertical deviation in primary position;* B, *+4 inferior oblique overaction in left eye on dextroversion; and* C, *+4 inferior oblique overaction in right eye on levoversion.*

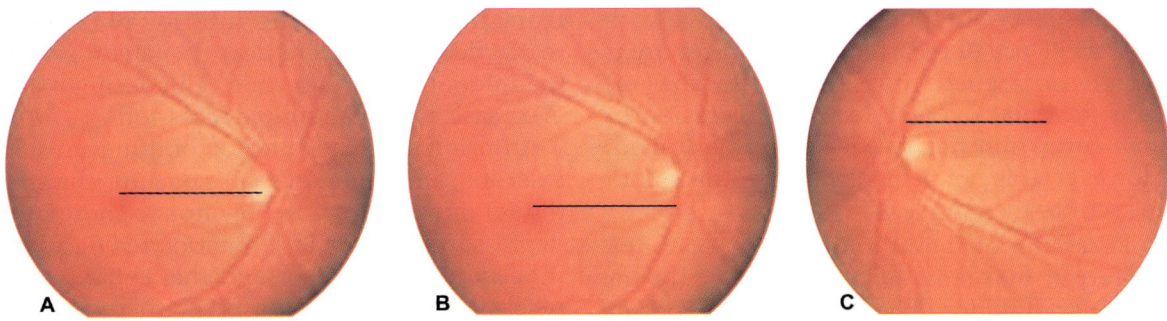

Fig. 11.2 *Fundus photograph showing relation of optic disc with foveola in a normal subject* (A) *and in a patient with inferior oblique overaction* (B) *direct view;* (C) *indirect ophthalmoscopic view.*

with primary as well as secondary inferior oblique muscle overaction (Fig. 11.2). However, *subjective excyclodeviation* (as demonstrated by double Maddox rod test, Hess screen test, the major amblyoscope or the Lancaster red-green test) is typically present in patients with SIOO (and extorsion is maximum in downgaze), when the onset is after 6 years of age, but is absent in patients with PIOO. Absence of subjective excyclodeviation in PIOO might be due to the development of some sensory adaptation in such patients owing to early onset of the condition.

8. *Forced duction test* is usually positive in primary as well as secondary inferior oblique overaction, indicating there by that both mechanical and innervational factors contribute to most inferior oblique overaction, including primary form.

Differential diagnosis

1. *Dissociated vertical deviation.* Inferior oblique overaction should be differentiated from dissociated vertical deviation (see pages 218 and 219).

2. *SIOOA.* Primary inferior oblique overaction can be differentiated from the secondary inferior oblique overaction as described in clinical features.

3. *Pseudo 'V' pattern* due to DVD, Duanes syndrome and large intermittent exotropia also needs to be differentiated from PIOOA.

Treatment

When hyperdeviation of the adducted eye becomes clinically significant, a weakening procedure on the inferior oblique muscle is indicated. Mostly, surgery is done for the functional reasons, that is, when the hypertropia produced by the overacting inferior oblique muscle presents an obstacle to fusion in lateral gaze or a V-pattern exists that prevents fusion in upward (V-exotropia) or downward (V-esotropia) gaze.

Inferior oblique weakening procedures that have been employed are as follows:

1. *Disinsertion,* i.e. cutting of the muscle from the globe near its insertion is an effective and easy technique. However, because of the unpredictable results and high rate of recurrences (>50%), this procedure is not much popular.

2. *Myectomy* involves excision of approximately 8 mm of inferior oblique muscle. This procedure is generally performed between the temporal border of inferior rectus muscle and insertion of the inferior oblique. It can also be performed nasally between the origin of inferior oblique and the nasal border of inferior rectus muscle. This procedure is also becoming unpopular because of unpredictable results, a high rate of recurrences (especially nasally performed myectomy) and occurrence of postoperative adhesive syndrome in some cases. However, temporally performed myectomy is still preferred by many surgeons especially for treating recurrent inferior oblique overaction. A unilateral myectomy will correct 5 to 20 PD of hypertropia.

3. *Denervation and extirpation,* i.e. excision of whole of the muscle with its Tenon's capsule covering after cauterisation of the neurovascular bundle has been reported to be effective with least incidence of recurrence. The procedure is reported to be effective in severe overaction (+4) or in residual overaction when recession or anteriorization has already been perfomed. However, it is not being considered necessary to sacrifice the muscle.

4. *Recession* of the inferior oblique is being preferred by many surgeons especially for secondary inferior oblique overaction and for cases with mild to moderate primary inferior oblique overaction. Recession of 6–10 mm can be performed as indicated. In this procedure, inferior oblique is detached from its insertion and is reattached to the sclera (along the lateral margin of the inferior rectus) at a site selected depending upon the amount of recession to be done. For example:

- *For a maximum recession of 12–14 mm,* anterior border of inferior oblique muscle is placed 4 mm behind the insertion line of inferior rectus muscle.
- *For 10 mm recession,* the anterior suture is placed 6 mm posterior to the lateral border of the inferior rectus muscle insertion and 4 mm temporal to the lateral border of the inferior rectus (approximately at the vortex vein), in this there occurs anteriorization of IO by 1–1.5 mm, that is why based on long-term follow ups it is said to be more powerful than 12–14 mm recession.

A recurrence rate to the tune of 15% is reported with simple recession. *The major advantage of the recession* is that it allows the weakening procedure to be titrated according to the severity of inferior oblique overaction as below:

- *For 1+ or 2+ overaction,* the inferior oblique muscle is recessed by 12–14 mm.
- *For 3+ overaction,* inferior oblique muscle is recessed by 10 mm.
- *For 4+ overaction,* 10 mm recession or full anterior transposition of IO is preferred.

5. *Recession with anterior transposition* is being considered more effective than simple recession. Therefore, it is recommended that this procedure may be preferable for large over-actions, particulary those associated with V-pattern due to primary inferior oblique overaction. In this procedure, after detaching

from the insertion, the inferior oblique is reattached to the sclera near the lateral end of the inferior rectus insertion. This technique is even easier than the simple recession.

Anteriorizing the inferior oblique muscle insertion, anterior to eyeball's equator changes the IO muscle from an elevator to more of a depressor. The more IO is anteriorized the more it becomes a depressor and this enhances its recession effect. Compared with recession, anteriorization decreases ocular elevation by approximately 15 PD more.

Graded IO anteriorization (as described below) works extremely well for both PIOOA and SIOOA:

- *+4 overaction:* Full anteriorization, up to the insertion line of temporal border of inferior rectus.
- *+3 overaction:* 1 mm posterior to IR insertion line
- *+2 overaction:* 3 to 4 mm posterior to IR insertion
- *+1 overaction:* 4 mm posterior and 1 mm lateral to IR insertion.

It is important to note that full anteriorization of the IO can be performed with a 'J' deformity of the new insertion, which can limit ocular elevation and produce a postoperative hypotropia worse in upgaze. The 'J' deformity is created when the posterior fibres of IO are anteriorized parallel or in front of inferior rectus insertion. This is seen mainly with U/L anterior transposition, so should be reserved for patients with appreciable hypertropia in upgaze or patients with superior oblique paresis with hypertropia >25 PD.

An anterior and nasal transposition procedure converts inferior oblique from an extorter to intorter and from an elevator to depressor, significantly improving large 'V' patterns.

Note. For surgical techniques of IO recession, *see* page 431.

Some observations about inferior oblique weakening

1. *Bilateral asymmetry.* If there is no superior oblique muscle paresis but there is a marked asymmetry of the overactions of the inferior oblique muscles, unilateral surgery on the muscle with the most marked overaction will often be followed by a significant degree of overaction in the unoperated eye. Therefore, bilateral inferior oblique weakening procedures are indicated for bilateral overaction, even if asymmetrical. However, inferior oblique muscles that are not overacting should not have a surgical weakening procedure. Further, recession of the inferior oblique can be graded depending upon the asymmetry.

2. Graded response. The response to any surgical weakening procedure on the inferior oblique is graded one, i.e. the larger overactions will show a greater response to the same amount of surgery.

3. Effect on associated horizontal deviation. When PIOO is associated with the V-pattern horizontal deviation, weakening of the one or even both inferior oblique muscles has little to no effect on the horizontal alignment in the primary position. Therefore, there is no need to make any adjustment in the amount of horizontal rectus surgery. Further, the weakening of the inferior oblique should be performed along with the horizontal muscle surgery and that there is no need to do two separate procedures. It has been observed that unilateral weakening of overacting inferior oblique in V-pattern strabismus can be expected to cause 5–10 prism dioptres and bilateral weakening 15–25 prism dioptres of eso shift in upgaze (decrease of an exodeviation or increase of an esodeviation) but almost little or no effect in primary gaze and downgaze.

4. Effect on associated vertical deviation. In cases with overaction of inferior oblique, secondary to paresis of ipsilateral superior oblique muscle, a weakening of that inferior oblique muscle could be expected to correct up to 15 prism dioptres of vertical deviation in primary position. The amount of vertical correction is roughly proportional to the degree of preoperative overaction. If the deviation is more than 15 PD, then additionally, the yoke contralateral inferior rectus should also be recessed (1 mm for every 3 PD deviation).

However, in cases with primary inferior oblique overaction neither unilateral nor bilateral weakening of this muscle has any significant effect on the vertical deviation in primary position.

5. Associated dissociated vertical deviation. When DVD is associated with inferior oblique overaction, the procedure inferior oblique recession with anterior transposition should be done. Since in most cases, this procedure alone can correct DVD, so any other surgical treatment for DVD should be deferred until later.

6. Effect on head tilt test and excyclodeviation. Weakening of inferior oblique in primary overaction does not produce a positive head-tilt test or any effect on subjective cyclodeviation. However, the objective excyclodeviation (as evidenced by indirect ophthalmoscopy) is either fully corrected or greatly reduced.

7. Recurrence of overaction is a common complication after weakening procedure. Its likelihood with a particular procedure in order of increasing frequency is as follows: Extirpation (least common), recession with anterior transposition, simple recession (15%), temporally performed myectomy, disinsertion, and nasally performed myectomy (33%).

SUPERIOR OBLIQUE OVERACTION

Superior oblique overaction, also referred to as *strabismus deorsoadductorius*, is now termed as *overdepression in adduction* (ODA). It is characterized by a downshoot of the eye in adduction.

Etiology

1. Primary overaction of the superior oblique muscle is of unknown etiology. Perhaps it may be due to mechanical or innervational causes or a combination of the two. It may occur as an isolated phenomenon or in association with exotropia or esotropia—often of A-pattern.

2. Secondary overaction of the superior oblique muscle is caused by a paralysis or paresis of either its antagonist muscle (ipsilateral inferior oblique muscle) or its yoke muscle (contralateral inferior rectus muscle). Rarely, it can also occur in cases with contracture of the contralateral superior rectus muscle, occasionally seen in conjunction with long-standing paralysis of the contralateral superior oblique muscle. Other causes of secondary overaction of the superior oblique, unrelated to paralysis are, Brown's syndrome and Duane's syndrome with co-contraction of the horizontal rectus muscles.

Clinical features

It is important to note that unlike superior oblique muscle, isolated palsy of inferior oblique is not much known and so is the secondary overaction of the superior oblique muscle. So much so that all bilateral superior oblique muscle overaction can be considered 'primary'. Anyhow, clinical features of primary superior oblique overaction (PSOO) versus secondary superior oblique overaction (SSOO) are as follows:

1. *Age of onset.* PSOO usually occurs by the age of 2–3 years while SSOO can occur at any age. SSOO occurs either spontaneously or few weeks to months following paresis of the ipsilateral inferior oblique muscle or contralateral inferior rectus muscle.

2. *Bilaterality.* PSOO is frequently bilateral although it can be asymmetric or rarely unilateral; while SSOO is occasionally bilateral.

3. *Downshoot of the eye in adduction* is the clinical characteristic of primary as well as secondary superior oblique overaction. That is with the eyes in lateral gaze and the abducting eye fixing the adducted eye downshoots or an exaggerated rotation of the eye occurs in the field of action of the superior oblique, i.e. the eye is over-depressed in adduction. Where the eyes are in lateral gaze and the adducting eye is made to fix, the abducted eye will be elevated and manifest as hypertropia on alternate cover test. Clinically, overaction of superior oblique can be graded on a scale of +1 to +4. In a +4 overaction, the cornea is directed straight down rather than down and in (Fig. 11.3).

4. *Associated horizontal deviation in primary position.* PSOO is commonly associated with either comitant exotropia (more common) or esotropia, usually of A-pattern (<10 PD in unilateral and >20 PD in bilateral SOOA). By contrast, SSOO is usually not associated with any form of concomitant deviation.

5. *Associated vertical deviation in primary position* is usually absent in PSOO. While vertical deviation (hypotropia) is characteristic of SSOO. Bilateral SOOA is associated with a small or no hypotropia in primary position, since the bilateral vertical deviations cancel each

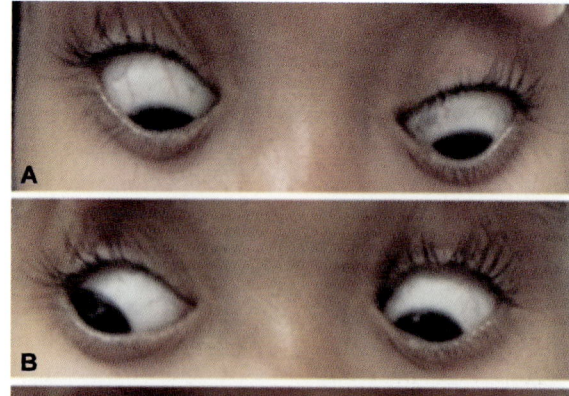

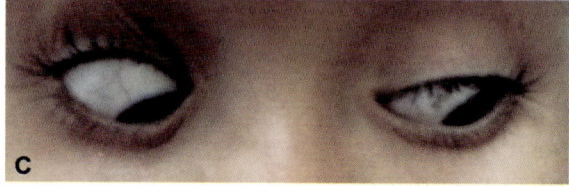

Fig. 11.3 *A patient with +4 overaction of superior oblique muscles.* A, *central downgaze;* B, *dextrodepression and;* C, *levodepression.*

other. However, reversing hypotropias in side gaze are typical, with a right hypotropia in left gaze and a left hypotropia in right gaze.

6. *Head tilt* in the direction of action of paralysed inferior oblique is typically present in patients with SSOO, when the onset is after 6 years of age (after visual maturity); while it is usually absent in patients with PSOO. Head tilting will not cause any difference in the amount of deviation in primary SOOA.

7. *Associated incyclodeviations.* Objective incyclodeviation, as evidenced by a disturbed relationship of the optic disc with foveola, can be demonstrated in both patients with primary as well as secondary superior oblique over-action. However, subjective incyclodeviation (as demostrated by double Maddox rod test, Hess screen test, the major amblyoscope or the Lancaster red-green test) is typically present in patients with SSOO, when the onset is after 6 years of age, but is absent in patients with PSOO.

8. *Forced duction test* is usually positive in both primary as well as secondary superior oblique overaction. An 'edge' of resistance is felt as the eye is passively rotated with forceps up and in (into the field of antagonist inferior oblique).

Differential diagnosis

1. *Brown syndrome* can be differentiated from primary SOOA, on a clinical basis as below:

- An ability to elevate the paretic eye in adduction effectively rules out Brown syndrome.
- In contrast to SOOA where hypotropia is maximum in downgaze, Brown syndrome is associated with a restriction of elevation thus causing a hypotropia that is greatest in upgaze.
- 'A' pattern in SOOA, while there is 'V' pattern in Brown syndrome. FDT +ve in Brown syndrome.

2. *Inferior oblique paresis.* There is ipsilateral SSOOA in which unlike PSOOA, there is positive head tilt test, hypotropia is greatest when patient looks up and in. The deviation worses in the gaze away from paretic eye. In IO palsy, the deviation worses with tilt toward the paretic eye because intorsion is impaired.

Treatment

In a patient with clinically significant ocular deviation or A-pattern associated with bilateral superior oblique overaction, a bilateral superior oblique weakening procedure is indicated, which can be accomplished as follows:

1. *Superior oblique tenotomy and tenectomy*: It is indicated for treating 'A' pattern strabismus and can correct 20 PD or more of A-pattern in the primary position and up to 45 PD in downgaze. The amount of correction achieved depends mostly on the size of preoperative pattern and the amount of SOOA. This can be done either nasally or temporally to the superior rectus muscle. Effectivity of superior oblique tenotomy increases, if performed closer to the trochlea; therefore, nasally performed operation gives more effect. This usually causes post-operative SO palsy and tortional diplopia in patients with fusion.

2. *Posterior tenectomy of superior oblique (PTSO)*: The anterior fibres of SO tendon are responsible for torsion, whereas the posterior fibres are implicated in downward rotation and abduction. This procedure is preferred over tenotomy in patients with bifoveal fusion because negligible extorsion is induced. This surgery can correct moderate A-pattern up to 20 PD with SOOA.

3. *Superior oblique lengthening by insertion of a silicone expander* or a non-absorbable suture is also an effective procedure. In fact several surgeons have proposed more controlled weakening by this procedure (rather than tenotomy) in patients with bifixation and normal stereopsis to eliminate the complications like torsional diplopia or symptoms of secondary superior oblique palsy with head tilt observed with simple tenotomy.

The weakening effect is graded by varying the length of the silicone that bridges the gap between the cut ends of the tendons. The spacer lengthens the tendon without altering the muscle mechanics at its insertion. This corrects 'A' pattern from 20 to 55 PD and also the SOOA associated with skew deviation.

Recommended length of spacer according to the magnitude of SOOA is as below.

- *+1 overaction:* 4 mm
- *+2 overaction:* 5 mm
- *+3 overaction:* 6 mm
- *+4 overaction:* 7 mm

Note. For surgical techniques of SO weakening, *see* page 433.

Some observations about superior oblique weakening

1. *Graded response.* The response to superior oblique tenotomy is graded one, i.e. the larger overaction will show a greater response to the same amount of surgery.

2. *Effect on associated horizontal deviation.* It has been observed by several surgeons that superior oblique tenotomy decreases the exotropia and increases the esotropia as shown in Table 11.1.

Since superior oblique tenotomy also influences the deviation in primary gaze; therefore, by experience, the surgeons must make adjustment for horizontal rectus muscle surgery when being contemplated simulta-neously. Alternatively, the tenotomies may be performed first and the horizontal muscle surgery can be taken later on. Of course, this will require two general anaesthesias.

Table 11.1 *Effect of superior oblique tenotomy on the associated horizontal deviation*

Procedure	Decrease in exotropia or increase in esotropia in prism dioptres		
	Upgaze	Primary gaze	Down-gaze
Unilateral tenotomy	None	8–10	20–25
Bilateral tenotomy	None	15	up to 70

3. *Effect on associated vertical deviation.* Secondary superior oblique overaction is almost always associated with vertical deviation in primary gaze and in its field of action. Superior oblique tenotomy is expected to correct almost full vertical deviation in the field of action of the muscle and of up to 15 PD in the primary gaze.

4. *Tortional diplopia, a positive head-tilt test and abnormal head posture* have been reported following bilateral superior oblique tenotomies performed for secondary superior oblique overaction in adults with a potential for single binocular vision. However, such problems are of no concern, if there is no potential for single binocular vision.

DISSOCIATED VERTICAL DEVIATIONS

Dissociated vertical deviation (DVD) is a comparatively ill-understood form of strabismus. That is why, it has been described under different names by the different workers. A few of the other names by which this condition has been described are: Alternating sursumduction, alternating hyperphoria, alternating hypertropia, alternating sursumvergence, occlusion hyperphoria, occlusion hypertropia, double hypertropia, dissociated vertical divergence, dissociated hyperdeviation and so on.

Dissociated vertical deviations are basically characterized by a hyperdeviation in one eye that is present while the other eye is fixing. The non-fixing eye is also extorted and slightly abducted. Thus, dissociated vertical devation (DVD) can be defined as an intermittent anomaly of the non-fixing eye consisting of upward excursion, excyclotorsion and lateral deviation.

The term dissociated vertical deviation is preferred because in it the two eyes are more independent of each other (dissociated movements) and do not follow the Hering's law of ocular motility, i.e. in contrast to a true vertical deviation, in DVD, the fellow eye does not exhibit refixation movement in the opposite direction.

Since the upward drifting of the non-fixing eye is often associated with lateral deviation and excyclotorsion, the term '*Dissociated strabismus Complex (DSC)*', has been suggested to denote all the components, i.e. dissociated vertical deviation (DVD), dissociated horizontal deviation (DHD) and dissociated torsional deviation (DTD).

ETIOLOGY

Exact etiology of the DVD is not known. Numerous theories have been put forward to explain the occurrence of DVD. A few such theories are mentioned below:

1. *Bielschowsky's theory of positive and negative subcortical vertical divergence centres.* Bielschowsky theorized that DVD occurs due to alternating and intermittent excitation of both subcortical vertical divergence centres. However, this theory has not been further substantiated.

2. *Theory of imbalance of binocular stimulation.* Spielmann postulated that DVD is caused by an imbalance of binocular stimulation. This theory explains the frequent occurrence of DVD in essential infantile esotropia and the occasional occurrence with sensory heterotropia. However, this theory does not explain the occurrence of DVD in patients with otherwise normal binocular functions.

3. *Brodsky theory.* According to this theory, DVD is a vestigial remnant of the dorsal light reflex of lower animals.

4. *Other theories* which have been put forward include:

• Theory of bilateral paralysis of the depressor muscles.

• Theory of defective mid-brain stimuli.

• Theory of two monocular conjugate mechanisms plus a binocular mechanism.

- Theory of defective monocular nasal retinal quadrant stimuli.
- Guyton's theory.

Thus many theories have been proposed to explain occurrence of DVD. However, findings of most of the theories could not be reproduced. Therefore, the exact etiology is still illusive. The lack of precise aetiologic information is further reflected by the plethora of terms which have been mentioned above to denote this condition.

CLINICAL FEATURES

1. Deviation. DVD is characterized by spontaneous occurrence of vertical deviation in either eye, when the patient is fatigued, or day dreaming (*manifest DVD*) or when fusion is interrupted by artificial means (*latent DVD*) (Fig.11.4). DVD is characterised by a slow upward drifting of the non-fixing eye. The vertically deviated eye is also extorted and slightly abducted.

2. Associations of DVD: DVD may also occur as an isolated phenomenon in patients with apparently normal binocular function. In general DVD may be associated with any congenital or acquired strabismus with motor fusion deficiency. Its common associations include:

Infantile esotropia is associated with DVD in over 75% cases. However, inspite of careful search, the condition is rarely diagnosed in infancy. It is usually diagnosed between 2 to 5 years of age. Mostly it becomes evident after the surgical alignment for horizontal squint has been done.

Infantile exotropia is also commonly associated with DVD. It has been described to occur as a part of a syndrome consisting of an A-pattern exotropia with overaction of the superior obliques and underaction of the inferior obliques (Fig. 11.5).

Excycloduction and latent nystagmus are frequently associated with DVD.

3. Head posture. Approximately, one-third of patients with DVD have a spontaneous abnormal head posture.

4. Laterality. DVD is frequently bilateral (alternating sursumduction) usually assymetric. Rarely it may be monocular.

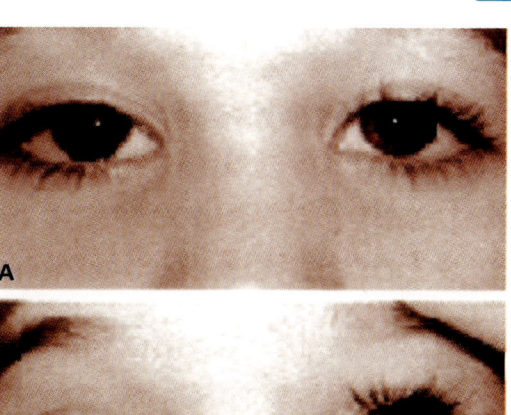
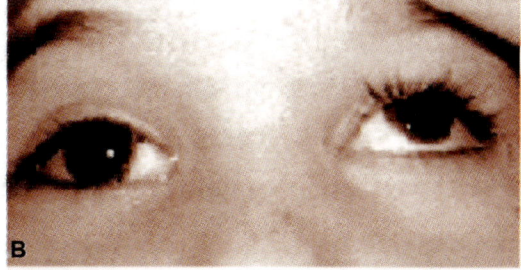
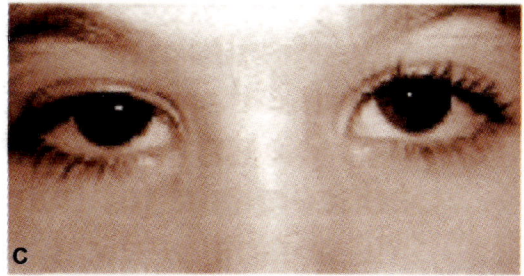
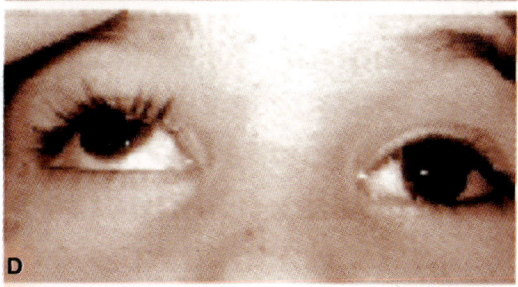
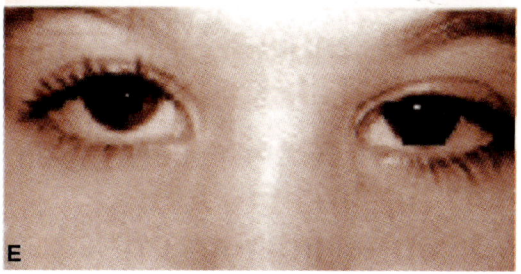

Fig. 11.4 *Dissociated vertical deviation. A, no initial deviation; B, left hypertropia with right eye fixing immediately after removal of the cover from the left eye; C, the left eye is drifting down; D, right hypertropia with left eye fixing immediately after removal of the cover from the right eye; E, right eye is drifting back to its original position.*

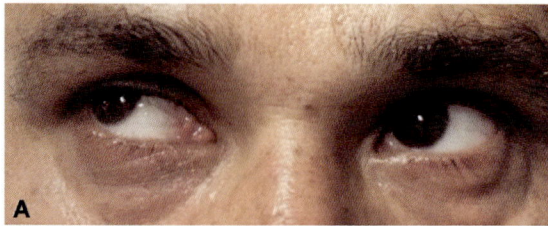

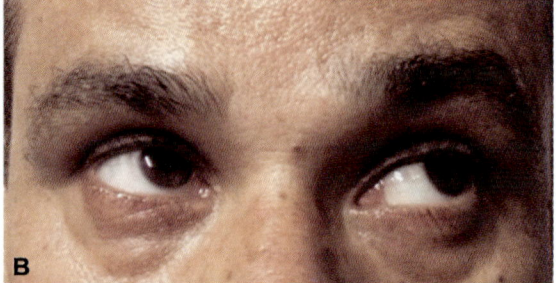

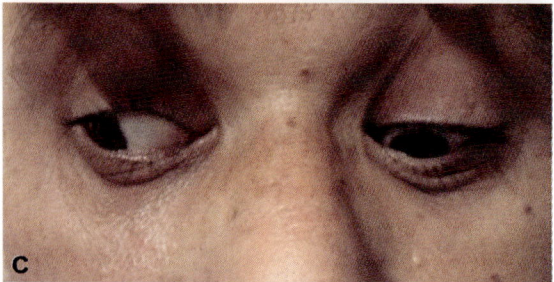

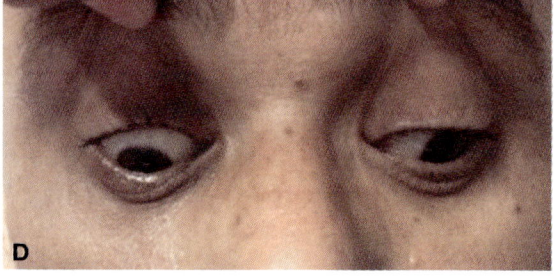

Fig. 11.5 *Dissociated vertical deviation with associated underaction of both inferior obliques (A and B) and overaction of both superior obliques (C and D).*

Monocular dissociated hyperdeviation may be seen in the presence of an intermittent exotropia. It is frequently found that when fusion is broken and the eye is deviated, the deviated eye develops a small hyperdeviation. This deviation is not associated with underaction of yoke muscles and is not present, when the deviated eye is not in abduction. It generally disappears following horizontal surgical correction.

Bilateral DVD or alternating sursumduction is a situation in which either eye elevates under cover

(double hyperdeviation). Not only does elevation takes place, but each eye tends to extort on occlusion and slowly depress and intort, when occlusion is removed. This deviation appears to be related to retinal illumination. It is important to note that in DVD when the hypertropic eye fixates, there is no corres-ponding hypotropia of the fellow eye (i.e. the eyes do not follow Hering's law of equal innervation). While in hypertropia, when the hypertropic eye fixates a target, the other eye moves downwards into a hypotropic position of equal magnitude.

Symmetric versus asymmetric DVD. Bilateral DVD may be symmetric or asymmetric. Degree of asymmetry of dissociated strabismus is determined by the magnitude of the deviation in primary position compared between the two eyes.

5. Comitance. DVD may be comitant or incomitant. The difference in the deviation of non-fixing eye between the primary and in all other gaze positions determines the degree of incomitance.

Comitant DVD. DVD that measures roughly the same (within ±7 PD) in primary position, adduction and abduction is called commitant DVD. This is the most common presentation.

Incomitant DVD refers to measurable disparity in the magnitude of DVD (>7 PD) between the primary position, abduction, and adduction. Incomitant DVD is usually associated with muscle dysfunction as below:

1. *DVD larger in the field of inferior oblique* of the non-fixing eye is characterized by following features:
   - *In primary position,* only DVD is seen.
   - *In adduction*, both true hypertropia and DVD are present.
   - *In abduction,* DVD is <5 PD.
   - *'V' pattern horizontal* deviation may be observed.

2. *DVD larger in adducted position* only, but DVD in abduction is >5 PD.

3. *DVD more in abduction* due to associated SOOA and 'A' pattern. As in the adducted position, SOOA causes more depression than the elevation occurring due to DVD so DVD increases in the abducted position.

Superior rectus contracture syndrome in DVD. Cases with marked asymmetric DVD, especially those with reduced visual acuity in one eye, can coexist with a superior rectus overaction/contracture syndrome in the non-fixing eye. In these cases, DVD is usually markedly decompensated and there occurs almost a permanent elevated position of the non-fixing eye which leads to shortening and contracture of the superior rectus. The presence of a co-existing superior rectus contracture syndrome in patients with marked asymmetric DVD should be suspected when the following clinical characteristics are present:

- *Hypertropia in the non-dominant eye* in all upgaze positions that is larger in supra-abduction.
- *Manifest hypertropia* in the non-dominant eye in primary position.
- *Positive Beilschowsky head tilt* test towards the affected side.
- *Hypertropia of the normal eye* when the non-dominant eye is fixing.
- *Larger hypertropia* when the non-dominant eye is rotated down and out.

Note. Patients with superior rectus contracture syndrome and DVD might need very large recessions of the superior rectus (up to 14 mm). It can be done in both eyes when symmetric DVD is seen but mostly asymmetric SR recession is required.

6. Binocular vision and sensory adaptations

- *Suppression* usually develops in patients with spontaneous DVD and thus eliminates diplopia.
- *Peripheral fusion* is often present in patients with DVD having a manifest deviation of 4D or less.
- *An absolute facultative central scotoma* in one eye, while both eyes are being used together for peripheral vision, is present even in patients having a latent DVD.

Hypotropic DVD

Hypotropic DVD is a rare condition. It is mostly unilateral and commonly associated with monocular visual deficits or high myopia. Although the nature of this intermittent slow downward ocular deviation is similar to that of hypertropic DVD, it should be considered a unique form of the dissociated strabismus complex. The downward drifts are not associated with any torsional movements and no nystagmus is observed.

DIAGNOSIS

1. *Cover-uncover test*

- *In patients with unilateral manifest DVD*, when the fixating eye is covered, there will occur a downward movement of the uncovered eye (but there will be no corresponding hypotropia of the covered eye).
- *In patients with alternate DVD*, either eye elevates under cover (double hyperdeviation) while the uncovered eye will move down to take fixation.
- *In patients with latent DVD*, there occurs no movement of the uncovered eye, but the eye under cover is elevated and moves downwards after it is uncovered (i.e. DVD is present only when the eyes have been dissociated).

2. *Spielmann's translucent occluder test* is better than the simple cover-uncover test for DVD. In a patient with latent DVD, through the translucent occluder, the eyeball is seen to upshift and there occurs characteristic slow drifting recovery on removing the occluder (Figs 11.6A and B). While in hypertropia associated with inferior oblique overaction, there occurs a refixation movement which is a fast saccade.

3. *Head tilt test.* Most patients with DVD show an increase in the size of DVD on contralateral head tilt (e.g. DVD in right eye increases with left head tilt). However, a few patients show converse response.

4. *Red glass (filter) test.* Red glass (filter) dissociates the two eyes and the eye behind the filter drifts up in a patient with DVD and the patient appreciates diplopia with red image being lower. The fact that a patient will localize the red image below the fixation light, regardless of whether the red glass is held before the right or left eye, clearly differentiates a DVD from other forms of cyclovertical deviations in which the red image is localized below or above the fixation light, depending on which eye fixates.

5. *Demonstration of Bielschowsky phenomenon.* In this test, one eye is covered with Spielmann translucent occluder (and is elevated undercover) while the other eye fixates (Fig. 11.6A). Then a photometric graded density neutral filter bar is placed before the fixing eye. In patients with DVD, as the filter with gradually increasing density is moved in front of the fixing eye, the elevated eye under cover will start moving downwards (Fig. 11.6C) and may go even below the primary position. When the filter bar is moved from positions of greater to lesser density the eye behind the cover will again elevate (Fig. 11.6D). Since Bielschowsky was first to note this intriguing observation, hence it is known by his name.

6. *Measurement of DVD*

i. *Prism base-down under the occluder test* can be useful in measuring DVD. In this test, prisms with base-down are placed in front of the deviating eye under the occluder and patient is asked to focus on the fixation target at 6 m distance. The occluder is then quickly shifted to the fixating eye allowing the previously dissociated and elevated eye to take up fixation. The alternate cover test is continued and base-down prism is added until no downward movement of the deviating eye is observed on switching occlusion. In the case of bilateral DVD, each eye is tested separately.

Grading of DVD, based on the degree, is as below:

- 1+ DVD: A small deviation (up to 9 PD)
- 2+ DVD: A moderate deviation (10 to 19 PD)
- 3+ DVD: A large deviation (>20 PD)

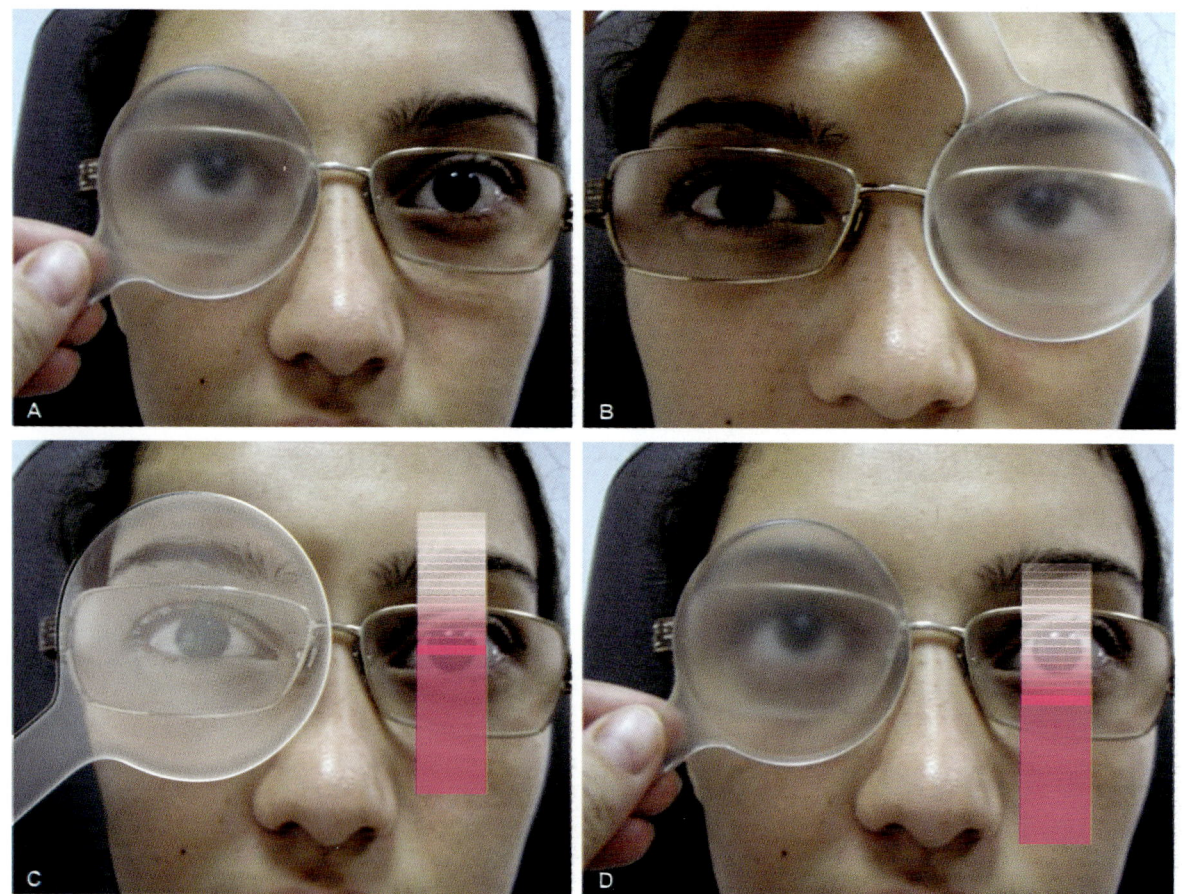

Fig. 11.6 *Detection of DVD using Spielmann's translucent occluder (A and B) and dimostration of Bielschowsky phenomenon (A, C and D).*

For a combined dissociated and a non-dissociated vertical deviation, i.e. in patients with DVD and true vertical deviation, measure the non-dissociated component by adding base-up prism over the non-DVD eye until the hypodeviation is neutralized during the alternate cover test. The next step is to measure the vertical deviation as previously described for dissociated vertical deviation. The actual dissociated vertical deviation measured is the difference between the two steps.

ii. *Modified form of Krimsky test* may be used to measure DVD in patients who cannot fix with deviating eye.

   For grading the full deviation on cover test, the occluder should be turned obliquely so that the eye remains occluded and at the same time examiner can look behind the occluder to grade deviation (Fig. 11.7). Alaternatively, a translucent occluder may be used to disrupt fusion while at the same time observing DVD undercover.

iii. An approximate grading of DVD may be done on cover test as follows:

• 1 + DVD: A small deviation
• 2 + DVD: A moderate deviation
• 3 + DVD: A large deviation

DIFFERENTIAL DIAGNOSIS

DVD must be differentiated from inferior oblique overaction as shown in Table 11.2.

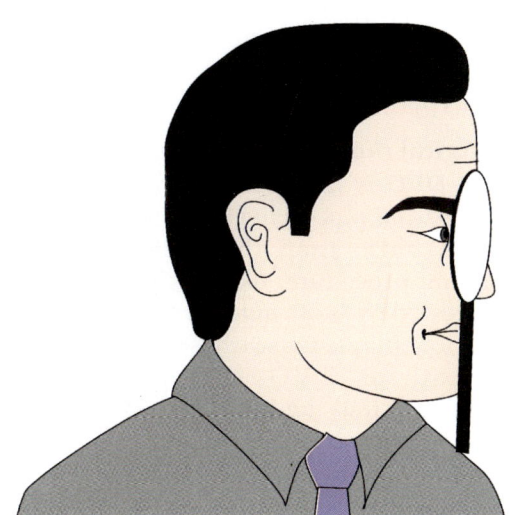

Fig. 11.7 *Technique of grading dissociated vertical deviation on cover test using occluder in tilted positon.*

Table.11.2 *Dissociated vertical deviation versus inferior oblique overaction*

Sr. no.	Feature	Dissociated vertical deviation	Inferior oblique over-action
1.	Hyper-deviation	Present in primary position in adduction and in abduction	Maximum in adduction, never in abduction
2.	Incyclo-duction on refixation	Present	Absent
3.	Speed of up-ward movement in deviating eye during refixation with non-deviating eye	Slow (2–200°/sec)	Rapid (200–400°/sec)
4.	Bielschowsky phenomenon	Present	Absent
5.	V-pattern	Absent	Present
6.	Superior oblique action	May overact	Usually underaction
7.	Pseudoparesis of contra-lateral superior rectus	Absent	Present
8.	Latent nystagmus	Often present	Absent
9.	External rotation of fundus on indirect ophthalmo-scopy (shown by an altered relation between fove-ola and optic disc)	Absent	Present

TREATMENT

A. *Non-surgical treatment* is not so effective in DVD. However, following measures may be useful:

I. *Conservative therapy to strengthen the fusional mechanisms* should be provided as below:

• *Optimal spectacle correction* should be prescribed. As the blurred vision may cause a latent DVD to become a manifest more frequently providing a clear images to both eyes encourages fusion

- *Correcting an associated horizontal deviation* either surgically or with prisms, promotes the possibility of peripheral fusion.
- *Treating amblyopia* by occlusion therapy also promotes peripheral fusion
- *Treating heterophorias* by orthoptics also promotes peripheral fusion.

II. *Conservative therapy in the form of changing the fixation pattern* by patching or optical means may be useful, especially in patients with asymmetric involvement or those accustomed to wearing glasses. For example, if a patient is having significant DVD of left eye while fixing with right eye and an insignificant DVD of right eye while fixing with left eye; a slight optical blurr induced in the right eye by addition of +2.0D lens will shift the fixation preference to the left and DVD may no longer be a cosmetic problem.

B. *Surgical treatment* is indicated, when DVD causes a significant cosmetic problem, i.e.:

- When large DVD manifests frequently or
- Anomalous head posture in present to control the DVD.

However, before contemplating surgery, it is important to differentiate DVD from over-action of the inferior oblique muscle (Table 11.2), since the surgical approach to these two conditions is different.

Note. Further, it should also be borne in mind that even the surgical treatment is also palliative, since currently no such surgical procedure is available that will completely cure this disorder.

Following surgical procedures have been tried by different workers:

I. Surgical procedures for comitant DVD

1. *Faden operation with superior rectus recession.* In this procedure, a 3–5 mm recession of the superior rectus muscle is combined with anchoring this muscle to the globe with a non-absorbable suture 12–15 mm posterior to its insertion (posterior fixation suture, or retroequatorial myopexy, or Faden operation). This procedure is more effective than SR recession alone, but recurrence occurring as late

as several years after an initial satisfactory result are reported by many workers. Botulinum toxin A injection into SR has been suggested as an alternative.

2. *Large recession of superior rectus muscle.* Unconventionally, large recession (7 to 10 mm) of superior rectus muscle has been suggested as effective treatment for DVD. Bilateral recession is indicated in bilateral cases of DVD. The asymmetric amount of surgery may be performed in the two eyes, when the deviation is asymmetric. Graded recessions, recommended based on the degree of DVD, are as below:

- *Grade I (up to 9 PD):* 5–7 mm
- *Grade II (10–19 PD):* 7–9 mm
- *Grade III (>20 PD):* 9–14 mm.

3. *Resection of the inferior rectus muscle* has also been suggested by some workers. Preferably, this procedure should be performed, if recurrences occur even after the large recession of superior rectus muscle. Recommended amount of resection of the inferior rectus muscle for DVD is 4 mm for small deviation, 6 mm for intermediate deviation and 8 mm for large angles. Resection of inferior rectus muscle may also elevate the lower eyelid.

4. *Recess-resect procedure.* A 4–5 mm recession of superior rectus muscle and 6 mm resection of inferior rectus muscle have also been recommended for treating large angle DVD. However, this procedure should be limited to those relatively infrequent patients who have a predominantly monocular vertical deviation with a hypertropia in primary position.

II. Surgical procedures for incomitant DVD

1. *When DVD is larger in the field of inferior oblique of the non-fixing eye, i.e in adducted position only,* then the inferior oblique weakening procedure, like IOAT is preferred. As suggested by Scott, anterior transposition of the inferior oblique muscle has been an effective treatment for DVD with IOOA. It is hypothesized that the IOAT procedure creates a vector for depression, and this antielevating force helps in controlling DVD. This procedure can create a limitation of elevation of the operated eye and may cause hypotropia in primary position when performed unilaterally.

It can also cause a restriction of elevation in abduction associated with Y or V pattern when performed bilaterally, particularly if the posterolateral fibres of the inferior oblique muscle are spread out laterally at the time of resuturing to the sclera. This complication was first called as *'antielevation syndrome'* (AES) by Kushner. IO transpostition more than 1 mm anterior to the inferior rectus muscle insertion as well as lateral spreading of the posterior fibres >2 mm at new insertion point are the risk factors to develop AES.

2. When DVD is larger in adducted position but significant in abduction (>5 PD) also. In these patients, both SR recession and IO weakening procedures are preferred.

3. When DVD is more in abduction due to associated SOOA and 'A' pattern, following procedures are required:

- *Bilateral SR recession* should be considered in patients with small degree of A pattern (up to 12 PD).
- *Additional SO weakening procedure* like posterior SO tenectomy is required with bilateral SR recession in patients with larger amounts of A-pattern (12–25 PD).

DISSOCIATED HORIZONTAL DEVIATION

Dissociated horizontal deviation (DHD) is defined as a change in the horizontal ocular alignment, unrelated to the accommodation, that is brought about solely by a change in the balance of visual input from the two eyes.

Characteristic features

- DHD usually manifests as spontaneous unilateral exodeviation or an exodeviation of greater magnitude in one eye during prism and alternate cover testing.
- Unlike in other forms of intermittent exotropia, the observed exodeviation is slow, variable and asymmetrical in the two eyes.

Assessment

- *To assess the horizontal dissociated deviation* (DHD), the same procedure as described for DVD is performed with base-in prism over the eye with DHD until no further inward movement of that eye is seen. Movement of the contralateral eye with this test can be ignored.
- *DHD may be distinguished from other horizontal strabismus* by lack of a corresponding exodeviation of the contralateral eye on alternate cover testing.

Treatment

DHD, depending upon the amount, is treated with LR recession of 3–8 mm on the affected side.

CYCLODEVIATIONS

Cyclodeviation (torsional strabismus) refers to a misalignment of the eyes around the antero-posterior axes.

CLASSIFICATION

A. Depending upon the constancy of deviation

1. Cyclophoria
2. Cyclotropia

Theoretically, the cyclodeviations have been classified into cyclophoria (latent cyclodeviation) and cyclotropia (manifest cyclodeviation); however, practically in most cases, no distinction can be made between a cyclophoria and a cyclotropia by means of the cover tests. Therefore, practically the cyclodeviations cannot be subdivided into latent and manifest forms.

B. Depending upon character of deviation

1. Excyclophoria and excyclotropia. The deviated eye is extorted, i.e. the eye is rotated around its anteroposterior axes in such a way that the superior portion of the vertical meridian (12 O'clock meridian) is torted temporally and the inferior portion of the vertical meridian (6 O'clock meridian) is torted nasally.

2. Incyclophoria and incyclotropia. The deviated eye is intorted, i.e. the eye is rotated around its anteroposterior axes in such a way that the superior portion of the vertical meridian (12 O'clock meridian) is torted nasally and the inferior portion of the vertical meridian (6 O'clock meridian) is torted temporally.

ETIOLOGY

In general, cyclodeviations result from an imbalance in the relationship between intorters (superior oblique and superior rectus) and extorters (inferior oblique and inferior rectus) of the eyeball under following situations:

1. *Paresis or paralysis* of any cyclovertical muscle, particularly oblique muscles (having larger torsional effect than vertical recti) is commonly associated with cyclodeviation. Cyclodeviation in such conditions is usually associated with a vertical deviation, but may also occur alone.

Bilateral excyclotropia secondary to closed head injury occurs due to bilateral superior oblique paralysis resulting from rupture of the anterior medullary velum, which is that area in the midbrain where the superior oblique fibres from both superior oblique nuclei decussate.

2. *Dissociated vertical deviations* are frequently associated with cyclodeviations.

3. *A- and V-pattern of horizontal strabismus* are also associated with cyclodeviations without an obvious paretic component.

4. *Horizontal deviations and simple hyperphorias* may also be associated with cyclodeviations, though rarely.

5. *Surgery on vertical recti or oblique muscles* may sometimes be complicated by cyclodeviations.

6. *Uncorrected oblique astigmatism* may also be associated with cyclodeviation.

7. *Other conditions* which have been reported to be associated with cyclodeviations include— endocrine ophthalmopathy, myasthenia gravis and plagiocephaly.

CLINICAL CHARACTERISTICS

Theoretically, one would expect that patients with cyclodeviations should have symptoms such as torsional diplopia, dizziness and difficulties in negotiating stair way, steps and streetcurves. However, in practice, most of the patients are asymptomatic, with the exception of paretic conditions of very recent onset, particularly traumatic unilateral or bilateral superior oblique paralysis. The reasons (factors) which have been put forward for most of the patients with cyclodeviations being asymptomatic are:

- Cyclofusion
- Suppression and ARC
- Physiologic adaptation
- Psychologic adaptation

1. *Cyclofusion.* It has been reported that cyclodisparity caused by cyclodeviations is mostly compensated by sensory cyclofusion which is very well developed in humans. Normal individuals can fuse up to 10°–15° of cyclodisparity in either direction, by vertical and cyclofusional movements. But only a few degrees of this disparity are offset by motor fusion.

The effectivity of sensory cyclofusion is well illustrated by comparing the testing of cyclodeviation by two different methods as below:

When tested with *Double Maddox rod test*, a patient shows cyclotropia. Same patients with well-developed cyclofusion, when tested with *Bagolini lenses* (after correcting the co-existing vertical and horizontal deviations, if any, with prisms), show that Maddox rod test which disrupts fusion reveals the exact amount of cyclotropia that can be measured exactly whereas the Bagolini lenses which do not disrupt fusion, test one's ability of cyclofusion.

2. *Suppression and anomalous retinal correspondence.* Some patients do not experience torsional diplopia due to development of suppression or anomalous retinal correspondence.

Note. It has been observed that even after occlusion of the non-paralysed eye, the patient does not see the visual environment tilted inspite of the fact that the affected eye is rotated around the anteroposterior axes. The cyclofusion and suppression or ARC also cannot explain this finding. Such a unique happening has been explained by the occurrence of physiological and psychological adaptation in patients with cyclotropia. These phenomena are described below.

3. *Physiologic adaptation.* It has been reported that to compensate for the image tilt in some patients with congenital or early acquired cyclodeviation, there occurs a physiologic adaptation in the form of spatial reorientation of the horizontal and vertical retinal meridians (Fig. 11.8). Perhaps such a physiologic adaptation has a neurophysiologic basis in the form of a change in orientation tuning of the striate cortical neurons. Further, it has also been

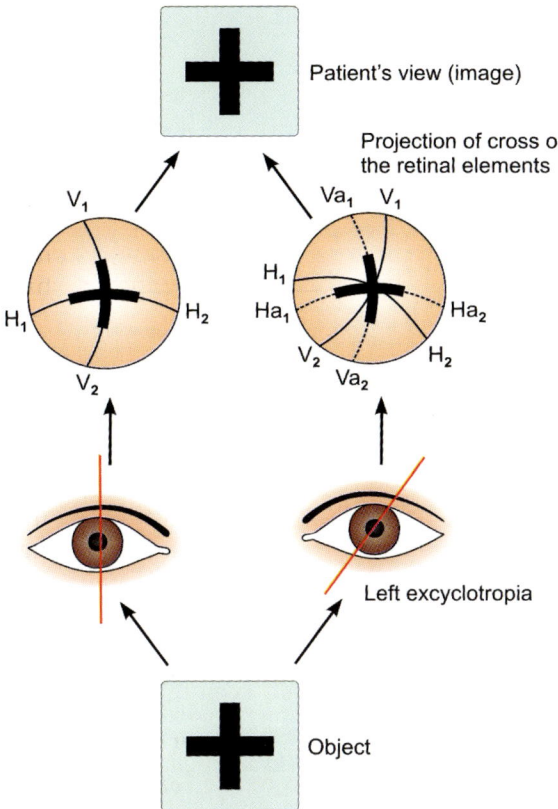

Patient's view (image)

Projection of cross on the retinal elements

Left excyclotropia

Object

Fig. 11.8 *Physiologic adaptation in the form of spatial reorientation of the horizontal and vertical retinal meridia in left eye with excyclodeviation. Note, image of a cross is no longer formed on the normal vertical (V_1–V_2) and horizontal (H_1–H_2) retinal meridia; but on the new vertical (Va_1–Va_2) and new horizontal (Ha_1–Ha_2) meridia.*

reported that this physiologic adaptation is reversible and after surgical treatment of cyclotropia, patient may get normal orientation after a brief period of seeing tilted environment.

4. *Psychologic adaptation.* A sort of psychologic adaptation due to empirical spatial clues may also help some patients with cyclotropia to be unaware of the tilted environment. The empirical spatial clues are based on the past experience of seeing the orientation of the familiar objects such as doors, windows, trees, etc. in the physical space. This fact is supported by the observation that patients with cyclotropia (diagnosed on Maddox rod test) who do not see the environment tilted may see a faintly illuminated horizontal line as tilted, when no other familiar visual clues are available.

DIAGNOSTIC TESTS

The deviated eye does not realign itself on covering the fixating eye, its position remains unchanged under monocular and binocular conditions. Therefore, cyclodeviations cannot be detected by routine objective examination. Therefore, tests for their diagnosis are specially done under following circumstances:

- When a patient complains of *tilting of images* (which is not very often).
- When the examiner notices a *torsional movement* of the eye on alternate cover test (only a very experienced and observent examiner can notice it).
- When there is a *palsy of a vertical muscle*, especially one of the two obliques. Associated vertical deviation is also noted.
- When it is detected while performing diplopia fields with Franceschetti method.

Diagnostic tests for cyclodeviations can be divided into subjective and objective tests.

Subjective diagnostic tests

The subjective tests can only be used for cyclodeviations beginning after visual maturation. Subjective tests include the following:

- Maddox double rod test
- Maddox double prism test
- Moddox wing test
- Major amblyoscope test
- Bagolini's striated lenses test
- Lancaster red-green test

1. *Maddox double rod test*. Maddox double rod test is a quantitative test to subjectively measure the cyclodeviation; but it cannot differentiate between cyclophoria and cyclotropia. It can be performed at distance and near.

Procedure. To perform this test, patient is asked to fixate a spotlight in a dark room. By means of a trial frame, a white Maddox rod is placed before the left eye, and a red Maddox rod before the right eye with their axes set at 90° (Fig. 11.9A). If no vertical deviation is present (which is not very often the case), a 6 D prism is placed with its base-down in front of one eye to assist the patient in observing the two lines easily (Fig. 11.9B). The results are interpreted as below:

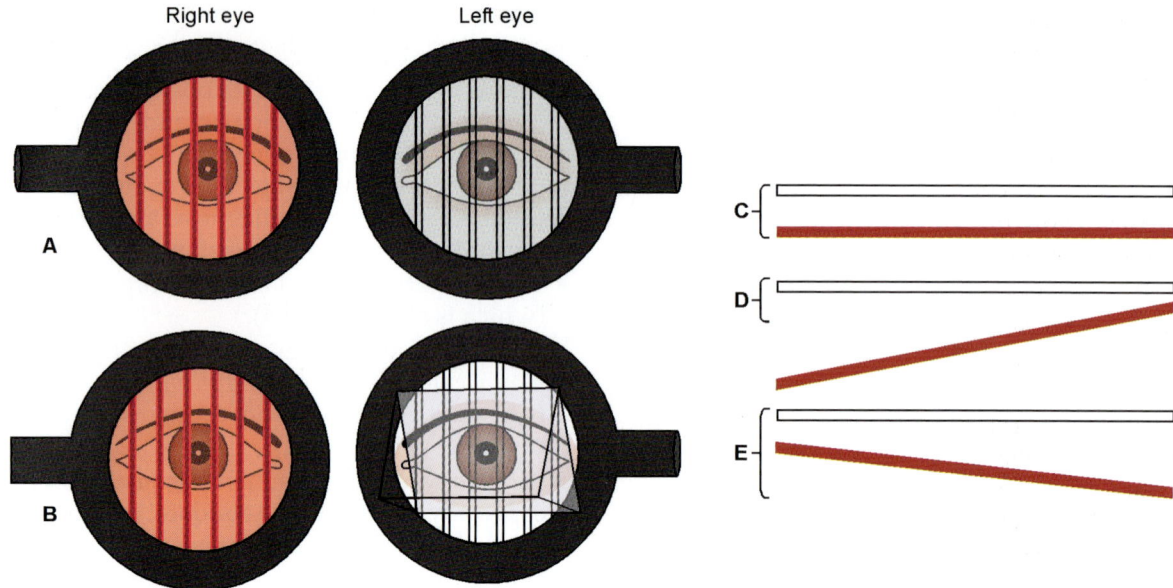

Fig. 11.9 *Double Maddox rod test (for explanation, see text).*

- If the two horizontal lines, one red and other white, observed by the patient are parallel, no cyclodeviation is present (Fig. 11.9C).
- If the red line is tilted outward(Fig. 11.9D), incyclodeviation is present and if the red line is tilted inward (Fig.11.9E), excyclodeviation is present in the right eye. The examiner than rotates the red Maddox rod inward or outward, respectively until the red and white lines are parallel. The amount of deviation is read in degrees on the trial frame. For example, if the red line which is tilted inward becomes parallel at the 100° position, indicates that patient has a 10° right excyclodeviation.
- Similarly, if cyclodeviation is present in left eye the white line will be tilted depending upon the type and degree of cyclodeviation.
- In the presence of bilateral cyclodeviation, e.g. in bilateral excyclodeviation in a patient with bilateral superior oblique palsy following closed head injury both the white and red lines will be tilted inward.

Note. It is important to note that with this test cyclodeviated eye will always be the non-fixing eye even when the patient fixes with the paretic eye. For example, if a patient with a left superior oblique palsy fixes with the left eye, the right eye will show the excyclodeviation on the double Maddox rod test, even though it is the normal eye.

Drawback of the double Maddox rod test

Double Maddox rod test is of value in substantiating and measuring cyclotropia since it disrupts the fusion. But, as it does not permit cyclofusion so it may be clinically insignificant under casual viewing which allows cyclofusion.

The small frame size of the maddox rods, available in most of the refraction trial boxes, makes it difficult, if not impossible, to examine for cyclodeviations in the peripheral field of vision. The cyclophorometer designed by Burian overcomes this problem but is not commercially available.

2. *Maddox double prism test.* Maddox double prism consists of two 4D prisms mounted base to base in a frame. It displaces the image in vertically opposite directions. To perform this test, patient is asked to fixate on a horizontal line drawn on a sheet of paper with the eye to be tested (e.g. say right eye) and the double prism is placed before the left eye. Patient sees three lines, central with the right eye and upper and lower with the left eye. The results of this test are interpreted as below:

- *No cyclodeviation* is present, when all the three lines are parallel.

- *Right incyclodeviation* is present, if the central line is tilted outward.
- *Right excyclodeviation* is present, if the central line is tilted inward.

Limitations
- This test can be performed only for near.
- Being a qualitative test, it cannot measure the cyclodeviation and cannot differentiate between cyclophoria and cyclotropia.

3. *Bagolini's striated lenses test.* Bagolini's striated lenses permit testing for cyclotropia under casual viewing conditions where cyclofusion take part. To perform this test, patient is asked to fixate a spotlight in a dark room. By means of a trial frame, the Bagolini's striated lenses are placed before both eyes with the axes of striations pointing towards the 90° mark. These lenses will produce an image of streak of light, perpendicular to the axes of striations without obstructing the surrounding fusible visual details (c.f. Maddox rods). The results of this test are interpreted as below:

- If the patient is able to fuse the two vertical lines that indicate that cyclotropia is fully compensated by cyclofusion.
- If the patient is unable to fuse the two vertical lines, the lenses are turned until fusion occurs and the amount and direction of the cyclotropia is read on the trial frames.

4. *Lancaster red green test.* This is the most complete test and has some advantages over other tests:
- It measures the torsional amplitude of each eye in nine different directions of gaze.

- It gives information about the pattern of cyclodeviation in each direction of gaze, and
- Measures cyclodeviation simultaneously along with the horizontal as well as vertical deviations.

5. *Synaptophore test* is also very useful for detecting and measuring the cyclodeviations.

Objective diagnostic tests

The objective diagnostic tests are useful for revealing any cyclodeviation, regardless of the age of onset (c.f. subjective tests). These tests include:
- Indirect ophthalmoscopy and fundus photography.
- Monocular visual field charting

1. *Ophthalmoscopy and fundus photography* Presence of cyclodeviation can be objectively evidenced by a disturbed relationship of the optic disc with foveola on indirect ophthalmoscopy and fundus photography. Normally, the foveola is aligned approximately with the junction of the middle and lower third of disc (Fig.11.10A). In excyclodeviation, fundus is rotated externally and the foveola appears to be situated below a line extending horizontally from just below the lower pole of optic disc (Fig.11.10B). In incyclodeviation, fundus is rotated internally and foveola appears to be situated above a line extending horizontally from the centre of the optic disc (Fig. 11.10C).

2. *Monocular visual field testing.* Evidence of objective cyclodeviation can also be found on monocular visual field charting which will show inward rotation of the blind spot in excyclodeviation and outward rotation of the blind spot in incyclodeviation.

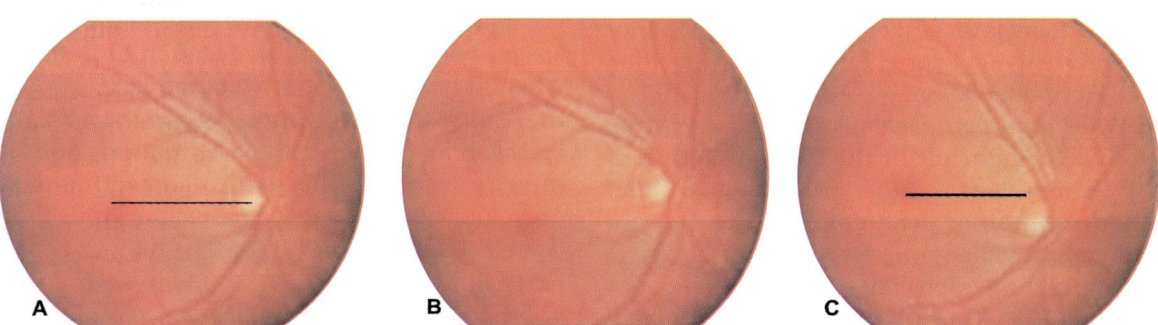

Fig. 11.10 *Fundus photograph showing relation of optic disc with foveola in a normal person (A), in a patient with excyclodeviation (B) and, in a patient with incyclodeviation (C).*

Interpretation of results of objective and subjective tests for cyclodeviation

1. *Objective tests'* results will always be positive in the affected (cyclodeviated) eye.

2. *Subjective tests'* results are affected by various factors such as cyclofusion, sensory adaptation, physiologic adaptation and psychologic adaptation. In patients with positive objective tests for cyclodeviation, subjective tests may be negative or reverse positive as follows:

i. *Negative subjective tests.* Subjective tests which do not produce dissociation of fusion such as Bagolini lenses test may be negative in patients with positive objective tests for cyclo-deviation. It indicates complete compensation of deviation by the cyclofusion.

ii. *Reverse positive subjective tests.* In contrast to that observed on objective tests for cyclodeviation; on the subjective tests, the cyclodeviated eye is always the non-fixing eye. This is true even when the non-fixing eye is normal and the opposite fixing eye has a paretic cyclovertical muscle and shows a cyclodeviation on objective tests. This has been explained by the assumption that perhaps a monocular sensorial adaptation takes place in the paretic, fixing eye.

TREATMENT

Only symptomatic (subjective) cyclodeviation (usually >5°) needs treatment, which is always surgical. The choice of surgery is as follows:

1. Treatment of subjective cyclodeviation associated with vertical deviation

i. *When a patient gets hyperdeviation and excycplodeviation* due to unopposed action of the inferior oblique following paralysis of homolateral superior oblique muscle, obviously the treatment is to weaken the offending inferior oblique. This will correct both hyperdeviation and excyclodeviation.

ii. *When a patient develops vertical deviation and cyclodeviation* in the field of action of paretic muscle (say superior oblique) without any overaction of the antagonist (i.e. inferior oblique); obviously the treatment of choice is tucking of the tendon of paretic muscle (superior oblique). Tucking of superior oblique will eliminate both hyperdeviation and excyclo-deviation occurring in its field of action.

iii. *A patient having bilateral superior oblique palsy* producing V-pattern esotropia and an excyclodeviation, needs bilateral tucking of the superior oblique to fully correct the entill problem.

2. Treatment of subjective cyclodeviation without associated vertical deviation

Such a proposition is of rare occurrence but often more difficult to handle; since a conventional weakening or strengthening procedure on cyclovertical muscle may correct the cyclo-deviation but it may produce an unwanted vertical deviation. Therefore, such surgical procedures should be performed which will exclusively affect the cyclodeviation. Following procedures have been described:

i. *Harada-Ito procedure* (anterolateral advance-ment of superior oblique tendon).

- This procedure, described in Japan, is becoming quite popular for correction of monocular aswellas binocular excyclodeviation due to palsy of superior oblique muscle.

- This procedure is based on the theoretical assumption that only the anterior part of the superior oblique tendon insertion is responsible for incyclodeviation of eye.

- This procedure basically consists of anterolateral advancement of the anterior part of the superior oblique tendon. This will result in shift of the line of pull in such a way that now on downgaze intorsion occurs which overcomes the extorsion without causing any vertical imbalance.

ii. *Nasal transposition of inferior rectus muscle.* This procedure has been suggested as an effective alternative for excyclodeviation in downgaze, where Harda-Ito procedure is not possible; for example, in patients with congenital absence of superior oblique tendon or in those where it has already been tenotomized.

iii. *Temporal transposition of the superior rectus muscle* may be added to nasal transposition of inferior rectus muscle for correcting the excyclotropia present in the primary position (*see* Fig. 15.18).

iv. *Temporal transposition of inferior rectus along with nasal transposition of the superior rectus muscle* has been found effective for correcting incyclodeviation.

v. *Other procedures* which have been reported to correct cyclodeviation without producing vertical or horizontal strabismus are:

- Slanting of the insertion of all rectus muscles.
- Vertical transposition of the horizontal rectus muscles (*see* Fig. 15.19).
- Transposition of the anterior aspects of the inferior and superior oblique tendons.

BIBLIOGRAPHY

1. Anderson, JR: Ocular vertical deviations and nystagmus, London, 1959. British Medical Association.
2. Bagolini, B, Campos, E, and Chiesi, C: Plagiocephaly causing superior oblique deficiency and ocular torticollis, Arch. Ophthalmol. 100:1093, 1982.
3. Bielschowsky, A: Die einseitigen und gegensinnigen ("dissoziierten") Vertikalbewegungen der Augen, Graefes Arch. Ophthalmol. 125:493, 1931.
4. Bielschowsky, A: Lectures on motor anomalies. Hanover NH, 1956, Dartmouth Publishing Co.
5. Burke, JP, Scott, WE, and Kutschke, PJ: Anterior transposition of the inferior oblique muscle for dissociated vertical deviation. Ophthalmology 100:245, 1993.
6. Duncan, L, and Noorden, GK von: Surgical results in dissociated vertical deviations, J Pediatr. Ophthalmol. Strabismus 21:25, 1984.
7. Esswein. MB, Noorden, GK von, and Coburn, A: Comparison of surgical methods in the treatment of dissociated vertical deviation, Am J Ophthalmol. 113:287, 1992.
8. Fink, WH, Surgery of the vertical muscles of the eye, ed. 2, Springfield, Ill., 1962, Charles C Thomas, Publisher, P. 369.
9. Guyton, DL and Noorden, GKvon: Sensory adaptations to cyclodeviations. In Reinecke. RD, editor: Strabismus, New York, 1978, Grune & Stratton, Inc.
10. Harada, M and Ito, Y: Surgical correction of cyclotropia, Jpn J Ophthalmol. 8:88, 1964.
11. Helveston, EM: Dissociated vertical deviaton: a clinical and laboratory study, Trans. Am Ophthalmol. Soc 78:734, 1980.
12. Herzau, V and Joos-Kratsch, E: Objective and subjective evaluation of xyclovergence and cyclofusion, Doc. Ophthalmol. 58:85, 1984.
13. Hooten, K, Myers E, Worall, R, and Stark, L: Cyclovergence: the motor response to cyclodisparity, Graefes Arch. Ophthalmol. 210:65, 1979.
14. Kii, T, Ogasawara, K, Ohba, M, Hotsubo, M, Sakai, N and Nakagawa, T: The effectiveness of the Faden operation on the superior rectus muscle combined with recession of the muscle for the treatment of dissociated vertical deviation, Acta Soc. Opthalmol. Jpn. 98:98, 1994.
15. Mumma, JV: Surgical procedure for congenital absence of the superior oblique, Arch. Ophthalmol. 92:221, 1974.
16. Noorden, GK von, Brown, DJ, and Parks,M: Clinical observations in cyclotropia. Presented at the American Orthoptic Council - American Association of Certified Orthoptists symposium at the American Academy of Ophthalmology and Otolaryngology, Dallas, September 16, 1973.
17. Noorden, GK von: Clinical observations in cyclodeviations, Ophthalmology 86:1451, 1979.
18. Noorden, GK von: Indications of the posterior fixation operation in strabismus, Ophthalmology 85:512, 1978.
19. Noorden, GK von, and Chu, MW: Surgical treatment options in cyclotropia, J Pediatr Opthalmol Strabismus 27:291, 1990.
20. Ogle, KN, and Ellerbrock, VJ: Cyclofusional movement, Arch. Ophthalmol 36:700, 1946.
21. Oliver, P, and Noorden, GK von: Excyclotropia of the nonparetic eye in unilateral superior oblique muscle paralysis, Am J Ophthalmol. 93:30, 1982.
22. Ruttum, M, and Nooden, GK von: Adaptation to tilting of the visual environment in cyclotropia, Am J Ophthalmol 96:229, 1983.
23. Spielmann, A: A translucent occluder for studying eye position under unilateral or bilateral cover test, Am. Orthopt J 36:65, 1986.
24. Spielmann, A: Les divergences verticales dissociees: exces de sursumversion lie a la fixation, Ophthalmologie 1:457, 1987.
25. Spielmann, A: The oblique Kestenbaum procedure revisited (sloped recession of the recti). In Lenk-Schafer, M, editor: Orthoptic horizons, Transactions of the Sixth International Orthoptic Congress, Harrogate, England, 1987, p. 433.

Chapter
12
Incomitant Strabismus

CLASSIFICATION

Incomitant squint is a type of heterotropia (manifest squint) in which the amount of deviation varies in different directions of gaze. Further, amount of deviation may also vary depending on which eye is fixing. Incomitant deviations include the following conditions:

1. *Vertically incomitant horizontal heterotropias* (A-, V-, X-, Y- and λ-pattern heterotropias)

2. *Paralytic strabismus*

i. *Paralytic esotropia*
- *Lateral rectus paresis or paralysis*
- *Divergence paralysis*

ii. *Paralytic exotropia*
- *Isolated medial rectus paresis*
- *Complete third nerve paralysis*
- *Paralysis of convergence*

iii. *Paralytic vertical deviation*
- *Single muscle paresis or paralysis*
  - *Superior oblique paralysis or paresis*
  - *Inferior oblique paralysis or paresis.*
  - *Superior rectus paralysis or paresis.*
  - *Inferior rectus paralysis or paresis.*
- *Part of complete third nerve paralysis.*
- *Supranuclear lesions.*

– *Double elevator paralysis.*
– *Double depressor paralysis.*

3. *Restrictive ocular motility defects*

A. *Restrictive strabismus due to misdirected muscle forces.*

1. *Congenital cranial dysinnervation disorders (CCDDs)*
2. *Congenital ectopic extraocular muscle insertion and/or pulley location*
3. *Displaced extraocular muscle*

B. *Restrictive strabismus due to mechanical restrictions*

1. Tight extaocular muscles
   - *Inelastic superior oblique in congenital Brown's syndrome*
   - *Thyroid ophthalmopathy*
   - *Entraped inferior rectus muscle in blowout fracture of orbital floor.*
   - *Monocular elevation deficiency (MED), caused by fibrotic IR muscle.*
   - *Strabismus fixus.*

2. Structural adhesions
   - *Fat adherence to extraocular muscles or sclera after strabismus surgery, retinal detachment surgery or periocular trauma*
   - *Congenital fibrotic bands*
   - *Acquired Brown's syndrome due to scarring/inflammation around, the trochlea*
   - *Conjuctival and Tenon's capsule scarring*

3. Orbital mass lesions
   - *Orbital tumours causing mass effect on the globe movements.*
   - *Glaucoma explant with large bleb causing mass effect.*

VERTICALLY INCOMITANT HORIZONTAL HETEROTROPIAS (A-, V-, X-,Y- AND λ-PATTARN HETEROTROPIAS)

TERMINOLOGY

The term vertically incomitant horizontal heterotropias refers to those horizontal deviations that change in magnitude with upgaze and downgaze. Urist introduced this concept to American literature in 1951 and Albert suggested the excellent descriptive terms A-pattern and V-pattern which are now accepted worldwide. In practice, the term vertically incomitant horizontal heterotropias has become synonymous with "A- and V-pattern". A few other patterns are also recognized as follows.

A-pattern horizontal heterotropia

An A-pattern designates a vertically incomitant horizontal heterotropia with increasing convergence (decreasing divergence) in upgaze and increasing divergence in downgaze. An A-pattern deviation is considered clinically significant, when the difference between upgaze and downgaze is at least 10 prism dioptres or more.

- *A-esotropia:* Esotropia will increase in upgaze and decrease in downgaze (Fig. 12.1).
- *A-exotropia:* Exotropia will decrease in upgaze and increase in downgaze (Fig. 12.2).

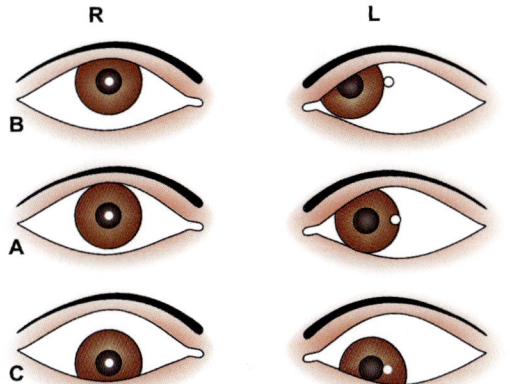

Fig. 12.1 *A-pattern esotropia. Note left esotropia in primary gaze (A) which increases in upgaze (B) and decreases in downgaze (C).*

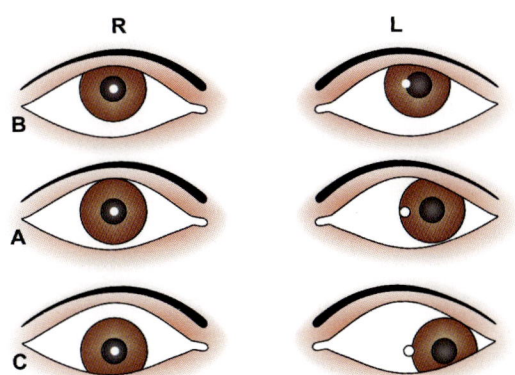

Fig. 12.2 *A-pattern exotropia. Note left exotropia in primary gaze (A) which decreases in upgaze (B) and increases in downgaze (C).*

V-pattern horizontal heterotropia

The V-pattern is present, when there is vertically incomitant horizontal deviation with increasing convergence (decreasing divergence) in downgaze and increasing divergence in upgaze. The V-pattern is considered clinically significant, only when it measures 15 prism dioptres or more difference between upgaze and downgaze.

- *V-esotropia.* The esotropia will increase in downgaze and decrease in upgaze (Fig. 12.3).
- *V-exotropia.* The exotropia will increase in upgaze and decrease in downgaze (Fig. 12.4).

Y-pattern horizontal heterotropia

Patients with Y-pattern have exotropia only in upgaze (Fig. 12.5).

λ(lambda)-pattern horizontal heterotropia

These patients have exotropia in downgaze only.

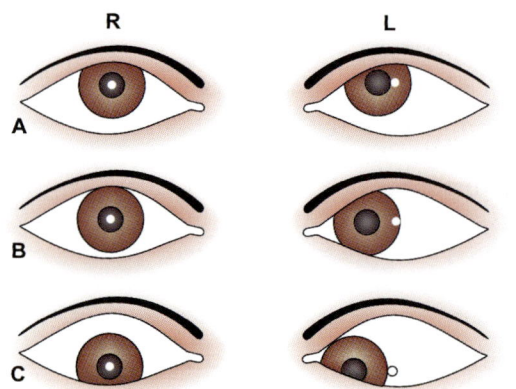

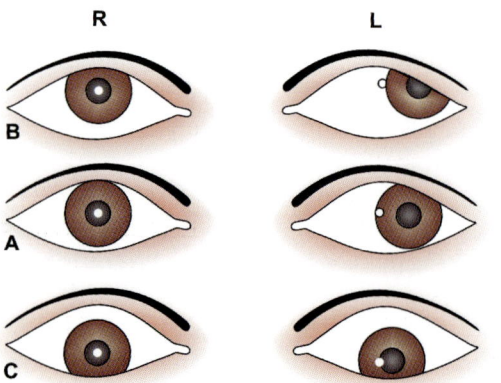

Fig. 12.3 *V-pattern esotropia. Note left esotropia (A) which decreases in upgaze (B) and increases in downgaze (C).*

Fig. 12.4 *V-pattern exotropia: Diagrammatic depiction of left exotropia (A) which increases in upgaze (B) and decreases in downgaze (C).*

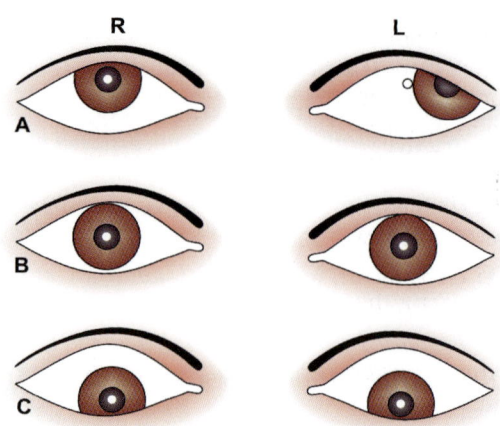

Fig. 12.5 *Y-pattern exotropia. Note left exotropia in upgaze (A) and no deviation in primary gaze (B) and downgaze (C).*

X-pattern horizontal heterotropia

These patients essentially have no deviation or only a small one in primary position, but a significant exotropia is present in upgaze as well as in downgaze (Fig. 12.6).

ETIOLOGY

Various theories have been put forward to explain the occurrence of A- and V-patterns. However, it has not been possible to explain the occurrence of such patterns in every case by any single aetiological factor. Perhaps different factors might be responsible in different cases. Each of the following conditions has been firmly documented as a cause of A- and V-patterns:

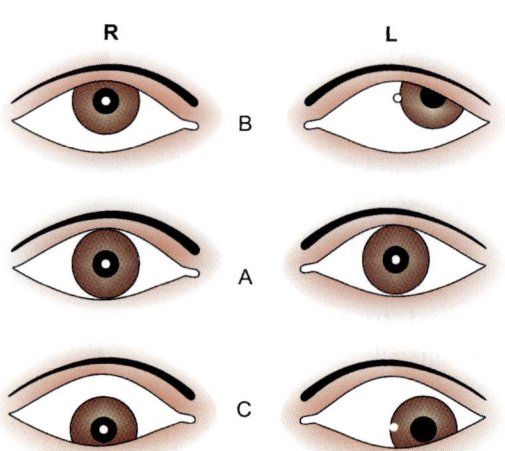

Fig. 12.6: X-*pattern* exotropia. Note no deviation in primary gaze (A) and exotropia in upgaze (B) and downgaze (C).

1. *Oblique muscle dysfunction.* Dysfunction of the oblique muscles is the most common clinical finding and surgery on these muscles has been eminently successfull in the elimination of these patterns. Following observations have been made:

- *Inferior oblique overaction* is frequently associated with V-patterns and surgical weakening of this muscle is effective in correcting the anomaly in most of such cases.
- *Superior oblique overaction* is often associated with A-patterns and surgical weakening of these muscles is effective in correcting the anomaly in majority of such patients.

Factors blamed for oblique muscle dysfunction are as follows:

- Innervational (primary or secondary overaction).
- Desagittalization of the muscle planes, i.e. disturbed parallelism of the superior and inferior oblique muscles.
- Anomalous insertion of oblique muscles.
- Ocular or orbital torsions.

The cause of oblique muscle dysfunction seems to be of secondary importance with regard to the management of these conditions. The main point is to search for the overacting or underacting oblique muscles. Unfortunately, there are some cases of A- and V-patterns that clearly do not show overaction of the obliques; and an alternative explanation and surgical treatment for these patients is necessary.

2. *Horizontal rectus muscle dysfunction.* Urist (1958) hypothesized that horizontal recti are responsible for A- and V-patterns as follows:

- *A-esotropia:* Underacting lateral recti.
- *A-exotropia:* Underacting medial recti.
- *V-esotropia:* Overacting medial recti.
- *V-exotropia:* Overacting lateral recti.

But, no convincing evidence has been presented to explain A- and V-patterns exclusively on a dysfunction of the horizontal recti.

However, surgically supraplacement and infraplacement of the medial and lateral recti are effective procedures for A-V-pattern, when not associated with overaction of the obliques.

3. *Vertical rectus muscle dysfunction.* Brown (1953) suggested that A-V-patterns may be caused by vertical rectus muscle dysfunction. However, this concept never gained popularity due to lack of any supporting evidence. Further, the horizontal transposition of the vertical recti proposed to correct A-V-pattern had also not been found very effective and thus not used today.

4. *Orbital factors.* It has been proposed that an apparent dysfunction of the oblique muscles unrelated to paresis of any cyclovertical muscle might be due to some structural orbital anomalies as evidenced by following observations of several workers:

- Patients with Alpert's syndrome or Crauzon's syndrome frequently show a V-pattern exotropia or esotropia with marked elevation of the adducting eye, which resemble the pattern caused by overacting inferior obliques.
- Patients with upward or downward slanting palpebral fissures may show A- and V-patterns.
- Orbital factors might be responsible for desagittalization of the muscle planes which in turn might be producing A- and V-patterns in some cases.

5. *Pulley abnormalities* in the form of heterotopia or laxity of the pulley have also been reported as a cause of 'A' and 'V' patterns. Diagnosis of pulley abnormalities is made on MRI orbital imaging. In such cases, surgery could be performed to stabilize or reposition the orbital pulley.

CLINICAL CHARACTERISTICS

Prevalence

Exact prevalence varies depending upon the criteria used to define the condition, degree of upgaze and downgaze used to test and the ethnic group tested. However, in general, between 15% and 50% of all strabismus cases have been reported to have associated A- or V-pattern in different studies. Common patterns found in clinical practice are V-esotropia, V-exotropia, A-esotropia and A-exotropia.

Symptoms and signs

Since fusion may have to be maintained for a long time in certain positions of gaze, so patients with

A- and V-patterns are more frequently troubled by:

- Intermittent transient diplopia, and
- Asthenopic symptoms.
- Abnormal head posture may be assumed to get rid of the symptoms. Chin is moved towards the apex of A- or V- in esotropia and away from the apex in exotropia as follows:
  - V-esotropia and A-exotropia chin may be depressed.
  - V-exotropia and A-esotropia chin may be elevated.

Sensory adaptations and amblyopia

- *Abnormal retinal correspondence* may also occur in patients with A-V-pattern. However, since the angle of deviation varies in different gazes, so will be the angle of anomaly. This is called covariation of the angle of anomaly.
- *Strabismic amblyopia* in A-V-pattern is as frequent as in other forms of horizontal strabismus. However, some patients with Y- and λ-patterns exotropia possess fusion potential in primary gaze, and so they will have less chances of developing strabismic amblyopia.

Clinical work-up

A detailed and thorough clinical work-up should be done as in any case of strabismus (page 100). However, points of special reference and interest are mentioned here.

a. *Measurement of deviation* is essential for diagnosis of A-V-pattern. Important points to be kept in mind are:

- Prism and alternate cover test should be employed for measurement.
- Measurements are done in extreme positions of gaze, using the proper refractive correction.
- Knapp stressed that false measurement can be best avoided by measuring the deviation at distance fixation.
- von Noorden, after detailed observations, has recommended that the best way to measure the deviation is at 33 cm fixation distance, with the refractive error fully corrected, and the eyes in position of 25° elevation and 35° depression while fixing on an accommodative target (Fig. 12.7).
- After measurement in upward gaze and downward gaze, A-V-pattern should be established, only if the difference in deviation between upward and downward gazes is as follows:

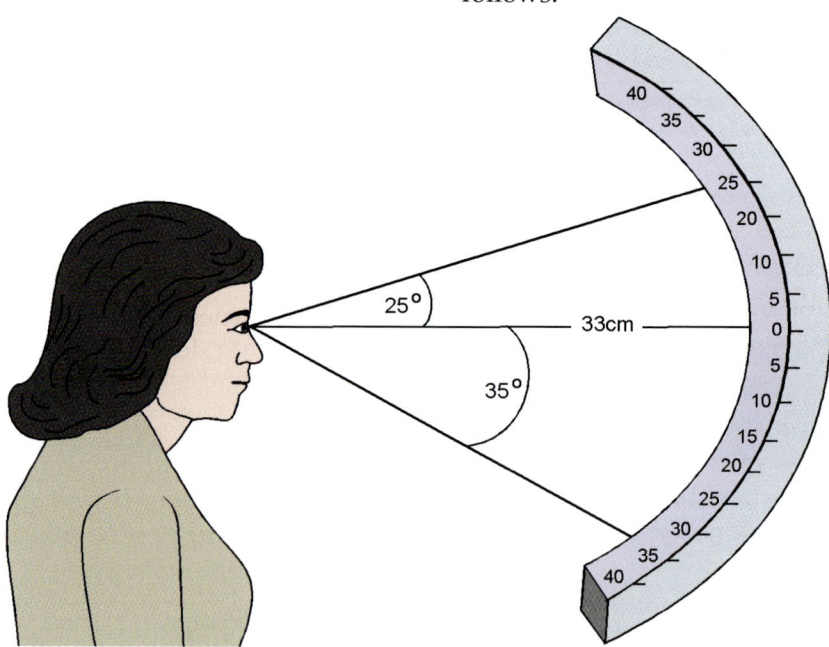

Fig. 12.7 *von Noorden's technique of measuring deviation with eyes in primary position, 25° elevation and 35° depression while fixing on an accommodative target to demonstrate A- and V-patterns.*

– For V-pattern, 15 prism dioptres or more, and

– For A-pattern, 10 prism dioptres or more.

b. Version test should be performed to note overactions and underactions of the oblique muscles. This is most important factor for planning the management of A-V-pattern.

c. Compensatory head posture should also be properly noted.

d. Binocular vision should be tested especially in the physiologically important positions of gaze, i.e. in the primary and downward (reading) positions to stress on the clinical significance of the vertical incomitance on the degree of interference with normal binocular function.

TREATMENT

Indications

Only clinically significant A-V-pattern needs to be treated for any of the following indications:

1. *To eliminate motor obstacles* in order to maintain, improve or regain comfortable single binocular vision;

2. *To improve the cosmetic appearance* of the patient; and

3. *To eliminate abnormal head position:* Chin elevation or chin depression.

Basic principles

1. While planning surgery, a special care should be taken for the functionally most important positions of gaze, i.e. primary and downgaze (reading).

2. *Overacting oblique muscles should be identified* with special attention and when discovered weakening of these muscles, surgery should be the first choice.

3. *Inferior oblique weakening has no effect on horizontal deviation* in primary position, so horizontal muscle surgery should be selected independently. Further, this procedure tends to be self-adjusting correcting all the V-patterns present without overcorrection.

4. *Superior oblique weakening may have some influence on the horizontal deviation in primary position,* so surgical procedure for the horizontal rectus muscle should be modified also according

to personal experience. Alternatively, horizontal rectus muscle surgery may be deferred for a later date.

5. When both the superior as well as inferior obliques are overacting, weakening of any oblique muscle is contraindicated.

6. *Vertical transposition or slanting of insertion of the horizontal recti* to correct A-V-pattern should be considered, only if the obliques are not overacting.

7. *Horizontal transposition of the vertical rectus muscles is an ineffective procedure* and so better avoided.

Surgical procedures

I. *Weakening of oblique muscles*

For technical facts about inferior oblique weakening, *see* page 431 and for superior oblique weakening, *see* page 433.

II. *Transposition of the horizontal rectus muscles*

Indications

1. As discussed earlier, vertical transposition or slanting of insertion of the horizontal rectus muscle for correction of A-V-pattern is to be considered, only if there is no associated overaction of the oblique muscle.

2. Occasionally, A-V-patterns may not be completely corrected or recur following weakening of the overacting oblique muscles, especially with inferior oblique recession. Such cases should be treated by extirpation of the overacting muscle (*see* page 431). However, if still there is residual A-V-pattern, then transposition of the horizontal rectus muscles may be tried.

Principles

1. *Medial rectus muscles* are always moved towards the direction of vertical gaze where the convergence is greater, i.e. upward in A-pattern and downwards in V-pattern. In other words, towards the apex of A- or V-pattern (Fig. 12.8).

2. *Lateral rectus muscles* are moved towards the direction of vertical gaze where the divergence is greater, i.e. upward in V-pattern and downwards in A-pattern (Fig. 12.8). In other words, towards the open or splayed portion of A or V.

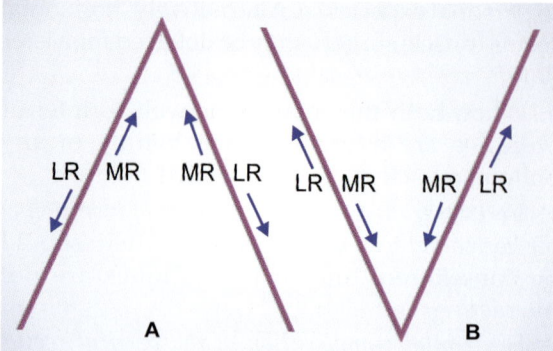

Fig. 12.8 *Direction of displacement of medial and lateral rectus muscles in weakening operations to treat A-pattern (A) and V-pattern (B) deviations.*

To remember, a useful mnemonic is MALE: Medial recti to the apex and lateral recti to the empty space.

Amount of transposition

Most of the surgeons prefer to move the insertion of the medial and lateral recti by half their width or 5 mm. Supraplacement or infraplacement by 5 mm will produce an approximate 15 and 20 prism dioptres change in the A- and V-patterns between upgaze and downgaze.

Mechanics of correction of A-V-pattern

1. When the medial recti are surgically transposed towards the apex of an A- or V-pattern, the arc of contact and therefore, the effective leverage of the medial recti will be reduced, when the eyes are moved in the direction of the apex. Hence the apex of A- or V-pattern will open. Conversely, when the eyes are moved towards the open or splayed portion of the A- or V-pattern, the arc of contact of the medial recti will be increased, and the leverage of these muscles will also be enhanced, and thus the open portion of the A- or V-pattern will close. Consequently, A- or V-pattern will be corrected.

2. When the lateral recti are transposed in the direction of the open or splayed portion of the A- or V-pattern and if now the eyes are moved in the same direction, the lateral recti will be less effective because of decreased leverage due to decrease in the arc of contact; consequently the open end of A- or V-pattern will close. Conversely, if the eyes are moved towards the

apex of A or V, the leverage of the lateral recti will be enhanced and the apical portion will open. Thus A- or V-pattern will be corrected.

III. *Horizontal transposition of the vertical rectus muscles*

Horizontal transposition of the vertical recti has been proposed as an alternative treatment. The superior recti are moved temporally and the inferior recti are moved nasally for an A-pattern and opposite for V-pattern. While this procedure is theoretically appealing, it is rarely performed today because of following reasons:

i. Most surgeons have not found it very effective.

ii. Since most patients with A-V-pattern also require horizontal muscle surgery for correction of the deviation in primary position; most surgeons prefer to transpose the horizontal rectus muscles rather than risk anterior segment ischaemia by operating on all four rectus muscles in the same session.

However, occasionally when vertical transposition of the horizontal rectus muscles is ineffective in correcting A-V-pattern, it may be worthwhile to try the horizontal transposition of the vertical rectus muscles.

Summary of treatment for the vertically incomitant horizontal strabismus

1. Treatment of V-pattern esotropia

i. *For correction of horizontal deviation in primary position:*

• Bilateral medial rectus recession, or

• Medial rectus recession and lateral rectus resection.

ii. *For correction of V-pattern:*

a. *Inferior oblique (IO) muscle weakening,* when overacting is done as below:

• Mild overaction: 6 mm IO recession

• Moderate overaction: 8 mm IO recession

• Severe overaction: 10 mm IO recession

• Markedly severe overaction: IO recession combined with anteropositioning (modified Elliot and Nankin method).

b. *Infraplacement of medial recti or infra-placement of MR and supraplacement of LR; or slanting their insertion.*

2. Treatment of A-pattern esotropia

i. *When superior oblique overaction is associated, bilateral tenotomy of superior*

- *Oblique muscles* should be performed and either bilateral medial rectus recession or recess-resect procedure should be performed for correction of horizontal deviation in the primary gaze after making adjustment for 10–15 prism dioptres which is corrected by bilateral superior oblique tenotomy. Alternatively, horizontal rectus muscle surgery may be deferred for a later date.
- *Transational recession of SO* (Prieto-Diaz procedure) may be performed for very severe overaction of SO muscle.

ii. *When superior oblique overaction is not present*, the treatment of choice is either bilateral medial rectus recession with supraplacement of the insertions; or combined supraplacement of the medial rectus and infraplacement of the lateral rectus muscle with a recess-resect procedure; or slanting their insertion.

3. Treatment of V-pattern exotropia

i. *If inferior oblique muscle overaction is present*, these muscles should be recessed and either a bilateral lateral rectus muscle recession or recess–resect procedure should be performed for the horizontal deviation in primary position.

ii. *When inferior oblique overaction is not present*, the treatment of choice is either bilateral lateral rectus muscle recession with supraplacement of the insertion or combined supraplacement of LR and infraplacement of MR with a recess-resect procedure; or slanting their insertion.

4. Treatment of A-pattern exotropia

i. *If superior oblique overaction is present*, its bilateral tenotomies should be performed. And keeping in mind the effect of superior oblique tenotomies on the horizontal deviation in primary position, either bilateral lateral rectus recession or a recess–resect procedure should be planned.

ii. *When superior oblique overaction is not present*, the treatment of choice is either bilateral lateral rectus muscle recession with infraplacement of the insertion or combined infraplacement of the LR and supraplacement of MR with a recess-resect procedure.

5. Treatment of Y-pattern exotropia

i. *No treatment is required*, when the patient fuses in primary position and downward gaze, has a normal head posture, and does not have double vision in upward gaze.

ii. *When chin elevation is present and there is associated overaction of the inferior oblique*; surgical weakening of both inferior oblique muscles will close the Y-pattern.

iii. *If the inferior obliques are not overacting*, supraplace the lateral recti without recessing or infraplace the medial recti without resecting.

6. Treatment of λ-pattern exotropia

Despite fusion in primary position, patients with λ-pattern exotropia may have considerable difficulty with near work (i.e. in downgaze). No horizontal surgery is indicated, but following procedures may be performed:

i. *If the superior obliques are overacting*, perform bilateral superior oblique tenotomies.

ii. *If the superior obliques are not overacting*, supraplace the medial recti without resecting or infraplace the lateral recti without recessing.

PARALYTIC SQUINT

Paralytic squit refers to ocular deviation resulting from complete or incomplete paralysis of one or more extraocular muscles. Complete paralysis is also called palsy and incomplete paralysis is called paresis.

ETIOLOGY

In many situations it may not be possible to pinpoint the cause. The lesion may be neurogenic (supranuclear, internuclear, nuclear, or infranuclear), myogenic or at the level of neuromuscular junction. The common causative lesions can be grouped as follows:

I. Neurogenic lesions

1. *Congenital lesions*. Hypoplasia or absence of nucleus is a known cause of third and sixth cranial nerves palsy. Birth injuries may mimic congenital lesions.

2. *Inflammatory lesions*. These may be in the form of encephalitis, meningitis, neurosyphilis or peripheral neuritis (commonly viral). Nerve trunks may also be involved in the infectious lesions of cavernous sinus and orbit.

3. *Neoplastic lesions.* These include brain tumours involving nuclei, nerve roots or intracranial part of the nerves; and intraorbital tumours involving peripheral parts of the nerves.

4. *Vascular lesions.* These are known in patients with hypertension, diabetes mellitus and atherosclerosis. These may be in the form of haemorrhage, thrombosis, embolism, aneurysms or vascular occlusions. Cerebrovascular accidents are more common in elderly people.

5. *Traumatic lesions.* These include head injury and direct or indirect trauma to the nerve trunks.

6. *Toxic lesions.* These include carbon monoxide poisoning, effects of diphtheria toxins (rarely), alcoholic and lead neuropathy.

7. *Demyelinating lesions.* Ocular palsy may occur in multiple sclerosis and diffuse sclerosis.

II. *Myogenic lesions*

1. *Congenital lesions.* These include absence, hypoplasia, malinsertion, weakness and musculofacial anomalies of extraocular muscles.

2. *Traumatic lesions.* These may be in the form of laceration, disinsertion, haemorrhage into the muscle substance or sheath and incarceration of muscles in fractures of the orbital walls.

3. *Inflammatory lesions.* Myositis is usually viral in origin and may occur in influenza, measles and other viral fevers.

4. *Myopathies.* These include, thyroid myopathy, carcinomatous myopathy and that associated with certain drugs. *Chronic progressive external ophthalmoplegia* (CPEO) is a bilateral myopathy of extraocular muscles, which may be sporadic or inherited as an autosomal dominant disorder.

III. *Neuromuscular junction lesion*

It includes myasthenia gravis. The disease is characterised primarily by fatigue of muscle groups usually starting with the small extraocular muscles, before involving other large muscles.

CLINICAL FEATURES

1. *Diplopia.* It is the main symptom of paralytic squint. It is more marked towards the action of paralysed muscle. It may be crossed (in divergent squint) or uncrossed (in convergent squint). It may be horizontal, vertical or oblique depending on the muscle paralysed. Diplopia occurs due to formation of image on dissimilar points of the two retinae (Fig. 12.9).

2. *Confusion.* It occurs due to formation of image of two different objects on the corresponding points of two retinae following misalignment of the visual axes of two eyes (Fig. 12.10).

3. *Ocular deviation.* In paralytic strabismus, the primary ocular deviation is incomitant and differs from the secondary deviation. However, with the passage of time there occurs spread of comitance.

Primary deviation. It is deviation of the affected eye, when the unaffected eye is used for fixation and is away from the action of paralysed muscle, e.g. if lateral rectus is paralysed, the eye is convergent.

Onset of paralytic ocular deviation may be of sudden as seen in trauma and vascular occlusions; or gradual as seen in tumours and multiple sclerosis.

Incomitance depending upon gaze. The angle of deviation changes with the direction of gaze. It

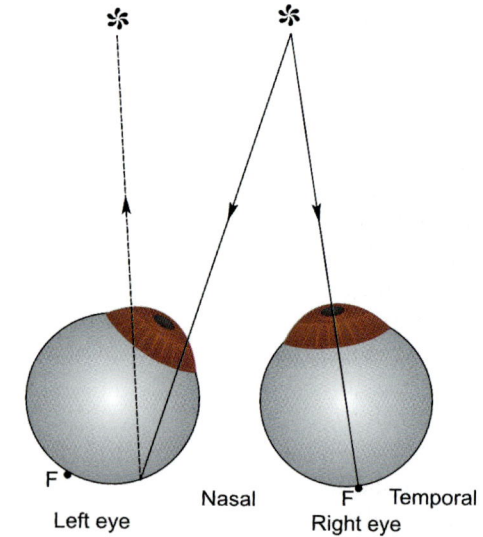

Fig. 12.9 *Uncrossed diplopia in a patient with left convergent squint.*

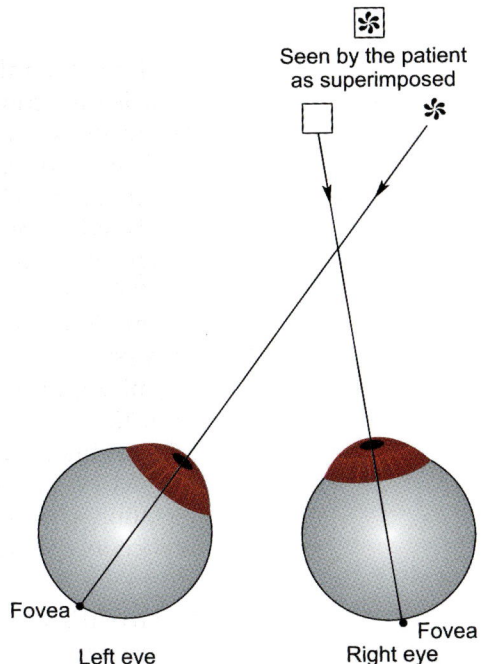

Seen by the patient
as superimposed

Fovea

Left eye

Fovea

Right eye

Fig. 12.10 *Confusion due to formation of image of two different objects on the corresponding points of two retinae.*

is greatest in the direction in which maximal activity is required for the involved muscle, i.e. in the diagnostic position of the muscle. For example, in a patient with paresis of right lateral rectus muscle during levoversion, no or little esotropia may be noted in right eye, while in primary position, right esotropia is marked, which will become maximum in dextroversion, i.e. deviation will be maximum in the field of action of right lateral rectus muscle.

Secondary deviation. It refers to deviation of the unaffected eye seen under cover, when the patient is made to fix with the affected eye. In a recently acquired ocular palsy, the secondary deviation is much greater than the primary deviation. This is due to the fact that the strong impulse of innervation required to enable the eye with paralysed muscle to fix is also transmitted to the yoke muscle of the sound eye resulting in a greater amount of deviation. This is based on Hering's law of equal innervation of yoke muscles.

In a long-standing ocular palsy, the secondary deviation is often much the same as the primary deviation because completion of the muscle sequelae leads to comitance.

Spread of comitance. A paralytic deviation undergoes several stages. The first stage is characterized by weakness of the paralyzed muscle during which secondary deviation is much more than the primary deviation as described above. Almost immediately following the paresis of an extraocular muscle, the direct antagonist begins to overact. A contracture of the antagonist muscle will develop within days to weeks, if the patient fixes with the unaffected eye. At this point, the deviation may become greater in the field of action of antagonist than it is in the field of action of weak agonist muscle. During the next stage, the deviation will spread into all fields of gaze and become increasingly comitant, i.e. there occurs a gradual spread of comitance to all fields of gaze. Ultimately, it may then no longer be possible to determine the nature of original deviation since the secondary deviation is often much the same as the primary deviation.

In most cases, spread of comitance occurs within a few weeks, months or even one to two years after the onset of paralysis. However, the spread of comitance is not a rule; in some cases of paralytic squint, it may not occur at all. Spread of comitance is quite common in infants with sixth nerve palsy, and ultimately patient may present with a comitant esodeviation.

4. *Ocular movements.* Restriction of ocular movements occurs towards the direction of action of the paralysed muscle/muscles. When the paralysis is of recent onset, a careful study of duction and version movements will make the diagnosis on the basis of incomplete movements in the field of action of the paralysed muscle. However, in long-standing cases, development of muscle sequelae such as contracture of the direct antagonist muscle and secondary inhibitional palsy of the contralateral antagonist muscle, present difficulties in the identification of the paralysed muscle. Under these circumstances, other tests like head-tilt test and Hess screen charting, etc. may be helpful in diagnosing the paralysed muscle.

5. *Past pointing.* Past pointing also described as *false projection* or *orientation* occurs due to increased innervational impulse conveyed to the paralysed muscle during movement in the direction of action of paralyzed muscle.

It can be demonstrated by asking the patient to close the sound eye and then to fix an object placed on the side of action of paralysed muscle. Patient will locate it further away in the same direction. For example, a patient with paralysis of right lateral rectus will point more towards right than the object actually is.

6. *Nausea, vertigo and dizziness.* Nausea, vertigo and dizziness result from diplopia, confusion and false localization. These symptoms are more prevalent in vertical and torsional diplopias than in horizontal diplopia. They do not occur in patients with congenital defects and disappear quickly in children. Adults adapt more slowly.

7. *Muscle sequelae.* Muscle sequelae refer to changes that take place in the extraocular muscles after some time of the paralysis or paresis of one or more of the extraocular muscles. The speed and extent to which they develop in different patients vary markedly. The exact reasons for this are unknown, but the speed and degree of their development depend partly on which eye the patient uses for fixation. Mostly, the patients use sound eye, however, sometimes the paretic eye may be used for fixation if: (1) it has better visual acuity, (2) it is originally dominant eye, or (3) fixation with paretic eye increases the separation of the double picture (due to secondary deviation) which causes less problem.

Muscle sequelae occur to much lesser degrees in patients with congenital paralysis as compared to the acquired paralysis. These occur more in paralysis due to lesions of the nerves than the lesions of muscles and include the following:

i. *Overaction of the contralateral synergistic (yoke) muscle.* Overaction of the yoke muscle develops quickly, when paretic eye is used for fixation and slowly, when the sound eye is used for fixation. This overaction of the yoke muscle is responsible for secondary deviation of the sound eye. With the passage of time, this overaction becomes habitual due to the development of spasm and contracture and remains, even if the original paresis should recover spontaneously.

ii. *Contracture of the direct antagonist.* After paralysis of a particular extraocular muscle, its direct antagonist is more or less unopposed and thus overact and is responsible for the primary deviation. Within a few weeks, the overacting muscle becomes spastic, contracting more and more leading to a greater angle of deviation. Eventually, this leads to a contracture, an organic change in the muscle in which muscle fibres are replaced by fibrous tissue.

iii. *Secondary inhibitional palsy of the contra-lateral antagonist muscle.* It is a manifestation of Hering's law of equal innervation. Since the direct antagonist of the paretic muscle is more or less unopposed, so it will require less than normal innervation for a particular extent of a movement. According to Hering's law, the same innervation will flow to its yoke muscle (which is contralateral antagonist of the paretic muscle). Consequently, the contralateral antagonist of the paretic muscle will exhibit a weakness; which has been called the secondary inhibitional palsy of the contralateral antagonist muscle. Perhaps the better term will be '*simulated weakness of the yoke's antagonist*' or PAY syndrome: pseudo-weakness of the antagonist of a yoke. This underaction of the yoke muscle of the antagonist occurs earlier and is more pronounced, when the paretic eye is used for fixation than when the sound eye is preferred for fixation.

The muscle sequelae developing following paresis of a particular muscle are shown in Table 12.1.

Figures 12.11 and 12.12 show the muscle sequelae occurring in a patient with right lateral rectus and left superior oblique muscles, respectively.

8. *Abnormal head posture.* An abnormal head posture is a common feature of the paralytic strabismus. A compensatory head posture does not necessarily develop in every patient with a paresis or paralysis of extraocular muscles. However, when present, it can aid in making the diagnosis.

Reasons for abnormal head posture. Abnormal head posture may be adapted for any of the following two reasons:

i. *To achieve binocular single vision.* Most frequently, an abnormal head posture is adapted to achieve binocular single vision, i.e. to avoid the troubling diplopia and/or confusion. For this purpose, the head is turned into the field of

Table 12.1 *Muscle sequelae following paresis of extraocular muscles*

Paretic muscle	Muscle sequelae		
	Overaction of contralateral synergistic (yoke) muscle	Contracture of directant antagonist muscle	Secondary inhibitional palsy of the contralateral antagonist muscle
Right lateral rectus	Left medial rectus	Right medial rectus	Left lateral rectus
Right medial rectus	Left lateral rectus	Right lateral rectus	Left medial rectus
Right superior oblique	Left inferior rectus	Right inferior oblique	Left superior rectus
Right inferior oblique	Left superior rectus	Right superior oblique	Left inferior rectus
Right superior rectus	Left inferior oblique	Right inferior rectus	Left superior oblique
Right inferior rectus	Left superior oblique	Right superior rectus	Left inferior oblique

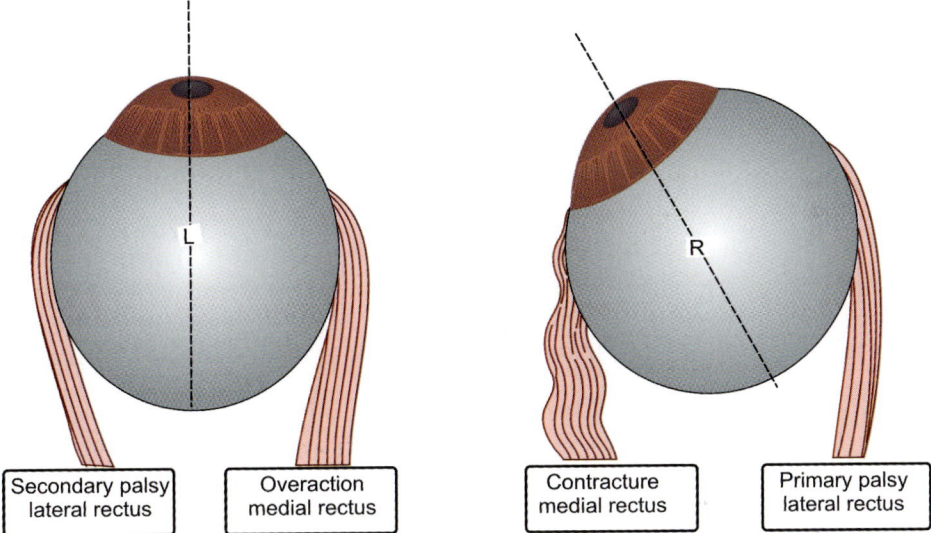

Secondary palsy lateral rectus | Overaction medial rectus | Contracture medial rectus | Primary palsy lateral rectus

Fig. 12.11 *Muscle sequelae following paralysis of right lateral rectus muscle.*

action of the paralysed muscle, and that the eyes are directed by the *doll's head phenomenon*. This process allows the patient to move his/her limited field of single vision so that it coincides with his/her egocentric (straight ahead) position. In other words, the patient can see the things in front of him/her as single.

ii. *To achieve wide separation of the two images.* Less frequently, patients with paralytic strabismus develop abnormal head posture in order to increase the separation between diplopic images. This occurs in patients who have no useful field of bifoveal single vision but suffer from the constant diplopia. Since they have no choice but to live with it, they attempt to separate

the double pictures as far as possible by turning the head in the field of paretic muscle. In this field, the deviation of the involved eye will be maximal and, thus, the 'true' and the 'false' image of objects in front will be maximally separated.

Components of abnormal head posture

A. *In horizontal rectus muscle palsy.* If one of the horizontally acting muscles (lateral or medial rectus) is involved, the abnormal head posture will consist of only one component, i.e. *face turn towards the action of paretic muscle.* For example, in a paresis of right lateral rectus muscle, there will be a face turn to the right side, and in a paresis of right medial rectus muscle, there will be a face turn to the left side.

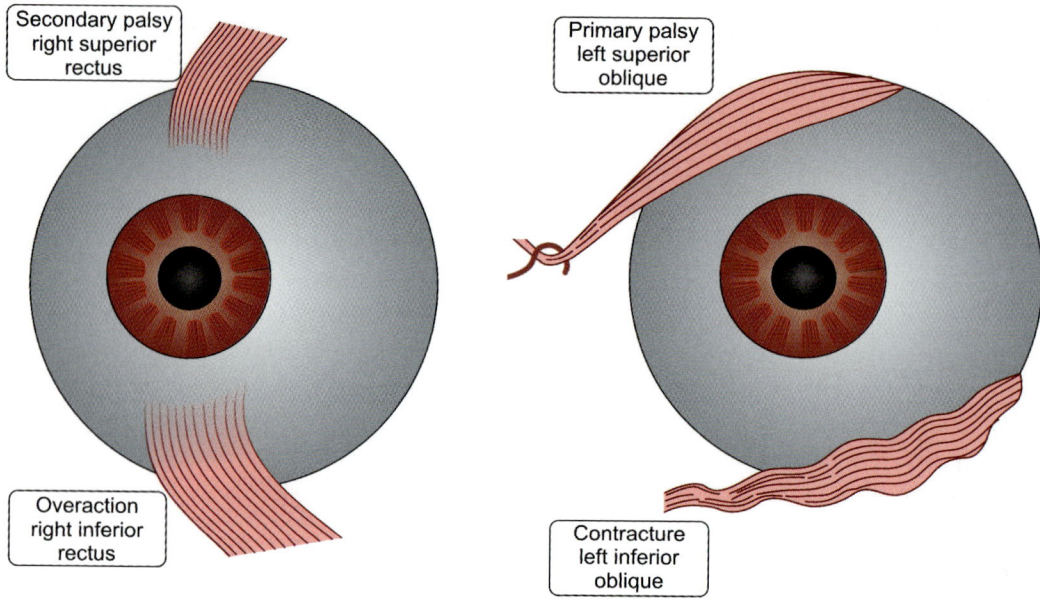

Fig. 12.12 *Muscle sequelae following paralysis of left superior oblique muscle.*

B. *In palsy of cyclovertically acting muscles.* The superior and inferior recti and the superior and inferior oblique muscles are cyclovertically acting muscles and contraction of any one of them alone would produce a combination of vertical, horizontal and torsional movements. If any one of these muscles is paretic, there will be three components of abnormal head posture as follows:

• Chin elevation or depression
• Face turn
• Head tilt

1. *Chin elevation or depression* occurs in paralysis/paresis of elevators or depressors of the eye, respectively. By doll's head pheno- menon, in chin elevation, the eyes move down and in chin depression, the eyes move up. In this way, the involved eye is brought out of the field of action of paretic elevator or depressor muscle.

2. *Face turn.* As mentioned above, face turn in the paresis of a horizontally acting muscle (medial or lateral rectus) is towards the action of the paretic muscle. However, in the paresis of one of the cyclovertically acting muscles, the face turn is such that the eyes are brought away from the field in which the muscle has its greatest vertical effect. Thus in the case of superior and inferior recti which have their maximal vertical effect in abduction, the face is turned so that the involved eye is adducted, when the patient looks straight ahead, i.e. in paresis of the vertical recti, the face will be turned towards the affected eye. Since the superior and inferior oblique muscles have their greatest vertical effect in adduction, the opposite is true for them and the face is turned so that the eye with the involved oblique is abducted, i.e. face is turned away from the affected eye (towards left in paresis of oblique muscle of right eye).

3. *Head tilt.* The head tilt occurs to compensate for the torsion or to help relieve the vertical separation of the double images as follows:

• In paresis of a oblique muscle, head tilt occurs to compensate the torsion caused by the direct antagonist of the paralysed muscle. For example, in paresis of right superior oblique, the head will tilt towards left to compensate for the extorsion caused by right inferior oblique muscle.

• In paresis of a vertical rectus muscle, the head tilt occurs to compensate the torsion caused by the contralateral antagonist of the paralysed muscle. For example, in paresis of right superior rectus, the head will tilt to the right to compensate for the extorsion of the left eye caused by overacting left inferior oblique muscle.

Diagnostic importance of abnormal head posture. The typical head posture adapted may be a pointer towards the paretic muscle especially in a fresh case of isolated muscle palsy.

Abnormal head postures assumed in paresis of extraocular muscle of right eye are as shown in Table 12.2.

As discussed above, it is not difficult to understand the different abnormal head postures that would theoretically occur as a result of the deficient eye movements caused by paralysis of individual muscle. However, in practice, conditions are not so clear because of the following factors:

- The paresis may be so slight that a partial compensation is already sufficient and the typical head posture may never develop.
- More than one muscle may be involved leading to a complex picture.
- Muscle sequelae and secondary changes may alter the original condition.

Ocular torticollis. The abnormal head posture adopted by the individuals with congenital and infantile paralytic squint is sometimes referred to as acquired ocular torticollis, because it resembles an orthopaedic deformity called congenital torticollis. In the later condition, the head cannot be straightened due to organic changes in the neck musculature. In contrast, the ocular torticollis is merely a functional position and the head can be straightened passively. In the early stages, if one eye is occluded, the patient with ocular torticollis will straighten the head. However, in late stages, secondary scoliosis may occur as a consequence of ocular

torticollis and because of it, patient's head may not straighten with monocular occlusion. Further, if secondary vertebral column changes have been allowed to develop, it may no longer be possible to correct the abnormal head posture even by surgically aligning the eyes.

Facial asymmetry due to atrophy of the lower side of the face is a feature of both long-standing ocular as well as congenital torticollis, so it cannot be considered a differentiating feature.

9. *Sensory adaptations*. Sensory adaptations such as suppression, abnormal retinal correspondence and amblyopia are, in general, less known with paralytic squint vis-a-vis concomitant squint; perhaps, because of the following reasons:

- Patients with paralytic squint can assume abnormal head posture to achieve a single binocular vision which may prevent the occurrence of suppression, ARC and amblyopia.
- Patients with paralytic squint have variable angle of deviation in various positions of gaze; while sensory adaptations usually develop in patients who have stable and constant angle of deviation.

With the passage of time, the deviation becomes increasingly comitant, as discussed under spread of comitance. Under such circumstances, the patient is unable to maintain fusion in any direction of gaze, and as a result, suppression, ARC and amblyopia become established.

Occurrence of comitance in paralytic squint is common but not universal. If the strabismus remains incomitant and onset is during childhood, diplopia in the paretic field of fixation may be prevented by *regional suppression.*

Amblyopia occurs in only those patients of paralytic squint who are unable to maintain simultaneous binocular vision in any direction of gaze and in whom paralysis occurs in early life. Further, sometimes, presence of amblyopia may cause confusion in the diagnosis of paralytic squint. This is because some patients, who prefer to fixate with the paretic eye because of certain reasons mentioned earlier, develop amblyopia in the non-paretic deviated eye.

Table 12.2 Abnormal head posture in extraocular muscle paralysis

Muscle paralysed	Components of abnormal head posture		
	Chin	Face turn	Head tilt
Right superior rectus	Elevation	Right	Right
Right inferior rectus	Depression	Right	Left
Right superior oblique	Depression	Left	Left
Right inferior oblique	Elevation	Left	Right
Right lateral rectus	–	Right	–
Right medial rectus	–	Left	–

■ INVESTIGATIONS OF INCOMITANT SQUINT

It should include: (1) evaluation from strabismic point of view and (2) investigations to find out the cause of incomitant squint, such as orbital ultrasonography, orbital and skull computerized tomographic scanning and detailed neurological investigations (which are beyond the scope of this chapter).

A detailed work-up of a strabismic patient is described on page 100. However, the salient points relevant to the paralytic strabismus are mentioned here in brief.

History

A detailed history should be taken with reference to following points:

1. *Subjective symptoms*
- *Diplopia.* Enquiry should be made to ascertain: Onset, constant/intermittent, distance at which diplopia is noticed, relative position of images, field where greatest separation of images occurs, any change since onset, does diplopia disappear, when eye is occluded.
- *Confusion.* It occurs due to formation of images of the different objects on the corresponding points of two retina.
- *Other subjective symptoms* which a patient with paralytic strabismus may experience are: Dificulty in focussing, headache, eye strain, general asthenopic symptoms and discomfort from abnormal head posture.

2. *Objective symptoms*
- Constant/intermittent deviation
- Abnormal head posture
- Ptosis, exophthalmos

3. *Any attributed cause*
4. *Any previous ocular problems and treatment taken*
5. *General health*
6. *Family history*

Inspection

1. Ocular posture
2. Abnormal head posture; note its exact components
3. Facial asymmetry
4. Ptosis, exophthalmos

Cover test

It should be carried out for near and distance; with and without abnormal head posture. The cover test will detect:

1. Presence of any manifest or latent deviation.
2. Type of deviation
3. Incomitance—primary versus secondary deviation
4. Normally fixing eye. Patient usually fixes with the nonaffected eye; but this may be influenced by visual acuity or dominant eye.

Ocular movements

Investigation of ocular movements is carried out while the patient watches a fixation target, i.e. moved from the primary position into each of the cardinal positions of gaze.

1. Version movements. The examiner compares the movement of the two eyes in all positions of gaze. Symmetric movement indicates that no defect is present. Unequal movements are seen in underactions, overactions and limitations.

2. Duction movements. Monocular movements are of value only in differentiating between a paresis and a total paralysis. Testing for ductions also helps to detect mechanical limitation of movements.

3. Doll's head movements and command movements testing is of particular use in supranuclear gaze palsies.

Measurement of deviation

1. Synoptophore method. Major amblyoscope is the best instrument for measurement of deviation in paralytic squint; since measurements are taken to compare the size of the deviation in each of the cardinal directions of gaze while each eye in turn is used for fixation. To make the comparison valid, it is extremely important that the fixation object be moved an equal distance from the primary position in each direction. For this, synoptophore can be adjusted so that the deviation can be measured while the patient is looking at an equal angle from the primary position in all directions of gaze.

2. Prism and cover test. It is an easy method, while carried out with the help of a prism bar. Measurements should be taken with and without abnormal head posture for near and distance fixation, fixing either eye. Measurements can be made in all the cardinal directions, but for comparison these are not considered very accurate. Since it is not possible to measure at an equal angle from the primary position in all directions; as is possible with the synoptophore.

3. *Measurement of torsional deviation* can be made with special slides on major amblyoscope, or on adapted Lees screen.

Note. In a paresis or paralysis of an extraocular muscle, the deviation will be greatest in the direction of maximal singular action of the muscle while the affected eye is fixating.

Diplopia test

For details, *see* page 121. Salient points are as follows:

- Tested with red/green goggles and a linear light, or without dissociation aids.
- Position of maximum vertical and horizontal separation of images and position of maximum torsion is noted.
- Distal image belongs to the affected eye.
- The results are recorded either by written description or as diplopia chart. Diplopia charts of paralysis of extraocular muscles of right eye and left eye are shown in Figs 12.13 and 12.14, respectively.

Bielschowsky three-step test (B3ST)

The classical head tilt test was proposed by Bielschowsky to differentiate between superior oblique palsy in one eye and superior rectus palsy in the contralateral side. However, presently in practice is the three step test as modified by Parks'. It is useful in diagnosing the paresis of any cyclovertically acting muscle. There are in total 8 cyclovertically acting muscles; 4 work as depressors of the eyes, and 4 work as elevators. The two muscles on each eye that are responsible for depression are the inferior rectus and superior oblique, and the two muscles on each eye that are responsible for elevation are the superior rectus and the inferior oblique.

As expected, at the onset of a cyclovertical muscle palsy, there will be limitation in the field of action of the paralysed muscle. Shortly thereafter, an overaction in the field of the antagonist muscle will be noted. With time, this overaction will produce a contracture of the antagonist. Thereafter, there will be spread of comitance, so that the amount of deviation will gradually increase and become approximately the same in the all fields of gaze. At this point, based on analysis of duction and version movements of the eye, the diagnosis of cyclovertical palsy becomes impossible. At this juncture, the *Parks' modification over Bielschowsky's head tilt* test can be quite useful. There are three steps of this test, each of which eliminates half of the remaining potential muscles, leaving only one muscle to be blamed after the three steps.

Procedure of three-step test

Step 1
- Perform cover-uncover test in primary position and determine which eye is hypertropic. If the patient's presenting sign is a hypodeviation, consider it hyperdeviation of the opposite eye. Step 1 reduces the number of affected muscles from 8 to 4.
- *A right hypertropia (RHT)* implies any of the following:
  – Weakness of depressors of right eye (RIR, RSO), or
  – Weakness of elevators of left eye (LIO, LSR).
- *A left hypertropia (LHT)* implies any of the following:
  – Weakness of depressors of left eye (LIR, LSO), or
  – Weakness of elevators of right eye (RIO, RSR).
- Let us assume, for example, the patient being examined has LHT. Draw an oval (with red lines) around the two possible muscle pairs responsible for LHT (Fig.12.15A).

Step 2
- Determine whether hypertropia (HT) is larger in right gaze or left gaze.
- If the LHT is larger in right gaze, it implies weakness of any of the 4 vertically acting muscles in right gaze:
  – RSR, RIR
  – LIO, LSO

- If the LHT is larger in left gaze, it implies weakness of any of the 4 vertically acting muscles in left gaze, i.e.
  – LSR, LIR
  – RIO, RSO

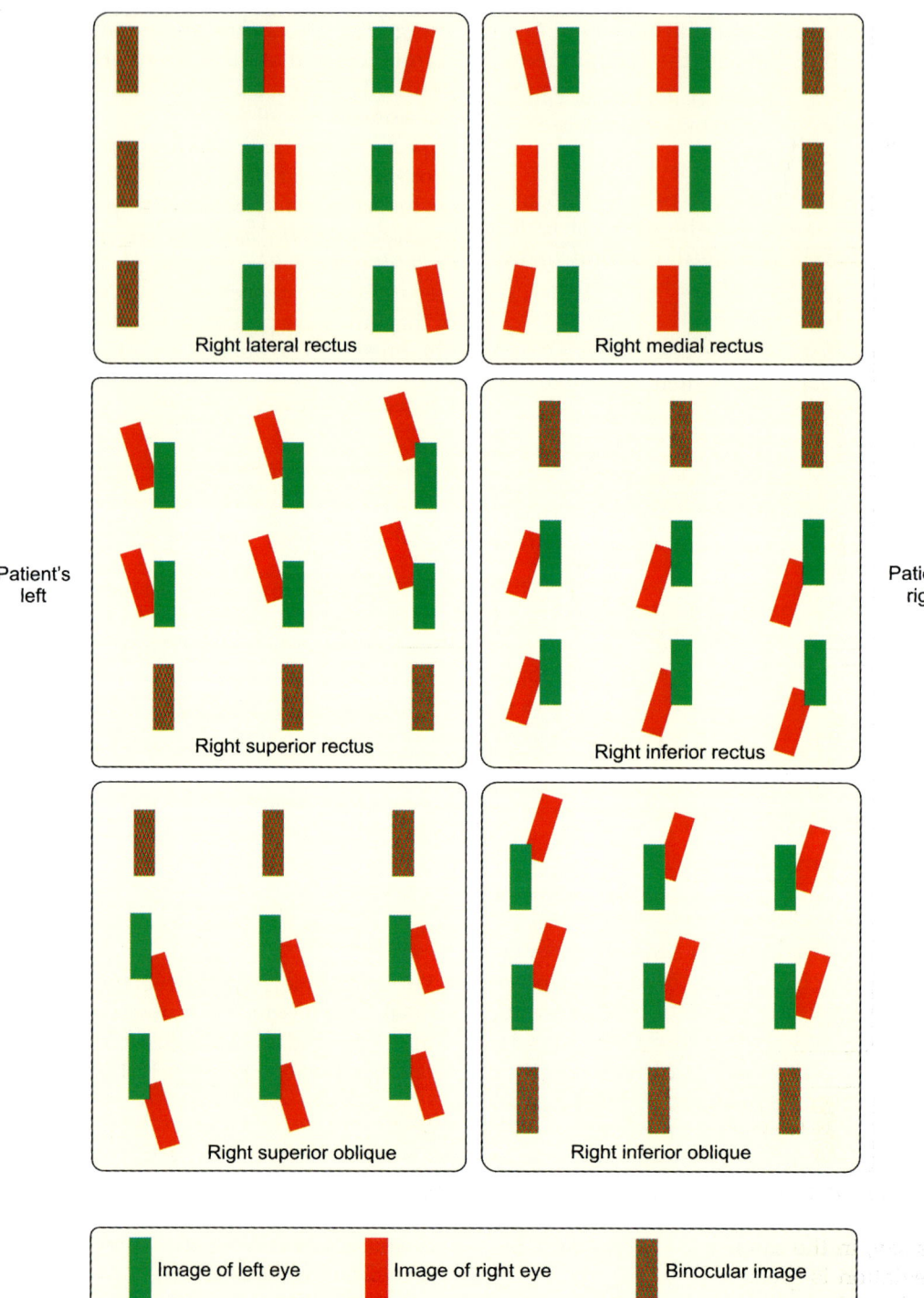

Fig. 12.13 *Diplopia charts (patient's view) of paralysis of extraocular muscles of the right eye.*

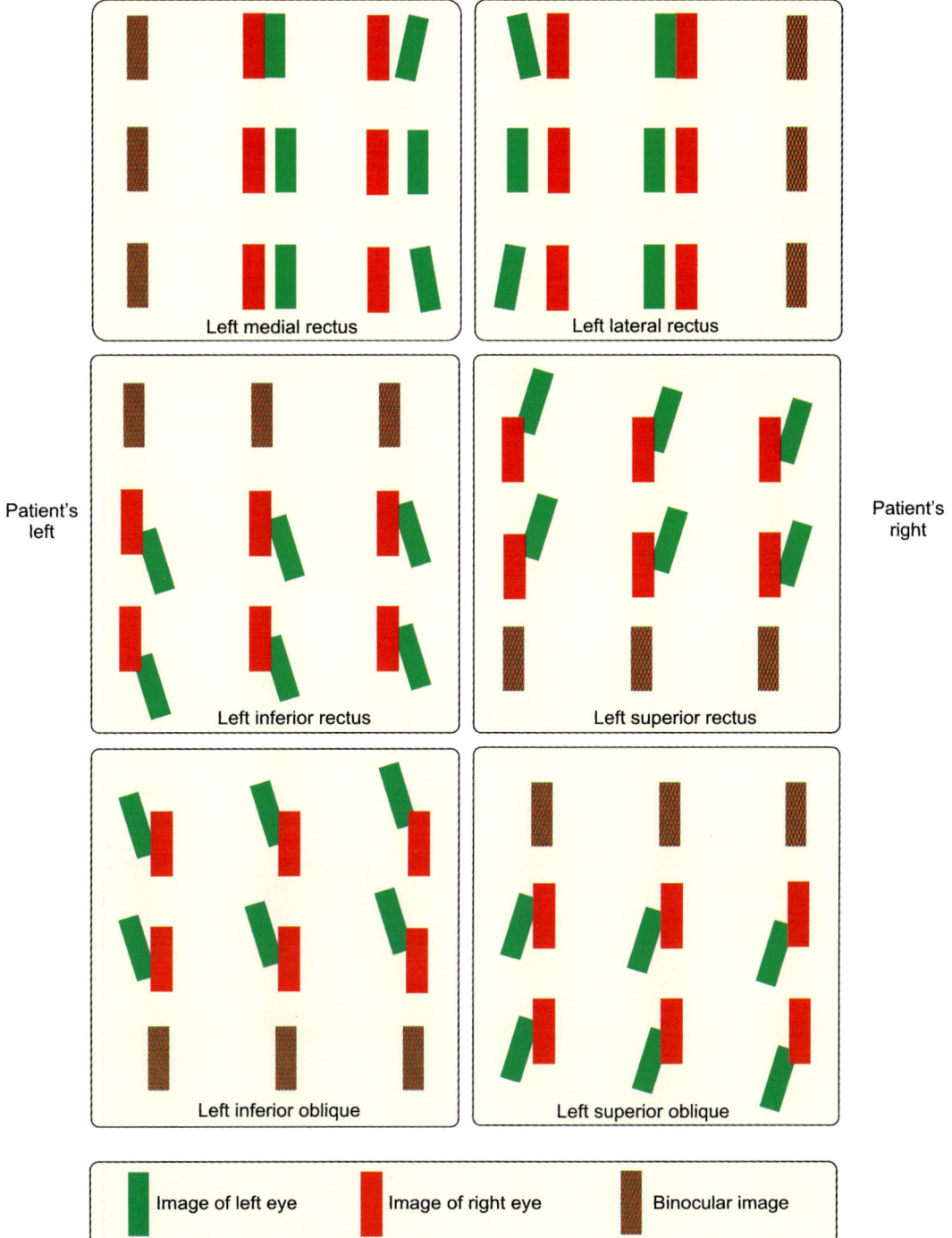

Fig. 12.14 *Diplopia charts (patient's view) of paralysis of extraocular muscles of the left eye.*

- Let us say, in the same patient having LHT, the deviation is greater in right gaze. Draw an oval (with green lines) around the two possible muscle pairs (Fig. 12.15B).

- Note that at this point, the paretic muscle must be either the LSO or RSR muscle, since they are the only muscles encircled twice (Fig. 12.15B).

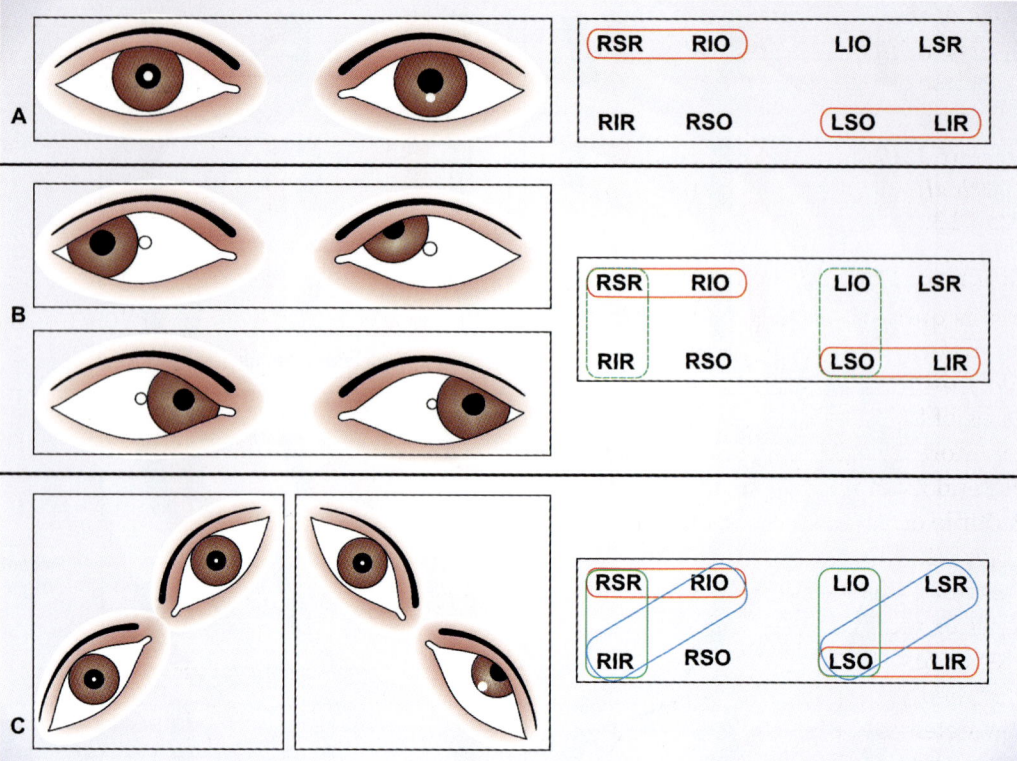

Fig. 12.15 *Bielschowsky's three-step test (B3ST) in a patient with left superior oblique paralysis. A, step 1; B, step 2; C, step 3 (for explanation, see text).*

Step 3

- Determine, if the HT is larger, when measured during head tilt to the left or right. For proper measurement, the base of the prism should be held parallel to the floor of the orbit and not parallel to the floor of the room. The Maddox rod and correcting prism should be held so that the line and base are parallel to the floor of orbit (Fig. 12.16).
- If the LHT is larger, when the head is tilted to the right, this implicates any of four muscles that act vertically in right tilt position, i.e. either intorters of right eye (RSR, RSO) or extorters of left eye (LIR, LIO).
- If the LHT is larger, when the head is tilted to the left, this implicates any of the four muscles that act vertically in left tilt position, i.e. either intorters of left eye (LSR, LSO) or extorters of right eye (RIR, RIO).
- Now, for the same individual, suppose that the vertical deviation is quite large, when the head is tilted to the left and is almost absent, when

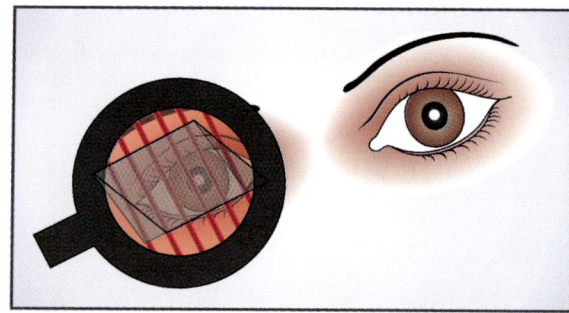

Fig. 12.16 *Measurement of deviation using Maddox rod and prism in a patient with right hypertropia. Note, head is tilted to the right and base of the prism is held parallel to the floor of the orbit. Maddox rod is held in such a way that the red line seen is also parallel to the floor of the orbit.*

the head is tilted to the right. Draw an oval (with blue lines) around the muscle implicated, i.e. (LSR, LSO, RIR, RIO) (Fig. 12.15C).
- Note that at this point, the LSO is the only muscle, i.e. surrounded by three ovals and is connected by the line that represents head tilt to the right (Fig. 12.15C).

Summary of the test shown in Fig. 12.15:

Step 1: LHT (LIR, LSO, RSR or RIO)

Step 2: Worse in right gaze (RSR or LSO)

Step 3: Worse in left tilt (LSO)

Results of B3ST in paralysis of various cyclovertically acting muscles are summarized in Table 12.3.

Limitations of Park's three-step test

This test is quite useful in general, but it is not always diagnostic and can be misleading, especially during following conditions:

- In cases of long-standing paresis.
- When more than one muscle are paretic, e.g.
  - Bilateral fourth nerve palsy
  - Multiple other muscle weakness
- In cases with restrictions.
  - Superior rectus overaction
  - Superior rectus contracture
  - Inferior restriction
- Dissociated vertical deviation (DVD)
- Pulley heterotopia
- Superior rectus palsy
- Skew deviation
- Prior extraocular muscle surgery

Quantitative measurement of extraocular muscle actions

The quantitative measurement of extraocular muscle action is most essential to comment about the paretic muscles and the pathological sequelae of the paralysis, viz. overaction, contracture and secondary inhibitional palsy.

Commonly employed tests to have a graphic record of the relative power of extraocular muscles in all directions of gaze are as follows:

- Hess screen test
- Lees screen test
- Lancaster red and green test

These tests are based on haploscopic principle and described in detail on page 121.

Uses of haploscopic tests

These tests are repeatable and their uses are as follows:

- Diagnose underactions and overactions of extraocular muscles and provide a good pictorial representation of muscle actions.
- Diagnose A- and V-phenomena.
- Diagnose mechanical/neurological palsy
- Diagnose congenital/acquired palsy
- Aid in plan of surgery—preoperatively
- Show effect of surgery—postoperatively.
- Provide an accurate and permanent record of change in state of ocular movements in subsequent visits and thereby form part of serial record of progress of palsy.
- Measure torsional movement with linear pointer (Dulley and Harden) or cyclotiltmeter (Brown).

Field of binocular fixation

It must be tested, wherever applicable, i.e. if patient has some field of binocular single vision. It provides, useful and repeatable information. The area of binocular single vision is opposite to the direction in which ocular motility is impaired.

The aim of treatment of muscle paralysis is to provide comfortable field of binocular fixation, i.e. the central field and lower quadrants.

For details of the test, *see* page 127.

Other tests

Other tests which can be carried out, if necessary, includes forced duction test, EMG, EOG, orbital ultrasonography and computerized tomographic scanning.

Table 12.3 *Results of Bielschowsky three-step head tilt test in paralysis of cyclovertically acting muscles*

Paralysed muscle	Bielschowsky head tilt test		
	Step 1 (hypertropia in primary gaze)	Step 2 (HT worse in left or right gaze)	Step 3 (HT worse on left or right tilt)
RSO	RHT	Left	Right
RIR	RHT	Right	Left
LIO	RHT	Right	Right
LSR	RHT	Left	Left
LSO	LHT	Right	Left
LIR	LHT	Left	Right
RIO	LHT	Left	Left
RSR	LHT	Right	Right

DIFFERENTIAL DIAGNOSIS OF INCOMITANT SQUINT

Differential diagnosis to be considered in patients with incomitant squint in general are as follows:

• Comitant (non-paralytic) versus incomitant (paralytic) squint.

• Congenital versus acquired palsies.

• Paralytic versus restrictive incomitant squint.

Comitant (non-paralytic) versus incomitant (paralytic) squint

As mentioned earlier, by and large, there arises no problem in differentiating comitant (non-paralytic) squint from the paralytic (incomitant) squint of recent onset. However, in patients with long-standing paralysis, there occurs spread of comitance and thus it becomes extremely difficult and at times even impossible to differentiate such a condition from the comitant squint. Anyshow, for a ready reference, the differences between paralytic and non-paralytic squint are depicted in Table 12.4.

Congenital versus acquired ocular palsy

Many a time, patients with congenital paralysis of an extraocular muscle may remain asymptomatic for decades because of either a strong fusion mechanism or by an unnoticed slight abnormal head posture. Such a patient, when reaches adult life, the chances are that, unless the latent deviation is small one, decompensation will begin to occur, especially between the ages of 30 and

S. no.	Feature	Paralytic squint	Non-paralytic squint
		Table 12.4 *Differences between paralytic and non-paralytic squint*	
1.	Age of onset	Any age	Usually in childhood
2.	Type of onset	Usually sudden, rarely may be slow or since birth	Usually gradual
3.	History of head injury	Common	Uncommon
4.	Diplopia	Usually present	Usually absent
5.	Ocular movements	Limited in the direction of paralysed muscle	Usually full
6.	False projection	It is common in palsy of recent onset, i.e. patient cannot correctly locate the object in space, when asked to do so in direction of paralyzed muscle. There occurs past pointing.	False projection is negative
7.	Head posture	A particular abnormal head posture may be present, depending upon the muscle paralysed.	Normal
8.	Nausea and vertigo	Usually present, due to confusion, diplopia and false projection	Absent
9.	Primary versus secondary deviation	Secondary deviation is more than primary deviation	Secondary deviation is equal to primary deviation
10.	Sensory adaptations (ARC, suppression, amblyopia)	Uncommon	Common
11.	Cyclotropia	Common with cyclovertical paresis	Uncommon, except in A- and V-patterns
12.	Muscle sequelae	Present in old cases	Absent
13.	Neurological findings or systemic diseases	May be present	Usually absent

40 years. The patient may notice that he/she is beginning to suffer from an intermittent diplopia, especially if he/she is tired, overworked, or suffering from ill health. Some of these patients may develop intermittent squint without diplopia due to suppression of the image of the deviating eye. Such patients may experience difficulty in focussing or have a feeling of using only one eye.

Under these circumstances, one needs to differentiate between cases of congenital paralysis with recent decompensation and those of acquired paralysis of recent onset. It is very essential, since in the former the treatment is invariably operative while the latter requires a diligent search for its cause by a complete medical and neuro-ophthalmologic evaluation and the appropriate treatment. Some of the chief differences between the congenital and acquired ocular palsies are summarized in Table. 12.5.

Paralytic versus restrictive incomitant squint

Incomitant ocular deviations are known both due to palsies as well as restrictions of extraocular muscles and are often confused with one another by even experienced examiners. Though, these are two distinct problems but mere measurement obtained with prism and alternate cover tests with either eye fixing do not differentiate between them, since in both, the secondary deviation is typically greater than the primary deviation. However, a differentiation between the two is most important for the successful treatment of incomitant deviation. It is unequivocal to state that the restrictions must be relieved first, before any other therapy, whether surgical or non-surgical to be effective.

Commonly employed tests to differentiate between palsies and restrictions are as follows:

1. *Passive forced duction test* (traction test)

As mentioned above, detection of associated restriction is most important for the successful therapy of an incomitant squint. Therefore, it is mandatory to carry out forced duction test (FDT) before any surgical therapy is undertaken.

S.no.	Feature	Congenital ocular palsy	Recent acquired ocular palsy
		Table 12.5 *Differences between congenital and acquired ocular palsies*	
1.	Onset of symptoms	Usually indefinite and intermittent	Usually definite and sudden
2.	Diplopia	Rare, intermittent diplopia in decompensation	Almost invariably present, but may be limited to paretic field
3.	Primary deviation	May be intermittent or constant angle of deviation may be large; but symptoms may be only slight	Usually constant Angle of deviation may be small and yet the symptoms may be pronounced
4.	Secondary deviation	Only slightly greater than the primary deviation (due to spread of comitance)	Usually much greater than the primary deviation
5.	Past pointing	Usually absent	Present
6.	Abnormal head posture	May persist on covering paretic eye because of secondary scoliosis and contracture of neck muscles	Disappears on covering paretic eye
7.	Facial asymmetry	Common with torticollis of long standing	Absent
8.	Amblyopia	May be present	Absent
9.	Forced duction test	May be positive due to contracture of antagonist	Negative
10.	Abnormal head posture in old photographs	May be present	Absent

Steps of the forced duction test (FDT)

i. *Anaesthesia.* In adults and cooperative elder children, FDT can be performed preoperatively under topical anaesthesia with 4% xylocaine instilled every 4 minutes for 4 times. In small and uncooperative children, FDT is done under general anaesthesia during surgery, taking an account of following points:

– To remove the effect of tonic innervational factors, the FDT should be performed, when patient has reached stage 3 of anaesthesia.
– If succinylcholine is to be used, preferably the FDT should be performed while the patient has received an inhalation anaesthetic by mask, but before intubation. Otherwise one will have to wait for at least 20 minutes till the contraction of the extraocular muscles caused by succinylcholine is over.
– Pancuronium, a nondepolarizing muscle relaxant, that does not alter the FDT, should be preferred over succinylcholine.

ii. *Grasping of the globe.* After proper anaesthesia, the globe should be grasped near the limbus with either a forceps without teeth or Pierse forceps to avoid tearing of the conjunctiva. Preferably, the globe should be held with the help of two forceps at right angle to the axis in which restriction is to be tested.

For example, in a patient with divergent squint (Fig. 12.17A), to distinguish between lateral rectus paralysis and mechanical restriction involving the medial aspect of the globe, the forceps should be applied at 6 and 12 O'clock positions (Fig. 12.17B).

iii. *Passive rotation of the globe.* After grasping, the globe should be rotated passively towards the direction of action of suspected weak muscle, e.g. into abduction in patients with lateral rectus weakness versus mechanical restriction involving medial aspect of the globe (Fig. 12.17C), taking following precautions:

– When FDT is being performed under topical anaesthesia, patient should be instructed to look at his/her hand held in the direction in which the eye is to be rotated by the forceps. This will help in avoiding the effect of tonic innervational factor.

– Care should be taken not to push the globe into the orbit posteriorly, since this may conceal a restriction of the movement resulting in a false negative FDT.
• To test the restrictions in the field of action of recti, the globe should be rotated, up, down, medially or laterally.
• To test the restrictions in the field of action of oblique muscles, the globe should be rotated both down and in, and up and in.

Note. FDT should be repeated at the time of surgery and also after completion of the surgery.

Interpretation of the results of FDT

1. *Forced duction test is labelled negative,* if no resistance is encountered during passive rotation and the examiner can rotate the globe to its full extent. A negative FDT implies that the motility defect is clearly caused by paralysis of the weak muscle.
2. *Positive FDT* is labelled, if a resistance is encountered during passive rotation of the globe. With a feeling of resistance, if the examiner can rotate the globe no further than the patient voluntarily can, the motility defect is purely due to mechanical restriction. However, with a feeling of resistance, if the examiner can passively rotate the globe beyond where the patient can voluntarily rotate it, but not to its full extent, the motility defect is a combination of mechanical restriction and agonist muscle weakness.

The restriction noted in the positive FDT may be one of the following types:

i. *Leash restriction* is caused by the mechanical factors such as marked scarring of Tenon's capsule and conjunctiva, contracture of an extraocular muscle and/or entrapment of muscle or its facial sheath on the side of globe opposite the limited field of rotation.

The globe can be passively rotated freely up to a point after which tethering effect of restriction does not allow the globe to move further any more. Such a restriction is not only felt but can also be seen as a taut string of conjunctiva (*String sign*).

ii. *Reverse leash restriction.* The tethering effect of restriction is similar to leash restriction as described above. However, the mechanical

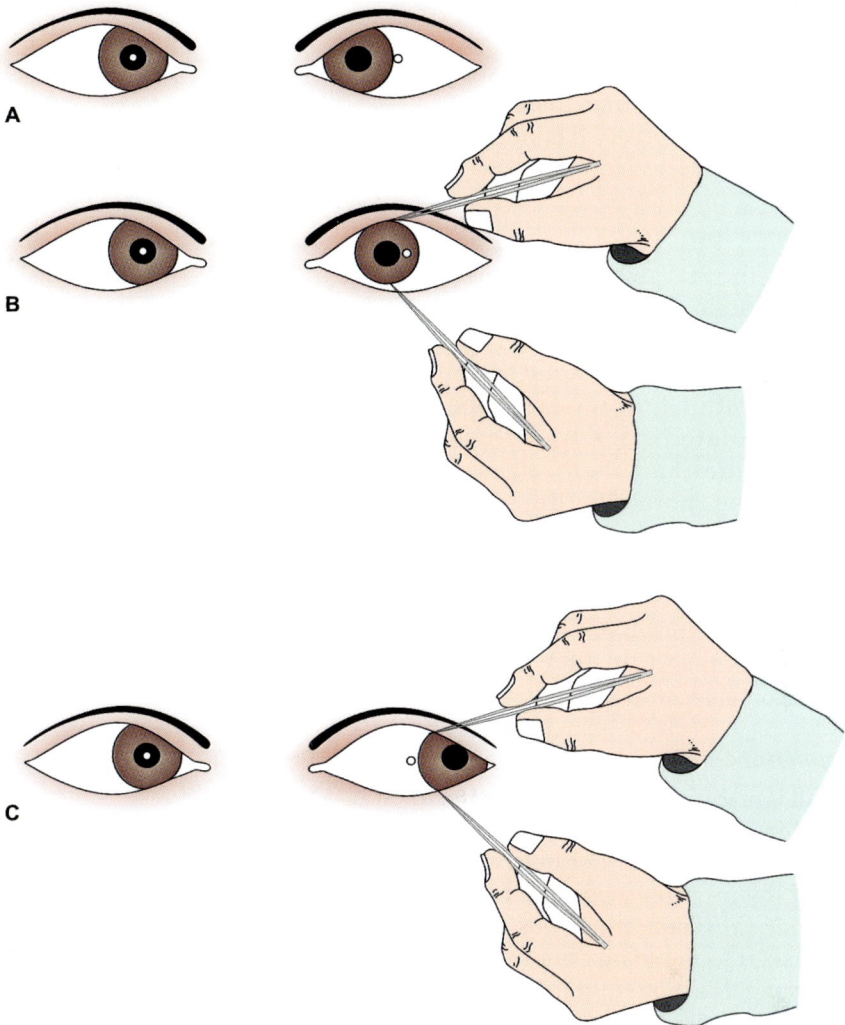

Fig. 12.17 *Technique of forced duction test (for explanation, see text).*

factors responsible for tethering are marked shortening of conjunctiva and Tenon's capsule, marked posterior scarring of orbital tissues or a tight posterior fixation suture used in Faden's operation on the same side of globe in which rotation is limited.

iii. *Elastic restriction* is caused by an early contracture of a muscle following paresis of its agonist, co-contraction of extraocular muscles due to effect of succinylcholine and orbital cellulitis. In contrast to the leash and reverse leash restriction (in which globe can be rotated to a point after which tethering effect of restriction does not allow the globe to move further any more), in elastic restriction, there occurs a partial resistance over the entire range of ocular movement which can be overcome by an increased force.

2. Exaggerated traction test

It is a modified forced duction test which is performed to estimate the tightness in superior oblique (SO) and inferior oblique (IO) muscles.

Procedure. For checking tightness of RSO, the eyeball is grasped near the limbus at 6 and 9 O'clock positions, as described in FDT. To perform this test, the eyeball is first pushed in the orbit and then elevated, adducted and rolled back and forth by extorting and intorting the globe across the tendon. During this manoeuvre, if the eyeball jumps across the tendon, tightness of the superior oblique is indicated.

Tightness of the inferior oblique is also tested in the similar manner, except that instead of elevating and adducting, the eyeball is pushed down and nasally.

3. Spring-back balance test

It is a continuation of the FDT, when performed under general anaesthesia. It is of specific use in patients who are suspected (after FDT) of having mechanical restriction and not a weak muscle. In this test, after holding near the limbus, eyeball is rotated back and forth vigorously for 2–3 times and then released suddenly. After settling, normally, the globe comes to rest in straight ahead position. However, in the presence of a significant mechanical restriction, the eyeball will be drawn towards the direction of the mechanical pull, e.g. the eyeball will be adducted, if the cause of mechanical restriction is located medially.

4. Active force generation test

In this test, eyeball is stabilized with the forceps applied at the limbus under topical anaesthesia and patient is asked to move his/her both eyes in the direction of the muscle to be tested. For example, if right lateral rectus muscle is to be tested, patient is asked to move his/her eyes in dextroversion. During this movement, the force generated by the contracting muscle of the eye being tested (e.g. Rt LR) is transmitted through the forceps to the examiner's fingers. From the feel of the transmitted force, examiner can judge subjectively whether the contracting muscle is weak or normal (Fig.12.18). For objectively quantifying this test, calibrated forceps are available which indicate the amount of force generated in grams. A normally acting muscle generates a force of 60–80 g in extreme gaze. This test is quite useful in diagnosing the weak muscle. However, it can only be performed in alert and co-operative patients.

5. Lid fissure changes on eye movements

• *Narrowing of lid fissure* along with globe retraction is seen in restrictive squints, as in Duane's retraction syndrome.

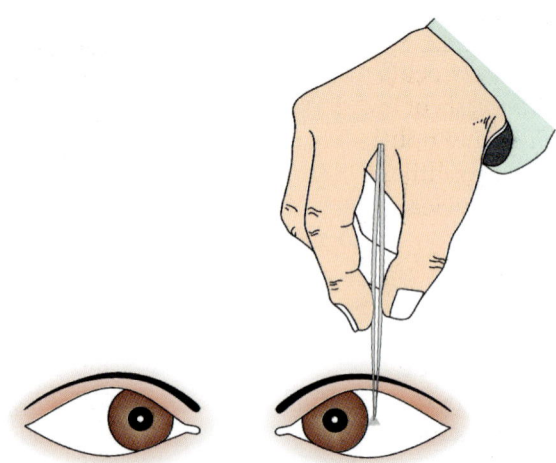

Fig. 12.18 *Technique of judging active force generated during ocular movement (muscle contraction). (For explanation, see text).*

• *Lid fissure widening* and a relative proptosis is noted in paralytic squint as the patient looks into the field of action of paretic rectus muscle.

6. Electro-oculographic measurement of saccadic velocity

Saccades are sudden, jerky conjugate eye movements, that occur as the gaze shifts from one object to another. These movements bring the object of regard quickly on the fovea with an average velocity of 250°/second in the field of action of the muscle concerned. Measurement of saccadic velocity with the help of specially designed electro-oculographic (EOG) recorder can help in differentiating muscle restrictions from the muscle weakness. The saccadic velocity is decreased in paretic muscle, while it is near normal in mechanical muscle restrictions.

7. Positional tonometry

It has been reported that intraocular pressure rises from the compression of a non-relaxing stiff muscle, when attempts are made to move the eye into the field of its antagonist. Perkin's hand-held applanation tonometer or Digilab Pneumo-tonometer can be used to measure the IOP in different gaze positions. A pressure increase of over 5 mm Hg in a particular field of gaze is indicative of a restriction.

CLINICAL VARIETIES OF OCULAR PALSIES

1. Isolated ocular muscle paralysis.
2. Paralysis of 3rd cranial nerve
3. External ophthalmoplegia
4. Total ophthalmoplegia
5. Internuclear ophthalmoplegia

ISOLATED OCULAR MUSCLE PALSIES

Superior oblique (4th nerve palsy) and lateral rectus (6th nerve palsy) are the most common muscles to be paralysed singly, as they have separate nerve supply. Isolated paralysis of the remaining four extraocular muscles is less known.

PARALYSIS OF FOURTH CRANIAL NERVE
(SUPERIOR OBLIQUE MUSCLE PARESIS)

The fourth cranial nerve (trochlear) is entirely motor in function and supplies only the superior oblique muscle of the eyeball. It differs from other cranial nerves in being:
- The only cranial nerve to arise from the dorsal aspect of the brain (midbrain);
- The only cranial nerve to cross completely on the other side (i.e. the trochlear nerve arises from the contralateral nucleus; and
- The longest and thinnest of all cranial nerves.
    The fourth cranial nerve palsy (superior oblique muscle paralysis) is the most common isolated cyclovertical muscle palsy encountered by the ophthalmologists. Fourth cranial nerve palsy may be unilateral or bilateral. Bilateral palsies are almost always acquired. Unilateral palsy (more common than bilateral) may be congenital or acquired.

Note. The applied anatomy of fourth cranial nerve (Page 12) should be reviewed before proceeding further.

Etiology

In order of frequency, following are the causes of fourth cranial nerve paralysis:

1. *Congenital paralysis* is quite frequent (about 40% cases). Congenital paralysis may result from a defect in the nucleus or the motor portion of the nerve (hypoplasia or even oplasia rarely).

    High definition magnetic resonance imaging (MRI) studies have identified two groups of congenital SOP:
- The most frequent type, present in 73% of cases, is a congenital cranial dysinnervation syndrome where the trochlear nerve is absent and results in secondary atrophy of the superior oblique muscle.
- The second type has a normal trochlear nerve and size of the superior oblique muscle, but has an abnormal laxity of superior oblique tendon.

Note. It has been reported that sometimes a spontaneous manifestation of fourth cranial nerve palsy in adult age might be due to decompensation of fusion mechanism in a patient with congenital palsy.

2. *Trauma* is another frequent cause of fourth nerve paralysis (about 34% cases). Because of the position of the trochlear nerves with respect to the tentorial edge, closed head injury (even minor) can result in fourth nerve palsy. Due to an impact in the area of anterior medullary velum, where the two nerves decussate, bilateral trochlear nerve palsies are quite common in head injury. Iatrogenic trauma, occurring after SO tenectomy and ethmoid sinus surgery, now has become rare due to refinment in the surgical techniques.

3. *Idiopathic.* In about 20% cases of 4th nerve palsy, cause could not be ascertained.

4. *Vascular and neurogenic* causes account for about 3 to 5% cases, seen in elderly age group, having acute onset and small angle hypertropia (<6 prism diopters).
- *Aneurysms and tumours* (trochlear Schwnomes and brain tumours) are rare causes.
- *Ocular myasthenia gravis* may present as an isolated unilateral superior oblique paralysis with an insidious course. Therefore, as a general rule, a patient who presents with an unexplained diplopia of any type should undergo a tensilon test.
- *Diabetic neuropathy* may occasionally involve the trochlear nerve. Therefore, in an undiagnosed case of 4th nerve paralysis, a glucose tolerance test should also be done to rule out diabetic cranial mononeuropathy.
- *Herpes zoster* can also be considered a potential etiologic agent.
- *Hydrocephalus* may be a cause of acquired unilateral or bilateral fourth nerve palsies.
- *Idiopathic intracranial hypertension* can also lead to fourth nerve palsies.

5. *Cavernous sinus and superior orbital fissure syndrome* may be considered a cause of 4th nerve paralysis in association with 3rd and 6th cranial nerves (*see* pages 312 and 328).

Clinical features

Clinical features in a patient with 4th nerve paralysis (Fig.12.19) are as follows:

1. *Cyclovertical deviation.*

When the patient fixates with normal eye, usually the involved eye is elevated, slightly adducted and extorted following weakness of the superior oblique muscle (Fig. 12.19K).

The hyperdeviation becomes more obvious, when the head is tilted towards ipsilateral shoulder (Bielschowsky head tilt test) (Fig. 12.19M). Depending upon severity, deviation seen is as below:

- *Mild cases* show hypertropia in down and adducted position.
- *Modirate cases* hypertropia in adduction only (without depression).
- *Severe cases* show hypertropia in primary position.

When the patient fixes with the paretic eye, the normal eye is hypotropic (depressed), adducted and extorted more than the primary deviation. Such a condition has been labelled as *fallen eye syndrome.*

In congenital cases, typically, parents may notice that one eye of this infant is higher than the other and that there is abnormal head posture.

2. *Abnormal head posture* occurs towards the action of paralysed superior oblique, i.e. chin is depressed, face is slightly turned towards the opposite side and the *head is tilted towards the opposite shoulder* (Fig. 12.19A). The degree of abnormal head posture is not always proportional to the size of the hypertropia. Compensatory head posture is the most common presenting sign of SO palsy.

- *In congenital SO palsy,* there is a large head tilt which is confirmed on the family album photography or FAT scan.
- *In bilateral acquired palsies,* there is a chin down posture to compensate for V esotropia.

Note. Rarely there may be head tilt towards affected side to increase separation of images and hence to ignore the second image.

3. *Facial asymmetry.* Another important clinical sign is facial asymmetry, which is a characteristic finding of congenital palsy. There occurs typical shallowing of mid-facial region between lateral canthus and the angle of the mouth on the side of head tilt. This is indication of long-standing SO palsy.

4. *Diplopia* is seldom noticed, if onset is during visual immaturity. However, when onset is after visual maturity, i.e. adult patients will experience homonymous vertical, diagonal or torsional diplopia. Image seen by the involved eye is lower, uncrossed and intorted. If principal complaint is of torsional diplopia then bilateral palsy should be suspected. Vertical separation increases while looking down, therefore, diplopia is particularly noticed by the patient while coming down the stairs. Further, such a patient may not have much problem as long as the eyes look above the horizontal plane.

5. *Ocular movements*. Three abnormalies may be observed:

- Ipsilateral SO under action is seen in patients with marked paresis or lax SO tendons.
- Ipsilateral IOOA is present in most of the cases.
- Contralateral SO overaction or pseudo SO overaction which are clinically indistinguishable due to decreased infraduction in abduction of the involved eye, there is apparent over depression of the fellow eye.

Note. Long-standing hypertropia can cause contracture of SR muscle which causes restrictions in depression and can be tested by forced duction test.

Ocular movements in a patient with superior oblique paralysis, e.g. of right eye, are affected as below:

- Movements of left eye are limited, when looking down and to right (Fig. 12.19H) (angle of deviation is also greatest in this direction).
- Overaction of left eye as looking up and to right (Fig. 12.19B).
- Overaction of right eye on looking down and to right (Fig. 12.19H).
- Underaction of right eye on looking up and to right (Fig. 12.19B).
- In a long-standing palsy with the paretic eye fixing, the inferior rectus of the hypotropic non-paretic eye can undergo hypertrophy, then contracture, resulting in limited elevation of the non-paretic eye on both ductions and

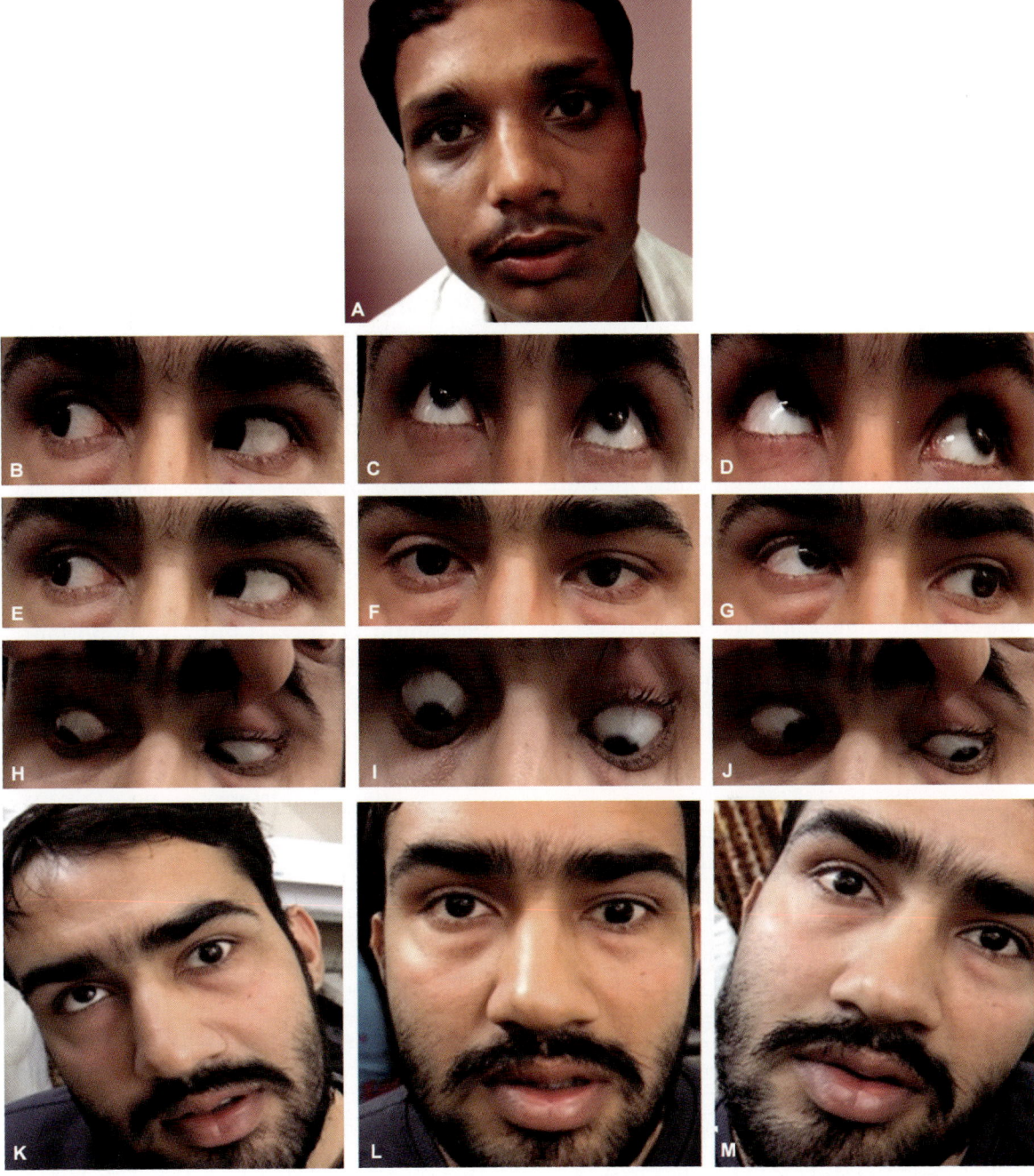

Fig. 12.19 *Left superior oblique palsy. A, Abnormal head posture, note head is tilted to the right shoulder, face is slightly turned to the right and chin is slightly depressed. B to J, Eyeballs in nine positions of gaze, note left hypertropia (F) which increases on right gaze (E). Also note left hypertropia (K) which increases on tilting the head to the left shoulder (M) and no change in hypertropia on tilting the head to the right shoulder (L). (Courtesy: Dr Kanwar Mohan)*

versions. The effect can simulate a double elevator palsy in the non-paretic eye, but this can be ruled out with the forced duction and head tilt tests.

Diagnosis

In the diagnosis of superior oblique palsy, one needs to consider the following:

- Differentiation of superior oblique paresis from other cyclovertical deviations.
- Unilateral versus bilateral superior oblique paresis.
- Congenital versus acquired superior oblique paresis.

Diagnosis of superior oblique paralysis

Differential diagnosis is made by performing following tests:

1. *Three-step test* The key to diagnose SO palsy is 3-step test which requires motility measurement in primary gaze, right and left lateral gaze and right and left head tilts (for details *see* page 293).

2. *Torsion* is usually measured objectively by indirect ophthalmoscope and subjectively by double Maddox rod test.

The following features are observed:

- *Congenital SO palsy* usually has no torsion.

- *Acquired SO palsy* is usually associated with complaints of subjective torsion.
- Cyclotorsion of <10° is seen in unilateral palsy and >10° in bilateral palsy.

3. *Hess screen* (Fig. 12.20) or Lancaster red/green test is useful for a meticulous follow-up of the patients.

4. *Diplopia charting* (Fig. 12.21) is also important as in all cases of acquired strabismus and should be done in all cases of SO palsy presenting with complain of vertical and diagonal diplopia.

5. *Measurement of ocular deviation* in all 9 diagnostic gaze positions, as well as in right and left head tilt is important in diagnosing and planning treatment for superior oblique palsy.

6. *Force duction test* should be done to look for SR contracture.

7. *Oblique traction test.* Intraoperative testing of SO is essential for evaluating patients with SO palsy, especially in young children where precise orthoptic measurement cannot be taken. This not only helps to identify the lax tendon that should be tucked but also importantly identifies tendon of normal length which should not undergo this procedure for the fear of brown syndrome.

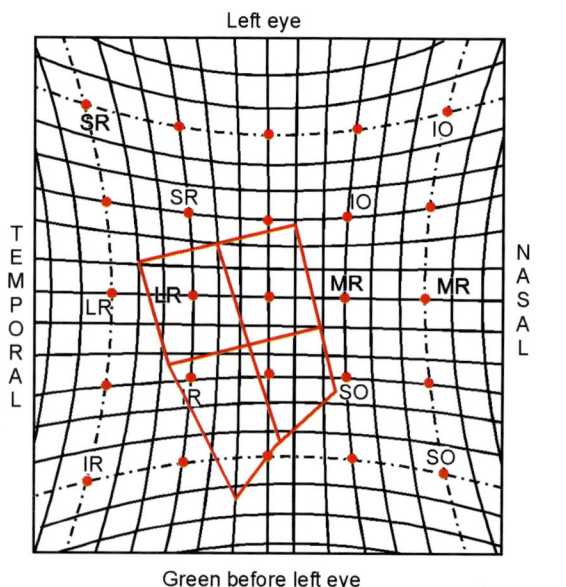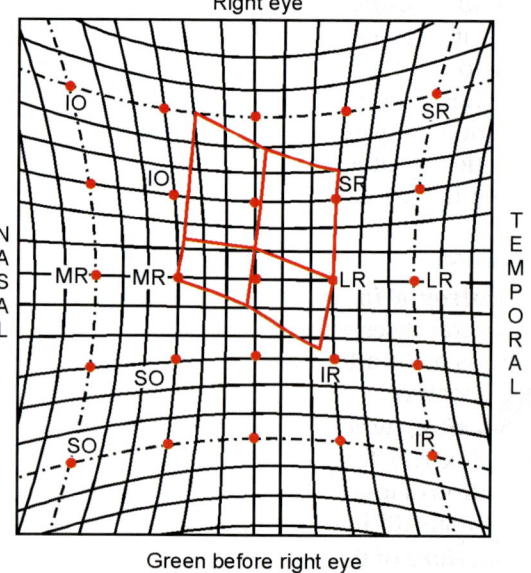

Fig. 12.20 *Hess chart of a patient with right superior oblique palsy.*

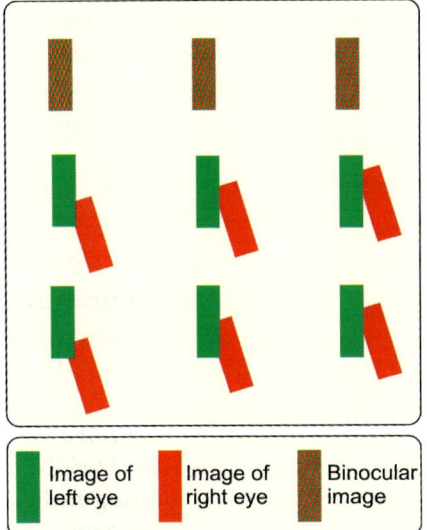

| Image of left eye | Image of right eye | Binocular image |

Fig. 12.21 *Diplopia chart of a patient with right superior oblique palsy.*

8. *Neuroimaging.* Most patients with isolated SO palsy do not need neurological workup. Indications of neuroimaging are:
- Fresh trauma
- Non-isolated, multiple palsies.
- Acquired palsy in absence of trauma.
- Presence of associated neurological sign.
- Younger patients presenting with acute symptoms

Modified Knapp and Moore's classification of superior oblique palsy. Depending upon the amount of hypertropia in different diagnostic positions of gaze, Knapp and Moore have classified common manifestations of superior oblique paralysis into 7 classes which has been modified by other workers by adding class VIII (Table 12.6).

Unilateral versus bilateral superior oblique palsy

1. *Esotropia in downgaze* is usually little in unilateral cases while in bilateral cases usually there is a V-pattern esotropia with chin down head posture.

2. *Torsion,* when measured by the double Maddox rod test, usually shows an excyclo-deviation of less than 10° in unilateral cases and more than 10° in bilateral cases.

3. *Ductions* of the superior oblique muscles are usually diminished in bilateral cases while in

Table 12.6 *Modified Knapp and Moore's classification of superior oblique palsy into eight classes*

Class	Pattern of deviation (e.g. in paralysis of LSO) Description	Diagrammatic depiction
I	HT is greatest when eye is elevated and adducted	
II	HT greatest when eye is depressed and adducted	
III	HT of equal magnitude in the entire paralysed field	
IV	HT of equal magnitude in the entire paralysed field and the entire inferior field (L-shaped or reverse L-pattern)	
V	HT is greatest in the entire inferior field	
VI	Underaction of both SO, overaction of both IO, V-pattern esotropia, bilateral positive Bielschowsky head tilt test	
VII	Canine tooth syndrome characterized by under-action of inferior oblique (acquired Brown's) and under-action of superior oblique. It usually occurs due to trauma in the area of the trochlea	
VIII	Comitant hypertropia but with positive head tilt test	

unilateral cases, actions may be normal or diminished.

4. *Head tilt test* is positive for the involved eye in unilateral cases, i.e. hypertropia increases on tilting the head towards ipsilateral shoulder. While, in bilateral palsies, tilting to either side will increase the hypertropia, i.e. right hypertropia on right tilt and left hypertropia on left tilt. Even after spread of comitance, the head-tilt test should be positive in fourth cranial nerve palsy.

Congenital versus acquired superior oblique palsy

Most patients are congenital, so facial asymmetry with old photographs showing head tilt, or asthenopia symptoms of long duration are sufficient to rule out acquired palsy. Following points are useful in differentiating congenital from acquired SO palsy:

1. *Amblyopia* is uncommon in acquired paresis but may be present in congenital ones.

2. *Excyclodeviation* and complaint of apparent tilting of objects are common in acquired cases.

3. *Abnormal head posture* may be traced to childhood from the old family photographs in patients with congenital palsy while not in those with acquired palsy.

4. *Presence of increased vertical vergence* may be the only suggestion of a previous palsy in some adult patients who develop spontaneous manifestations of 4th nerve palsy due to decompensation of fusion mechanism in old case of congenital palsy.

5. *Long, redundant or floppy superior oblique tendon* seen during surgery may indicate a congenital palsy.

Table 12.7 summarizes the differences between congenital and acquired superior oblique palsy.

Differential diagnosis

1. **Thyroid ophthalmopathy** is a chronic restrictive disease in which:

- IR muscle, which is most commonly involved (positive on FDT).
- Signs of proptosis, lid lag, lid retraction, lagophthalmos.
- Signs of active disease, i.e. chemosis, orbital congestion are seen.

- On imaging, enlargement of muscle belly is seen.

2. **Brown syndrome**. In it, there is underaction of ipsilateral IO whereas in SO palsy, there is ipsilateral IOOA.

3. **Primary IOOA**. It is usually seen with infantile esotropia. There is absence of hyperdeviation in the primary position, lack of torsion and negative head tilt test.

4. **Skew deviation** is an acquired, acute, hyperdeviation which may or may not be comitant. Presence of neurologic signs refers to brainstem or cerebellum involvement.

Treatment

I. General principles of therapy are same as described in therapy of paralysis of sixth (page 313) and third (page 332) nerves.

II. Non-surgical treatment

1. **Amblyopia**, when present, should be treated first; if the patient is a child, surgery is usually indicated.

2. **Segmental membrane prisms** or **segmental occlusion** of the lower third of the spectacle lens before the paretic eye with semiopaque Scotch tape may be tried till surgery is undertaken.

3. **Alternate occlusion** or occlusion of the sound eye may be performed to create visual comfort in patients in which binocular single vision cannot possibly be restored by any means.

4. **Prisms** may be used to overcome diplopia in small, symptomatic, comitant or nearly comitant deviations that do not have a symptomatic

Table 12.7 *Differences between congenital and acquired superior oblique palsy.*		
Features	Congenital SO palsy	Acquired SO palsy
Diplopia	No complain of diplopia, only intermittent vertical diplopia in decompensated palsy	Usually complain of vertical, diagonal or torsional diplopia with incomitant hypertropia
Torsion	There is no measurable subjective torsion	Excyclotorsion usually seen more so in bilateral palsy
Head tilt	Present since infancy (old photographs)	Anytime later following the onset
Traction test	Lax SO tendon confirmed by traction test intraoperatively	SO traction test is normal
Facial asymmetry	Facial asymmetry is usually present	There is no facial asymmetry
Fusional amplitudes	Significantly increased (16–30 prism diopters)	Normal (2–3 prism diopters)
Amblyopia in the involved eye	May be present	Usually absent

torsional component. If this alleviates the symptoms, surgery is not warranted.

III. Surgical treatment. Surgical treatment is indicated for a:

- Significant abnormal head posture,
- Vertical deviation, or
- Diplopia.

A significant head tilt is the main indication for surgery in children younger than age 5, as it is thought that the uncorrected torticollis will lead to progressive facial asymmetry.

Surgical approach employed should take into consideration:

- Presence of SR contracture,
- SO laxity, and
- Degree of torsion.

Various surgical schemes have been recommended. Knapp and von Noorden's modified approach depending upon the class of paresis is summarized in Table 12.8.

Based on the degree of deviation (hypertropia) and status of muscle sequelae following paresis of SO muscle, the line of surgical management is summarized below:

Hypertropia is ≤20 PD

One muscle surgery as below:

- IO weakening—if IOOA
- SR recession—if contracture of SR positive
- SO tuck—if SO tendon laxity
- Contralateral IR recession—if no SR contracture and no SO tendon laxity

Hypertropia >20 PD

Two muscle surgery, i.e. ipsilateral IO weakening + any of the following:

- SR recession—if contracture of SR positive
- SO tuck—if SO tendon laxity
- Contralateral IR recession—if no SR contracture and no SO tendon laxity.

Other recommendations are:

1. *Superior oblique muscle* tuck is a hard procedure to quantitate. It is best employed:

- When the deviation is greatest in opposite downgaze and so muscle is moderately to markedly underacting.
- For acquired bilateral SO palsy or weakness.

- To reduce or eliminate the head tilt in congenital SO palsy that presents in early childhood.

2. *Anterior temporal displacemet of the anterior half of the SO muscle tendon* **(Harada-Ito procedure)** is indicated as an alternative to SO tuck, when the deviation is primarily torsional. This procedure does not correct any vertical deviation in primary position, but corrects the excyclo-deviation and the abducting weakness of the SO muscle in downgaze.

- *Intraoperative adjustment of Harada–Ito procedure is possible by visualizing objective torsion of the fundus using indirect ophthalmoscope.*
- *Postoperative adjustment of Harada–Ito procedure has also been described using adjustable sutures.*

3. *Fell's modification of Harada-Ito procedure* involves disinserting the anterior fibres of the superior oblique tendon and transposing them 8 mm posterior to the superior insertion of the lateral rectus muscle.

4. *Bilateral Harada-Ito procedures* are indicated in some cases of bilateral fourth nerve palsy.

LATERAL RECTUS PARALYSIS

The abducent (sixth cranial) nerve is a small and pure motor nerve that supplies the lateral rectus muscle. Isolated lateral rectus muscle paralysis (sixth cranial nerve paralysis) is next common to isolated paralysis of superior oblique muscle.

Note. Applied anatomy of sixth cranial nerve (page 16) should be reviewed before proceeding further.

Etiology

A. Congenital sixth nerve palsy due to hypoplasia of its nucleus or developmental anomaly in the motor nerve fibres is quite rare.

- *Congenital absence of the 6th nerve nucleus and aplasia of the nerve* is associated with Duane's syndrome (congenital cranial dysinnervation disorder).
- *Congenital horizontal gaze palsy* due to involvement of gaze centre may be confused with congenital 6th nerve palsy.
- However, sixth cranial nerve paresis occurring shortly after birth had been reported and

Table 12.8 *Knapp's and von Noorden's surgical schemes for left superior oblique muscle paresis*

Modified knapp's class of paresis	Pattern of deviation	Muscle sequelae associated with LSO palsy	Recommended surgical treatment
Class I	Maximum HT in dextroelevation	Overaction of ipsilateral IO (LIO)	Weakening of ipsilateral IO (LIO)
Class II	Maximum HT in dextrodepression	Underaction of paretic LSO	
		a. If laxity of SO tendon (grade III and IV laxity)	Tuck of ipsilateral SO (LSO) or recession of contralateral inferior rectus (RIR)
		b. If no laxity of SO tendon and IO overaction present	Weakening of ipsilateral IO (LIO)
Class III	*HT equal* in entire paralysed field (all dextroversion position)	Weakness of paretic SO (LSO) with overaction of ipsilateral IO (LIO)	
		a. If HT ≤20 PD	Weakening of ipsilateral IO (LIO)
		b. If HT >20 PD with	
		• SO tendon laxity	LIO weakening + LSO tuck
		• No SO tendon laxity	LIO weakening + RIR recession
Class IV	HT equal in entire paralysed field and inferior field (i.e. dextroposition and downgaze positions (L-shaped)	Contracture of ipsilateral SR (LSR)	
		a. If deviation <20 PD	LSR recession + LIO weakening
		b. If deviation >20 PD with	LSR recession + LIO weakening
		• SO tendon laxity	weakening + LSO tuck
		• No SO tendon laxity	LSR recession + LIO weakening + RIR recession
Class V	HT maximum in all downgaze positions	Long-standing SO palsy with spread of comitance	
		a. If SO tendon laxity	LSR recession + LSO tuck or RIR recession
		b. If with IO overaction	LSR recession + LIO weakening
Class VI	V-pattern esotropia with reversing Bielschowsky head tilt test	Bilateral SO palsy (underaction) with bilateral IO overaction	
		a. If torsion ≤15°	Bilateral IO weakening
		b. If torsion >15°	Bilateral IO weakening + B/L Harada-Ito procedure or B/L IR recession
Class VII	HT in all downgaze position, primary position and in dextroversion	Underaction of inferior oblique and superior oblique (acquired Brown's syndrome) Usually occur due to trauma in trochlear area (canine tooth syndrome)	
		• If aligned (no deviation) in primary position	No procedure
		• If ipsilateral hypertropia	Recess contralateral IR (RIR)
		• If ipsilateral hypotropia	Explore trochlea to release restriction
Class VIII	Comitant hypertropia but with positive head tilt test	Spread of comitance	
		• If IO overaction	LIO weakening
		• If tight SR	LSR recession
		• If lax SO tendon	SO tuck or RIR recession

Aim of surgical treatment is to correct the incomitant esotropia, improve abduction, provide a useful field of binocular single vision and to eliminate the abnormal head posture.

Recommended surgical measures are as below:
I. Recess-resect operation. A supra maximal (12–16 mm) recession of the antagonist medial rectus with about 8–10 mm resection of the lateral rectus muscle is often a successful first operation in most patients with incomplete paralysis. This procedure often provides a useful field of binocular single vision and eliminates the abnormal head posture.

- In case a mild paresis is still present, *weakening of the contralateral medial rectus muscle* with or without Faden procedure may be considered as a second operation.
- *Adjustable suture surgery* may be helpful for final adjustments in co-operative patients with paralytic squint.

II. Muscle transposition procedures recommended for a complete paralysis of lateral rectus muscles. Medial rectus recession should also be combined especially, when there is medial rectus contracture. Forced duction test is useful in discovering MR contracture.

1. *Jensen's procedure combined with the medial rectus recession* is useful by balancing the partially active forces. In the Jensen's procedure, the superior rectus, inferior rectus muscles and the paralysed lateral rectus muscle are split for 8–10 mm from their insertion backwards with the help of a muscle hook. Then the superior half of the lateral rectus is united with the lateral half of the superior rectus and the inferior half of the lateral rectus with the lateral half of inferior rectus with the help of a non-absorbable suture (e.g. 5–0 Mersilene). The knot should be tied near the equator (Fig. 15.22).

2. *Hummelscheim operation.* In this procedure, after spliting the superior and inferior recti, their lateral halves are disinserted and sutured to the tendon of lateral rectus muscle. This operation is *rarely done nowadays* and is thus mainly of historical interest.

3. *Berens and Girard procedure.* In this procedure, the full inferior and superior rectus tendons are disinserted and sutured with the tendon of lateral rectus at its insertion. This procedure combined with a recession of the medial rectus is recommended by von Noorden in children with complete paralysis of sixth cranial nerve.

4. *Carlson and Jampolsky transposition procedure.* In this procedure, medial rectus muscle is spared. After splitting the vertical recti, their temporal halves are inserted under the lateral rectus. It is essential to separate the halves of the vertical recti to the deepest point toward the apex of the orbit, allowing the transposed parts of the vertical recti to slide toward the LR, which also minimises vertical deviations. This procedure reduces the angle of deviation below 10PD, improves abduction, prevents relapses, and also prevents anterior segment ischemia.

5. *Superior rectus transposition with MR recession* have also shown good results in literature. This procedure is successfully tried in lateral rectus palsy and also in abduction deficit conditions like Duane's syndrome and Mobius syndrome, especially if hypertropia is also associated. It may induce vertical deviation also.

III. Contralateral medial rectus muscle recession with or without Faden operation can be considered an option for the residual lateral rectus abduction deficit and/or residual esotropia, often the above surgical measure.

MEDIAL RECTUS PARALYSIS

Isolated medial rectus paralysis is extremely rare, yet do occur, often without any satisfactory explanation.

Etiology

Exact etiology of this rare entity is not known. However, trauma and vascular disorders may be implicated in occasional cases.

Clinical features

1. *Incomitant exotropia* occurs in the primary position in the involved eye (Fig. 12.26A) due to unopposed action of the lateral rectus. The exotropia increases in gaze towards the paralysed medial rectus (Fig. 12.26B). The

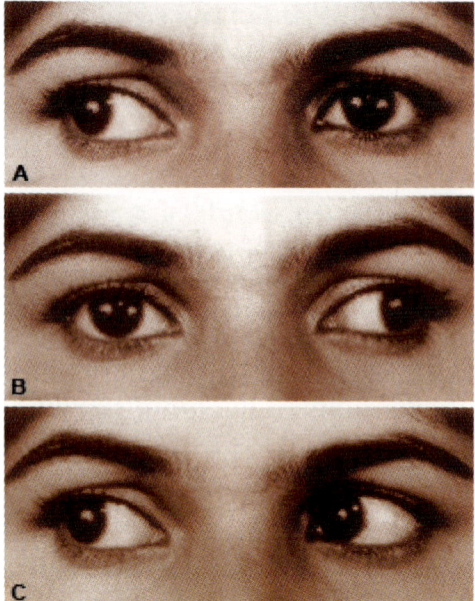

Fig. 12.26 *A patient with right medial rectus paralysis having right exotropia in primary gaze (A) which increases in left gaze (B) and the patient becomes orthotropic in right gaze (C).*

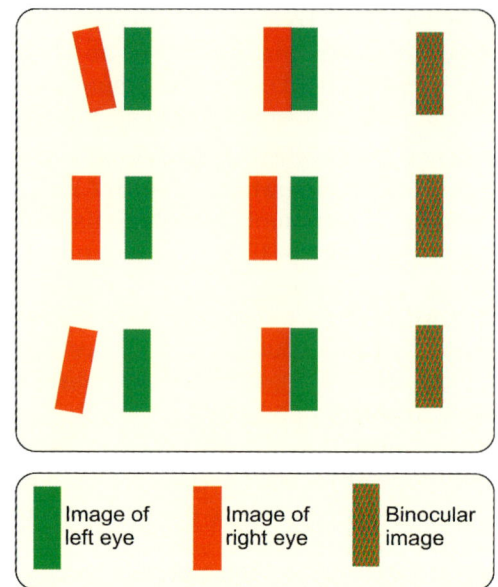

Fig. 12.27 *Diplopia chart of a patient with right medial rectus palsy.*

patient becomes orthotropic in the opposite gaze (Fig. 12.26C).

- *Secondary deviation* in the uninvolved eye, when the patient fixates with the paretic eye is larger than the primary deviation.

2. *Abnormal head posture* is frequently associated with incomitant exotropia. Face is turned towards the action of the paralysed medial rectus.

3. *Diplopia.* A crossed horizontal diplopia with maximal image separation while looking towards opposite side and during near fixation is appreciated (Fig. 12.27).

4. *Ocular movements* in a patient with paralysis of medial rectus (e.g. of right eye) affected are as below:

- Adduction in right eye is limited.
- Overaction of right eye on dextroversion
- Overaction of left eye on levoversion
- Underaction of left eye on dextroversion.

5. *Hess screen charting* is as shown in Fig. 12.28.

Differential diagnosis

Isolated medial rectus palsy should be differentiated from internuclear ophthalmoplegia (*see* page 333).

Treatment

1. *Conservative treatment* is similar to that of lateral rectus palsy (page 314).

2. *Surgical treatment,* when indicated, consists of:

- *Recession of the antagonist lateral rectus* combined with resection of the involved medial rectus. The amount of surgery depends upon the size of deviation.
- *Vertical rectus transposition* to the medial rectus muscle is also recommended as an alternative procedure.

INFERIOR RECTUS MUSCLE PALSY

An isolated paralysis of the inferior rectus muscle is extremely rare condition.

Etiology

1. *Congenital.* Inferior rectus palsy, a rare entity, is often congenital.

2. *Acquired.* Occasionally, inferior rectus palsy may be due to an injury of the orbit (either at the time of injury or at the time of repair of the orbital floor fracture), myasthenia gravis, vascular diseases and following a peribulbar or retrobulbar anaesthesia for any intraocular surgery.

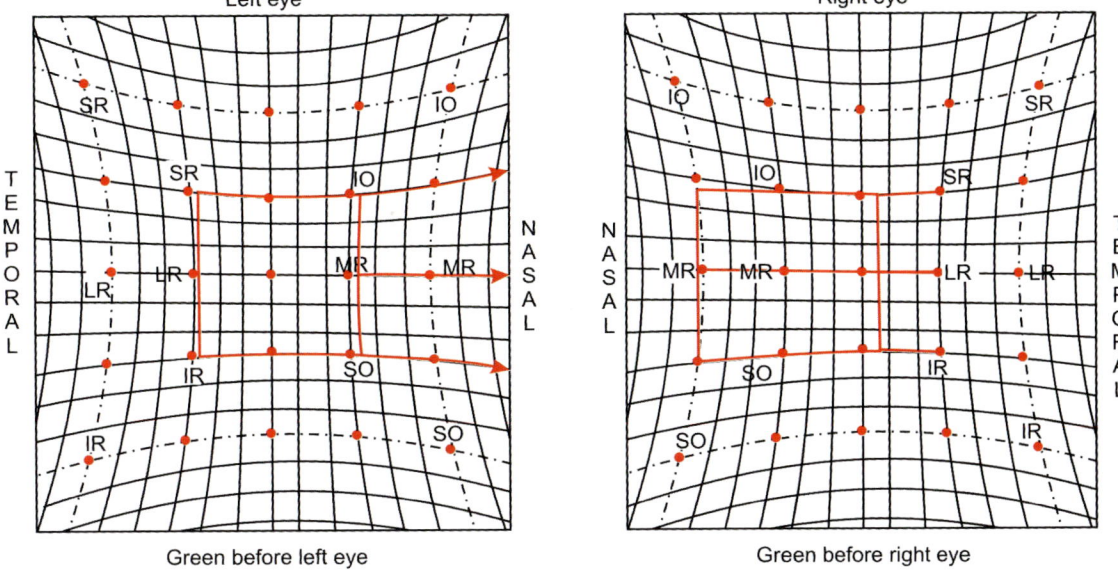

Fig. 12.28 *Hess chart of a patient with right medial rectus paralysis.*

Clinical features

1. Deviation. In primary position, the involved eye is hypertropic and slightly intorted due to the unopposed action of the antagonistic superior rectus muscle (Fig. 12.29A). When patient fixates with the paretic eye, secondary deviation in the opposite eye consists of depression and intorsion more than the primary deviation.

2. Pseudoptosis can be appreciated in the normal eye, when patient fixates with the paretic eye. This occurs because of the drooping of the upper lid associated with moving down of the globe.

3. Widening of palpebral fissure may be seen in the paretic eye, when patient fixates with the normal eye. This occurs due to upward movement of the upper eyelid associated with the elevation of the globe.

4. Abnormal head posture is often present and consists of slight chin depression, face turn and head tilt towards the affected side (Fig. 12.29B).

5. Diplopia (Fig.12.30). Image seen by the involved eye is lower, crossed and extorted; vertical separation increases, when looking down and to the same side; extorsion increases, when looking towards the opposite side.

6. Ocular movements in a patient with inferior rectus palsy (e.g. of right eye) are affected as below (Fig. 12.29 I to IX):

- *Movements of right eye* are limited, when looking down and right (Fig. 12.29 VII).
- *Overaction of right eye* on looking up and to right (Fig. 12.29 I).
- *Overaction of left eye* on looking down and to right (Fig. 12.29 VII).
- *Underaction of left eye* on looking up and to right (Fig. 12.29 I).

7. Hess screen pattern seen in right inferior rectus palsy is shown in Fig. 12.31.

Treatment

1. Conservative treatment is similar to as described for lateral rectus palsy (page 314).

2. Surgical treatment, when indicated should be planned depending upon the size of the deviation and results of forced duction test (FDT) as below:

i. *Recession of the superior rectus* should be performed, if FDT shows restriction of this muscle.

ii. *Resection of inferior rectus* is preferred, when FDT is negative and deviation is small.

iii. *Resection of inferior rectus and recession of the superior rectus* should be combined, if the

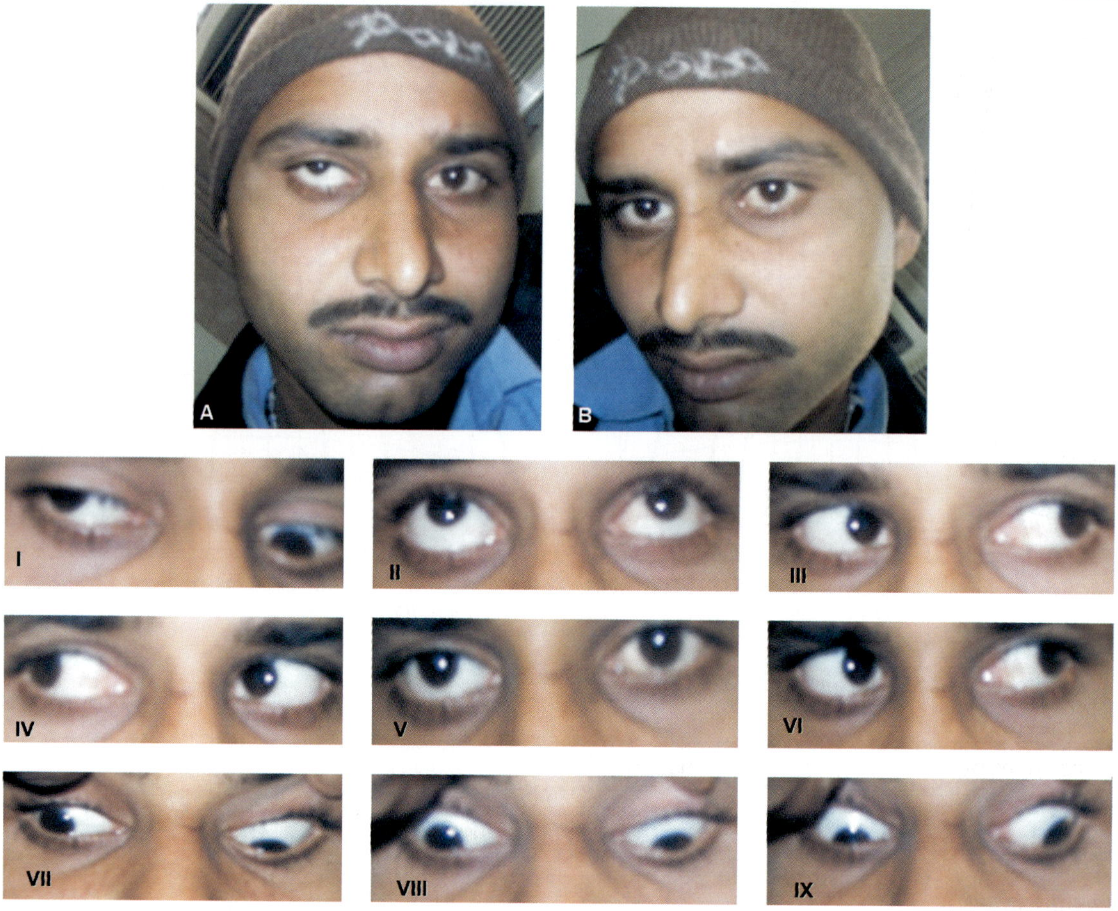

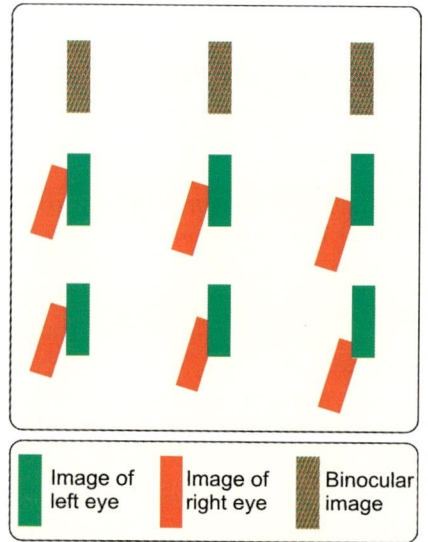

Fig. 12.29 *A patient with right inferior rectus paralysis: A, Right hypertropia with left eye fixating; B, Abnormal head posture; and I to IX, Ocular movement in nine positions of gaze (Courtesy: Dr Subhash Dadeya).*

| Image of left eye | Image of right eye | Binocular image |

Fig. 12.30 *Diplopia chart of a patient with right inferior rectus paralysis.*

deviation is large. This surgery can correct up to 30–40D of vertical deviation in the primary position.

iv. *Other options* include IR plication, reverse Knapp, IO anterior transposition.

SUPERIOR RECTUS PARALYSIS

An isolated paralysis of superior rectus muscle is a rare entity. Since the superior division of the third cranial nerve innervates both superior rectus and levator muscle, so weakness of superior rectus may be associated with weakness of levator and thus a ptosis in the affected eye.

Etiology

1. *Congenital.* Isolated superior rectus muscle palsy is usually congenital.

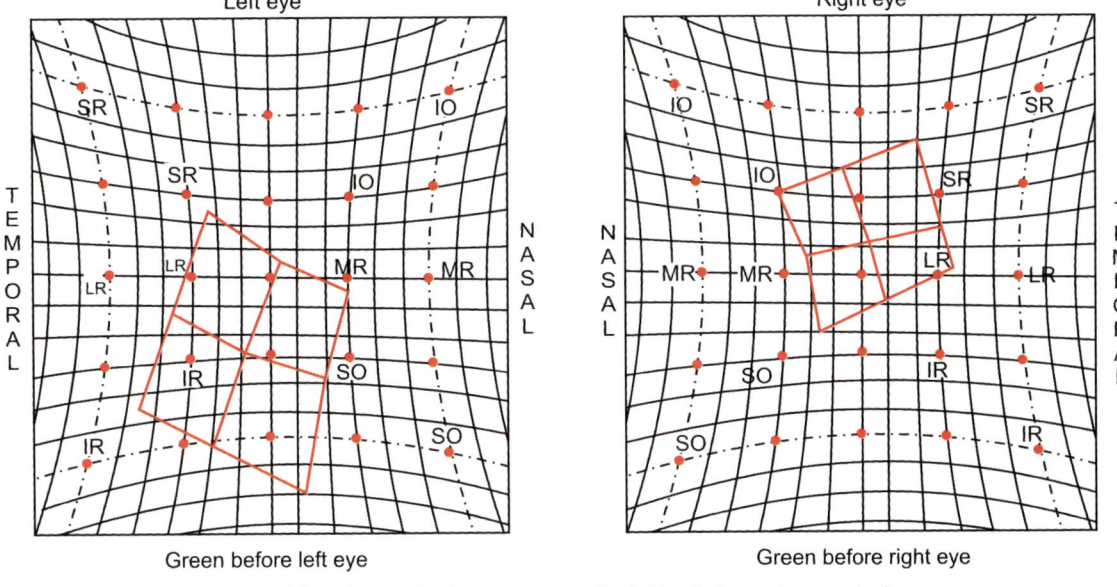

Fig. 12.31 *Hess chart of a patient with right inferior rectus paralysis.*

2. *Acquired.* SR palsy may be secondary to trauma (e.g. after a bridle suture during cataract surgery) or occasionally be associated with vascular disorders and viral infections.

Clinical features

1. *Deviation.* When the normal eye is fixing, the paretic eye is hypotropic in primary position (Fig. 12.32A). Usually, there is no vertical deviation in adduction. The inferior rectus overacts and consequently objective excyclodeviation develops which can be detected by indirect ophthalmoscopy or by plotting the blind spot in the visual field. Subjective cyclodeviation is typically absent, since in most cases the condition is congenital. When patient fixates with the paretic eye the normal eye is hypertropic, slightly abducted and slightly extorted; more than the primary deviation (Fig. 12.32B).

2. *Ptosis* may be associated in the affected eye, if LPS is also weak.

3. *Pseudoptosis* may be associated with the hypotropic globe in primary position (Fig. 12.32A). It must be differentiated from the true ptosis. Pseudoptosis disappears, when the patient fixates with the paretic eye.

4. *Abnormal head posture* is not always present in patients with superior rectus palsy. However,

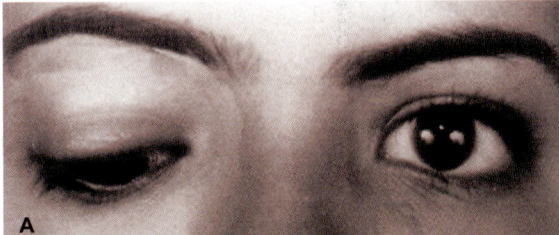

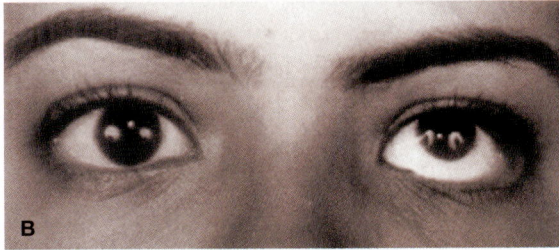

Fig. 12.32 *A patient with right superior rectus paralysis and pseudoptosis and hypotropia in the affected eye while fixating with the left nonaffected eye (A). When fixating with the paretic right eye, pseudoptosis disappears and the nonparetic left eye becomes hypertropic (B).*

in some recent cases, chin may be elevated, face turned to the same side and head tilted towards the normal side. In most patients, after sometimes, head is tilted towards the same side due to overaction of the yoke muscle (opposite inferior oblique).

5. *Diplopia* may be present in recent cases only. For example, in a patient with paralysis of right

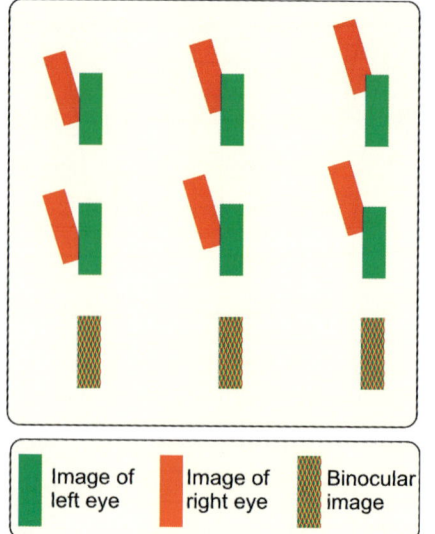

| Image of left eye | Image of right eye | Binocular image |

Fig. 12.33 *Diplopia chart of a patient with right superior rectus palsy.*

- Movements of right eye are limited, when looking towards up and right.
- Overaction of right eye on looking down and to right.
- Overaction of left eye on looking up and to the right.
- Underaction of left eye on looking down and to right.

7. Hess screen charting pattern seen in right superior rectus palsy is shown in Fig. 12.34.

Differential diagnosis

1. Primary superior rectus palsy needs to be differentiated from the inhibitional palsy of the superior rectus (contralateral antagonist) secondary to weakness of the superior oblique muscle of the opposite eye.

2. Paretic weakness of the superior rectus should be differentiated from the restrictive limitation of movements following entrapment of inferior rectus and/or soft tissue in fracture floor of the orbit and contracture of inferior rectus following myositis, after cataract surgery, ocular epibulbar anaesthesia.

Forced duction test, active force generation test and saccadic velocity test are quite useful in differentiating paretic limitation from restrictive limitation of movements (page 300).

superior rectus, image seen by the involved eye is higher, crossed and intorted (Fig. 12.33). Vertical separation increases, when looking up and to the right; intorsion increases, when looking to left.

6. Ocular movements in a patient with right superior rectus muscle paralysis are affected as below:

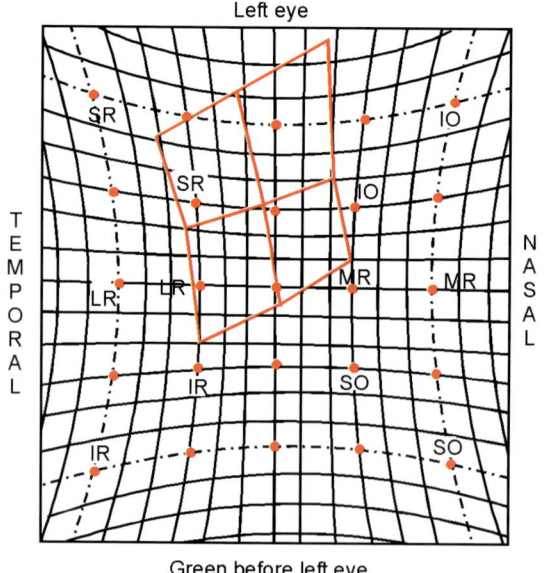

Green before left eye

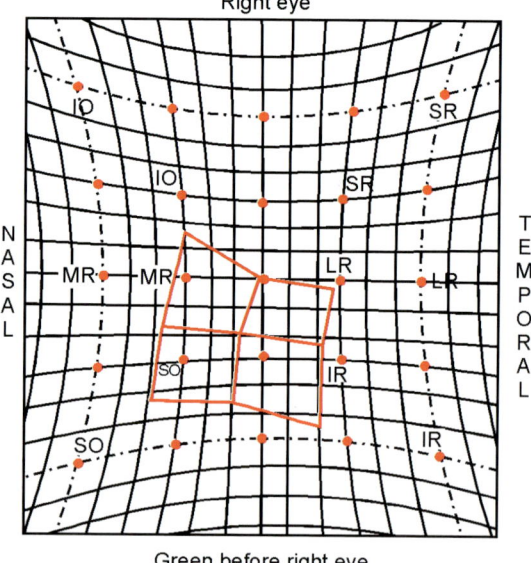

Green before right eye

Fig. 12.34 *Hess chart of a patient with right superior rectus palsy.*

Treatment

1. *Conservative treatment* is on the general lines (page 314).

2. *Surgical treatment* of isolated superior rectus muscle paralysis, depending upon the size of deviation, is as follows:

i. *Recession of inferior rectus* by 4 mm is sufficient for a deviation up to 15^Δ.

ii. *Recession of inferior rectus* by 4 mm combined with 4 mm *resection of superior rectus* may correct a vertical deviation of $30–40^\Delta$ in primary position.

iii. *Weakening procedure on the inferior oblique* of the non-paretic eye may be required in addition to the recess-resect procedure, when the deviation is more than 40^Δ.

INFERIOR OBLIQUE PALSY

Isolated inferior oblique palsy is the least common of all extraocular muscle palsies.

Etiology

Inferior oblique palsy may be congenital or acquired. *Acquired disorders* like stroke, syphilis and myasthenia gravis and trauma can also cause IO palsy.

Clinical features

1. *Deviation.* When fixing with the normal eye, patient will have hypotropia of the involved eye (Fig. 12.35A) and when fixing with the paretic eye, patient will have hypertropia of the normal eye in the primary position. The greatest deviation occurs, when the patient attempts to elevate the adducted paretic eye (Fig. 12.35B). The deviation worsens with horizontal gaze into the field of action of affected IO or with head tilt towards the side opposite the paretic eye.

2. *Abnormal head posture* consists of chin elevation, head tilt towards the paralyzed side, and the face is turned towards the uninvolved side, i.e. away from the side of palsy.

3. *Bielschowsky head tilt test* is positive on tilting the head towards the normal side.

4. *Diplopia* is usually not a complaint, since in most of the cases, onset is congenital. However, in a recent acquired case image seen by the paretic eye is higher, uncrossed and extorted;

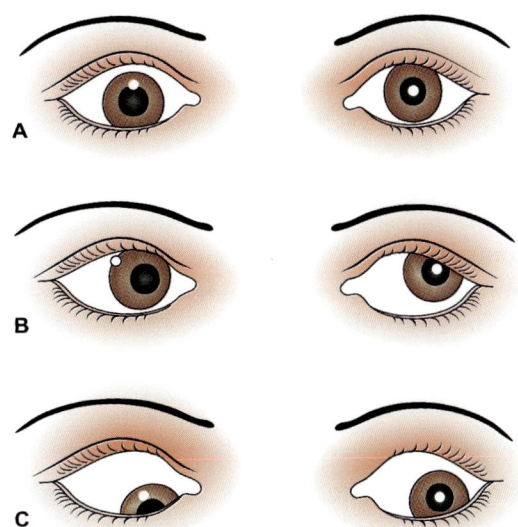

Fig. 12.35 *Right inferior oblique palsy. Note:* A, *right hypotropia in primary gaze;* B, *underaction of right inferior oblique on levoelevation and* C, *secondary overaction of right superior oblique on levodepression.*

vertical separation increases, when looking up and to left; extorsion increases, when looking to right (Fig. 12.36).

5. *Ocular movements* in a patient with paralysis of inferior oblique muscle, say of right side, will be affected as below:

- *Underaction of right inferior oblique,* i.e. movements of right eye are limited, when looking up and to left (Fig. 12.35B).

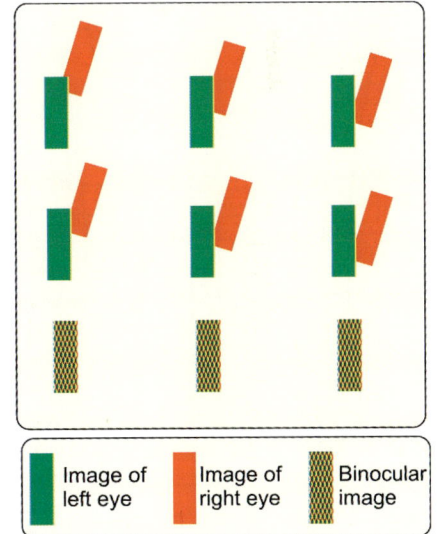

Image of left eye	Image of right eye	Binocular image

Fig. 12.36 *Diplopia chart of a patient with right inferior oblique palsy.*

- *Secondary overaction* of right superior oblique, i.e. overaction of right eye on looking down and to left (Fig. 12.35C).
- Overaction of left eye on looking up and to left.
- Underaction of left eye on looking down and to left may occur due to inhibitional palsy of contralateral IR.

6. *An objective incyclodeviation* is evidenced on indirect ophthalmoscopy.

7. *Hess screen charting* in a patient with inferior oblique palsy is shown in Fig. 12.37.

Differential diagnosis

Brown's superior oblique sheath syndrome can be differentiated from inferior oblique palsy as below:

- In Brown's syndrome the involved eye is frequently depressed more severely in adduction than it is with inferior oblique paralysis.
- *Overaction of superior oblique* is minimal or absent in Brown's syndrome.
- *Forced duction test* is positive in Brown's syndrome.
- *'A' pattern* is typically present with inferior oblique palsy, whereas a 'V' pattern in typical of Brown syndrome.

Treatment

1. *Conservative treatment,* when required, is on the general lines (page 314).

2. *Surgical treatment* is frequently indicated since in most cases, onset is congenital. Aims of surgery are to correct abnormal head posture, to correct deviation in primary position and to treat diplopia. The general principle of strengthening the weak muscle and weakening the strong muscle is not applicable in cases with inferior oblique palsy; since most workers have reported that inferior oblique resection or advancement is usually unsatisfactory. Surgery has to be individualized approach depending on amount of vertical deviation, spread of comitance and degree of increase in deviation in ipsilateral gaze. Therefore, recommended treatment is as below:

i. *Superior oblique tenotomy* should be performed in the involved eye, when superior oblique overaction is marked, i.e. weakening of ipsilateral antagonist.

ii. *Recession of the superior rectus (i.e. weakening of contralateral yoke muscle, and resection of the inferior rectus (i.e. strengthening of contralateral antagonist) of the normal eye is recommended, when there is not much overaction of the superior oblique muscle in the*

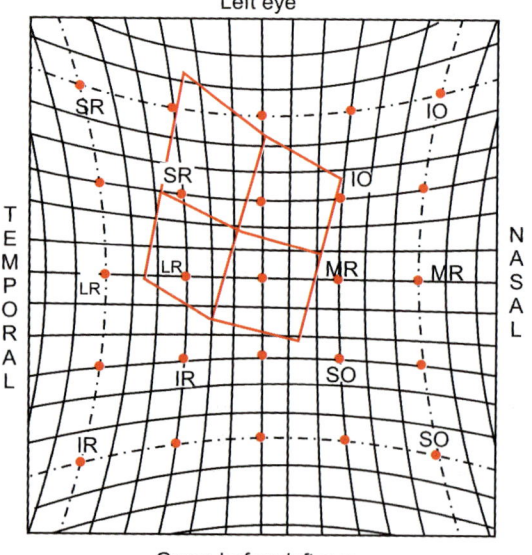

Green before left eye

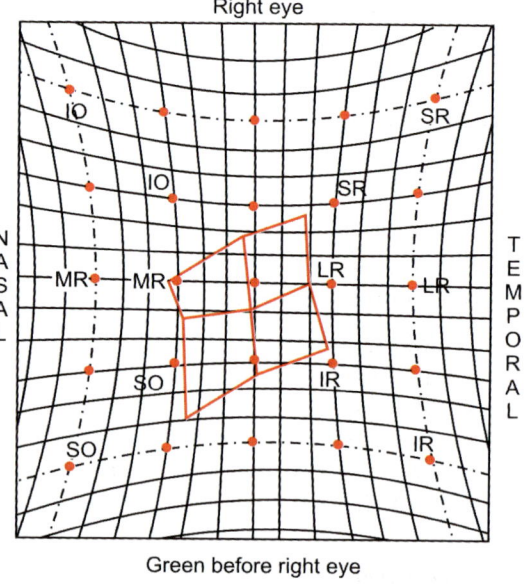

Green before right eye

Fig. 12.37 *Hess chart of a patient with right inferior oblique palsy.*

involved eye. Though, this procedure will not improve the action of the inferior oblique muscle, it will restore comitance in the paretic field of gaze.

DOUBLE ELEVATOR PALSY (MONOCULAR ELEVATION DEFICIENCY)

The term 'double elevator palsy', literally means paralysis of both elevators (superior rectus and inferior oblique) of the same eye; resulting in a clinical condition characterized by elevation deficiency in the entire range of upward gaze, i.e. in primary gaze, in adduction as well as in abduction. In the literature, many cases have been reported with similar clinical characteristics (i.e. limitation of elevation in entire upgaze) occurring due to mechanical restrictions involving the inferior aspect of the globe (without any associated palsy of elevators). Even some cases with mixed etiology have also been reported. Keeping in view the above, it will be better to use the term *'Monocular elevation deficiency (MED) syndrome'*, for the patients having such an elevation deficiency.

Etiological types of monocular elevation deficiency

Monocular elevation deficiency may be either congenital or acquired. Depending upon the underlying factors responsible, the monocular elevation deficiency can be classified into following three groups:

1. Double elevator weakness. This entity is characterized by:

i. Negative forced duction test,

ii. Reduced force generation of elevators (evidence of paralysis), and

iii. Reduced saccadic velocities in upgaze movements of affected eye.

Etiology of the combined weakness (paresis) of superior rectus and inferior oblique of the same eye is not known exactly and is difficult to explain even anatomically. Possible explanations given for the two types (congenital and acquired) of double elevator weakness are as follows:

a. *Congenital elevator weakness.* There are two views about it:

i. One view is that basically weakness of the elevation is caused by a superior rectus palsy of long-standing and that due to spread of comitance the field of action of inferior oblique is involved.

ii. Other workers have suggested it to be a supranuclear elevation insufficiency. Supranuclear MED is characterized by intact or mildly reduced vertical saccadic velocity below midline and absent velocity above midline with Bell's phenomenon being usually present. While in SR palsy the vertical saccades are slowed both above and below the midline and Bell's phenomenon is absent.

b. *Acquired elevator weakness* is usually sudden in onset and nearly muscular in origin. It has been suggested by some workers that vascular insufficiency in a penetrating vessel to the pretectum is the likely cause of a postulated unilateral supranuclear lesion just rostral to the oculomotor nuclear complex.

2. Mechanical restriction to elevation of globe is another cause of monocular elevation deficiency. This group is characterized by:

• Positive forced duction to elevation,

• Normal active force generation (no muscle paralysis), and

• Normal saccades of the superior rectus.

Etiology. Its reported causes are:

• *Congenital or acquired* fibrosis involving the soft tissue in the inferior aspect of the globe.

• *Anomalous insertion* of the inferior rectus muscle.

Note. Other forms of mechanical restrictions such as those associated with fractures of the orbital floor and endocrine myopathy also cause elevation deficiency, but cannot be included as the cause of restrictive form of 'monocular deficiency syndrome'. In fact, these are well established separate entities and need to be differentiated for management point of view.

3. Combination of restriction and weakness. Monocular elevation deficiency in this group is caused by inferior rectus restriction and also weak elevators. This group is characterized by:

• Positive forced duction in elevation (evidence of restriction).

- Reduced force generation of elevators of involved eye (evidence of paralysis).
- Reduced upward vertical saccadic velocities in involved eye (evidence of paralysis).

Clinical features

I. Vertical deviation, head posture, diplopia and ptosis are the cardinal features of monocular elevation deficiency. Manifestation of these features depends upon the presenting pattern.

Depending upon the fixation pattern adapted by a particular patient (because of many known and unknown factors), following three presentation patterns are known in patients with monocular elevation deficiency:

1. Binocular fixation. Some patients prefer to keep their head tipped backward and maintain a binocular fusion. In fact, the posture adopted by these patients moves the eyes, by means of the "dolls head phenomenon", into the field of action of the depressors of the globe. Visual acuity is usually normal in these patients.

However, when these patients hold their head erect in primary position, there may occur:

i. *Hypotropia* of the affected eye, and

ii. Vertical *diplopia*

2. Fixation with uninvolved eye. These patients have following features:

i. *Hypotropia* in involved eye (Fig. 12.38E)

ii. *Pseudoptosis* accompanying hypotropia (Fig. 12.38E). (The ptosis disappears, when the patient fixates with the paretic eye (Fig. 12.38F).

iii. *True ptosis* due to associated LPS weakness, may be present in 50% of cases. True ptosis does not resolve when patient fixes with paretic eye. Pseudoptosis and true levator weakness may also occur simultaneously.

iv. *Amblyopia* of the affected eye with a visual acuity of 6/60 or less.

v. *Diplopia* is absent.

3. Fixation with involved eye. Because of certain predispositions, some patients prefer to fix with the involved eye. These patients present with following features:

i. *Hypertropia* of normal eye which is greater due to secondary deviation (Fig. 12.38F).

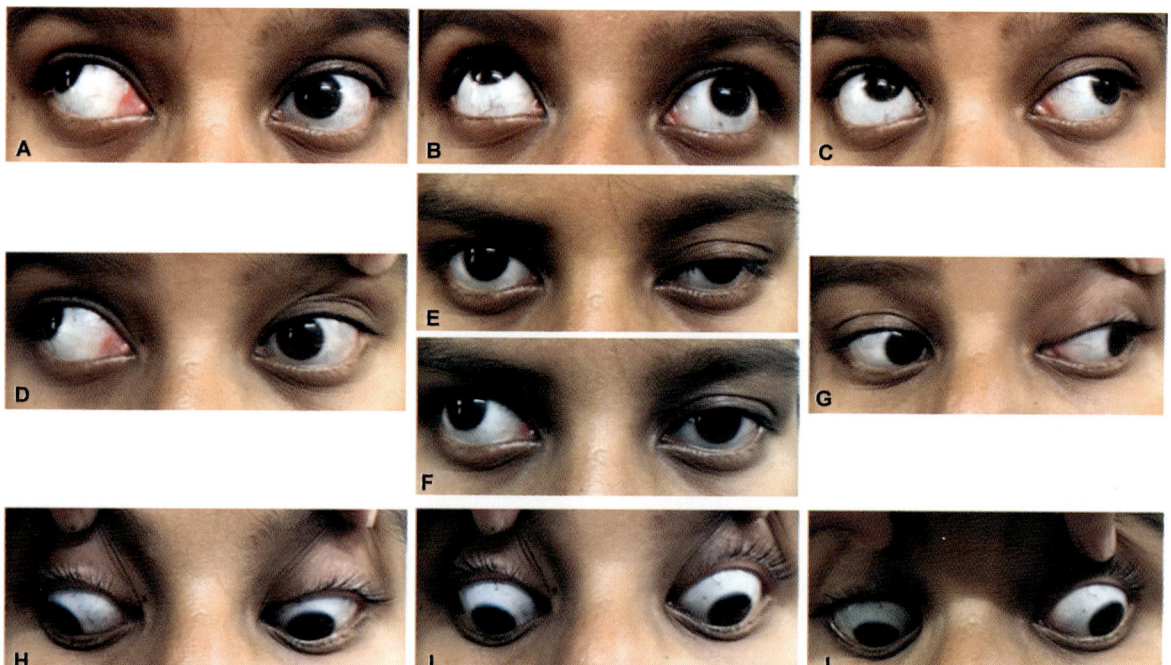

Fig. 12.38 *Monocular elevation deficiency of the left eye. Note: limitation of elevation in upgaze (B), on levoelevation (C), and dextroelevation (A). Note left ptosis in primary gaze when fixing with normal eye (E) and marked hypertropia due to secondary deviation in normal right eye when fixing with the paretic right eye (F).*

ii. *Visual acuity* in the normal eye may be reduced.

iii. *True ptosis* due to associated weakness of LPS may be present.

II. Limitation of elevation (in adduction as well as in abduction, both on versions and ductions) beyond midline, is the main clinical characteristic of this condition (Fig. 12.38 A to C).

III. Other clinical characteristics

i. *An extra or deep lower lid fold* on the affected side may be seen in patients with inferior rectus muscle restriction.

ii. *Bell's phenomenon* is usually very poor or absent in the eye with inferior rectus muscle restriction as compared to the eye without inferior rectus muscle restriction.

iii. *Positional tonometry* performed with applanation tonometer shows a rise in IOP of more than 3 mm Hg in 15° upward gaze as compared to that in primary gaze in patients with restrictive limitations. No such significant increase in IOP occurs in paretic weakness.

Differential diagnosis

Congenital elevator weakness should be differentiated from:

- Brown's syndrome
- Congenital fibrosis of inferior rectus muscle.
- Vertical Duane's syndrome
- Congenital absence of SR
- Congenital palsy of superior division of 3rd nerve.

Acquired elevator weakness should be differentiated from:

- *Blow-out fracture* of orbital floor with incarceration of inferior rectus muscle.
- *Thyroid ophthalmopathy* with inferior rectus myopathy.
- Acquired fibrosis of IR
- *Anomalous insertion* of inferior rectus muscle.
- *Abnormal accessory muscle* between annulus of Zinn and the posterior part of the globe.

Treatment

Indications of treatment include:

- Large vertical deviation in primary position with or without ptosis, and
- Significant abnormal head posture.

Surgical procedures recommended are as follows:

1. *Knapp's procedure* is useful in patients with elevator weakness without any restrictive involvement. In this procedure, medial rectus and lateral rectus muscles of the involved eye are transposed to a position near the insertion of the superior rectus muscle (Fig. 15.21).

2. *Recession of the inferior rectus muscle* is recommended in the presence of inferior restriction for a vertical deviation up to 18–20D.

3. *Recession of the inferior rectus muscle plus resection of the superior rectus* is indicated, when in the presence of inferior restriction, the deviation is more than 18 to 20D.

4. *Recession of inferior rectus with Knapp's procedure* may be required in patients with MED due to combined restriction as well as weakness of elevation. It is best to perform the operation in two stages. In the first stage, IR recession should be done and at a later stage, if required, Knapp's procedure should be done. The second procedure should be done after 4 months to prevent anterior segment ischemia. However, if both procedures are performed in same sitting then ciliary vessel sparing procedure should be preferred.

Note. Knapp's procedure usually corrects 20–35 PD of hypotropia in primary position. Knapp procedure after IR recession usually has greater effect.

5. *Augmented transposition* using posterior fixation suture should be done for large hypotropia >35 PD, with no IR restriction.

6. *Modified Knapp's.* If horizontal deviation is also present then recess-resect and also transpose the MR and LR muscles.

DOUBLE DEPRESSOR PALSY

The term 'double depressor palsy' literally means paralysis of both depressors (inferior rectus and superior oblique) of the same eye resulting in a clinical condition characterized by depression deficiency in the entire range of downward gaze, i.e. in primary gaze, in adduction as well as in abduction.

Etiology

The exact etiology of this rare congenital condition is not known. Further, even anatomically it is not possible to explain the involvement of two muscles innervated from different nuclei. It has been suggested that the condition double depressor palsy might result from any of the following situations:

1. *A long-standing inferior rectus palsy* with spread of comitance to the field of the ipsilateral superior oblique muscle.
2. *A long-standing inferior rectus palsy* and secondary superior rectus contracture.
3. *A long-standing superior oblique palsy* with spread of comitance to the ipsilateral inferior rectus muscle.

Clinical features

1. Deviation. The paretic eye is *hypertropic in* primary position, when the normal eye is fixing (Fig. 12.39A I and B V).

2. Ocular movements. Ductions are limited in the entire lower field of gaze (Fig. 12.39A II to IV and BVII to IX) and normal in all other gaze positions.

Differential diagnosis

Double depressor palsy should be differentiated from mechanical restriction. Forced duction test and saccadic velocity measurements are helpful in differentiating paresis from mechanical restrictions.

Treatment

1. Inverse Knapp's procedure is useful in patients having a definite weakness. In this procedure, lateral and medial recti are

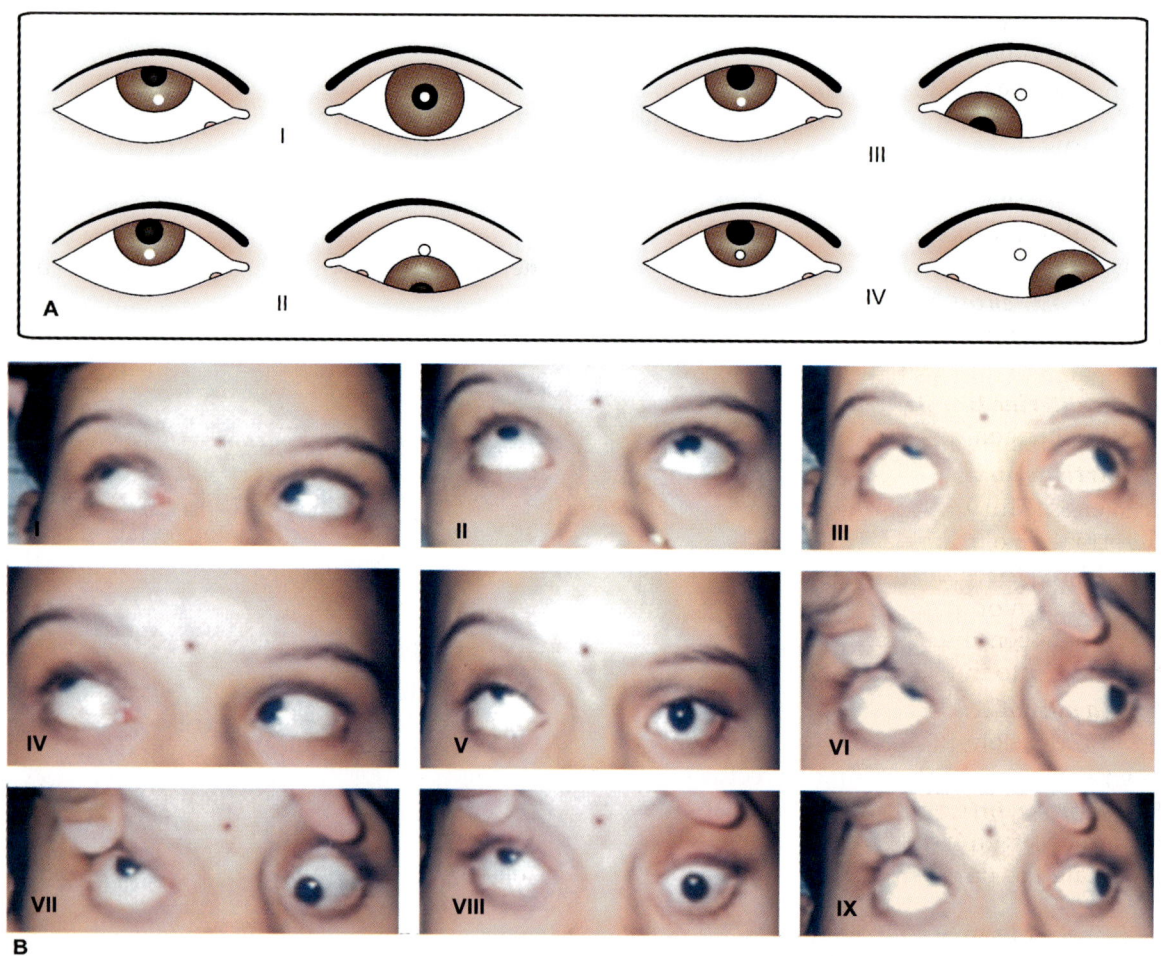

Fig. 12.39 *Double depressor palsy right eye: A, Diagrammatic representation; and B, clinical photograph in nine positions of gaze (Courtesy Dr Shubhang Bhave). Note right hypertropia in primary position (A I and B V) and limitation of depression in central downgaze (A II and B VIII), dextrodepression (A III and BVII) and levodepression (A IV and B IX).*

disinserted and reattached near the insertion of inferior rectus.

2. *Recession of the superior rectus muscle* may be performed in patients with superior mechanical restrictions.

TOTAL THIRD NERVE PARALYSIS

The third cranial (oculomotor) nerve is entirely motor in function. It supplies all the extraocular muscles except lateral rectus and superior oblique. It also supplies the intraocular muscles namely—sphincter pupillae and ciliary muscle.

Total paralysis of third cranial nerve may be congenital or acquired. While acquired paralysis of third nerve is of common occurrence, the congenital palsies are uncommon.

Note. Applied anatomy of third nerve and its nucleus should be reviewed before proceeding further (*see* page 12).

ETIOLOGY

A. Congenital third cranial nerve palsy

It has been reported to occur due to following causes:

1. *Developmental* aplasia or hypoplasia of the third nerve nucleus or the nerve is extremely rare.

2. *Intrauterine trauma* has been mentioned as a cause of congenital third nerve palsy.

3. *Birth trauma.* It is believed that most congenital third nerve palsies are caused by deformation of the soft skull of the fetus by the moulding forces during labour. Probably, compression of the third nerve occurs at some point between the brainstem and the entry of the nerve into the cavernous sinus.

4. *As a part of cerebral palsy.* Third nerve palsy may occur as one of the components of cerebral palsy.

5. *Infantile intracranial infections* such as encephalitis and meningitis have also been implicated as possible causes.

B. Acquired third nerve palsy

The causes which can involve the third nerve at various levels with their peculiar features are as follows:

1. *Nuclear lesions*
- Lesions involving purely the third nerve nucleus complex are relatively uncommon.
- *Common causes* include vascular diseases, demyelination, primary tumours and metastasis.
- Lesions involving *entire nucleus* cause an ipsilateral third nerve palsy with ipsilateral sparing and contralateral weakness of elevation.
- Lesions involving *paired medial rectus* sub-nuclei (ventromedial nucleus) cause a wall-eyed bilateral internuclear ophthal-moplegia (WEBINO), characterised by defective convergence and adduction.

2. *Fascicular lesions*
- *Causes* are similar to nuclear lesions.
- *Benedikt's syndrome* characterised by ipsilateral third nerve palsy associated with tremors and jerky movements of the contra-lateral side, occurs due to lesions at the intermediate level of the midbrain. Third nerve paralysis occurs due to involvement of fasciculus as it passes through the red nucleus.
- *Weber's syndrome.* In it fascicular part of the nerve is involved, while passing through the cerebral peduncle. The syndrome is characterised by ipsilateral third nerve palsy, contralateral hemiplegia and facial palsy of upper motor neuron type.

3. *Lesions involving basilar part of the nerve*
- As the nerve runs in the subarachnoid space at the base of skull unaccompanied by any other cranial nerve, *isolated third nerve palsies are* frequently basilar.
- *Causes:* (1) *Aneurysms* at the posterior communicating artery cause isolated third nerve palsy with involvement of pupil. (2) *Extradural haematoma* which may cause tentorial pressure cone with downward herniation of the temporal lobe this compresses the third nerve as it passes over the tentorial edge (Fig. 12.40). Initially there occurs fixed dilated pupil, which is followed by a total third nerve palsy. (3) *Diabetes* causes isolated 3rd nerve palsy with sparing of the pupillary reflexes.

4. *Lesions involving intracavernous part of the nerve*
- Because of its close proximity to other cranial nerves, intracavernous third nerve palsies

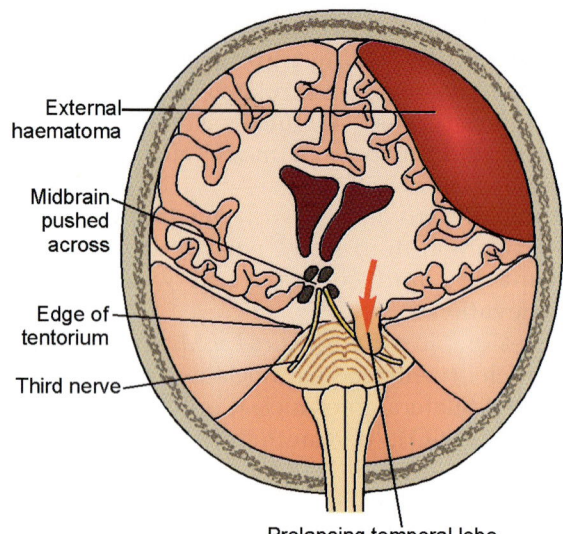

External haematoma

Midbrain pushed across

Edge of tentorium

Third nerve

Prolapsing temporal lobe

Fig. 12.40 *Mechanism of third nerve palsy in extradural haematoma.*

are usually associated with involvement of the fourth, the sixth nerve, and the first division of the trigeminal nerve.

- In intracavernous 3rd nerve palsy, pupil is spared. Sometimes, pupil may be constricted owing to involvement of sympathetics.
- *Causes:* (1) *Pituitary apoplexy* may cause a third nerve palsy as a result of haemorrhagic infarction of a pituitary adenoma (e.g. after child birth), with lateral extension into the cavernous sinus. (2) *Intracavernous lesions* which may cause a third nerve palsy include aneurysms, meningiomas, carotid cavernous fistulae and Tolosa-Hunt syndrome (granulomatous inflammation).

5. Lesions of the intraorbital part of the nerve
- May cause isolated extraocular muscle palsies or may involve either superior division or inferior division or both divisions.
- Involvement of superior divison of 3rd nerve is commonly associated with other cranial nerve palsies, whereas involvement of inferior divison of 3rd nerve is frequently isolated.
- *Causes:* Orbital tumours, pseudotumours, trauma, viral illness and vascular diseases.

6. Neuropathic processes which can involve the third nerve after it leaves the midbrain are as follows:

- *Vascular causes* of third nerve palsy include diabetes and hypertension. Diabetic cranial mononeuropathy is a well-known cause of third cranial nerve palsy. It is characterized by rapid onset, periocular pain, pupil sparing with complete resolution within 2–3 months without development of aberrant regeneration.
- *Herpes zoster ophthalmicus* can involve the third nerve by means of contiguous spread from the ophthalmic division of the fifth cranial nerve to other cranial nerves or they pass through superior orbital fissure.
- *Ophthalmoplegic migraine* may cause partial or complete 3rd nerve palsy especially in children under 10 years. It is characterized by periocular pains, nausea and vomiting followed by ophthalmoplegia.
- *First syndrome,* characterized by a bilateral, progressive and painless ophthalmoplegia, is another neuropathic cause of third nerve palsy. It is a variant of Gullian-Barre syndrome. It may be associated in the bilateral peripheral facial weakness.

Clinical groups of causes of third nerve palsy

Causes of isolated third nerve palsy can be summarized as below:

1. *Idiopathic.* In about 25% cases, cause is not known.

2. *Vascular diseases.* Diabetes and hypertension are the common medical causes of pupil sparing isolated third nerve palsy.

3. *Trauma* is also an important cause of isolated third nerve paralysis. Mechanism of third nerve involvement by an extradural haematoma is shown in Fig. 12.40.

4. *Aneurysm* at the junction of the posterior communicating artery with the internal carotid artery is an important cause of isolated, painful third nerve palsy with involvement of the pupil. Other causes of painful third nerve palsy are migraine, Tolosa-Hunt syndrome and diabetes.

5. *Miscellaneous.* Other rare causes include tumour, vasculitis associated with collagen disorder, syphilis and tuberculosis.

Causes of third nerve palsy in children
- Congenital (40–50%)
- Traumatic

- Inflammatory
- Post-viral syndromes
- Migraine
- Neoplasms (rarely)

Causes of third nerve palsy in adults
- Aneurysm
- Diabetes
- Neuritis
- Trauma
- Infection
- Tumour (rare causes)

Causes of pupil sparing third nerve palsy.
Vascular causes such as diabetes and hypertension which affect the vasa nervorum often cause pupil sparing third nerve palsy. On the other hand, compressive lesions usually cause pupil dilatation due to compression of pial vessels.

CLINICAL FEATURES
Clinical features of complete third nerve paralysis can be described as below:

- General features
- Congenital versus acquired paralysis
- Features due to aberrant regeneration.
- Cyclic oculomotor paralysis.

General clinical features
Depending upon the anatomical basis, in general, clinical features of a case of total third nerve palsy (Fig. 12.41A and B) are as follows:

1. *Ptosis.* It occurs due to paralysis of the levator palpebrae superioris muscle.

2. *Ocular deviation.* Eyeball is turned down, out and slightly intorted due to actions of the lateral rectus and superior oblique muscles.

3. *Ocular movements* (Fig. 12.42) are restricted due to paralysis of the various muscles as below:

- Adduction—due to medial rectus
- Elevation—due to superior rectus and inferior oblique
- Depression—due to inferior rectus
- Extorsion—due to inferior rectus and inferior oblique.

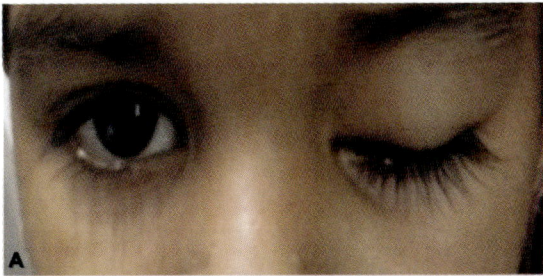
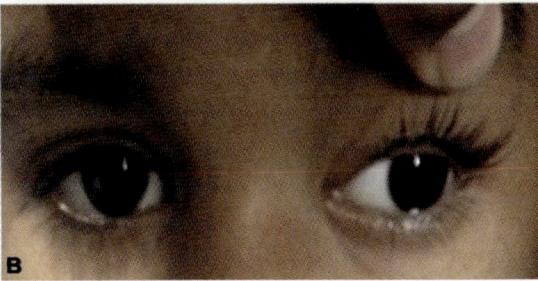

Fig. 12.41 *A patient with third cranial nerve paralysis showing ptosis* (A) *and divergent squint* (B).

4. *Pupil is fixed and dilated* due to paralysis of the sphincter pupillae muscle. However, in pupil sparing lesions, it is normal.

5. *Accommodation* is completely lost due to paralysis of the ciliary muscle. However, in pupil sparing lesions, it is normal.

6. *Diplopia.* A crossed horizontal diplopia with slight vertical misalignment elicited on manually raising the eyelid occurs due to paralytic divergence squint with associated slight intorsion and downward rotation.

7. *Abnormal head posture.* If the pupillary area is uncovered, to avoid diplopia, head is moved in a position consistent with the direction of action of paralyzed muscles, i.e. face is turned on the opposite side, head is tilted towards the affected side and chin is slightly elevated.

Clinical features: congenital versus acquired third nerve palsy

1. **Age.** Congenital third nerve palsy is more frequently seen in children, while acquired is more common in adults.

2. **Intraocular muscles** are usually not involved in congenital third nerve palsy.

3. **Ptosis** is variable in congenital third nerve palsy, but, some degree of lid drooping is usually present while, in most acquired cases there is complete drooping of the upper lid.

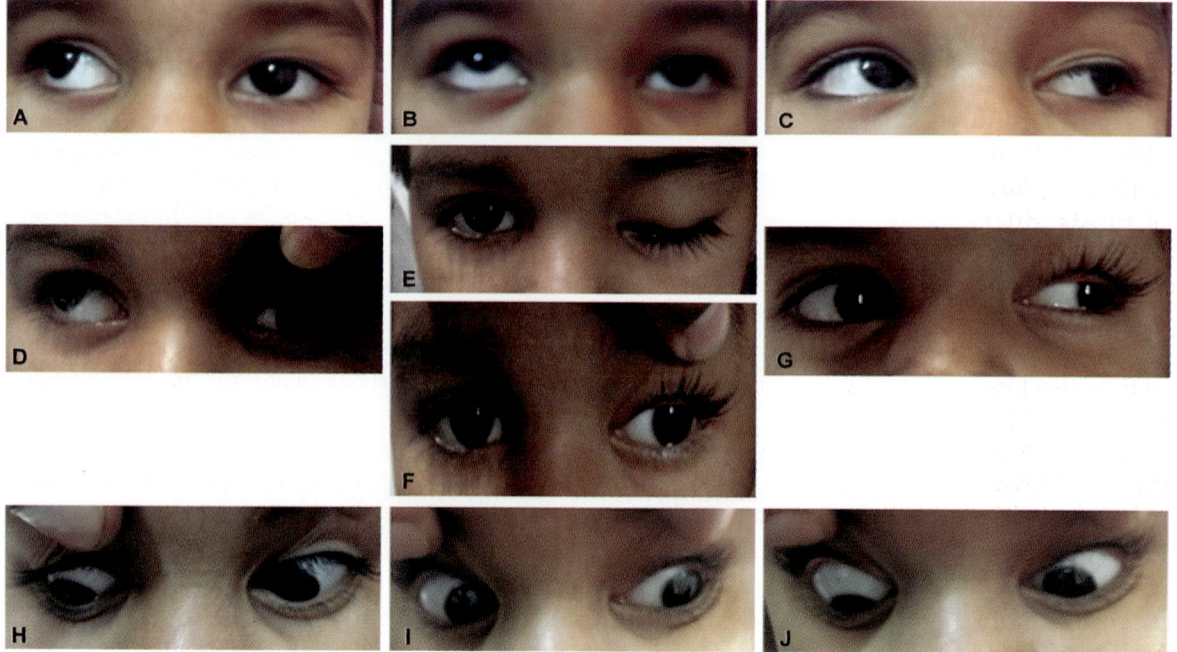

Fig. 12.42 *Ocular movements and nine positions of gaze in a patient with right third nerve paralysis.*

4. Suppression and amblyopia are quite common in congenital paralysis. However, it is often surprising to note good visual acuity in the affected eye, because it is expected that the patient always uses the normal eye and the affected eye will have deep amblyopia. Probably visual acuity is maintained because the patient uses the paretic eye in the down and out position, a position in which nose precludes the use of normal eye. As a result, most patients with congenital third nerve palsies have only a small degree of amblyopia, approximately 6/18 to 6/24.

5. Aberrant regeneration is more frequently seen in congenital palsy.

Features due to aberrant regeneration of third nerve

Aberrant regeneration can occur following congenital or acquired third nerve palsy. It may occur even without a preceding oculomotor paralysis in patients with a slowly growing intracavernous meningioma or with a carotid aneurysm. Aberrant regeneration is thought to result from a miswiring of axons from the proximal portion of the nerve into the peripheral segment of the nerve. The misdirection syndrome (aberrant regeneration) follows more commonly in a compressive injury of the oculomotor nerve, e.g. those associated with birth trauma.

Features due to aberrant regeneration of third nerve (all of which may not necessarily be present in a given patient) are as follows:

1. *Pseudo-Graefe's sign.* It refers to elevation of the upper lid on attempted downgaze. It perhaps occurs due to miswiring of the nerve fibres originally meant for inferior rectus with the nerve fibres going into levator palpebrae superioris.

2. *Widening of the palpebral fissure* on adduction and narrowing of the fissure on abduction.

3. *Pseudo-Argyl Robertson pupil.* It refers to a dilated fixed pupil that does not react to direct or consensual light stimulation but does react slightly on convergence and also on adduction.

4. *Retraction of the upperlid* occasionally may be accompanied by contraction of the pupil.

5. *Eyeball may be retracted* and adducted on attempted upgaze.

Cyclic oculomotor paralysis

It is the rarest but an interesting form of third nerve paralysis which is usually congenital in origin. As the name implies, it is characterized by an alternate paresis and spastic contraction of the extraocular and intraocular muscles supplied by the third cranial nerve. The spastic phase is shorter than the paretic phase. The two phases continue to alternate even in sleep but disappear in deeper stages of anaesthesia.

1. *Paretic phase* is characterized by occurrence of ptosis, dilatation of pupil, impairment of accommodation, weakness of adduction, weakness of vertical movements and an outward turning of the globe.

2. *Spastic phase* is characterized by contraction of the muscles—beginning with adduction and elevation of the lid. It is followed by pupillary constriction and improvement in accommodation. Ultimately, the eye may return to primary position to be followed, shortly by the paretic phase.

MANAGEMENT

Management of third cranial nerve palsy remains the most difficult, incomplete and least satisfying. In general, the management includes investigations, treatment of the cause, conservative treatment and surgical treatment.

Investigations

Third nerve palsy of acute onset, especially if non-pupil sparing, should be subjected to through neuro-ophthalmic evaluation and be investigated with prompt and appropriate neurologic studies.

1. *Magnetic resonance imaging (MRI) and carotid angiography.* Probably, it is best to perform MRI in such cases and then proceed further as below:

  a. *In children below 10 years of age regardless of the state of pupil,* if MRI is normal, carotid angiography is not essential because of the less likelihood of aneurysm.

  b. *In patients above 10 years of age with pupil involvement,* if MRI shows a mass compatible with an aneurysm or even if MRI is normal, perform carotid angiography to rule out aneurysm.

  c. *In patients above 10 years of age with* pupil sparing, if MRI is normal, a thorough medical evaluation should be conducted. In patients of vasculopathy age group (>40 years), hypertension and atherosclerosis should be

taken care of. Further, diabetic mononeuropathy should always be ruled out by glucose tolerance test in patients with pupil sparing third nerve palsy.

All such patients should be observed frequently and if pupil is involved or signs and symptoms of subarachnoid haemorrhage develop immediately, angiography is required to rule out aneurysm.

2. *Tensilon test.* One should remember the dictum that any unexplained cause of diplopia or ptosis requires a Tensilon test to exclude myasthenia gravis.

3. *ESR.* In patients of more than 55 years of age with symptoms of polymyalgia rheumatica, ESR estimation should be done. If ESR is found high, then temporal artery biopsy should be performed to rule out temporal arteritis.

Treatment of the cause

If on investigation, a definite cause of third nerve palsy such as intracranial aneurysm, diabetes, myasthenia gravis, etc. is found, patient should be referred to neurosurgeon or neurophysician depending upon the indication. However, if no surgical cause is found, patients should be managed conservatively followed by extraocular muscle surgery, if required.

Conservative treatment

1. *Observations.* Like any other paralytic squint, wait and watch for the self recovery should be done at least for 6–8 months. During this period, patient should be followed every 6 weeks, and at each follow-up visit, following examinations should be done.

• Measurement of exotropia and hypotropia with prism for cover test.
• Diplopia charting.
• Hess charting.

2. *Amblyopia* is frequently associated with third nerve paresis in paediatric patients and must be sought and treated aggressively. Therefore, surgical treatment to raise the ptotic lid is needed urgently in children. Alternate patching should be done to prevent occurrence of amblyopias.

3. *Diplopia* is difficult to treat with prisms, because of its variable nature.

- *Complete ptosis* is useful in preventing diplopia in visually mature patient. Therefore, ptosis surgery should be deferred until after the eye has been straightened.
- *Alternate patching* is required to prevent diplopia in visually mature patients with incomplete ptosis. Opaque contact lens or blurred spectacles can be used as alternative to patching.

4. Botulinum toxin. Use of botulinum toxin is another nonsurgical option in the acute phase of partial third nerve paresis. This is, especially useful in cases of isolated involvement of MR muscle. It paralyses the antagonist LR temporarily and thus neutralizes horizontal deviation in the primary position. It also prevents contracture of LR muscle. After recovery of the injected muscle, the remaining vertical deviation may need to be corrected by prisms or surgical therapy. Some patients may not need surgery later on. Use of botulinum toxin for vertical muscle imbalance is rarely indicated, as SR should not be injected as ptosis can occur if toxin is placed into the levator—SR complex.

5. Vitamin B-complex may be used as neurotonic.

6. Systemic steroids may hasten the recovery in patients with non-specific inflammation. Further, in patients with temporal arteritis or rheumatological disorder, high doses of steroids are recommended.

Surgical treatment

General principles

1. *Wait and watch approach.* Like any other paralytic squint at least 6–8 months should elapse before performing any surgical treatment to straighten the eye.

2. *Surgery should be undertaken continuously* in patients with complete palsy and good binocular visual function, since elevation of the lid and incomplete realignment without useful single binocular fields may produce incapaci-tating diplopia.

3. *Surgery for third nerve paralysis is challenging and the outcome must be discussed* with the patient. Associated factors such as the presence of ptosis, pupillary involvement, amblyopia, aberrant regeneration, poor Bell's phenomenon, superior oblique (SO) overaction, and lateral rectus (LR) contracture may further complicate the matter. Further, it should be explained to the patient or parents that several operations will most likely be necessary to straighten the eyes and both patience and understanding are important throughout the course of treatment. It should also be emphasized to the patient that inspite of multiple operations, one can achieve functional and cosmetic correction only in primary position and not in different gazes.

Goals of surgery

- To improve alignment in primary gaze.
- To produce or enlarge some degree of binocular single vision.

Surgical procedures

Surgery should be contemplated, only if the strabismus measurement and diplopia remain stable for 3 months (i.e. partial recovery has stabilized). It usually occurs after 6–8 months of paralysis.

Aim of surgery is to give alignment in the two important positions, i.e. primary and downgaze.

Planning for the appropriate surgical procedure must be dictated by the severity of the weakness of the muscles as follows:

1. Surgery for exotropia (lateral rectus recession and medial rectus resection)

- *In an incomplete palsy*, recess-resect procedure should be planned as done for comitant exotropia.
- *In complete paralysis*, Helveston and many others have advised supramaximal recession of lateral rectus (14–16 mm) and resection of medial rectus (8–14 mm), to align the eye in primary position. But this has limited success as overtime chronic contracture of LR and elongation of resected muscle, causes exotropic drift again.

  Myectomy of LR muscle to accomplish a super-maximal weakening effect of abduction in patients with complete third nerve palsy has also been recommended. However, this often results in recurrence of exotropia.
- *Adjustable sutures* during recess-resect procedure are quite useful in co-operative patients.

2. Surgery for hypotropia include:

- *Supraplacement of horizontal recti during recess-resect procedure* is preferred by some surgeons.
- *Superior oblique tenotomy* is preferred by some surgeons over the supraplacement of horizontal recti.
- *Inferior rectus recession with resection of superior rectus* is preferred by some surgeons to correct hypotropia is ease with preserved patial function of vertical recti. But a caution is required about the possibility of anterior segment ischaemia.
- *Faden recession of contralateral vertical recti* is also helpful in correcting the vertical misalignment in primary position or downgaze.

3. Transposition of superior oblique tendon. If eye remains still exotropic after 3 months of above procedures, in this situation, a further adduction effect can be obtained by transposition of the insertion of the superior oblique tendon to a point 2 to 3 mm anterior to the medial side of superior rectus insertion. Transposition procedure is meant to create a tonic adducting force to the globe to keep it in primary position rather than produce any true adductive force during horizontal gaze. This is a difficult procedure.

Thus, transposition of superior oblique tendon may be considered in a patient with acquired third nerve palsy, only if the following conditions are met:

- Palsy is complete
- Involved eye is fixing eye.
- Maximum recess-resect surgeries on the horizontal recti have failed to restore the globe to primary position.

4. In case of palsy of inferior division of 3rd nerve. Transposition of lateral rectus muscle to the site of insertion of inferior rectus muscle and transposition of superior rectus muscle to medial rectus area, combined with tenotomy of superior oblique to align the eye in primary position should be carried out. This also helps to correct intorsion and provides a vector force in the direction of palsied muscle.

5. In case of palsy of superior division. Knapp's procedure should be carried out (*see* page 440).

6. Anchoring of the lateral rectus to periosteum of lateral orbital wall by non-absorbable. 5-0 mersilene suture along with 8-0 mm of medial rectus resection has also been recommended for alignment of globe in the primary position.

7. Surgery for ptosis. Once the paralytic strabismus is treated maximally, the paralytic ptosis is treated with frontalis sling, taking care that the globe is not overly jeopardized because of impaired or absent Bell's phenomenon. Ptosis should be corrected only to cover half of the cornea with relaxed brow. Protective measures to avoid exposure keratopathy must be taken.

INTERNUCLEAR OPHTHALMOPLEGIA

Internuclear ophthalmoplegia results from a lesion of the medial longitudinal fasciculus (MLF) and that is why, is also known as MLF syndrome. It is a supranuclear disorder described on page 372.

EXTERNAL OPHTHALMOPLEGIA

External ophthalmoplegia refers to paralysis of all extraocular muscles sparing the intraocular muscles.

TOTAL OPHTHALMOPLEGIA

Total or complete ophthalmoplegia refers to paralysis of all extraocular muscles including LPS and intraocular muscles, viz., sphincter pupillae and ciliary muscle. It results from combined paralysis of third, fourth and sixth cranial nerves. It is a common feature of orbital apex syndrome and cavernous sinus syndrome.

RESTRICTIVE OCULAR MOTILITY DEFECTS

Restrictive strabismus is a type of incomitant squint characterized by limitation of movements due to causes other than paralytic. In such cases limitation of ocular movements is out of proportion to the amount of deviation in the primary position.

Causes of restrictive strabismus can be arranged in two groups:

A. Restrictive strabismus due to misdirected muscles forces.
B. Restrictive strabismus due to mechanical restriction.

A. RESTRICTIVE STRABISMUS DUE TO MISDIRECTED MUSCLE FORCES

Misdirected muscle foreces that work against the normal agonist muscle function as seen in following conditions:

1. *Congenital cranial dysinnervation disorders (CCDDs)*, e.g. Duane's retraction syndrome.
2. *Congenital ectopic extraocular muscle insertion and/or pulley location.*
3. *Displaced extraocular muscle*, e.g.
   - Superior displacement of medial rectus as seen in craniosynostosis.
   - Slippage of lateral rectus muscle as seen in some patients of high myopia with large posterior staphylloma.
   - Iatrogenic displacement of muscle as reported after inferior oblique anteriorization.

CONGENITAL CRANIAL DYSINNERVATION DISORDERS

Congenital cranial dysinnervation disorders (CCDDs) encompass a group of disorders that result from developmental errors in innervation of the ocular and facial muscles and not from primary dysfunction of the muscles themselves. The CCDDs can be classified as below:

I. *CCDDs primarily affecting horizontal ocular motility*
   - Duane's retraction syndrome (DRS)
   - Horizontal gaze palsy with progressive scoliosis (HGPPS)

II. *CCDDs primarily affecting vertical ocular motility*
   - Congenital fibrosis of extraocular muscles (CFEOMs) type 1, 2 and 3
   - Congenital ptosis

III. *CCDDs primarily affecting facial muscles with associated ocular motility defects*
   - Congenital facial weakness (CFP)
   - Moebius syndrome

I. CCDDs PRIMARILY AFFECTING HORIZONTAL OCULAR MOTILITY

These disorders resut from developmental anomalies of sixth cranial nerve and/or its nucleus, and include:

- Duane's retraction syndrome (DRS), and
- Horizontal gaze palsy with progressive scoliosis (HGPPS).

DUANE'S RETRACTION SYNDROME

Duane's retraction syndrome is a common entity. Stilling (1887) was probably the first person to describe this condition followed by Turk (1890). In 1905, Alexander Duane defined the retraction syndrome to consist of six characteristic features and since then his name has been attached with this syndrome. However, European literature prefers to refer to it as *'Stilling-Turk-Duane' retraction syndrome*. The syndrome in its classic form is characterized by the following features:

- Limitation of abduction and/or adduction
- Retraction of globe on adduction
- Narrowing of palpebral fissure on adduction and widening on abduction.
- Frequently, upshoot or downshoot of eye on attempted adduction.

Etiology

Currently, it is believed that Duane's syndrome is *a congenital cranial dysinnervation disorder (CCDD)* of brainstem origin rather than occurring due to structural anomalies of the muscles as thought earlier.

Paradoxical innervation of the horizontal rectus muscles is the main etiological factor. Electromyographic (EMG) studies have shown that most cases of DRS have paradoxical innervation of the horizontal rectus muscles as shown in Fig. 12.43 and explained under the pathogenesis of ocular features individually (page 336–338).

Paradoxical innervation is there for both LR and MR rectus muscles, so both co-contract during abduction and adduction resulting in:

- *Abduction*—limitation
- *Adduction*—limitation
- *Palpebral aperture*—narrowing in primary position as well as in adduction and abduction.
- *Globe* retraction.

Probable cause of dysinnervation is:
- *Embryopathy*, i.e. developmental disturbance is responsible for dysinnervation. This fact is

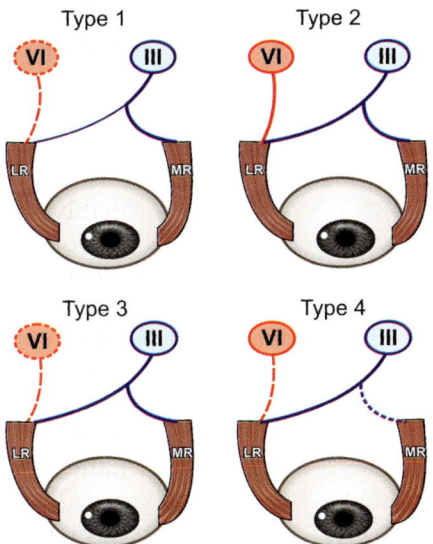

Type 1 Type 2

Type 3 Type 4

Fig. 12.43 *Right eye illustration of potential innervation patterns in different types of Duane syndrome. VI indicates fibres of the sixth cranial nerve. III indicates fibres of the third cranial nerve. Dashed lines indicate hypoplastic or absent nerve fibres. Thin lines indicate relative decreased innervation.*

corobarated by the type of associated systemic anomalies as well as the frequent association of Duane's syndrome in well documented cases of thalidomide embryopathy.

• *Hereditary* basis for the anomaly has also been suggested on the basis of familial occurrence

with dominant inheritence pattern of the syndrome.

Classification of Duane's syndrome

Duane's retraction syndrome (DRS) has been classified by various workers (Brown 1950, 1958; Lyle and Bridgeman 1959, Huber, 1974). However, to avoid confusion only the most commonly accepted Huber's classification is given here.

Huber's classification is not only most useful one clinically, but is well supported by electromyographic documentation. Huber classified Duane's syndrome into three types I, II, III and recently type IV has also been added (all associated with paradoxical innervation) as given below:

Duane's type I is the most common (78%) followed by type III (15%) and type II is the least common variety. A manifest ocular deviation in primary position may or may not be present in Duane's retraction syndrome. Huber's classification though most useful clinically, does not tell about the associated type of deviation. Khurana (1988) has modified Huber's classification by dividing each type into three subtypes depending on the deviation in primary position, viz. a, b and c for esotropia, exotropia and orthotropia, respectively (Table 12.9). This

Type	Subtype	Eye in primary position	Other features
	Ia	Esotropic	Marked limitation of abduction Almost normal adduction
I	Ib	Exotropic	Narrowing of palpebral fissure on adduction
	Ic	Orthotropic	Retraction of globe on adduction
	IIa	Esotropic	Marked limitation of adduction, almost normal adduction
II	IIb	Exotropic	Narrowing of palpebral fissure on attempted adduction
	IIc	Orthotropic	Retraction of globe on attempted adduction
	IIIa	Esotropic	Marked limitation of abduction
III	IIIb	Exotropic	Marked limitation of adduction Narrowing of palpebral fissure on attempted adduction and abduction
	IIIc	Orthotropic	Retraction of globe on attempted adduction and abduction

Table 12.9 *Khurana's modification over Huber's classification of Duane's retraction syndrome*

minor modification has made the Huber's classification complete and more specific.

Clinical features

Clinical features of Duane's syndrome can be discussed as: (I) General features, (II) Features related to ocular motility defect, (III) Associated ocular abnormalities, and (IV) Associated systemic abnormalities.

I. General features

1. *Females* are more frequently involved than males.
2. *Left eye* is more commonly affected (75%) than the right.
3. *Bilateral* involvement is less frequent (20%) than unilateral occurrence.
4. *Sporadic cases* are most common, but familial occurrence with dominant inheritance pattern has also been reported.

II. Characteristic of different types of Duane's syndrome

Characteristic ocular features of DRS types I, II, III have been described along with the pathogenesis (*see* page 336–338)

Duane's retraction syndrome type I

Pathogenesis. Electromyographic studies have revealed that on attempted abduction, there is lack of innervation to the LR causing marked limitation of abduction and on attempted adduction, along with MR, the LR also gets innervation (paradoxical).

Characteristic features of type I DRS (Fig. 12.44), thus, are:

In primary position eye may be orthophoric, esotropic (more common) or exotropic.

On attempted abduction since LR muscle does not receive innervation, so:
- *Abduction* is limited markedly,
- *Palpebral fissure* is normal or slightly widened, and
- *Globe* is slightly protused. This happens as a result of relaxation of both LR and MR muscles during abduction.

On attempted adduction, since along with MR, LR also gets anomalous innervation, so due to contraction of MR and LR:
- *Adduction* is present but limited, due to co-contraction of MR and LR
- *Palpebral fissure* becomes narrow, and
- *Globe is retracted,*
- *Upshoot or downshoot* of the globe may occur due to slippage caused by co-contraction of MR and LR

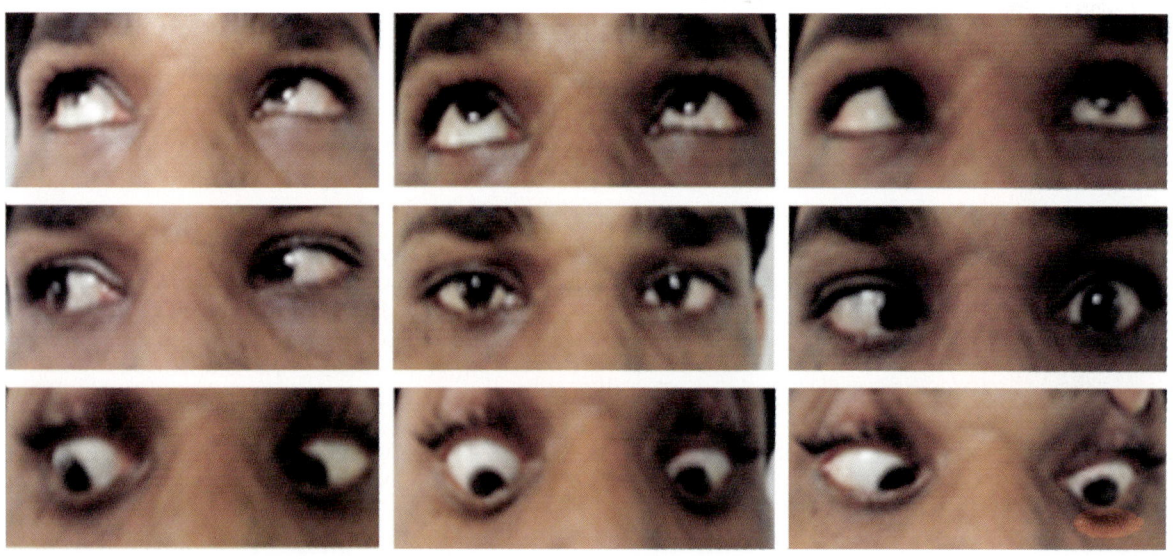

Fig. 12.44 *Type I Duane's retraction syndrome left eye with mechanical upshoot.*

Duane's retraction syndrome type II

Pathogenesis. Electromyographic studies have demonstrated that:

- *On abduction*, the LR receives normal or subnormal innervation.
- *On adduction*, LR also gets innervation (paradoxical) along with MR. Adduction and other features similar.

Characteristic features of type II DRS (Fig. 12.45) are:

In primary position, eyeball may be orthophoric, esotropic or exotropic (more common).

On attempted abduction

- *Abduction* is normal or there may be slight limitation due to subnormal innervation and/or associated MR contracture.
- *Palpebral aperture* remains normal or slightly widens.

On attempted adduction due to co-contraction of MR and LR:

- *Adduction* is limited
- *Palpebral aperture* becomes narrow, and
- *Globe* is retracted.

Duane's retraction syndrome type III

Pathogenesis. Paradoxical innervation is present for both LR and MR muscles.

Characteristic features. There occurs co-contraction of LR and MR both during attempted adduction and abduction resulting in:

- Marked limitation of adduction as well as abduction along with associated
- Narrowing of palpebral aperture, and
- Marked retraction of the globe
- Upshoots and downshoots are frequently present (Fig. 12.46).

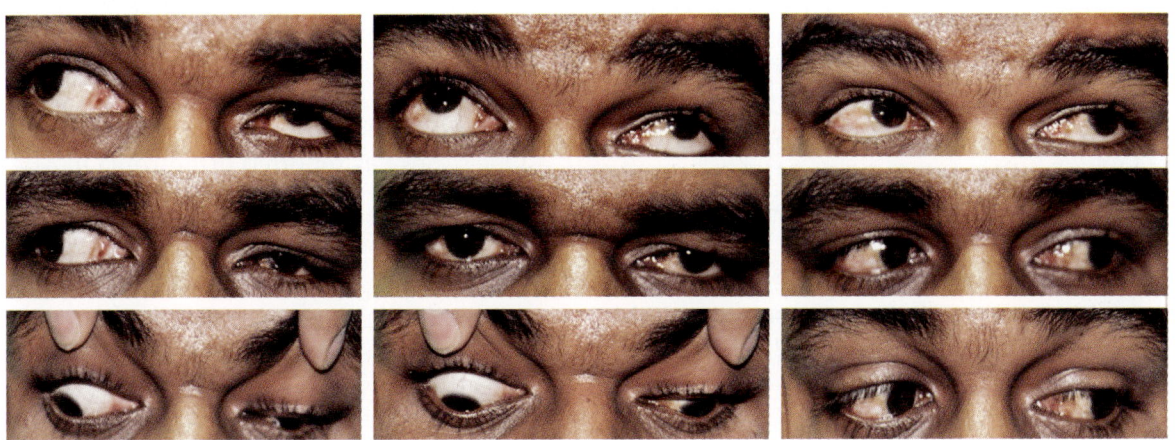

Fig. 12.45 *Type II Duane's retraction syndrome left eye (Courtesy: Dr Kanwar Mohan).*

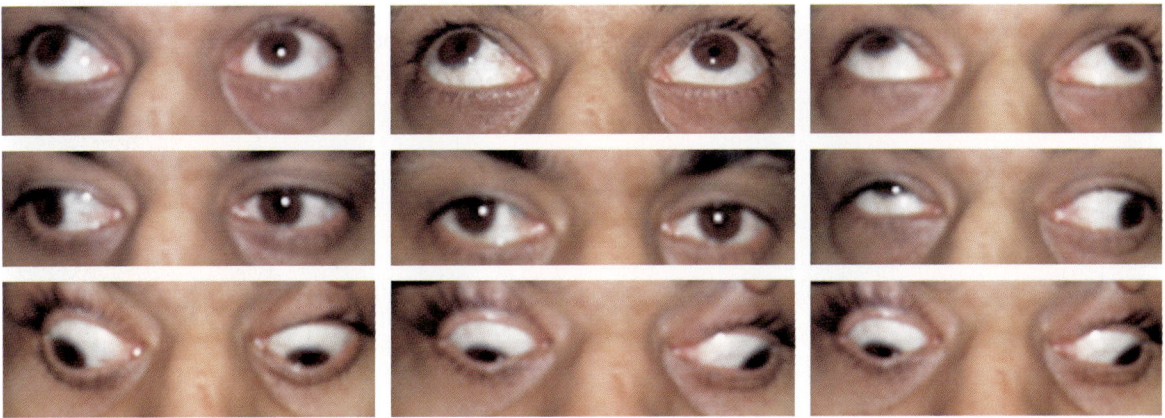

Fig. 12.46 *Type III Duane's retraction syndrome left eye with innervational upshoot.*

Type IV Duane syndrome

Type IV Duane syndrome has also been called as simultaneous abduction, synergistic divergence, the "splits", and perversion of the extraocular muscles by various workers from time to time. (Wilcox et al, 1981 and Wagner et al 1987). Schliesser et al (2016) have recommended that synergistic divergence (Fig. 12.47), a rare entity with features similar to those of Duane syndrome, should be classified as Type IV Duane syndrome as it has unique findings and an innervation pattern different from the other three types.

Pathogenesis. In the case of simultaneous abduction, the oculomotor nerve sends nerve fibres to the lateral rectus and the signal causes the eye to abduct and co-contract when it should simply adduct.

Characteristic features of Type IV Duane syndrome include (Fig. 12.47):
- Exotropia in primary gaze,
- Face turn opposite the involved eye,
- Essentially full abduction of the involved eye,
- Absent adduction of involved eye with simultaneous abduction in gaze opposite the involved eye, and
- Narrowing of the palpebral fissure.

Associations of type IV Duane reported include:
- Abnormal MRI—midbrain finding,
- Goldenhar syndrome,
- Cerebral palsy,
- Nystagmus, and
- Anisometropia

Treatment Weakening by recession of the tight lateral rectus is the key treatment in these patients.

Inverse Duane's syndrome

Inverse Duane's syndrome has the following features:

On abduction there occur
- *Abduction limitation* either due to co-contraction of MR along with LR muscle (congenital inverse Duane's syndrome) or due to some fibrosis or entrapment of MR along the medial orbital wall following trauma (acquired inverse Duane's syndrome).
- *Palpebral aperture* narrowing, and
- *Globe* retraction.

On adduction, the LR relaxes normally so following features are noted:
- *Adduction* may be normal or slightly limited especially in acquired cases due to fibrotic bands.
- *Palpebral aperture* usually remains normal, and *Globe* also remains within normal position.

III. Other ocular features

1. *Horizontal deviation.* The eyeball in primary position may be esotropic, orthotropic or exotropic.
   - One series has reported orthotropia in 31% cases, esotropia in 53% cases and exotropia in 16% cases.
   - *Esotropia* has been reported to occur most frequently with type I, followed by type III and type II.
   - *Exotropia* is associated more commonly with type II than types I and III.
   - *Orthotropia* is more frequent with type III than types I and II.

   Deviation should be measured in both habitual head position and forced straight head primary position both for distance and near and also in up, down and lateral gazes. The poor

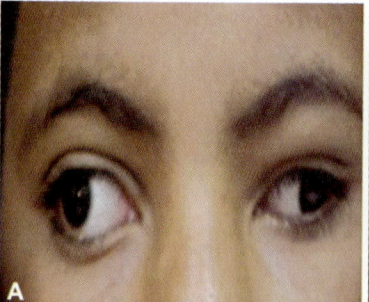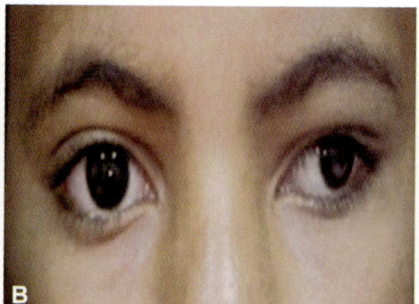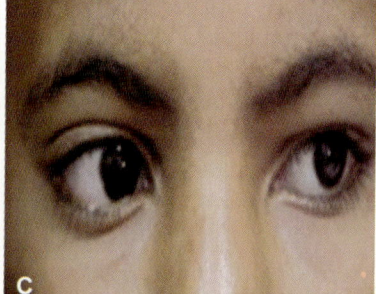

Fig. 12.47 *Photograph of patient with type IV Duane syndrome.*

abducting saccade in affected eye undercover makes the test less accurate, so the prisms should be placed in front of the affected eye and fellow eye should be observed under partial cover. The deviation in esotropic patients is usually less than 30 PD in unilateral cases with the non-affected eye fixing. However, in bilateral non-fusing Duane's or unilateral Duane's fixing with the affected eye there may be large degree of esodeviation.

Patterns: A large incidence of increased anomalous innervation of LR in elevation or depression explains the frequent observation of V, A or X pattern in these patients.

Y or lambda patterns are seen in patients with anomalous LR recruitment only in upgaze or downgaze, respectively. Bilateral Duane's with fusion often displays A-pattern. In DRS, the patterns are not due to oblique dysfunction but by co-contraction of lateral and vertical muscles.

2. Vertical deviations are often present with characteristic *upshoot or downshoot,* when the affected eye is adducted. These occur more frequently in severe anomalous lateral rectus recruitment. Two types of upshoots and downshoots have been described;

a. *Mechnical upshoots and downshoots* are reported to result from a tight lateral rectus muscle (leash effect). In this condition, the affected eye begins to adduct normally and then suddenly upshoots or downshoots.

b. *Innervational upshoots and downshoots* are reported to result from misinnervation of the vertical recti muscles. In this condition, there occurs a progressively increasing vertical deviation of the affected eye as it starts adducting.

Electromyographic studies have also demons-trated an abnormal synergistic innervation between the medial rectus and the superior and inferior oblique muscles in some cases; and this may also explain the upshoot or downshoot in adduction, i.e. frequently seen in this syndrome. Gradual upshoots may be due to superior rectus contracture or inferior oblique overaction (IOOA).

3. Abnormal head posture. Unilateral cases are frequently accompanied by a head turn for fusion. So DRS patients usually have normal binocularity in a preferred fusing position by means of compensatory head posture despite the incomitance. The face turn is towards the affected eye in eso Duane and away from affected eye in exo Duane.

4. Diplopia is complained very infrequently despite the fact that prevalence of deviation in primary position is quite common. This may be because of either face turn to achieve fusion or occurrence of suppression.

5. Sensory adaptations. Patients who suppress also develop abnormal retinal correspondence and amblyopia.

IV. Associated ocular abnormalities

• *Anisometropia with hyperopia* is a frequent association and may even be the cause of amblyopia in some cases. Therefore, refraction is very important especially in children. However, more recent studies have shown that anisometropia in Duane's syndrome is no higher than the normal population.

• *Other ocular abnormalities* which have been associated with Duane's syndrome include optic nerve hypoplasia, morning glory syndrome, congenital ptosis, nystagmoid movements, congenital cataract, heterochromia iridis, persistent hyaloid arteries, choroidal colobomas, districhiasis, pupillary anomalies, keratoconus, microphthalmos and many others.

V. Associated systemic abnormalities

Some of the systemic abnormalities which have been reported to be associated with Duane's retraction syndrome are as follows: Klipple-Feil syndrome, Goldenhar's syndrome, facial hemi-atrophy, cervical spina bifida, umbilical hernia, polydactly, Chiari I malformations, sensori-neural hearing deficits and Wildervank syndrome or cervico-oculoacoustic syndrome (combination of Duane's syndrome, sensori-neural hearing loss and Klippel-Fiel anomaly of the spine).

Diagnosis

• Duane's retraction syndrome is usually diagnosed on version tests by its typical signs. Carefully look for anomalous vertical movements also, as this is important in determining the surgical strategy. There is a curved outward rotation pattern uniquely characteristics of Duane's which shows complete absence of abduction (–4) in horizontal gaze, while more outward rotation in upgazes and downgazes due to anomalous innervation in upgaze and downgaze.

- *Adduction saccadic velocity* can be reduced in the affected eye in all types of Duane's syndrome.
- *Abduction saccadic velocity* is reduced only in type I and III.
- *Measuring the eyelid fissure in abduction and adduction* to determine the degree of globe retraction. This represents an indirect sign of amount of anomalous innervation to LR muscle. A greater degree of anomalous innervations is correlated with an increased amount of globe retraction.
- *Force duction and force augmentation tests.* The two components responsible for abduction limitation are: amount of normal innervation to LR and degree of contracture of MR. These can be differentiated by force duction test and force augmentation test which compares the voluntary abduction end point with possible extension of this end point by forcing further abduction manually with forceps. This proves the paralysis of agonist and no contracture of antagonist.

Force generation test also helps to determine the active force generated by LR. Adduction limitations which are usually seen in patients with severe anomalous innervation to LR that prevents the eye from moving into adduction. This can be determine by force degeneration test described by Romero Apis.

In this test, the patient is asked to look halfway between the primary position and full adduction and then, eye is moved further into adduction while the patent is asked to further adduct the eye. Resistance caused by co-contracting LR in adduction can be appreciated at this point. Then the patient is asked to abduct the eye and grasping at temporal limbus, the examiner attempts to adduct the eye. Then note that if resistance has disappeared as now in abduction, LR does not receive abnormal innervation.

- Rarely, an acquired form of Duane's retraction syndrome *(Pseudo-Duane's syndrome)* may occur as a result of scarring following muscle surgery or other surgery involving the conjunctiva and Tenon's capsule and thus need to be differentiated from true Duane's syndrome.

Management

Non-surgical measures Refractive error and/ or amblyopia, when present, should be treated first, on general lines (*see* page190)

Surgical treatment in Duane's retraction *Indications* include:
- An abnormal head posture,
- A significant deviation in the primary position,
- Marked globe retraction, or
- Marked upshoots and downshoots.

General observations. In general, disappointing results of surgery have been reported for this condition. Therefore, better one should not operate, when binocular single vision is present in primary position of gaze or if it can be maintained with a slight head turn.
- *Further, no set rules exist for surgical treatment of Duane's syndrome* and that planning in each case should be made individually taking into consideration the coexisting horizontal and vertical deviations.
- *Rough guidelines*, recommended, are described briefly.

I. *Management of Eso-DRS*

Esotropia is classically more common in DRS type I where LR innervation is normal in abduction and anomalous in adduction. Sometime esotropia may also occur in DRS type II and type III. Depending upon the findings eso-DRS can be managed as below.

Management of esotropia

1. *MR recession of affected eye* may be effective in small angle esotropia (<20 PD) in primary position in patients with mild DRS (cases with minimum anomalous LR activity and normal LR in adduction).

2. *Assymetric bilateral MR recession* with more recession of the fellow good eye (even up to 9 mm depending upon the amount of deviation)

is indicated in cases with large esotropia (>20 PD).

Advantage of asymmetric MR recession is that it produces a fixation dures without fear of adduction deficiency in the good eye. In addition to correcting esotropia in primary position, it will also decrease the likelihood of MR contracture of the affected eye through the fixation dures of the good eye which leads to a continuous inhibition of the MR of the affected eye.

Management of associated globe retraction

LR recession of the affected eye along with asymmetric MR recession may be helpful in cases of esotropia with severe globe retraction, due to anomalous LR.

Management to improve abduction

Superior rectus transposition (SRT) or vertical rectus transposition (VRT) to the lateral rectus is useful to achieve abduction force in cases where there is no severe anomalous LR recruitment and there is marked abduction deficit (–3 to –4). These procedures help to improve the abduction and also less MR recession is required to correct the exotropia. *SRT* has decreased risk of anterior segment ishaemia, but may induce vertical incomitance.

Balanced partial VRT, is therefore, preferred over SRT by many surgeons.

Management of upshoots and downshoots

1. *Faden operation (posterior fixation suture) with or without recession of the lateral rectus muscle* 14 mm posterior to its insertion has been advocated in patients with marked upshoots or downshoots of mechanical type. (Leash phenomenon).

2. *Y-splitting of the lateral rectus muscle.* In case of upshoots and downshoots, Y-split with LR recession of the affected eye can be done in addition to treating esotropia. The LR is split from its insertion as far posteriorly as possible, spreading the muscle halves 10 mm up and 10 mm down (20 mm between them). This is also followed by LR recession 5–10 mm to negate the resection effect created by splitting the muscle halves.

II. *Management of exo-DRS*

Patients with exo-DRS, usually have anomalous LR innervation in adduction and normal or subnormal LR innervations in abduction. There may be associated globe retraction and upwards and downshoot. Depending upon the situation, following measures used:

1. *LR recession* (supramaximal) of the affected eye may be useful for correcting exotropia amd globe retraction.

2. *LR periosteal fixation* has been reported to be effective in correcting exotropia, and anomalous head posture, and improving adduction (as PF wards off the anomalous activity of LR). Further, it can be combined with *partial VRT* to improve abduction in patients with subnormal LR innervation.

3. *LR recession with Y-split* is an option for exotropia with upshoot and downshoot in cases with normal LR activity.

III. *Management of ortho-DRS*

These patients are usually orthotropic in primary position but there is severe globe retraction with upshoots and downshoots.

Symmetrical recession of MR and LR of the affected eye with adjustable sutures on one muscle and Y-split of LR is a good option in such cases.

Management of Y and lambda patterns in DRS

Such patients usually have:
- Less deficient abduction,
- Anomalous LR innervation only in vertical gazes
- No globe retraction, and
- Adduction in the involved eye is worse in upgaze.

Bilateral LR recession with elevation of tendons in Y-pattern and downshift in lambda pattern is the procedure of choice.

Bilateral SR recession in Y-pattern and bilateral IR recession in lambda pattern can also be considered.

HORIZONTAL GAZE PALSY WITH PROGRESSIVE SCOLIOSIS

Etiology and genetics

Horizontal gaze palsy with progressive scoliosis (HGPPS) is a rare autosomal recessive disorder with the locus on chromosome 11 (11q 23–25). The condition is thought to result from agenesis of the abducens nucleus including both alpha motar neurons and interneurons.

Clinical features

- *Congenital horizontal gaze palsy* with progressive scoliosis (HGPPS), as the name indicates, is characterized by complete absence of conjugate horizontal gaze and childhood onset progressive scoliosis.
- *Vertical eye movements and convergence* are preserved.
- There are no associated ptosis and other somatic abnormalities.
- Some patients may have nystagmus, esotropia, and/or retraction on adduction.

MRI scan of brain in patients with HGPPS shows hypoplasia of pons, absence of facial colliculi, butterfly configuration of medulla and deep midline pontine cleft (split pons sign).

II. CCDDs PRIMARILY AFFECTING VERTICAL OCULAR MOTILITY

These disorders result from the developmental anomalies of third and fourth cranial nerves or their nuclei. These include:
- Congenital fibrosis of extraocular muscles (CFEOMs), and
- Congenital ptosis.

CONGENITAL FIBROSIS OF EXTRAOCULAR MUSCLES

Congenital fibrosis of extraocular muscles (CFEOMs) refers to a group of disorders that result from primary dysinnervation of oculomotor and/or trochlear innervated extra-ocular muscles. The genetic loci for the CFEOMs phenotypes are known as FEOM. Till date, three CFEOMs and four FEOM loci have been defined.

CFEOM 1 phenotype

Genetics. It is an outosomal dominant disorder with main locus FEOM 1, on chromosome 12.

Primary defect. In this condition is of superior division of oculomotor nerve.

Clinical features include bilateral (Fig. 12.48A).:
- *Congenital ptosis,*
- *Globe infraducted* in primary position
- *Gaze restriction* is noticed in upgaze as well as horizontal gaze.
- *Misdirected eye movements* in the form of marked synergistic convergence on attempted upgaze.
- *Forced duction test* is often positive in upgaze.
- *Marcus Gunn jaw winking* phenomenon is noticed in 30–40% cases.

CFEOM 2 phenotype

Genetics. Autosomal recessive disorder with main locus, FEOM 2, on chromosome 11.

Primary defect is in the development of both the oculomotor and trochlear nuclei.

Clinical features (Fig. 12.48B).
- *Ptosis* is often severe
- *Exotropia* is usually of large angle
- *Ocular movements,* horizontal as well as vertical are severely restricted.

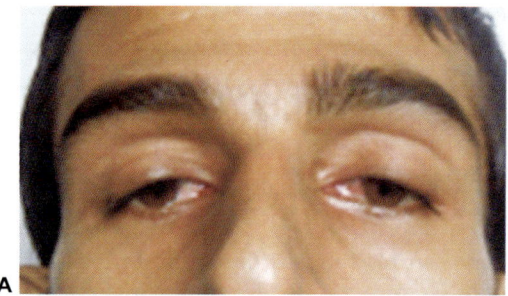

A

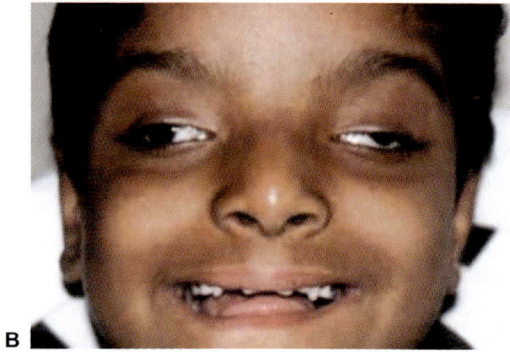

B

Fig. 12.48 *Congenital fibrosis of extraocular muscles (CFEOM): A, Type I and B, Type II*

CFEOM 3 phenotype

Genetics. Inheritance is autosomal dominant with incomplete peneterance. The main locus is the FEOM 3 on chromosome 16.

Primary defect in the development of oculomotor nucleus is variable.

Clinical features are variable:
- *Forced duction test* is usually positive
- Misdirected eye movements or globe retraction are rarely seen.

Differential diagnosis

CFEOMs should be differentiated from:
- Monocular elevation deficiency,
- Brown's syndrome,
- Congenital progressive external ophthalmoplegia (CPEO), and
- Duane's retraction syndrome.

III. CCDDs PRIMARILY AFFECTING FACIAL MUSCLES WITH ASSOCIATED OCULAR MOTILITY DEFECTS

These disorders result from the abnormalities in the development of the facial nerve and/or nucleus. These include:
- Congenital facial weakness, and
- Möbius syndrome

MÖBIUS SYNDROME

The eponym Möbius syndrome refers to congenital bilateral abducent paralysis associated with congenital facial palsy with variable other associations.

Etiology and genetics

Möbius syndrome is being considered a heterogeneous group of congenital disorders caused by developmental defects related to a variety of insults such as ischaemia, toxic effects of prenatal used drugs such as misoprostol, benzodiazepines.

To date, two phenotypes with responsible genotypes reported are:
- MBS 1 phenotype with the locus 13q12.2–13, and
- MBS 4 phenotype with the locus 1p22.

Clinical features (Fig. 12.49)

- *Abduction* is usually limited in both eyes.
- *Gaze palsy* may be there

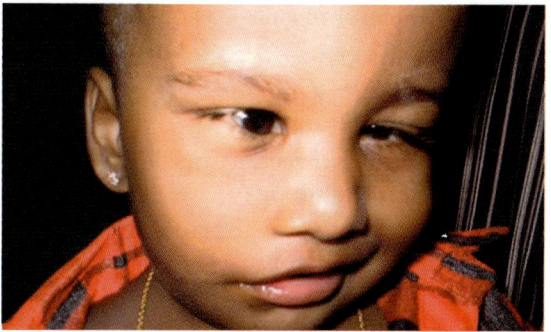

Fig. 12.49 *A child with mobius syndrome (Courtesy: Dr. Kalpana and Dr. Sandra).*

- *Deviation.* Usually eyes are straight in primary position, a few patients may have esotropia
- *Facial weakness* is characterised by:
  - Mask-like facies with mouth constantly held open.
  - Eyelids cannot be closed completely.

Associations include:
- *Paralysis or hypoplasia* of tongue due to involvement of hypoglossal nerve with speech and swallowing difficulties are extremely common.
- *Other cranial nerves* which can be involved are 3rd, 4th, 9th, and 10th.
- *Craniofacial anomalies* which may be associated are epicanthal folds, microstomia, micrognathia and external ear defects.
- *Limbs abnormalities* include webbed fingers and toes, suppernumerary digits, club foot and syndactyly.
- *Deafness and mental retardation* are also reported.
- *Congenital heart defects* such a ventricular septal defect are also reported.
- *Respiratory defects* with tachypnoea and other respiratory difficulties occur in some patients.

Management

- *Prevention of exposure keratitis* due to facial weakness may be done by tarsorrhaphy.
- *Esotropic patients*, though rare, may be managed by MR recessions with or without LR resection.

B. RESTRICTIVE STRABISMUS DUE TO MECHANICAL RESTRICTIONS

Restrictive strabismus due to mechanical restrictions may be caused by:

I. *Tight extaocular muscles,* as occurs in:

- Inelastic superior oblique in congenital Brown's syndrome
- Thyroid ophthalmopathy
- Entrapped inferior rectus muscle in blow-out fracture of orbital floor.
- Monocular elevation deficiency (MED), caused by fibrotic IR muscle.
- Strabismus fixus.

II. *Structural adhesions,* e.g. as seen in:
- Fat adherence to extraocular muscles or sclera after strabismus surgery, retinal detachment surgery or periocular trauma
- Congenital fibrotic bands
- Acquired Brown's syndrome due to scarring/inflammation around, the trochlea
- Conjunctival and Tenon's capsule scarring

III. *Orbital mass lesions,* e.g.
- Orbital tumours causing mass effect on the globe movements.
- Glaucoma explant with large bleb causing mass effect.

Note. A few of the conditions are described here.

TIGHT EXTRAOCULAR MUSCLES

BROWN'S SYNDROME

Brown syndrome refers to mechanical restriction (a significant limitation) of elevation in adduction caused by an overly taut superior oblique tendon of the same eye. On version testing, the condition mimics an inferior oblique palsy except that a V-pattern is present in contrast to A-pattern associated with inferior oblique palsy.

Etiology

The condition may be congenital or acquired. Originally, Brown divided the syndrome into true sheath syndrome (now congenital) and simulated sheath syndrome (now acquired).

1. *Congenital Brown's syndrome* is presently thought to be caused by a congenitally taut superior oblique tendon (short and inelastic tendon). Originally, Brown thought that these cases occur due to congenitally shortened anterior sheath of the superior oblique tendon; the theory which has not been proved by subsequent workers. In fact, Parks observed that the superior oblique tendon sheath does not exist at all and that the term 'superior oblique tendon sheath syndrome' introduced by Brown is a misnomer.

2. *Acquired Brown's syndrome* is presently thought to be caused by an acquired taut superior oblique tendon, secondary to following conditions:
- *Tenosynovitis* of the superior oblique trochlear apparatus.
- *Trauma to the trochlear region* in any form may cause this abnormality. The '*canine tooth syndrome*' of Knapp also falls into this category. Surgical trauma has emerged as another cause of acquired Brown's syndrome (traumatic Brown's syndrome).
- *Rheumatoid nodules* on the superior oblique tendon posterior to the trochlea. Association with other autoimmune diseases like SLE, Sjögren syndrome and Graves' ophthalmopthy is also reported.
- *Retrotrochlear thickening* of the tendon or anomalies of the trochlea itself may lead to impaired slippage of the tendon through the trochlea.
- Idiopathic

Clinical features

Congenital cases (also known as true or primary syndrome) are constant and unilateral in 90% percent of patients. Most acquired cases are intermittent and more likely to improve spontaneously. The syndrome is rarely seen in adults. The clinical features of this syndrome can be divided into main consistent features and less important variable features.

Main consistent clinical features include the following (Fig. 12.50):

1. *Elevation is limited significantly,* characteristically in adduction and present in abduction. There may or may not be mild limitation of elevation in midline. Degree of limitation is same on versions and ductions.
2. *Overaction of superior oblique* is characteristically *absent* which normally would be found with a paretic inferior oblique muscle.
3. *Divergence* in upgaze producing a V-pattern.

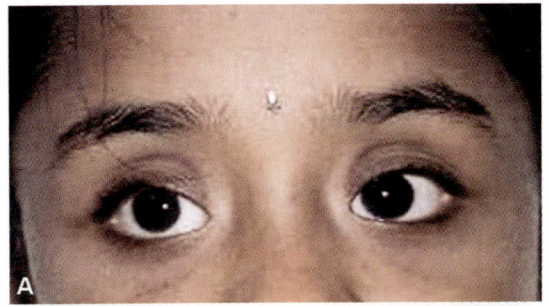
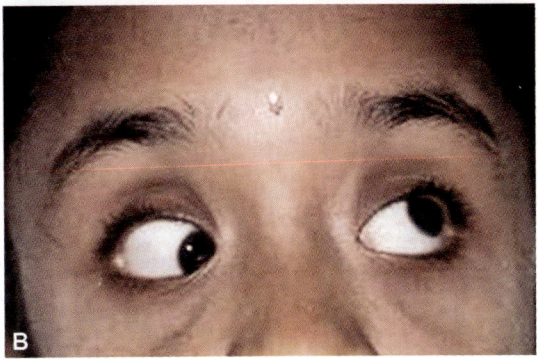

Fig. 12.50 *Brown's syndrome right eye:* (A), *Note limitation of elevation in right eye which is marked in adducted position* (B) *(Courtesy: Dr Kalpana an Dr Sandra).*

4. *Forced duction test is positive on attempts* to elevate the adducted eye; but is negative on attempts to elevate the abducted eye.

Less important and variable clinical features include:

1. *Downshoot* in adduction.
2. *Widening of the palpebral fissure* on adduction.
3. *Straight eyes in primary* position are present in most patients but a few may have hypotropia.
4. *Compensatory head posture* (chin up) may be present in patients with hypotropia.
5. *An audible click* may be produced when such patients are able to elevate their adducted eye. Some observers have even used the term *'superior oblique click syndrome'* for such patients.
6. Inflammatory signs like superonasal orbital pain, and tenderness may be present in acquired cases.

Bilateral Brown's syndrome, when present, exihibits 'V' pattern exotropia. Rest features being similar to unilateral cases.

Grading of Brown's syndrome

Eutis et al have graded Brown's syndrome into mild, moderate and severe (Table 12.10).

Brown plus syndrome, is the term used by Jampalesky for the cases having vertical deviation in the primary position or in adduction, with or without compensatory head posture.

Table 12.10 *Grading of Brown's syndrome (Eutis et al)*

Grade	Restriction of elevation in adduction	Downshoot in adduction	Hypotropia in primary position
1–Mild	+	–	–
2–Moderate	+	+	–
3–Severe	+	+	+

Differential diagnosis

1. *Inferior oblique paralysis versus Brown's syndrome*

- *Limitation to elevation in adduction* is greater on testing for ductions than versions in inferior oblique paralysis, while in Brown's syndrome, it is equal.
- *Overaction of the superior oblique muscle* is typically absent in Brown's syndrome, while it is present in inferior oblique palsy.
- *Forced duction test* is positive in Brown's syndrome, while it is negative in inferior oblique palsy.
- *Park's 3-step test* is positive in inferior oblique palsy.

2. *Other conditions with restriction of elevation*

which need to be differentiated from the Brown's syndrome are double elevator palsy, fracture of the orbital floor, Graves' ophthalmopathy and congenital fibrosis of the inferior rectus muscle. In all these conditions, elevation is equally restricted in adduction, primary gaze and in abduction; while in Brown's syndrome, elevation is restricted only in adduction.

Management

1. *Conservative treatment.* Acquired cases should be observed, since spontaneous improvement has been reported. These cases depending upon the situation may need:
- Range of eye motility exercises (elevation and adduction exercises).

- Steroids either orally or by injection near the trochlea in inflammatory cases.
- Correction of the underlying cause, when possible such as trauma to the trochlea.

2. Surgical treatment. Results of the surgery for this entity are controversial and, therefore, surgery should only be undertaken in severe (grade 3) cases of Brown's syndrome, i.e. in the presence of:

- A significant cosmetically disfigurement head tilt; or
- Severe and constant congenital Brown syndrome that threatens binocularly and development of amblyopia
- A large hypotropia, in primary position or
- Unacceptable downshoot in adduction.

Surgical procedures recommended are as follows:

1. *Superior oblique tenotomy.* It is a simple, safe and effective procedure in treating Brown's syndrome. However, about 50% cases develop symptoms of superior oblique paralysis which can be managed by *recession of either ipsilateral inferior oblique or contralateral inferior rectus.*

2. *Superior oblique tenectomy.* To avoid the risk of superior oblique palsy, Parks recommends performing a 6 mm superior oblique tenectomy within the intermuscular septum along the nasal border of superior rectus.

3. *Superior oblique weakening with a silicone expander* has also been advocated by Wright in 1991 to prevent superior oblique palsy following tenotomy. This procedure involves expanding the length of the tendon using a silicone spacer usually silicone retinal 240 band. The weakening effect is graded by varying the length of the silicone that bridges the gap between the cut ends of the tendon. In a Brown syndrome 6–7 mm expander is recommended. A *chicken suture* can be placed in lieu of an expander to retain the cut-ends of superior oblique tendon together. However, this procedure is difficult and cumbersome. Such a procedure may actually be more relevant in cases with superior oblique overaction (Brown plus).

4. *Other superior oblique weakening* or lengthening procedures such as:

- *Chicken suture* in nasal half of tendon or
- *Loop suture* at the insertion may also be tried.

THYROID OPHTHALMOPATHY

This term is coined to denote typical ocular changes which include lid retraction, lid lag, and proptosis. These changes have also been labelled as: Endocrine exophthalmos, malignant exophthalmos, dysthyroid ophthalmopathy and ocular Graves' disease (OGD).

Etiopathogenesis

It may be a part of Graves' disease (the syndrome consisting of hyperthyroidism, goitre and eye signs) or may be associated with hypothyroidism or even euthyroidism. Thus, a direct causative connection between the thyroid dysfunction and the ocular changes remains elusive. There is an increasing evidence to suggest that Graves' ophthalmopathy has an autoimmune etiology. Most data presently support the postulate that an autoantigen is coexpressed in the thyroid gland and orbital fibroblast. This antigen is recognised by the circulating T cell lymphocytes. Activating the T cells (CD4 cell) trigering an immune response. The activated T cells secrete various cytokines, interferon, interleukin L-alpha and tumour necrosis factor (TNF), which cause proliferation of fibroblasts in the orbit and production of glycosaminoglycans (GAGs).

Presence of mucopolysaccharides, predo-minantly hyaluronic acid, together with interstitial oedema and inflammatory cells accounts for the proptosis, and swelling of extraocular muscles.

Clinical features

1. Lid signs. These are: (i) retraction of the upper lids producing the characteristic staring and frightened appearance (Dalrymple's sign), (ii) *Lid lag* (von Graefe's sign), i.e. when globe is moved downwards, the upper lid lags behind, (iii) fullness of eyelids due to puffy oedematous swelling (Enroth's sign), (iv) difficulty in eversion of upper lid (Gifford's sign), (v) infrequent blinking (Stellwag's sign).

2. Conjunctival signs. These include deep injection and chemosis.

3. Pupillary signs. These are of less importance and may be evident as inequality of dilatation of pupils.

4. Ocular motility defects. These range from convergence weakness (Mobius's sign) to partial or complete immobility of one or all of the extrinsic ocular muscles. Severe restrictive myopathy occurs due to lymphocytic infiltration of the extraocular muscles and varying amounts of oedema, inflammation and fibrosis.

- The most common ocular mobility defect is a *unilateral elevator palsy*, Fig. 12.51 caused by involvement of the inferior rectus muscle followed by *failure of aduction* due to involvement of medial rectus muscle.
- Thus, thyroid (endocrine) myopathy is a common cause of *acquired vertical deviation* in adults, especially females. It is a rare cause of acquired vertical deviation in children.

5. Exophthalmos. It is a common and classical sign of the disease. As a rule, both eyes are affected; but it is frequent to find one eye being more prominent than the other. Even unilateral proptosis is not uncommon. In majority of cases, it is self-limiting.

6. Exposure keratitis and symptoms of ocular surface discomfort. These include sandy or gritty sensation, lacrimation and photophobia. Corneal exposure has been attributed to upper lid retraction, exophthalmos, lagophthalmos, inability to elevate the eyes and a decreased blink rate.

7. Optic neuropathy. It occurs due to direct compression of the nerve or its blood supply by the enlarged rectus muscles at the orbital apex. It may manifest as papilloedema or optic atrophy with associated slowly progressive impairment of vision.

American Thyroid Association (ATA) classification

ATA has classified Graves' ophthalmopathy, irrespective of the hormonal status into following classes characterised by the acronym 'NOSPECS'

Class 0 : **N**o signs and symptoms.

Class 1 : **O**nly signs, no symptoms (signs are limited to lid retraction, with or without lid lag and mild proptosis).

Class 2 : **S**oft tissue involvement with signs (as described in class-1) and symptoms including lacrimation, photophobia, lid or conjunctival swelling).

Class 3 : **P**roptosis is well established.

Class 4 : **E**xtraocular muscle involvement (limitation of movement and diplopia).

Class 5 : **C**orneal involvement (exposure keratitis).

Class 6 : **S**ight loss due to optic nerve involvement with disc pallor or papilloedema and visual field defects.

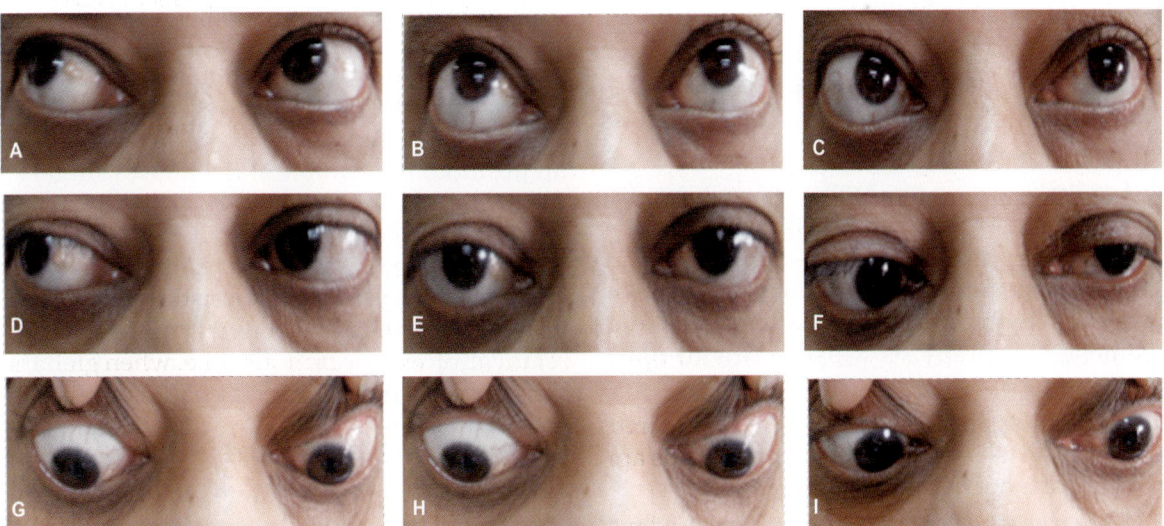

Fig. 12.51 *A patient with Graves' ophthalmopathy depicting limitation of left superior rectus muscle due to involvement of left inferior rectus muscle.*

For practical purposes, it has been described as *'early'* (which include ATA class 1 and 2) and *'Late Graves' ophthalmopathy'* (class 3 to 6).

Investigations

1. *Thyroid function tests.* These should include: serum T3, T4, TSH and estimation of radioactive iodine uptake.

2. *Positional tonometry.* An increase in intraocular pressure in upgaze helps in diagnosis of subclinical cases.

3. *Ultrasonography.* It can detect changes in extraocular muscles even in class 0 and class 1 cases and thus helps in early diagnosis. In addition to the increase in muscle thickness, erosion of temporal wall of orbit, accentuation of retrobulbar fat and perineural inflammation of optic nerve can also be demonstrated in some early cases.

4. *Computerised tomographic scanning.* It may show proptosis, muscle thickness, thickening of optic nerve and anterior prolapse of the orbital septum (due to excessive orbital fat and/or muscle swelling).

Management of Graves' ophthalmopathy

It is in addition to and independent of the therapy for the associated thyroid dysfunction; as the later usually does not alter the course or ophthalmic features. The treatment modalities employed are as follows:

1. Topical artificial tear drops in the day time and ointment at bedtime are useful for relief of foreign body sensation and other symptoms of ocular surface drying.

2. Guanethidine 5% eyedrops may decrease the lid retraction caused by overaction of Muller's muscle.

3. Systemic steroids may be indicated in acutely inflamed orbit with rapidly progressive chemosis and proptosis with or without optic neuropathy.

4. Immunosuppressive drugs may be required to control acute inflammation when steroids are not effective or contraindicated.

5. Radiotherapy (2000 rads given over 10 days period). It may help in reducing orbital oedema in patients where steroids are contraindicated.

6. Lateral tarsorrhaphy should be performed in patients with exposure keratopathy (with mild to moderate proptosis) not responding to topical artificial tears.

7. Prismatic glasses may help to relieve the mild diplopia in primary position or rending gaze. But since the deviation is usually very incomitant, prism often does not alleviate the diplopia in all positions of gaze.

8. Surgical orbital decompression: It should be performed, only when systemic steroids and radiotherapy have proved ineffective in patients with marked proptosis associated with severe exposure keratopathy and/or optic neuropathy with imminent danger of permanent visual loss.

The most commonly employed technique is *'two wall decompression'* in which part of the orbital floor and medial wall are removed.

9. Extraocular muscle surgery. It should be carried out for left out diplopia in primary gaze, after the congestive phase of disease is over and the angle of deviation is constant for the last 6 months.

Recession of the affected muscle (inferior rectus, medial rectus or superior rectus as the case may be) is the primary surgical treatment. Strengthening procedure should be avoided. Extraocular muscle surgery may eliminate diplopia in primary gaze but rarely restores normal motility because of the restrictive myopathy that typifies Graves' ophthalmopathy.

Adjustable suture surgery may help optimize the alignment and rotations in these difficult cases. Since late overcorrection frequently occurs, especially with large inferior rectus recessions, slight undercorrection (fusion with a slight chin-up position) is desirable at the time of surgery.

10. Cosmetic surgery for persistent lid retraction. It consists of levator and Muller's muscle recession. Recently, implantation of scleral grafts has become a popular technique.

11. Blepharoplasty. It may be performed by removal of excess fatty tissue and redundant skin from around the eyelids.

ORBITAL BLOW-OUT FRACTURE

These are isolated communited fractures which occur, when the orbital walls are pressed indirectly. Blow-out fractures mainly involve orbital floor and medial wall.

Etiology

These generally result from trauma to the orbit by a relatively large, often rounded objects, such as tennis ball, cricket ball, human fist (Fig. 12.52) or part of an automobile. The force of the blow causes a backward displacement of the eye and an increase in intraorbital pressure with a resultant fracture of the weakest point of the orbital wall, usually this point is the orbital floor, but this may be the medial wall also.

Classification

1. *Pure blow-out fractures.* These are not associated with involvement of the orbital rim.
2. *Impure blow-out fractures.* These are associated with other fractures about the middle third of the facial skeleton.

Clinical features

- *Periorbital oedema and blood extravasation* in and around the orbit (e.g. subconjunctival ecchymosis) are initial lesions. This may mask certain signs and symptoms seen later.
- *Emphysema* of the eyelids occurs more frequently with medial wall than floor fractures. It may be made worse by blowing of nose. *Paraesthesia and anaesthesia* in infraorbital nerve distribution (lower lid, cheek, side of nose, upper lip and upper teeth) are very common.
- *Ipsilateral epistaxis* as a result of bleeding from maxillary sinus into the nose is frequently noted in early stages. *Proptosis* of variable degree may also be present initially because of the associated orbital oedema and haemorrhage.
- *Enophthalmos.* After about 10 days, as the oedema decreases, the eyeball sinks backward and somewhat inferiorly resulting in enophthalmos. Three factors responsible for producing enophthalmos are: (a) escape of orbital fat into the maxillary sinus; (b) backward traction on the globe by entrapped inferior rectus muscle and (c) enlargement of the orbital cavity from displacement of fragments.
- *Diplopia* also becomes evident after decrease in oedema. It typically occurs in both up- and downgaze (double diplopia) due to entrapment of soft tissue structures in the area of the blow-out fracture (floor more commonly than medial wall).

The presence of muscle restriction can be confirmed by a positive *'forced duction test'.*

- *Restricted elevation,* restricted depression may occur in fracture floor of the orbit.
- *Pseduo-Duane's refraction syndrome* (or acquired inverse-Duane's syndrome), presentation may occur in fracture of medial wall of the orbit.
- *Saccadic eye movement testing* is sometimes helpful to determine whether ocular movement limitation is because of a restrictive process or a paretic process.
- *Associated severe ocular damage* is rare. This is because a 'blow-out fracture' is nature's way of protecting the globe from injury. Nevertheless the eye should be carefully examined to exclude the possibility of intraocular damage.

Radiological examination

1. *Plain X-rays.* The most useful projection for detecting an orbital floor fracture is a nose-chin (Water's) view. The common radiological findings are—fragmentation and irregularity of the orbital floor; depression of bony fragments and 'hanging drop' opacity of the superior maxillary antrum from orbital contents herniating through the floor (Fig. 12.53).

2. *Computerised tomography scanning and magnetic resonance imaging.* These are of greater value for detailed visualisation of soft

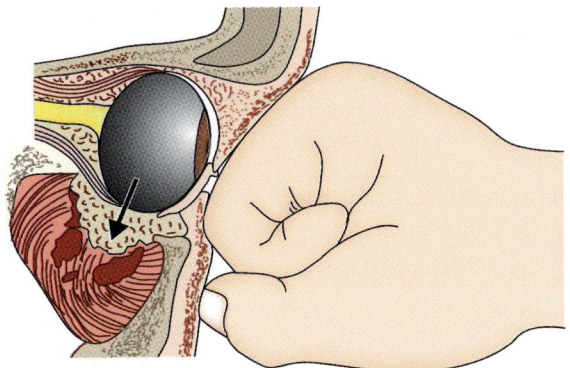

Fig. 12.52 *Mechanism of blow-out fracture of the orbital floor.*

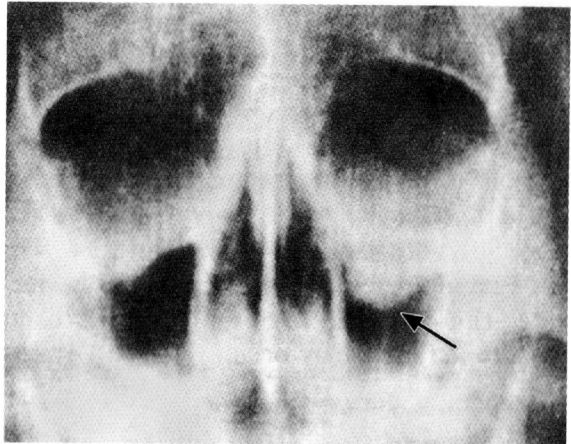

Fig. 12.53 *Plain X-ray orbit (AP view) showing herniated orbital contents (arrow) with blow-out fracture of the orbital floor.*

tissues. Coronal sections are particularly useful in evaluating the extent of the fracture.

Management

Surgical repair to restore continuity of the orbital floor may be made with or without implants. It may not be required in many cases.
- *Optimal time for surgery*, when indicated, is after 10–14 days of injury.
- *Indications of surgical intervention* include:
  - Diplopia not resolving significantly in the early days after trauma
  - A fracture with a large herniation of tissues into the antrum
  - Incarceration of tissues in the fracture with resulting globe retraction and increased applanation tension on attempted upward gaze; and
  - Enophthalmos greater than 3 mm.
  Any of these factors, alone or combined, could indicate that early orbital repair is necessary.

Residual strabismus after 3–6 months of injury can generally be corrected by using standard eye muscle surgical techniques:
- Recession of inferior is done first
- Resection of superior rectus may also be done, if required.

STRABISMUS FIXUS

In strabismus fixus, fibrosis involves the horizontal recti and the involved eye is fixed in extreme position. It may be unilateral or bilateral. It occurs in two forms—convergent and divergent.

Strabismus fixus convergence is more common.

Etiology. Strabismus fixus convergence (SFC) can be congenital or acquired.
- *Congenital* cases are more common. In such cases, lateral rectus palsy with medial rectus fibrosis has been described as the cause.
- *Acquired* cases though rare, are reported to be due to myopic myositis and amyloidosis of the lateral rectus muscle.

Clinical features Patient's eyes are fixed in extreme convergent position and he/she cannot abduct either eye past the midline (Fig. 12.54). It can be differentiated by forced duction test from bilateral sixth nerve palsy.

Treatment of strabismus fixus convergence includes:
- *Medial rectus recession.* Supramaximal recession with silicon expanders have been reported to give good functional and cosmetic results.
- *Loop myopaxy of LR and SR* to the sclera in superotemporal part with non-absorbable suture or silicon sling is also reported to give reasonable good results in cases with tight MR.
- *Disinsertion of MR and resection of LR* has also been described.
  In addition, recession of the medial conjunctiva and Tenon's capsule may be needed to bring the eyes in the centre in primary position.

Strabismus fixus divergence is comparatively rare condition characterized by fixation of eyes in extreme divergence.

Surgery for divergent strabismus fixus is just reverse of the strabismus fixus convergence.

CONGENITAL TIGHT INFERIOR RECTUS MUSCLE

- In some children, a congenital hypotropia occurs accompanied by marked limitation of upgaze.
- The condition may be unilateral or bilateral and in some cases there may be fibrosis of the levator muscle as well. Probably, the condition is a variant of generalized fibrosis.

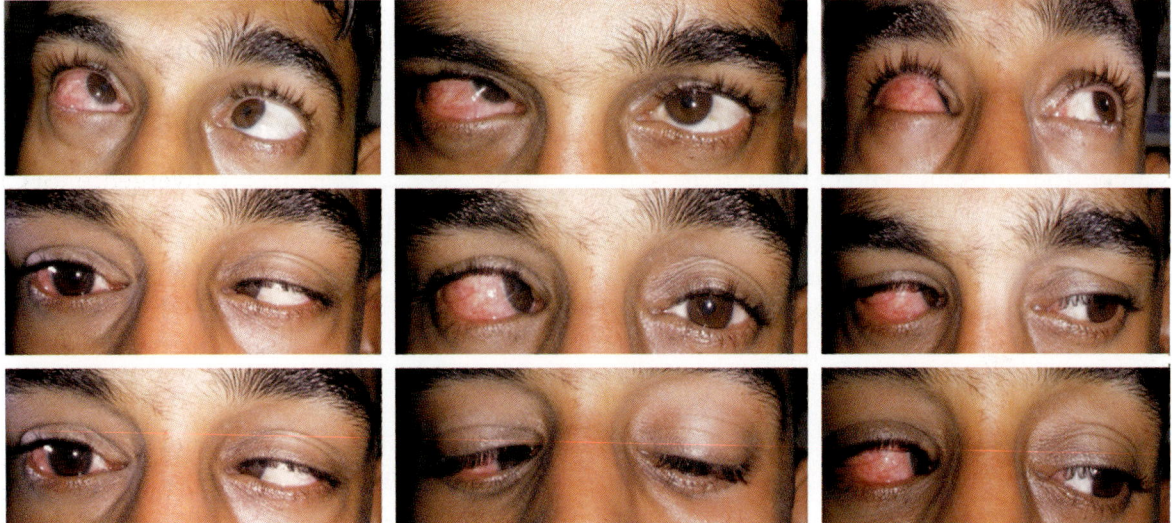

Fig. 12.54 *Strabismus fixus convergence*

- Forced duction test reveals an inferior restriction.
- Surgical exploration reveals a tight inferior rectus which is adherent to the globe.
- Treatment consists of release of globe adhesions and a maximal inferior rectus recession, to relieve the restriction in upward rotation.

STRUCTURAL ADHESIONS

ADHERENCE SYNDROME

Clinical features. Two types of adherence syndrome, the lateral adherence syndrome and superior adherence syndrome, have been reported to occur due to developmental abnormal fascial connections.

- In the *lateral adherence syndrome,* an abnormal fascial connection is seen between the muscle capsule of the lateral rectus and inferior oblique, which produces limitation of ocular rotation in the field of lateral rectus muscle.
- In the *superior adherence syndrome,* an abnormal fascial connection exists between the superior rectus and tendon of the superior oblique, causing limitation of rotation in the field of superior rectus muscle.

  Treatment consists of severing of all the adhesions after disinsertion of the lateral or superior rectus muscle. To comfirm that, all the adhesions have been removed, after the surgery, eye should be rotated medially for lateral adherence syndrome and inferiorly for superior adherence syndrome.

TIGHT LATERAL RECTUS SYNDROME

Causes This syndrome is probably seen most commonly in association with a long-standing large angle exotropia. Large bimedial recession followed by contracture of the lateral recti has also been implicated as a cause.

Clinical features The tight lateral rectus syndrome is characterized by bilateral restriction of the eyes on attempted adduction and an apparent overaction of all the four obliques.

- *Forced duction test* shows restriction of both the lateral recti, an observation which helps in differentiating it from bonafide oblique overaction.

Treatment consists of recessions of the lateral recti combined with temporal conjunctival recession. Medial rectus, resection or advancement may be required.

CONTRACTURE OF EXTRAOCULAR MUSCLES

- *Contracture of antagonist extraocular muscle* is of common occurrence after paralysis of an agonist extraocular muscle, that with time produces a restriction.
- *Treatment* consists of recessing the antagonist muscle.

ADHESIVE SYNDROME

- Adhesive syndrome or cicatricial strabismus refers to a restrictive type of strabismus which occurs following squint surgery, most commonly after inferior oblique myectomy done at the insertion end of the muscle.
- It is thought to result from a fibrous and fatty proliferative inflammatory response following surgical entry of the portion of Tenon's capsule and fat into the wound.
- Hypotropia is associated with an inferior restriction or forced duction test.

POSTOPERATIVE SCARRING

Postoperative scarring of the conjunctiva and extraocular muscles may occur producing restrictions. Treatment consists of recession of the affected muscles and conjunctiva.

Postoperative scarring of the Tenon's capsule has been reported to produce an L-deformity of inferior oblique, J-deformity of rectus muscle and cicatricial advancement of a rectus muscle.

- *L-deformity of the inferior oblique* occurs following accidental incorporation of the inferior oblique into the insertion of lateral rectus muscle during resection surgery on it.
- *J-deformity of a rectus muscle* refers to postoperative pull of the belly of the recessed muscle forward over the insertion site. It occurs due to the 'purse-string' pulling action of Tenon's capsule following an insufficient surgery on it.
- *Cicatricial advancement* of a rectus muscle also results from an insufficient surgery on the intermuscular membrane and Tenon's capsule. The 'purse-string' action of the insufficiently separated Tenon's capsule pulls the new insertion of the muscle back to its original insertion.

Treatment consists of re-exploration to define the problem and release the restriction.

ORBITAL MYOSITIS

Causes: The clinical spectrum of orbital myositis can be seen in the following conditions:
- Idiopathic orbital inflammatory disease (IOID)
- Autoimmune myositis

- Cysticercosis of extraocular muscles
- Mild grade orbital cellulitis.

Clinical features include:
- Ocular pain
- Conjunctival congestion
- Proptosis
- Ptosis may also occur in some cases
- Deviation of the involved eye and diplopia
- Restriction of eye movements (positive forced duction test).

Investigations helpful in diagnosis include:
- Orbital ultrasonography
- CT scan/MRI imaging of the orbit and head (to rule out suspected neurocysticercosis).

Treatment
- *Systemic steroids* are useful in idiopathic orbital inflammatory diseases and autoimmune myositis.
- *Oral albendazole*, under cover of steroids is useful in cysticercosis.
- *Antibiotics and anti-inflammatory drugs* are needed in mild grade orbital cellulitis.

BIBLIOGRAPHY

1. Adler FH: Superior oblique tendon sheath syndrome of Brown. Arch. Ophthalmol. 48:264, 1959.
2. Aebli R: Retraction syndrome. Arch. Ophthalmol. 10:602, 1933.
3. Afifi AK Bell. WE, and Menezes, AH: Etiology of lateral rectus palsy in infancy and childhood J Child.Neurol, 7:295, 1992.
4. Ahluwalia BK, Gupta NC, Goel SR and Khurana, AK: Study of Duane's retraction syndrome. Acta Ophthalmol. 66:728, 1988.
5. Albert DG: Personal communication. In Parks, MM: Annual review: strabismus. Arch. Ophthalmol. 58:152, 1957.
6. Arimoto H: Ocular findings of thalidomide embryopathy. Jpn J Clin Ophthalmol. 33:501, 1979.
7. Bahn RS and Heufelder, AE: Pathogenesis of Graves ophthalmopathy. N Engl J Med 329:1468, 1993.
8. Bell JA, Fielder AR and Viney S: Congenital double elevator palsy in identical twins. J Clin Neuro Ophthalmol. 10:32, 1990.
9. Berens C and Girard, L: Transplantation of the superior and inferior rectus muscles for paralysis

of the lateral rectus muscle. Am J Ophthalmol. 33:1041, 1950.

10. Berlit P: Isolated and combined pareses of cranial nerves III, IV and VI. A retrospective study of 412 patients. J. Neurol. Sci. 103:10, 1991.

11. Bielschowsky, A:2 Die Motilitatsstorungen der Augen. In Axenfeld, T, and Elschnig, A, editors: Graefe Saemisch's Handbuch der gesamten Augenheikunde, ed. 2, vol. 8, Berlin, 1939, Julius Springer.

12. Bielschowsky A: Lectures on motor anomalies, Hanover, NH, 1943 (reprinted 1956). Dartmouth College Publications.

13. Boyd. TAS, Leitch, GT, and Budd, GE: A new treatment for "A" and "V" patterns in strabismus by slanting muscle insertions: a preliminary report. Can. J Ophthalmol. 6: 170, 1971.

14. Breinin G: The physiopathology of the A- and V-patterns. In Symposium: the A- and V-patterns in strabismus. Trans Am Acad Ophthalmol. Otolaryngol. 57:157, 1953.

15. Brosky MC, Pollock SC and Buckley EG: Neural misdirection in congenital ocular fibrosis syndrome: Implications and pathogenesis. J Pediatr. Ophthalmol, Strabismus 26:159, 1989.

16. Brown HW: Congenital structuralmuscle anomalies. In Allen, JH, editor: Strabismus ophthalmic symposium I. St. Louis, 1950, Mosby- Year Book. Inc., p. 205.

17. Brown HW: Isolated inferior oblique paralysis. Analysis of 97 cases. Trans. Am. Ophthalmol. Soc, 55:415, 1957.

18. Brown HWL: Congenital structural anomalies of the muscles. In Allen, JH editor: Strabismus ophthalmic symposium II, St. Louis, 1958, Mosby-Year Book, Inc., p. 391.

19. Brown HW: True and simulated superior oblique tendon sheath syndromes. Doc. Ophthalmol. 34: 123, 1973.

20. Brown HW: Vertical deviations. In Symposium, strabismus. Trans. Am. Acad Ophthalmol. Otolaryngol. 57:157, 1953.

21. Brown WB: Isolated inferior oblique paralysis. Trans Am. Ophthalmol. Soc. 55:415, 1957.

22. Burke JP, Ruben JB and Scott WE: Vertical transposition of the horizontal recti (Knapp procedure) for the treatment of double elevator palsy: effectiveness and longterm stability. Br. J Ophthalmol. 76:734, 1992.

23. Burian HM and Van Allen MW: Cyclic oculomotor paralysis. Am. J Ophthalmol. 55:529, 1963.

24. Costenbader FD: Introduction. In Symposium: the A- and V-patterns in strabismus. Trans. Am. Acad. Ophthalmol. Otolaryngol. 68:354, 1964.

25. Dotti MT, Federico A, Palmeri S, and Guazzi GC: Congenital oculo-facial paralysis (Moebius syndrome) evidence of dominant inhertance in two families. Acta Neurol. 11:434, 1989.

26. Duane A: Congenital deficiency of abduction associated with impairment of adduction, retraction movements, contraction of the palpebral fissure and oblique movements of the eye. Arch. Ophthalmol. 34:133, 1905.

27. Duane RD, Schatz NJ and Caputo AR: Pseudo Duane's retraction syndrome. Trans. Am. Ophthalmol. Soc. 74:122, 1976.

28. Duke-Elder S and Wybar K: System of ophthalmology, vol. 6: Ocular motility and strabismus, St. Louis, 1973, Mosby-year Book, Inc., p. 736 ff.

29. Esswein MB and Noorden GK von: Paresis of a vertical rectus muscle after cataract surgery. Am J Ophthalmol. 116:424, 1993.

30. Fells P and Collin JRO: Cyclic oculomotor palsy. Trans. Ophthalmol. Soc. UK 99:192, 1979.

31. Fink WH: The A and V syndromes. Am. Orthopt. J. 9:105, 1959.

32. Fitzsimmons R, Lee J and Elston J: The role of botulinum in the management of sixth nerve palsy. Eye 3:391, 1989.

33. Fitzsimmons R, Lee JP and Elston J: Treatment of sixth nerve palsy in adults with combined botulinum toxin chemodenervation and surgery. Ophthalmology 95:1535, 1988.

34. Gobin MH: Sagittalization of the oblique muscles as possible cause for the "A", "V", and "X" phenomena. Br J Ophthalmol. 52:13, 1968.

35. Gopal KSS: Acquired double depressor palsy. Indian J. Ophthalmol. 36:35, 1988.

36. Gottlob L, Catalano RA and Reinecke RD: Surgical management of oculomotor nerve palsy. Am J Ophthalmol. 111:71, 1991.

37. Guyton D: Exaggerated traction test for the oblique muscles. Ophthalmology 88:1035, 1981.

38. Hardesty HH: Diagnosis of paretic vertical rotators. Am.JOphthalmol. 56:811, 1963.

39. Helveston EM: A new two step method for the diagnosis of isolated cyclovertical muscle palsies. Am. J. Ophthalmol. 64:914, 1967.

40. Helveston EM, Krach D, Plager DA and Ellis FD: A new classification of superior oblique palsy based on congenital variations in the tendon. Ophthalmology 99:1609, 1992.

41. Huber A: Electrophysiology of the retraction syndrome. Br J Ophthalmol. 58:293, 1974.

42. Jampolsky A: Oblique muscle surgery of the A- and V-pattern. J Pediatr. Ophthalmol. 2:31, 1965.

43. Jampolsky, A: Surgical leashes and reverse leashes in strabismus surgical managemnet. In Symposium on strabismus: transactions of the New Orleans Academy of Ophthalmology, St. Louis, 1978, Mosby-Year Book. Inc., p.244.

44. Khawam E, Scott A and Jampolsky A: Acquired superior oblique palsy. Diagnosis and management. Arch. Ophthalmol, 77:761, 1967.

45. Knapp P and Moore S: Diagnosis and surgical options in superior oblique surgery. Int. Ophthalmol. Clin. 16:137, 1976.

46. Knapp P: Diagnosis and surgical treatment of hypertropia, Am, Orthopt. J. 21:29, 1971.

47. Knapp P: Vertically incomitant horizontal strabismus: the so-called A and V syndrome. Trans. Am. Ophthalmol. Soc, 57:666, 1959.

48. Knapp P: A- and V-patterns. In Symposium on strabismus. Transactions of the New Orleans Academy of Ophthalmology, St. Louis, 1971, Mosby - Year Book, Inc., p 242.

49. Kodsi SR and Younge BR: Acquired oculomotor, trochlear, and abducent cranial nerve palsies in pediatric patients. Am. J. Ophthalmol. 114:568. 1992.

50. Manners RM, O'Flynn E and Morris RJ: Superior oblique lengthening for acquired superior oblique overaction. Br J Ophthalmol. 78:280, 1994.

51. Metz HS: Saccadic velocity measurements in strabismus. Trans, Am. Ophthalmol. Soc. 81:630, 1983.

52. Metz HS, Scott AB and Scott WE: Horizontal saccadic velocities in Duane's syndrome. Am. J. Ophthalmol. 80:901, 1975.

53. Noorden GK von, Awaya S and Romano PE: Past-pointing in paralytic strabismus. Am. J Ophthalmol. 71:27, 1971.

54. Noorden GK von and Hansell R: Clinical characteristics and treatment of isolated inferior rectus paralysis, Ophthalmology 98:253, 1991.

55. Noorden GK von, Murray E and Wong SY: Superior oblique paralysis. A review of 270 cases. Arch. Ophthalmol. 104:1771, 1986.

56. Noorden GKvon and Ruttum M: Torticollis in paralysis of the trochlear nerve. Am Orthopt. J 33: 16, 1983.

57. Noorden GK von, Tredici TD and Ruttum M: Pseudo-internuclear ophthalmoplegia after surgical paresis of the medial rectus muscle. Am J Ophthalmol. 98:602, 1984.

58. Noorden GK von and Olson CL: Diagnosis and surgical management of vertically incomitant horizontal strabismus. Am J Ophthalmol. 60:434, 1965.

59. Olivier P and Noorden GK and Excyclotropia of the nonparetic eye in unilateral superior oblique muscle paralysis. Am. J. Ophthalmol. 93:30, 1982.

60. Olivier P and Noorden GK von: Results of superior oblique tenectomy in inferior oblique paresis. Arch. Ophthalmol. 100-581, 1982.

61. Parks MM: Isolated cyclovertical muscle palsy. Arch. Ophthalmol. 60: 1027, 1958.

62. Parks MM: The weakening surgical procedures for eliminating overaction of the inferior oblique muscle. Am J Ophthalmol, 73:107, 1972.

63. Roper-Hall G and Feibel RM: Measurement of the field of binocular single vision in the evaluation of incomitant paralytic strabismus. Am. Orthopt. J 24:77, 1974.

64. Rush JA and Younge BR: Paralysis of cranial nerves III, IV, and VI: causes and prognosis in 1,000 cases. Arch. Ophthalmol. 99:76, 1981.

65. Ruttam M and Noorden GK von: Orbital and facial anthropometry in A- and V-pattern strabismus. In Reinecke, RD, editor: Strabismus II, New York, 1984, Grune & Stratton, Inc,., p. 363.

66. Scott WE and Kraft SP: Classification and surgical treatment of superior oblique palsies: I. Unilateral superior oblique palsies. Tran sactions of the New Orleans Academy of Ophthalmology, New York, 1986, Raven Press, P. 15.

67. Scott WE and Kraft SP: Classification and surgical treatment of superior oblique palsies: II. Bilateral superior oblique palsies. Transactions of the New Orleans Academy of Ophthalmology, New York, 1986, Raven Press, p. 265.

68. Scott AB and Stella SL: Measurement of A- and V-patterns. J. Pediatr. Ophthalmol. 5:181, 1968.

69. Stilling J: Untersuchungen iiber die Entstehung der Kurzsichtigkeit, Wiesbaden, 1887, J.F. Bergmann, P. 13.

70. Turk S: Bemerkungen zu einem Falle von Retraction des Auges. Cbl. Pract. Augenheilk. 23:14, 1899.

71. Urist MJ: Horizontal squint with secondary vertical deviations. Arch. Ophthalmol. 46:245, 1951.

72. Urist MJ: Recession and upward displacement of the medial rectus muscles in A-pattern esotropia. Am J Ophthalmol. 65:769, 1968.

73. Villaseca A: The A and V syndromes. Am. J. Ophthalmol. 52:172, 1961.

74. Wilson ME and Hoxie J: Facial asymmetry in superior oblique muscle palsy. J Pediatr. Ophthalmol. Strabismus 30: 315, 1993.

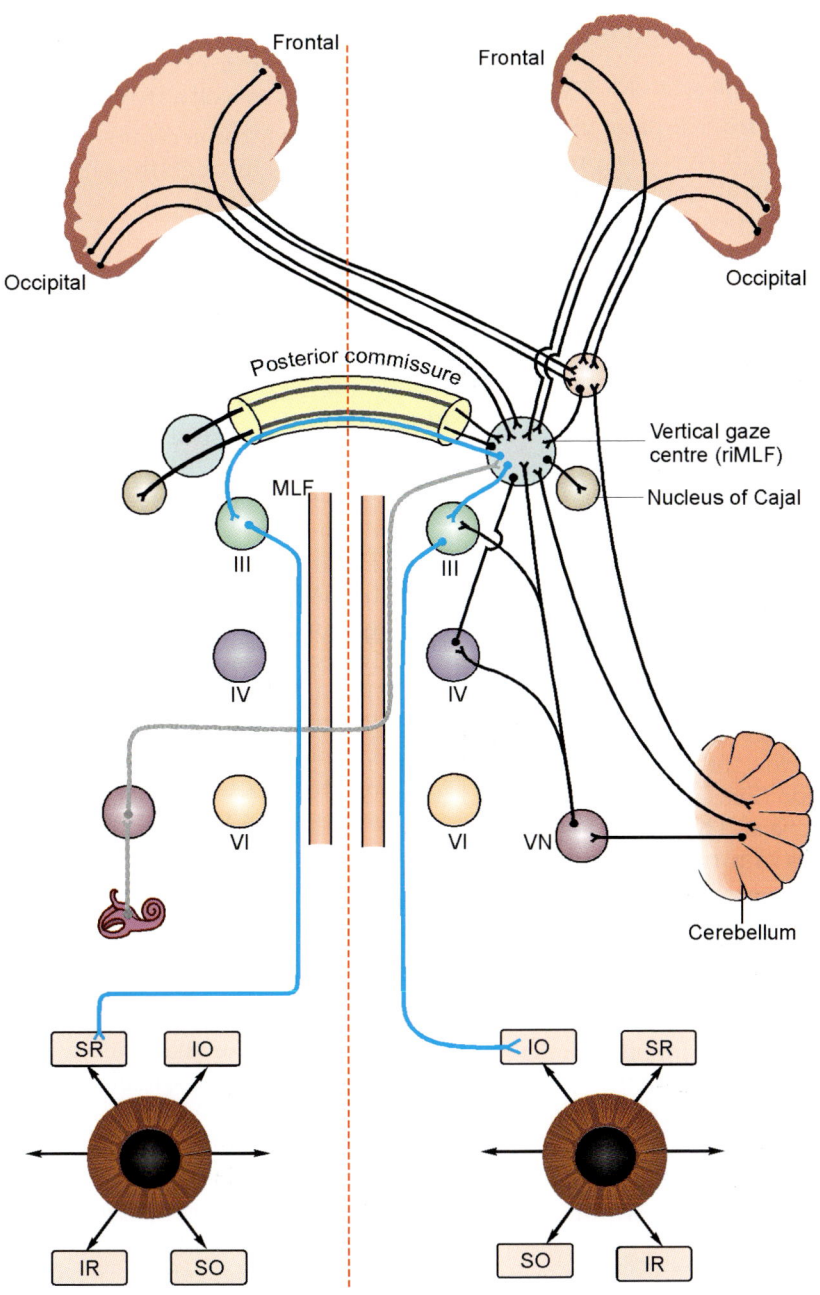

Fig. 13.4 *Pathway for vertical gaze (upgaze) saccadic eye movements.*

- Superior colliculus
- Vestibular apparatus
- Cerebellum
- Medial longitudinal fasciculus

1. Paramedian pontine reticular formation

Horizontal gaze centre. The paramedian pontine reticular formation (PPRF) is the primary centre responsible for generating horizontal conjugate gaze. The PPRF is positioned ventral to the medial longitudinal fasciculus (MLF). It extends from the level of the trochlear nerve nucleus to the abducens nerve nucleus (Fig. 13.1).

- *Afferent connections.* Most afferent connections to the PPRF are through the vestibular nucleus. It receives signals from both the frontal cortical areas concerned with generation of saccades and ipsilateral occipitoparietal cortical area concerned with generation of pursuits directly (for voluntary movements) and through the superior colliculus (for involuntary movements). Vestibular input for horizontal eye movements comes from the contralateral vestibular apparatus by way of the vestibular nuclei. An axon from the vestibular nucleus crosses to the opposite abducens nucleus, where it innervates a motor neuron and an internuclear neuron for horizontal gaze in the opposite direction (Fig. 13.2).
- *Efferent connections.* The centre for horizontal gaze movements in turn is connected with the homolateral abducent nucleus present next to it. The axons of the internuclear neurons of the abducent cross the midline and travel through the medial longitudinal fasciculus (MLF) of the opposite side to that part of nucleus of the oculomotor nerve which innervates the medial rectus muscle (Figs 13.2 and 13.5). Therefore, impulses from this centre produce contraction of the homolateral lateral rectus muscle and the opposite medial rectus, hence binocular gaze movements to the side of the stimulated centre.

2. Rostral interstitial nucleus of medial longitudinal fasciculus

Vertical gaze centre. The vertical gaze centre is the rostral interstitial nucleus of the medial longitudinal fasciculus (riMLF) located at the level of upper pole of the red nucleus. Slightly caudal to the riMLF and directly connected to it lies the interstitial nucleus of Cajol (INC). This nucleus contains neurons which appear to be involved in vertical gaze holding and vertical pursuit.

- *Afferent connections.* The vertical gaze centre (riMLF) receives impulses from both the frontal and occipital cortical ocular motor centres as well as from the superior colliculus.
- *Efferent connections.* The riMLF nucleus projects through the posterior commissure to its equivalent on the other side of the mesencephalon as well as directly to the nuclei of III and IV cranial nerves supplying the extraocular muscles concerned with the vertical movements (Figs 13.3, 13.4 and 13.6).

3. Posterior commissure

Dorsal and rostral to the riMLF is the posterior commissure, a fibre tract that contains some scattered neuronal cell bodies. Lesions in this region produce abnormalities of upward gaze. It is likely that the fibres for upward gaze leave the riMLF and pass through this region before reaching the oculomotor and trochlear nuclei. Involvement of the posterior commissure may be part of the dorsal midbrain syndrome (Parinaud syndrome). In this syndrome, there is impairment of upwardly directed saccades or, in extreme cases, loss of all vertical movement. Other signs include pupillary mydriasis and light-near pupillary dissociation, corectopia, and convergence-retraction nystagmus.

4. Convergence and divergence centre

At present, nothing is known about the location of a subcortical divergence centre. In fact, there is no evidence that such a centre exists at all. Similarly, a subcortical centre for convergence also may not exist at all and convergence as well as divergence may be purely cortical functions. However, clinical evidence points that the pretectal area is probable site for the subcortical convergence centre; since lesions in this area abolish convergence. The impulses to the so-called convergence centre come from the frontal and the occipital ocular motor centres. Convergence occurs only upon simultaneous bilateral stimulation of either the frontal or the occipital motor centres. These impulses are relayed to the nuclei of both third nerves which innervate the medial recti muscles (Fig. 13.8).

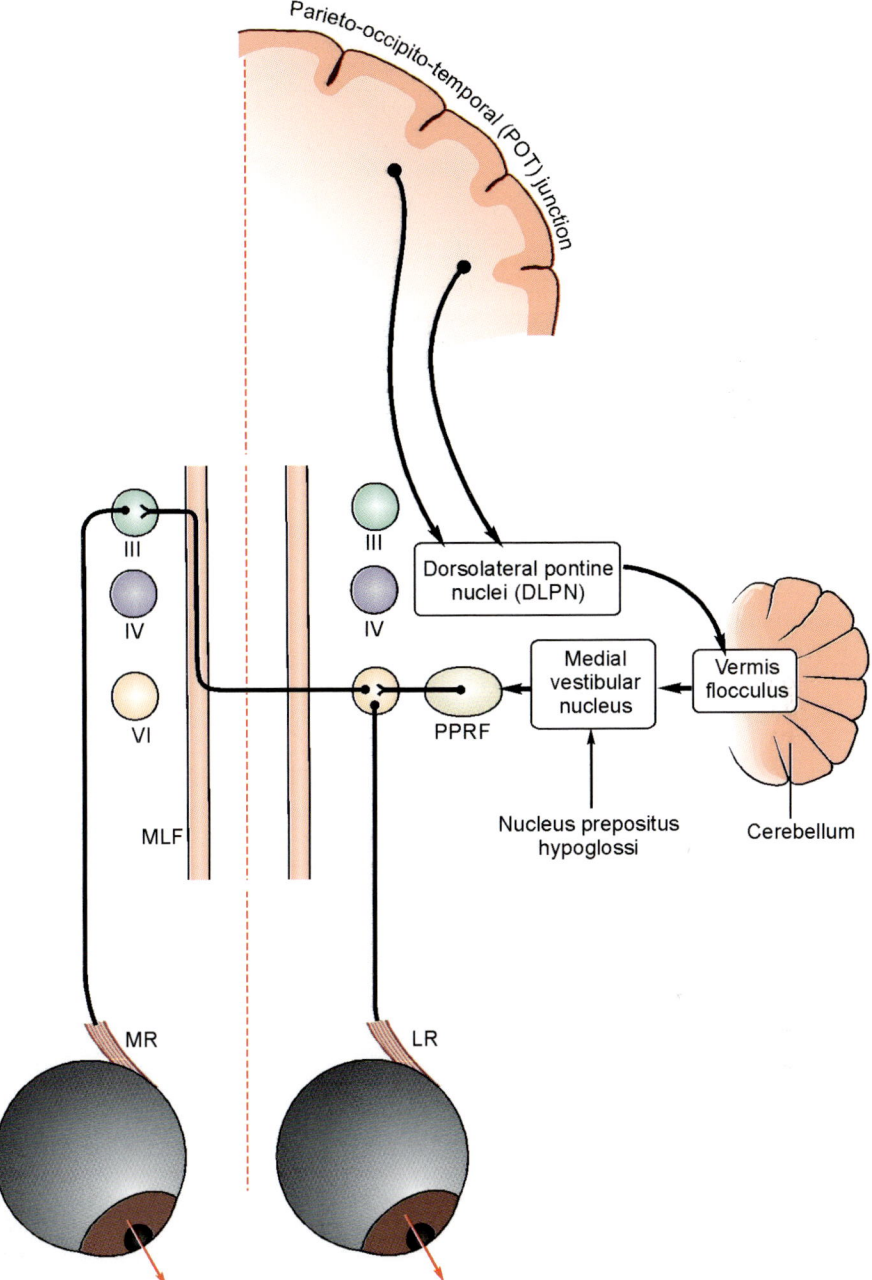

Fig. 13.5 *Neural pathway of horizontal pursuit eye movements.*

5. Superior colliculus

These structures in the dorsal midbrain play a role in both ocular motor and sensory function. The superior colliculus receives visual input directly from branches of retinal ganglion cell axons. Visual input also comes indirectly from the visual cortex, the parietal and frontal lobes, and the substantia nigra. There are efferent projections to the brainstem premotor areas. The superior colliculus can generate visually directed saccades independently and may play a role in the control of pursuit eye movements. In primates, ablation of both FEFs and both superior colliculi is necessary to produce permanent saccadic defects.

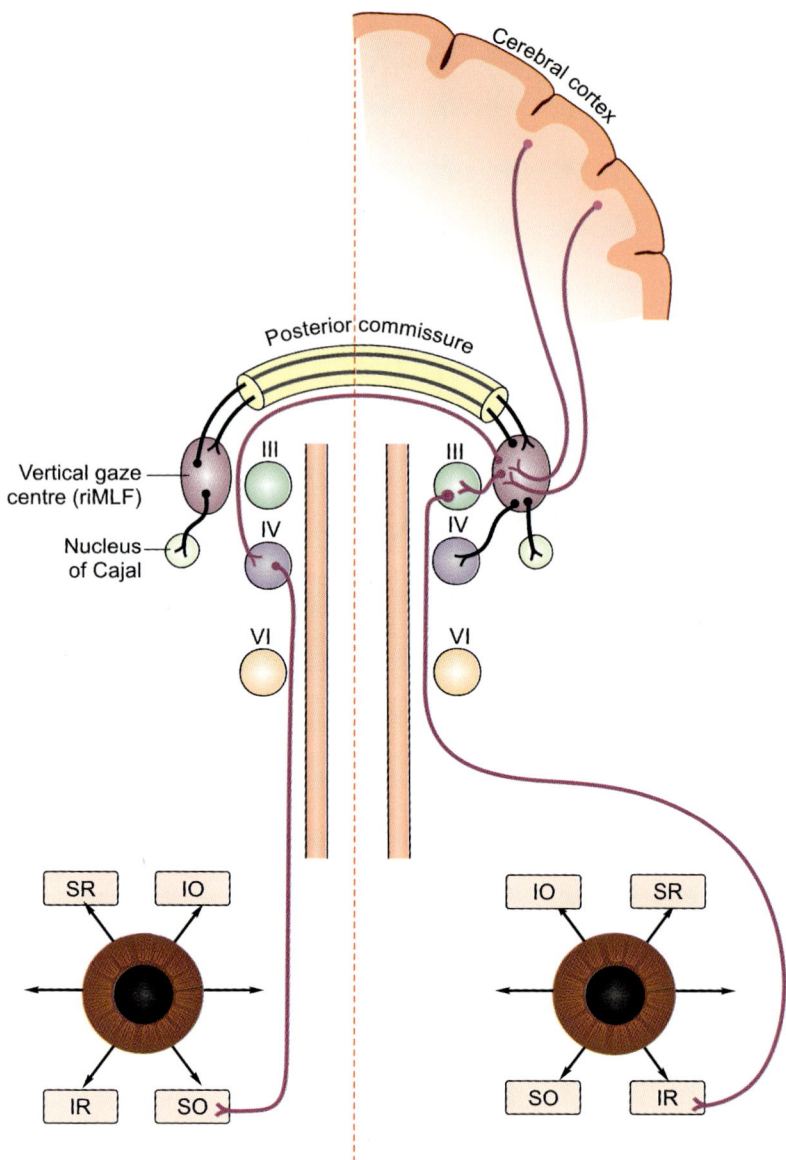

Fig. 13.6 *Neural pathway of vertical persuit (downgaze) eye movements*

6. Vestibular apparatus

Reflex eye movements that compensate for changes in the position of head or body originate from the vestibulum. They are called statokinetic reflexes. If, for instance, the head is turned to the left, the eyes perform an involuntary compensatory movement to the right which allows continuous fixation of the object. These reflexes are innate and unconditioned, occurring even in blind. The vestibular apparatus is a receptor specialized to sense changes of equilibrium and position. It is part of the inner ear and is comprised of three semicircular canals, the sacculus and the utriculus, all of which belong to the membranous labyrinth. The apparatus derives its name from the vestibulum, which is the bony cavity housing the utriculus and the sacculus.

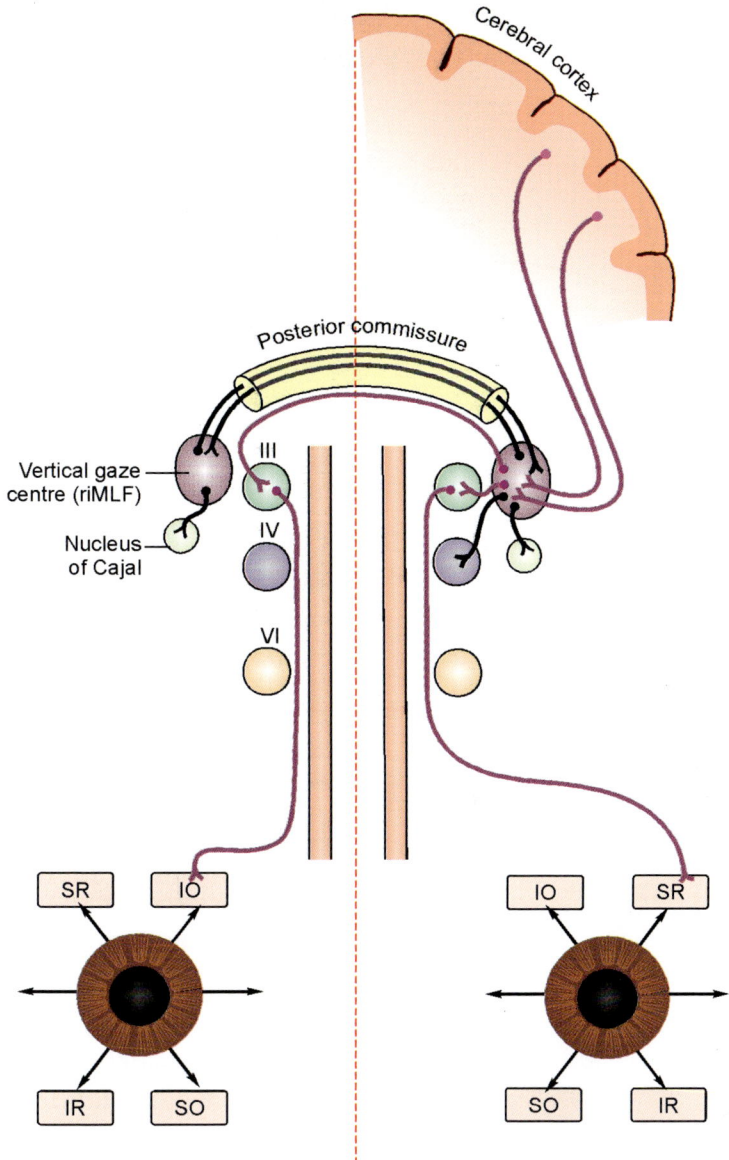

Fig. 13.7 *Neural pathway of vertical persuit (upgaze) eye movements.*

Semicircular canals

The semicircular canals contain receptor organs called cristae that sense movements of the head. Each of the canals is oriented perpendicular to the other two so that a three-dimensional structure is formed roughly coinciding with the horizontal, vertical, and frontal planes. The canals are filled with a watery fluid, the endolymph. When the head moves, the endolymph is subjected to inertia and exerts a

certain pull on the sensory hair of the cristae. This stimulus excites the receptor cells and elicits a nerve impulse that is transmitted through the vestibular nerve (part of nerve VIII) to the vestibular nuclei in the brainstem.

Sacculus and utriculus

The sacculus and the utriculus each contains a macula that functions in a manner similar to that of the cristae of the semicircular canals. Whereas

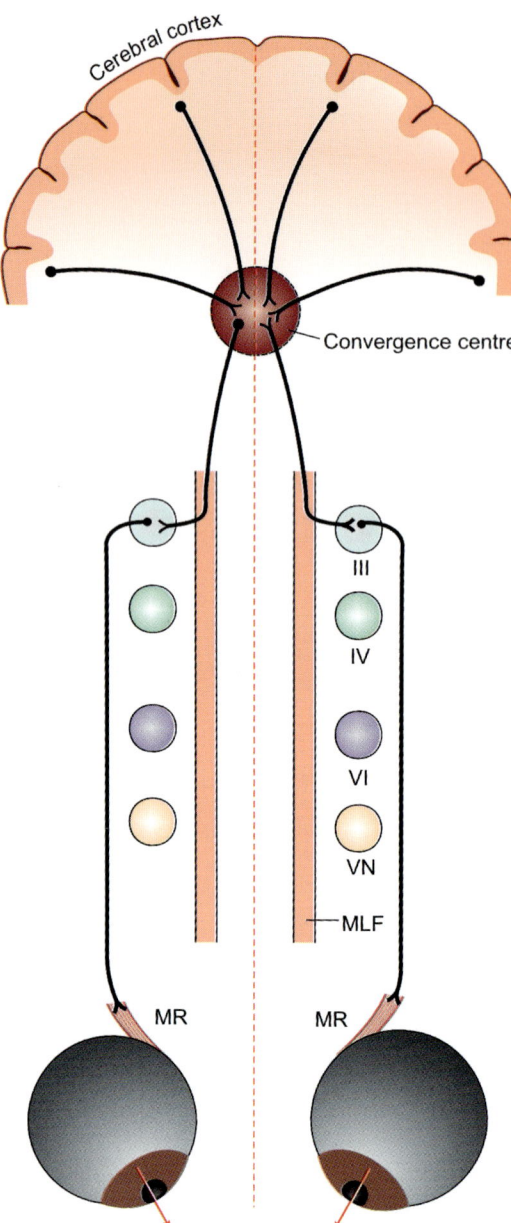

Fig. 13.8 *Presumptive pathway of convergence.*

the cristae respond to head movements (statokinetic reaction), the macula of the utricle responds to gravity (static reaction). On top of each macula rests a gelatinous plate into which protrudes hair from the surface of the macula. The plates, which contain mineral crystals, follow the force of gravity and slide to which ever side is dependent, thereby pulling on the hair. This leads to stimulation of the terminal branches of the vestibular nerve that supply the maculae. The function of the sacculus is not known.

Vestibular nerve

The vestibular nerve (part of nerve VIII) enters the brainstem at the level of the lower end of the pons and terminates in the vestibular nuclei. The vestibular nuclei, in turn, are connected directly to the abducens nuclei and to the nuclei of the ocular motor nerves through the medial longitudinal fasciculi (Figs 13.3–13.7). Stimulation of a labyrinth or of a vestibular nerve causes conjugate deviation of the eyes to the opposite side. Depending on the nature of the stimulus, the eyes may remain in the deviate position or a nystagmus may result. A nystagmus is an oscillatory movement of the two eyes. Both eyes turn in the same direction and are suddenly pulled back into the primary position by a fast, jerky movement, where upon the cycle begins again with conjugate deviation. Usually, the first phase of nystagmus, the conjugate deviation, is distinctly slower than the second phase in which the corrective movement takes place. Diagnostically, vestibular nystagmus can be produced to test the integrity of the vestibular reflex mechanism. For this, the patient is either submitted to rotation on a revolving chair (rotatory vestibular nystagmus) or his/her external auditory canals are irrigated with hot or cold water (caloric vestibular nystagmus).

7. Medial longitudinal fasciculus

The medial longitudinal fasciculus (MLF) is a fibre tract that extends from the spinal cord to the oculomotor nerve nucleus. It contains primarily ascending fibres, the majority of which arise in the superior and medial vestibular nuclei. The MLF is in close proximity to the ocular motor nuclei and influences both ipsilateral and contralateral nuclei.

Functions of MLF. The medial longitudinal fasciculus plays an important role in the pathway of ocular movements. Its main functions can be summarized as follows (Fig. 13.9):

• It connects the oculomotor nuclei with one another.

• It transmits signals from the subcortical–horizontal gaze centre for the horizontal versions to the opposite medial rectus muscle.

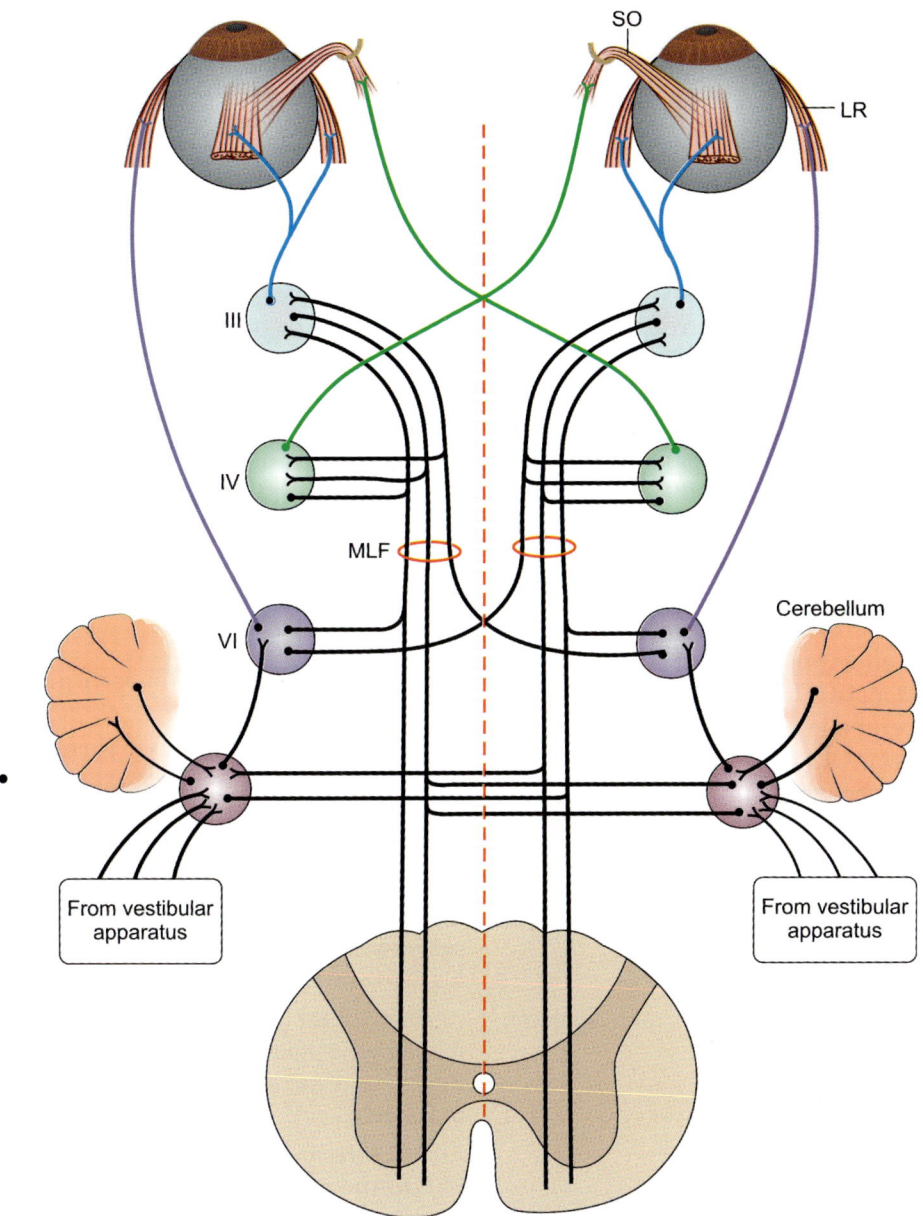

Fig. 13.9 *Connections of medial longitudinal fasciculus (MLF).*

- It transmits impulses originating from the vestibular nucleus (in response to statokinetic stimulation) to the ocular motor nuclei as well as to nucleus innervating muscles of head and neck.

- It relays signals from the proprioceptors of the head and neck muscles to the ocular motor nuclei.

Lesions of MLF. An abnormality of the MLF causes problems with horizontal and vertical gaze co-ordination of the two eyes. The clinically most important connection passing through the MLF links the contralateral abducens nucleus with the ipsilateral medial rectus subnucleus. Abnormalities of this tract produce an internuclear ophthalmoplegia. Such a lesion produces slowed or complete loss of adduction of the ipsilateral eye and abducting nystagmus of the fellow eye.

8. Cerebellum

The cerebellum appears to be involved in the immediate modulation of ongoing eye movements, as well as in the long-term adaptive processes that compensate for ocular motor dysmetria. The cerebellum controls and adjusts the size of saccades. The latter ability is essential for maintaining accurate ocular motor performance during growth and aging, during and after ocular motor disease, or even while using spectacles. For instance, the use of aniso-metropic spectacles produces a varying anisophoria in different directions of gaze, which must be compensated in each direction of gaze.

Hemicerebellectomy produces ipsilateral saccadic and contralateral pursuit defects, while total cerebellectomy creates persistent saccadic dysmetria and abolishes smooth pursuit. The cerebellum has numerous connections to nuclear and supranuclear ocular motor centres.

SUPRANUCLEAR EYE MOVEMENT SYSTEMS

Following supranuclear eye movement systems have been recognized:

- Saccadic system
- Smooth pursuit system
- Vergence system
- Vestibular system
- Optokinetic system
- Position maintenance system

All these systems perform specific functions and each one is controlled by a different neural system but share the same final common path, i.e. the motor neurons that supply the extraocular muscles.

SACCADIC SYSTEM

Saccades are sudden, jerky conjugate eye movements that occur as the gaze shifts from one object to another. Thus they are performed to bring the image of an object quickly on the fovea. Though normally voluntary, saccades may be involuntary aroused by peripheral, visual or auditory stimuli. The saccades include:

- Horizontal saccades, and
- Vertical saccades.

Detailed features of saccadic eye movements are described on page 34.

Neural pathway
Cortical areas

The pathway originates in the premotor cortex of the frontal motor area. From there, the fibres for voluntary saccades pass directly and for involuntary saccades through the superior colliculus to the contralateral horizontal gaze centre in PPRF (Fig. 13.2).

Pathways involved in the cortical generation of saccades

It appears that there are three pathways involved in the cortical generation of saccades:

i. ***Ventral pathway.*** The ventral pathway projects by way of the posterior portion of the anterior limb of the internal capsule and the medial part of cerebral peduncle to reach the pons, where there is a partial decussation and termination in the PPRF.

ii. ***The dorsal pathway*** passes from the FEF through the thalamus, the pulvinar, the pretectal nuclei, and the superior colliculus to reach the brainstem.

iii. ***The intermediate pathway*** extends from the FEF to the rostral ocular motor nuclei and the interstitial nucleus of Cajal.

Brainstem pathway

Recent evidence suggests that the saccades (horizontal as well as vertical) are generated by groups of neurons located in the brainstem and are controlled by higher frontal system (for voluntary saccades) and collicular system (for involuntary saccades). The brainstem neurons concerned with generation of saccades form the final premotor circuits. These neurons are of three types:

- Excitatory burst neurons (EBN)
- Inhibitary burst neurons (IBN), and
- Pause neurons (PN).

Brainstem pathway for saccades is described below.

Pathway for horizontal saccades

For horizontal saccades, the excitatory neurons are located in horizontal gaze centre in paramedian pontine reticular formation (PPRF) and project to the ipsilateral abducens nucleus. The axons from these cells synapse in the abducens nucleus on motor neurons that innervate the ipsilateral lateral rectus and on the interneurons that innervate contra-lateral medial rectus subnucleus by way of the contralateral MLF (Fig. 13.2).

Pathway for vertical saccades

For the vertical saccades, the excitatory neurons are located in the vertical gaze centre formed by rostral interstitial nucleus of medial longitudinal fasciculus (riMLF) and other neurons in the region of posterior commissure.

- *For downward saccades* (Fig. 13.3), the activated neurons in the riMLF send impulse directly through the fibres that synapse upon the inferior rectus subnucleus of the ipsilateral IIIrd nerve and contralateral IVth nerve

nucleus for superior oblique muscles. riMLF nuclei of both sides are connected by a commissure which projects into the interstitial nucleus of Cajal (INC) and to the ipsilateral IIIrd nerve nucleus.
- *For upward saccades* (Fig. 13.4), the activated neurons in the riMLF send impulse through the fibres that synapse upon the inferior oblique subnucleus of the ipsilateral IIIrd nerve; and through the fibres which pass via posterior commissure and synapse upon the superior rectus subnucleus of the contra-lateral IIIrd nerve.

Activities of brainstem involved in generation of saccades neurons

As mentioned above, three types of neurons are involved in generation of saccades: Excitatory burst neurons (EBN), inhibitory burst neurons (IBN) and pause neurons (PN). These neurons generate saccades by a 'pulse-step' innervation system (Fig. 13.10). The 'pulse' is created by sudden firing of the neurons to the extraocular muscles. After the eyeball is moved to the new position; to keep it in the same position, sustained contraction of the muscle is required. This is called a step and is affected by tonic contraction of muscles due to continuous discharge from neurons.

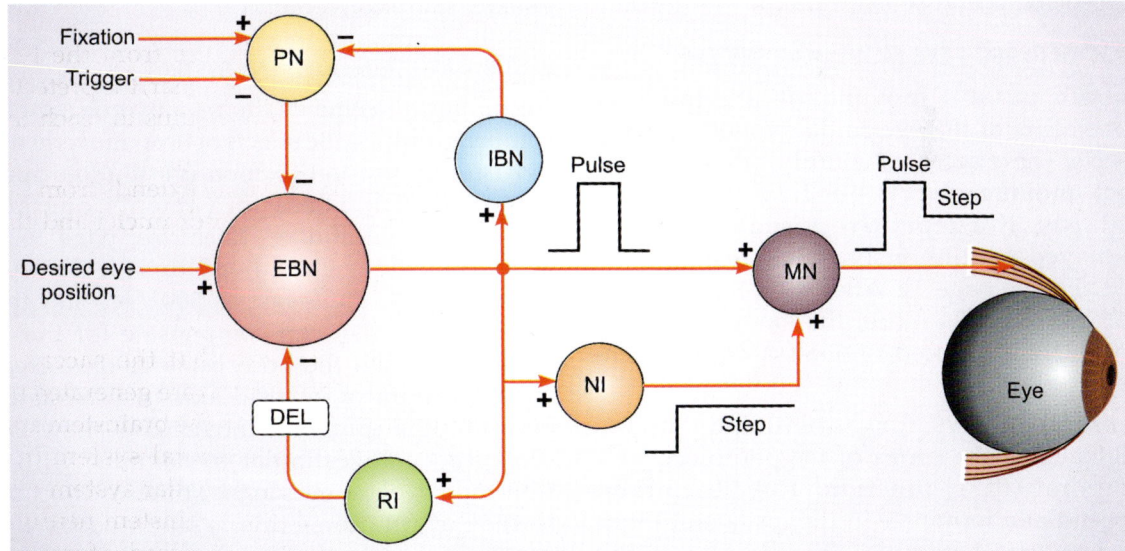

Fig. 13.10 *Showing relation between the three sets of neurons (excitatory burst neurons, pause neurons and inhibitory burst neurons) concerned with generation of saccades.*

Excitatory burst neurons

The excitatory burst neurons (EBNs) discharge at high frequencies just prior to and during the saccades and provide the eye velocity commands known as the pulse (Fig. 13.10). Burst cells discharge, only when there is need for a fast eye movement and do not discharge during fixation, pursuit or vergence eye movements.

The EBNs send impulses to the neurons of cranial nerve nuclei supplying to yoke muscles for the gaze movements.

Inhibitory brust neurons (IBNs)

The inhibitory burst neurons (IBNs) send impulses through the medullary reticular formation to the neurons of cranial nerve nuclei supplying to the antagonist muscles of the yoke muscles for the concerned gaze movement and thus inhibit these muscles and allow the gaze movement to occur.

Their firing rate is inversely proportional to the excitatory burst cells

Pause neurons

These neurons discharge tonically, except just before and during saccades, when they pause. They appear to exert an inhibitory influence on the burst neurons preventing extraneous saccades occurring during fixation. These cells inhibit the burst cells within the ipsilateral PPRF. These cells are important during fixation and smooth pursuit. Abnormalities of these cells lead to opsoclonus and ocular flutter.

SMOOTH PURSUIT EYE MOVEMENT SYSTEM

Smooth pursuit movements are tracking movements of the eye as they follow moving objects. These occur voluntarily, when the eyes track moving objects but take place invo- luntarily, if a repetitive visual pattern is displayed continuously. Their features are described on page 34. When the velocity of the moving object is more, the smooth pursuit movement is replaced by small saccades (catch- up saccades).

Neural pathway for pursuit movements originates in the cortex of the perito-occipito- temporal (POT) junction. The fibres then descend and terminate in the ipsilateral PPRF for horizontal pursuits (Fig. 13.5) and the ipsilateral mesencephalic reticular formation for the vertical pursuits (Figs 13.6 and 13.7); and

then possibly directly to the ocular motor nuclei. The right occipital lobe, therefore, controls pursuits to the right and the left occipital lobe those to the left. The cerebellum is closely associated with normal pursuit movements. The FEF and the superior colliculi paly a modulating role in the production of pursuit eye movements by POT junction. Lesions in the POT area produce ipsilateral pursuit defects.

VERGENCE MOVEMENT SYSTEMS

Vergence movements allow focussing of an object which moves away from or towards the observer or when visual fixation shifts from one object to another at a different distance. Vergence movements are very slow (about 20°/ sec) disjugate movements. They have a latency of about 160 msec. Different types of vergence movements are described on page 35.

Neural pathway. The exact neuroanatomical substrate is not known. Stimulation of parieto- occipital region (area 19 or 22) provokes vergence movements in monkeys. Premotor signals are thought to originate in the mesenchephalic reticular formation with separate population of cells for convergence and divergence. The fibres travel then to the relevant cranial nuclei (Fig. 13.8). This link seems to course outside the MLF, since the MLF lesions usually spare convergence.

VESTIBULAR EYE MOVEMENT SYSTEM

Vestibular movements are usually effective in compensating for the effects of head movements in disturbing visual fixation (vestibulo-ocular reflex—VOR). These movements operate through the vestibular system (*see* page 362). Most rotations of the head do not involve angular rotations as fast as 300°/sec and the vestibular system can compensate for these. However, when the body is rotated at great speeds around a vertical axis (e.g. a skater performing a spin), eye movements show the so-called oculovestibular nystagmus, with a slow motion of the eyes in the opposite direction to that of rotation—this is initiated by the vestibular mechanism—followed by a quick jerky binocular 'return' movement in the direction of rotation. This sequence is repeated as long as the angular acceleration lasts. It is likely that the fast component of nystagmus is mediated by mechanisms similar to those responsible for saccades.

OPTOKINETIC SYSTEM

This system helps to hold the images of the seen world steady on the retinae during sustained head rotation. This system becomes operative, when the vestibular reflex gets fatigued after 30 seconds. The optokinetic response is evoked by rotation of the visual field before the eyes. It consists of a movement following the moving scene, succeeded by a rapid saccade in the opposite direction. In fact, the transient head rotation stimulates both the vestibulo-ocular reflex with a latency of only 10 ms and the optokinetic reflex with a latency of 70 ms. However, during sustained rotation with eyes open, the vestibulo-ocular reflex ceases while the optokinetic system maintains a steady discharge from the vestibular nuclei to sustain the compensatory optokinetic nystagmus.

POSITION MAINTENANCE SYSTEM

This system helps to maintain a specific gaze position by means of rapid micromovements called 'flicks' and slow micromovements called 'drifts'. This system coordinates with other systems.

Neural pathway for this system is believed to be the same as for saccades and smooth pursuits.

SUPRANUCLEAR DISORDERS OF EYE MOVEMENTS

INTRODUCTION

Anatomic background and site of lesions

As described above, the supranuclear pathways connect the frontal lobe, occipital lobe and cerebellum with the mesencephalon, i.e. midbrain and pons (containing the nuclei controlling the extraocular muscles and the centres for horizontal and vertical conjugate gazes). The pathway transmitting impulses from the frontal lobe centres to the mesencephalon may be referred to as *frontomesencephalic pathway* and that connecting occipital lobe centres with

mesencephalon as *occipitoparieto-mesencephalic pathway.*

Supranuclear disorders thus result from the lesions involving the cortical centres or the lesions interrupting the frontomesencephalic pathway, occipitoparietomesencephalic pathway, cerebellar pathways, centres for horizontal and vertical conjugate gazes and medial longitudinal fasciculus. Thus, the supranuclear ocular motility disturbances result from interruption of the neural pathway before they reach the eye movement generators.

Characteristic of supranuclear disorders

The basic characteristic of supranuclear lesions (other than those interrupting vergence mechanism and the medial longitudinal fasciculus) are that

- *Both eyes are affected equally* and that the disturbance is one of deficient or defective conjugate eye movements.
- *They usually do not produce diplopia* because both eyes are equally involved.

List of common supranuclear disorders

Some of the common supranuclear disorders are as follows:

- Oculormotor apraxia
- Horizontal conjugate gaze paralysis
- Internuclear ophthalmoplegia
- One-and-a-half syndrome
- Vertical conjugate gaze paralysis
- Skew deviation
- Cogwheeling
- Ocular dysmetria, ocular flutter and opsoclonus
- Double elevator paralysis
- Nystagmus, and
- Comitant squint. (It is considered the most common supranuclear disorder. It is being presumed that the comitant squint represents primarily a deficiency in the vergence movement mechanism).

Differentiating supranuclear from nuclear and infranuclear lesions

In patients with gaze palsy, following tests can be used to know whether the eyes can be moved reflexively in the direction of the paresis.

1. *Oculocephalic (doll's eye) reflex test*. Patient's head is tilted forward by 30 degrees and asked to fixate a distant target. Patient's head is then rotated in the direction opposite to the gaze palsy and movements of the eyes are noted. Since this test uses direct projections from the vestibular system to the oculomotor nuclei, gaze palsies caused by lesion of the cerebral cortex can be typically overcome. However, in prenuclear nuclear or infranuclear lesions, the doll's eye reflex does not overcome the palsy.

2. *Vestibulo-ocular reflex (VOR) testing*. To perform VOR test, patient's head is tilted by 60 degrees and the external auditory meatus is irrigated with either cold or warm water to stimulate the horizontal semicircular canal. In patients with supranuclear gaze palsies the stimulation causes the eye to slowly deviate resulting in nystagmus with fast (corrective) phase to the opposite side with cold stimulation and same side with warm stimulation (to remember the mneumonic COWS: Cold-Opposite; Warm-same).

OCULAR MOTOR APRAXIA

A total loss of voluntary conjugate gaze in all directions is known as oculomotor apraxia. In order to bring their eyes into the desired gaze position, patients with oculomotor apraxia characteristically have a head thrusting movement. Oculomotor apraxia can be congenital or acquired.

Congenital ocular motor apraxia

Etiopathogenesis

Congenital ocular motor apraxia (COMA) is a rare disorder of unknown etiopathogenesis. It is more common in boys than girls and may be familial.

- *Agenesis of the corpus callosum* and hydro-cephalous have been reported to be associated with some cases.
- *Mass lesions of cerebellum compressing* the rostral part of the brainstem have been reported in many infants presenting with oculomotor apraxes.

Clinical features

Clinical features include:
- An inability to generate normal, voluntary horizontal saccades. In early infancy, blindness may be suspected because of the inability to fixate or follow objects.
- Changes in horizontal fixation are made by a head thrust that overshoots the target followed by a rotation of the head back in the opposite direction once fixation is established.
- Vertical saccades and random eye movements are intact.
- Vestibular and optokinetic nystagmus are impaired.
- Reading can be difficult with this condition.
- Developmental delay, especially motoric, may be present.

Differential diagnosis

Congenital ocular motor aparaxia (COMA) need to be differentiated from 'Familial horizontal gaze palsy with scoliosis'(HGPS). HGPS is an autoimmune recessive disorder characterized by paralysis of horizontal gaze since birth, progressive scoliosis, impaired OKN and VOR reflexes, but intact convergence and vertical eye movements.

Acquired ocular motor apraxia

Bilateral lesions of the frontoparietal cortex have been reported to be associated with the acquired oculomotor apraxia. It needs to be differentiated from the conditions that affect the generation of voluntary saccades, including metabolic and degenerative diseases such as Huntington's chorea.

HORIZONTAL CONJUGATE GAZE PARALYSIS

Horizontal conjugate gaze paralysis refers to equal paralysis of same sided horizontal movement in both eyes, i.e. either levoversion or dextroversion is deficient or defective.

Site of lesion

As described earlier, the frontal lobe is connected with the mesencephalon through the frontomesencephalic pathway. This pathway descends into the internal capsule and is thought to cross completely at the level of fourth nerve nucleus (Figs 13.2–13.4). It is primarily involved in the saccadic eye movement system.

A destructive lesion in the cortical centre or frontomesencephalic pathway above decussation (Fig. 13.11A) produces defects in conjugate gaze to the opposite side. Lesions below the decussation (Fig. 13.11B) produce defects in conjugate gaze to the same side as the lesion. Lesions involving 6th nerve nucleus (1 in Fig. 13.14) and PPRF (2 in Fig. 13.14) can also produce horizontal gaze palsy on the same side. It is important to note that since the area of the frontal lobe concerned with horizontal eye movements is so large, small lesions of the frontal lobe rarely affect conjugate horizontal gaze.

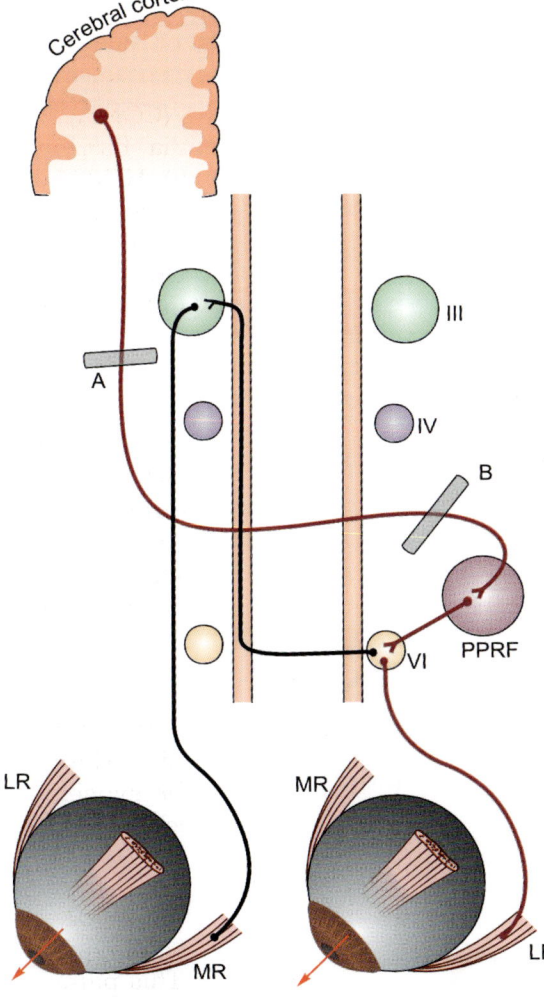

Fig. 13.11 *Site of lesions producing conjugate paralysis to the opposite side* (A) *and the same side* (B).

Efferent fibres from the occipital lobe connecting the mesencephalon from the occipitoparietomesencephalic pathway. This pathway also crosses to the opposite side at the level of 4th nerve nucleus. Lesions involving this pathway will also produce conjugate movements to the opposite side or same side depending upon the site of lesions similar to frontal lobe lesions. However, the conjugate paralysis caused by lesions of occipitoparietal pathway is of lesser magnitude than that caused by lesions involving the frontal voluntary system.

Causes of conjugate paralysis

1. Vascular lesions producing infarctions or haemorrhages.
2. Inflammatory lesions
3. Tumours

Clinical features

As described above, when the frontomesence-phalic tract is interrupted by a lesion above the crossing, there is a deficit of rapid eye movements to the opposite side; thus the right sided lesion will affect:

1. Saccades to the left.
2. The fast phase of the optokinetic nystagmus, when it is to the left.
3. The fast phase of caloric or vestibular nystagmus when it is to the left.
4. On looking to the left, there may be a gaze paretic nystagmus with the fast phase to the left with varying amplitude and rhythm.
5. Gaze paralysis and conjugate deviations caused by hemispheric lesions are usually transient, probably due to compensation from the contralateral uninvolved hemisphere. While, paralysis resulting from lesions in the brainstem are less marked but last as long as the lesion exists since no compensation of function occurs.
6. Lesions causing gaze paralysis (e.g. infarction, haemorrhages and tumours) also produce severe neurologic signs such as hemiplegia and thus the eye signs are usually over-shadowed.

INTERNUCLEAR OPHTHALMOPLEGIA

Internuclear ophthalmoplegia (INO) results from a lesion of the medial longitudinal fasciculus

(MLF) that interrupts fibres passing from the subcortical centre for horizontal gaze of one side to the nucleus of the third nerve on the other side (Fig. 13.12A). It is the only supranuclear defect that does not result in a gaze paralysis.

Etiology

- *Disseminated sclerosis* is the most common cause of bilateral INO.
- *Cerebrovascular accident and brain tumour* can also cause bilateral INO.
- *Infarct of small branch of the basilar artery* is usually associated with unilateral INO.

Clinical features

Unilateral INO. As is clear from the Fig. 13.11, patient with unilateral INO on version movements will exhibit:

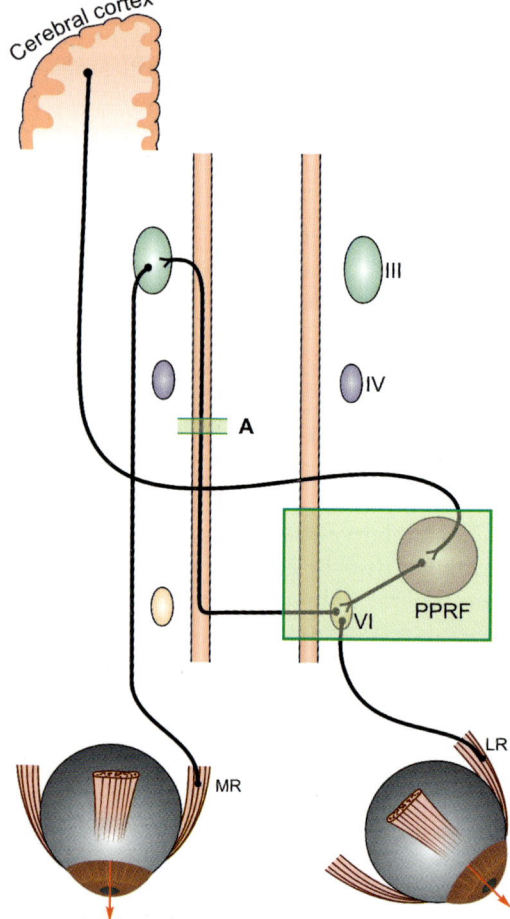

Fig. 13.12 *Site of lesion (A) producing internuclear ophthalmoplegia.*

- Tropia in the involved side.
- *Limitation of adduction* on the involved side (Fig. 13.13A) and
- *Normal abduction* of the opposite eye (Fig. 13.13B).
- *Nystagmus* is associated with abduction of the opposite side. Nystagmus in INO is a secondary response to the weakness of adduction and not caused directly by the central defect.
- *Convergence* is normal in many patients and thus both eyes adduct normally to fixate a near object.
- *Skew deviation* of some degree may be noted with the eye ipsilateral to the lesion slightly higher than the other.

Bilateral INO is more frequent than unilateral INO. Depending upon the site of lesion, other cranial nuclei and convergence mechanism may also be involved.

Differential diagnosis

1. *Isolated medial rectus palsy* needs to be differentiated from the INO.

2. *Pseudointernuclear ophthalmoplegia* should be distinguished from the true INO. Pseudo-INO, i.e. a condition characterised by limitation of adduction and nystagmus of the abducting eye caused by lesions other than lesions of MLF, such as:

- That occurring due to myasthenia gravis
- That following recession and retroequatorial posterior fixation of both medial rectus muscles.

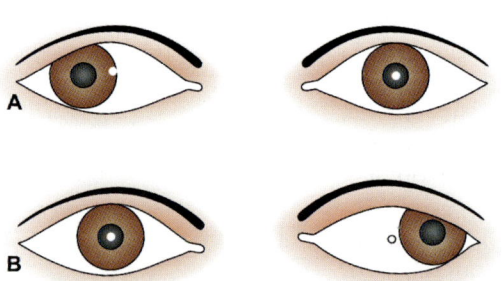

Fig. 13.13 *Diagrammatic depiction of right internuclear ophthalmoplegia. Note right exotropia in primary position (A) and limitation of adduction in the right eye with normal abduction in the left eye (B).*

Treatment

Unfortunately, still there is no effective treatment for INO.

ONE-AND-A-HALF SYNDROME

One-and-a-half syndrome (paralytic pontine exotropia) consists of a unilateral internuclear ophthalmoplegia and a contralateral-horizontal gaze palsy.

Etiology

An extensive caudal lesion in the pons can affect the horizontal gaze centre and the adjacent MLF, resulting in a palsy of both medial rectus muscles and one lateral rectus (i.e. gaze palsy plus INO) (Fig. 13.12B and 4 in Fig. 13.14). Causes include demyelination, vascular, tumour and inflammation.

Features

The main clinical and diagnostic features are as follows: The only remaining horizontal movement is abduction by the unaffected lateral rectus, which is associated with the typical abducting nystagmus. When the patient attempts to fixate with this eye in the primary position, the nystagmus will reduce or cease. There is, therefore, a palsy of conjugate gaze on one side and an INO on looking to the other side. A marked compensatory head posture may be adopted to achieve fixation with the preferred eye. Although complete 'one-and-a-half' syndromes are rare, partial or incomplete syndromes are more common. They can be diagnosed on clinical assessment. A Hess chart is useful in monitoring the condition. However, care must be taken in its interpretation, as synergist muscles are affected in patients with lesions involving the horizontal gaze centre as well as the MLF (partial one-and-a-half syndrome). Since the basis of the Hess chart is a comparison of action of synergistic muscles, the test is comparing abnormal with abnormal and, if viewed in isolation, the gaze palsy element may be missed.

VERTICAL CONJUGATE GAZE PARALYSIS

Vertical conjugate gaze paralysis refers to paralysis of either upward gaze or downward

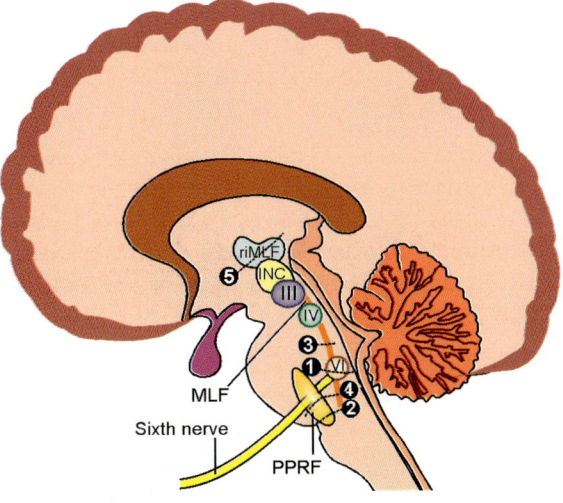

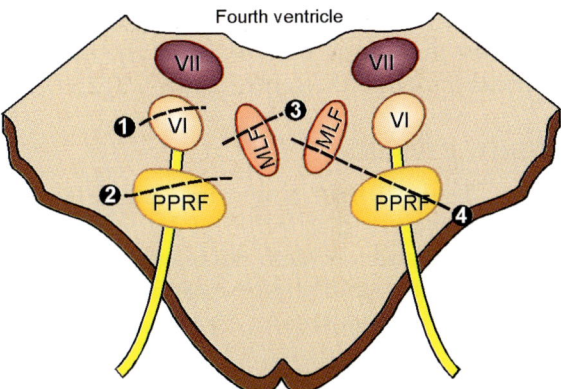

Fig. 13.14 *Site of lesions producing supranuclear disorders. Horizontal gaze palsy may result from lesion involving 6th nerve nucleus (1) and PPRF (2); Internuclear ophthalmoplegia results from a lesion of medial longitudinal fasciculus (3), one-and-a-half syndrome results from a lesion involving both the MLF and PPRF (4); and vertical gaze palsy may result from a lesion involving riMLF (5).*

gaze or both upward and downward gazes equally in both the eyes.

Site of lesion, causes and clinical features

As mentioned earlier (page 360), the vertical gaze centres (riMLF) are located at the level of upper pole of red nucleus and that a vertical version occurs only upon simultaneous stimulation from both the hemispheres. Therefore, vertical gaze paralysis will occur, if there is a lesion of similar extent in each hemisphere involving riMLF (5 in Fig. 13.14). Further, the fact that paresis of upward gaze may occur while the downward gaze is unaffected and vice versa, indicates that there must be some separation of the two centres anatomically.

The upgaze palsy is typically caused by lesions involving the posterior commissure and characteristically occurs in Parinaud's dorsal midbrain syndrome. The most common cause of a Parinaud's syndrome is a pinealoma in which deficiency of upward gaze is associated with pupillary abnormalities.

The downgaze palsy is less common and occurs, when both sides of the midbrain tegmentum posterior to the red nucleus are damaged. Downgaze palsy is frequently associated with convergence paresis and thus it can be assumed that perhaps the convergence centre and the pathway mediating convergence are in close approximation to the centre for downgaze.

SKEW DEVIATION

Skew deviation is a vertical strabismus resulting from a disruption of input into the oculomotor and trochlear nuclei. Cyclotorsion is often a feature and other symptoms and signs of central nervous system disease are usually present.

Etiology

Skew deviation arises from a peripheral or central imbalance of otolith inputs to the oculomotor and trochlear nuclei.

Structures involved in the pathogenesis of skew deviation include: The middle ear and the vestibular nerve; the vestibular nuclei in the brainstem; the cerebellum; the medial longitudinal fasciculus; the interstitial nucleus of Cajal in the midbrain.

Features

The features of skew deviation are: A vertical strabismus, which can be transient or permanent. Transient deviations are common in unilateral internuclear ophthalmoplegia. A deviation, which may be concomitant or incomitant. Incomitant skew deviation must be differentiated from a cyclovertical muscle palsy, and typically resembles a unilateral or bilateral

inferior rectus muscle or a unilateral superior rectus underaction. Incyclotorsion of the hypertropic eye. This is similar to one-half cycle of see-saw nystagmus and reflects the common occurrence of both disorders with lesions involving the interstitial nucleus of Cajal. Other signs of central nervous system disease, usually, involving the brainstem and cerebellum. The strabismus can be monitored using a Hess chart.

COGWHEELING

Defects in slow pursuit tracking to the opposite side may be produced by lesions affecting one occipital lobe. These pursuit movements may be interrupted by saccadic movements; this sign is known as cogwheeling. A lesion interrupting the occipitoparieto-mesencephalic pathway above the decussation in the midbrain will cause a breakdown in tracking or following objects to the opposite field. When the lesion is below the crossing of fibres, the defect is to the same side.

OCULAR DYSMETRIA, OCULAR FLUTTERS AND OPSOCLONUS

Ocular dysmetria. It is a defect in the saccadic eye movement mechanism believed to be caused by lesions of the cerebellum and cerebello-mesencephalic pathway. Normally, when a patient is asked to make saccadic movement from one target to another, there is a small undershoot and a precise end point is reached. In ocular dysmetria, there is tendency of both eyes to overshoot the object of regard, and small oscillations occur until a stable endpoint is reached.

Ocular flutter. It refers to rapid horizontal oscillations of the eyes in primary position. It is thought to be related to fixation difficulties.

Opsoclonus. It refers to a sequence of saccadic eye movements that may be in either direction but are predominantly horizontal. These movements are spontaneous and may show a rhythm to their amplitude and frequency.

BIBLIOGRAPHY

1. Bender MB: The oculomotor decussation. Am J Ophthalmol 54:591, 1962.

2. Bizzi E: Discharge of frontal eye field neurons during eye movements in unanesthetized monkey. Science 157:1588, 1967.

3. Bizzi E: Discharge of frontal eye fields neurons during saccadic and following eye movements in unanesthetized monkey. Exp Brain Res 6:69,1968.

4. Daroff RB: Control of ocular movement. Br. J Ophthalmol 58:217, 1974.

5. Daroff RB: Physiologic, anatomic and pathophysiologic considerations of eye movements. Trans Ophthalmol Soc UK 90:410, 1970.

6. Gay AJ, Newman NM, Keltner JL., Stroud MH: Eye Movement Disorders. St Louis. CV Mosby Co. 1974.

7. Weber R. Daroff RB: The metrics of horizontal saccadic eye movements in normal humans. Vision Res 2:921, 1971.

Chapter

14

Nystagmus and Related Oscillations

NYSTAGMUS

DEFINITION AND FEATURES

Definition

Nystagmus comes from the Greek word *nystagmos* (to nod) and may be defined as repetitive, to and fro involuntary movement of one or both eyes that is initiated by a slow phase (drift). The movements which are not regular and rhythmic are called *nystagmoid movements*.

Features of nystagmus movements

1. *Type of waveform* Eye movements that point the retinal fovea at an object of interest are called *foveating* and those that move the fovea away from the object are called *defoveating*. In nystagmus, each cycle of movement is usually initiated by an involuntary, defoveating drift of the eye away from the object of interest, followed by a return movement. Based on the characteristics of defoveating and foveating movements, the nystagmus may be of pendular or jerky type.

- *Pendular nystagmus*, in which both the defoveating and refoveating movements are slow (non-saccadic), and of equal velocity in each direction (Fig. 14.1A). It may be horizontal, vertical, oblique, rotatory or mixed.

• *Jerk nystagmus* is characterized by the slow defoveating movement in one direction and fast refoveating movement (saccadic) component in the other direction; the later being a recovery phenomenon aimed at refixation. The direction of jerk nystagmus is defined by the direction of fast component (phase). For instance, if the fast phase beat to the right, this is called *right beating* nystagmus. Likewise the jerk nystagmus may be left, up, down or rotatory.

Waveform can further be characterized and documented by the nature of the slow phase as shown in Fig. 14.1B to E.

2. Direction. Direction or plane of nystagmus can be horizontal, vertical, oblique, torsional or mixed. For a jerk nystagmus, the direction is described according to the fast phase. For simplicity of recording, the direction of nystagmus in case notes the following method may be used:

a. *Pendular nystagmus*
  • Horizontal ←→
  • Vertical ↕
  • Rotatory ⌣
  • Oblique ⬊⬈

b. *Jerk nystagmus with quick phase*
  • To the right ←—
  • To the left —→
  • Up ↑
  • Down ↓
  • Right rotatory (anti-clockwise) ⌐
  • Left rotatory (clockwise) ⌐
  • Oblique up to right ↖ or left ↗
  • Oblique down to right ↙ or left ↘

3. Conjugacy. Nystagmus may be of conjugate, disconjugate or dissociative type.

• *Conjugate nystagmus.* Binocular nystagmus with symmetric direction, amplitude and rate in both eyes.
• *Disconjugate nystagmus.* Monocular or binocular with different directions and frequencies in two eyes.
• *Dissociative nystagmus refers to* unidirectional but assymetrical nystagmus in two eyes. Such type of nystagmus is seen in internuclear ophthalmoplegia.

4. Amplitude. The amplitude is measured in degrees and represents the extent of movement between the start of drift away from fixation and the start of corrective movement in the opposite direction. The amount of movement should be approximately equal. In majority of cases, the amplitude increases, when the patient looks in the direction of the fast phase (*Alexender's law*). When the patient looks in the opposite direction, the amplitude reduces, the oscillation ceasesor the direction of the nystagmus may reverse. There are very few exceptions to this rule, but in some cases of vertical nystagmus, the amplitude increases on looking in the direction of the slow phase.

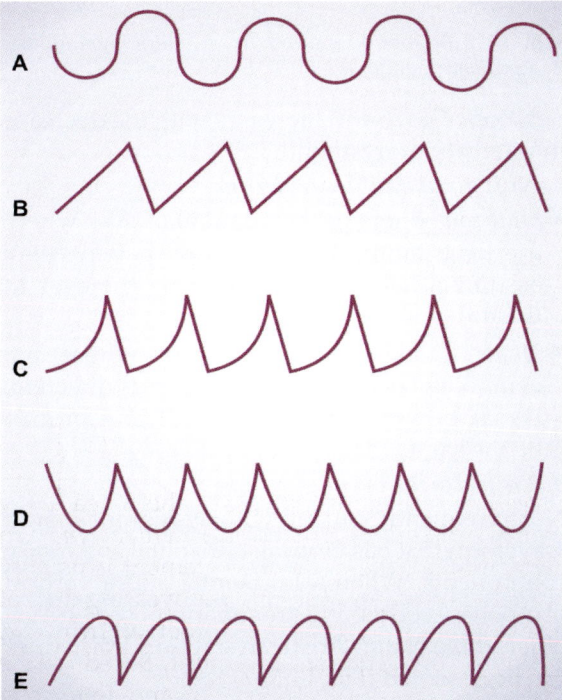

Fig. 14.1 *Waveform characteristics of pendular nystagmus (A) and, jerk nystagmus (B to E). (B) Jerk nystagmus with slow components of constant velocity; (C) Jerk nystagmus with slow components of exponentially increasing velocity; (D) Jerk nystagmus with slow components of exponentially increasing velocity with extended foveation periods that follow slow movements; (E) Jerk nystagmus with slow components of exponentially decreasing velocity.*

Grading of amplitude. The amplitude is graded as small, medium or large as below:

- *Fine (small)*—excursions less than 3°
- *Medium*—excursions between 5° and 15°
- *Coarse (large)*—excursions more than 15°

A dissociated nystagmus has different amplitudes in both eyes. Subtle forms of nystagmus, due to low amplitude or inconsistent presence, require prolonged observation over 2–3 minutes. Low amplitude nystagmus may be detected only by viewing the patient's retina with an ophthalmoscope. In case records amplitude is recorded by the thickness of arrows or increasing lines in arrows, e.g.

- Small >———➤ or ———➤
- Medium »———➤ or ———➤➤
- Large »»———➤ or ———➤➤➤

5. *Frequency.* Frequency of nystagmus refers to number of beats, i.e. to-and-fro movements per second.

Grading and recording of frequency. It is done into low (slow), moderate and high (fast):

- Low (Lo): 1–2 Hz
- Moderate (M): 3–4 Hz
- High (H): > 5 Hz

6. *Intensity.* Intensity of nystagmus is the product of amplitude and frequency.

Grading of intensity. Nystagmus of each type may be seen in the primary position or it may be made apparent, only when the visual axes are deviated. On these grounds, nystagmus may be graded as to its intensity into:

Recording of frequency

- *First degree nystagmus.* In it, the movements occur only in that direction of the gaze in which the quick phase occurs.
- *Second degree nystagmus.* In it, the movements are also present in the primary position.
- *Third degree nystagmus.* In it, movements are also present in the direction of the gaze to the side opposite to that of the quick phase.

7. *Foveation period.* It is the period in the waveform where eye velocity is at minimum and thus visual acuity is maximum (Fig.14.2). The foveation period is maximum in the null

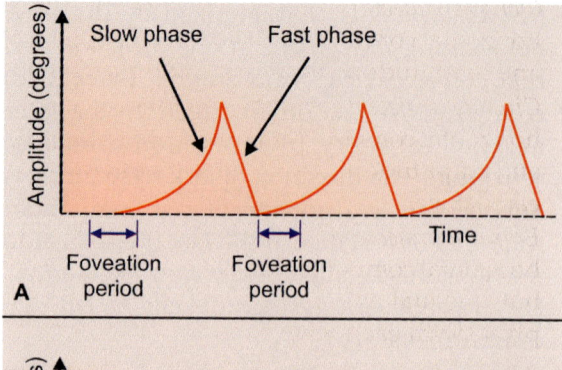

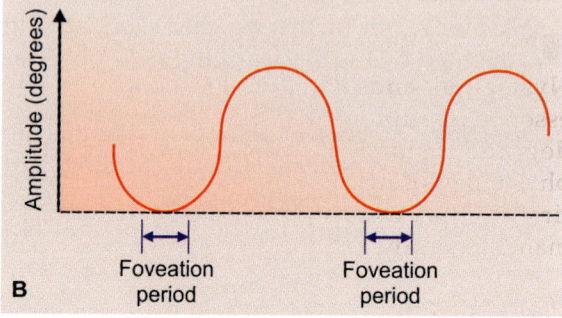

Fig. 14.2 *Foveation period in:* A, *Jerk nystagmus;* B, *Pendular nystagmus.*

position of gaze and increases with the decrease in intensity of nystagmus.

8. *Null zone and neutral zone*

- *Null zone* refers to the position of eyes where a jerk nystagmus is absent. Some patients may assume a head posture to bring the eyes in the null zone.
- *Neutral zone* is the point from where fast component of nystagmus changes its direction. It may be different than the null zone or may be the same.

9. *Trajectories of nystagmus*

Not infrequently patients with nystagmus show a waveform that has vertical, horizontal and rotary components. When a horizontal and a vertical component coexist and are superimposed on each other, three characteristic nystagmus trajectories can be observed (Fig. 14.3):

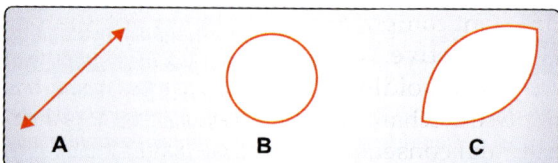

Fig. 14.3 *Trajectories of nystagmus:* A, *Oblique;* B, *Circular:* and C, *Elipticle.*

a. *Oblique trajectory* occurs when vertical and horizontal components are of equal frequency and amplitude and in phase with each other.

b. *Circular trajectory* occurs when vertical and horizontal components are of equal frequency and amplitude and are 90°, out of phase with each other.

c. *Eliptical trajectory* occurs when vertical and horizontal components are of equal frequency but unequal amplitudes and are 90° out of phase with each other.

PATHOPHYSIOLOGY OF NYSTAGMUS

Nystagmus and other related conditions in essence disrupt steady fixation and thereby degrade vision. To understand the pathophysiology of nystagmus, we must, therefore, first look at what are the mechanisms that maintain steady fixation.

Mechanisms that work together to maintain a steady gaze

1. *Fixation*, which has two distinct components:

a. The visual system's ability to detect retinal image drift and program corrective eye movements; and

b. The suppression of unwanted saccades that take the eye off target.

2. *Vestibulo-ocular reflex (VOR)*, by which eye movements compensate for head movements at short latency during natural activities, especially locomotion. The proprioceptors of the vestibular system are the semicircular canals of the inner ear, which respond to changes in angular acceleration due to head rotation4.

3. *Neural integrator*, ability of the brain to hold the eye at an eccentric position in the orbit against the elastic pull of the suspensory ligaments and extraocular muscles. A gaze-holding network called the neural integrator generates this signal. The cerebellum, ascending vestibular pathways, and oculomotor nuclei are important components of the neural integrator.

For effective working of the performance, three gaze-holding mechanisms are tuned by adaptive mechanisms (*recalibration*) that monitor the visual consequences of eye movements.

A nystagmus is caused by defect in any of above mechanisms or their adaptive tuning. In other words, nystagmus occurs due to disturbances in the sensory or motor systems responsible for neuromuscular coordination of the extraocular muscles, which in turn provides a steady fixation under normal circumstances.

* *Sensory system* consists of the retina, the vestibular system and the proprioceptive endorgans of the cervical musculature.

* *Motor system* is formed by the extrinsic ocular muscles innervated by the oculomotor cranial nerves. The *cerebellum* controls the muscle tone and facilitates the smooth operation of the reflex responses involved.

CLASSIFICATION

Many classifications have been proposed for the nystagmus, and so, the reader will find different classifications in different books. It is important to note here that the terms motor and sensory nystagmus are no longer being considered. National Eye Institute Workshop has developed a new classification in 2001 called the classification of eye movement abnormalities and strabismus (CEMAS). In this volume, a simple classification has been adopted by slightly modifying CEMAS as below:

A. *Physiological nystagmus*

1. Optokinetic nystagmus
2. Endpoint nystagmus (eccentric gaze nystagmus)
3. Physiological vestibular (caloric or rotational) nystagmus
4. Voluntary nystagmus

B. *Pathological nystagmus*

I. *Early onset (childhood) nystagmus*

1. *Infantile nystagmus syndrome* (includes old names such as 'congenital', 'motor', 'sensory', idiopathic and nystagmus blockage)

2. *Fusion maldevelopment nystagmus* syndrome (old names "latent, manifest latent," nystagmus blockage)

3. *Spasmus nutans syndrome*
   * Without optic pathway glioma
   * With optic pathway glioma

II. *Acquired nystagmus.* This group includes various forms of nystagmus acquired after infancy, which can be further classified as follows:

1. *Nystagmus associated with diseases of visual system*
   - Ocular jerk nystagmus
   - Vertical nystagmus
   - See-saw nystagmus
   - Acquired pendular nystagmus

2. *Vestibular nystagmus*
   - i. Peripheral vestibular nystagmus, e.g. Menière and drug toxicity nystagmus
   - ii. Central vestibular nystagmus
     - Downbeat
     - Upbeat
     - Torsional
     - Horizontal
   - iii. Periodic alternating nystagmus

3. *Nystagmus due to disorders of gaze holding*
   - Gaze-evoked nystagmus
   - Dissociated nystagmus (ataxic nystagmus)
   - Bruns' nystagmus
   - Convergence-retraction nystagmus
   - Centripetal and rebound nystagmus

Note. Only a very brief account of the various types of nystagmus is given here just as a passing reference. For detailed accounts, the readers should consult certain standard textbooks on neuro-ophthalmology.

PHYSIOLOGICAL NYSTAGMUS

1. Optokinetic nystagmus. It is a physiological jerk nystagmus induced by presenting to gaze the objects moving serially in one direction; such as strips of a spinning optokinetic drum. The eyes will follow a fixed strip momentarily and then jerk back to reposition centrally to fix up a new strip. Similar condition occurs while looking at outside things from a moving train.

OKN is used for:

- Assessment of vision in young infants and uncooperative adults.
- Reversal of OKN is seen in infantile esotropia syndrome and congenital nystagmus (now called infantile nystagmus syndrome).
- Asymmetry/absent vertical OKN is diagnostic of neurological/neurometabolic lesions and warrants neuroimaging in children with nystagmus.

2. End-point nystagmus. It is a transient fine jerk horizontal nystagmus seen in normal persons on extreme right or left gaze.

3. Physiological vestibular nystagmus. It is a jerk nystagmus which can be elicited by stimulating the tympanic membrane with hot or cold water. It forms the basis of caloric test. If cold water is poured into right ear, the patient develops left jerk nystagmus (rapid phase towards left) while the reverse happens with warm water, i.e. patient develops right jerk nystagmus. It can be remembered by the mnemonic 'COWS' (Cold-Opposite, Warm-Same).

Physiological vestibular nystagmus can also be elicited with head rotation (which is utilized for vision assessment in young infants). Dampening of physiological nystagmus should occur in 5–10 seconds after stopping the rotation. If it does not, it means that there exists significant visual impairment.

PATHOLOGICAL NYSTAGMUS

A. EARLY ONSET (CHILDHOOD) NYSTAGMUS

The three most common forms of nystagmus seen in childhood begin in infancy and are, therefore, not congenital. These include:
1. Infantile nystagmus syndrome
2. Fusion maldevelopment nystagmus syndrome
3. Spasmus nutans syndrome

1. Infantile nystagmus syndrome

Infantile nystagmus syndrome (INS) is the new name given in the CEMAS system for the old 'congenital nystagmus, motor and sensory nystagmus.'

Etiology. It may be: (I) *idiopathic* or (II) *associated with sensory deprivation* due to any of the following causes:
- *Retinal diseases*, such as retinoblastism, retinopathy of prematurity (ROP), persistant hyperplastic primary vitreous (PHPV)
- *Ocular albinism*, characterized by iris transillumination defects and foveal hypoplasia.
- *Aniridia, i.e.* bilateral near total congenital iris absence.
- *Leber's congenital amaurosis,* characterized by markedly abnormal or flat electroretinogram bilateral congenital toxoplasmosis and bilateral macular hypoplasia.

- *Other causes* include, bilateral congenital cataract, achromatopsia, congenital stationary night blindness, bilateral optic nerve hypoplasia.

Characteristic features. It is characterized by erratic waveform with or without roving eye movement associated with reduced visual acuity due to above mentioned conditions.

CEMAS criteria for INS is summarized below:

- Infantile onset
- Ocular motor recordings show diagnostic (accelerating) slow phases
- Wave forms may change in early infancy,
- Head posture usually evident by 4 years of age.
- Vision prognosis dependent on integrity of sensory system.

Symbolic recording of an idiopathic case of INS is shown in Fig. 14.4.

Common associated findings
- Conjugate, horizontal-torsional, increases with fixation attempt
- Progression from pendular to jerk
- Family history often positive

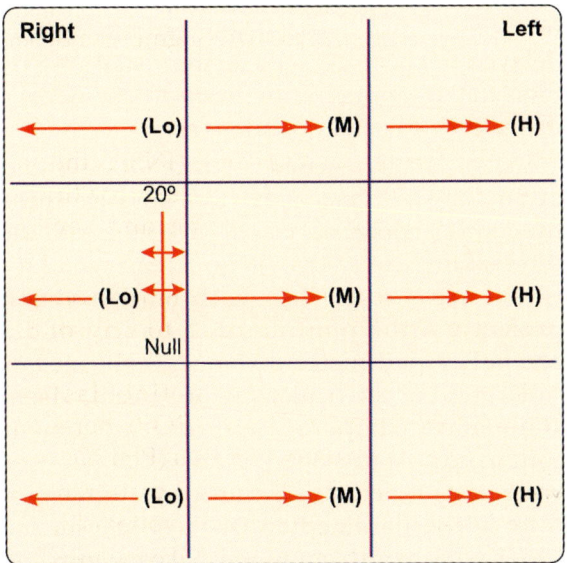

Fig. 14.4 *Symbolic recording of a case of idiopathic infantile nystagmus syndrome (INS) depecting left beating horizontal jerk nystagmus of medium amplitude and moderate frequency in primary position. Intensity of nystagmus increases in left gaze and decreases in right gaze. There is null zone in right gaze with pendular waveform.*

- With or without normal visual acuity due to associated sensory system deficits (e.g. albinism, achromatopsia) associated strabismus or refractive error
- Null and neutral zones present,
- Associated head posture or head shaking may exhibit a "latent" component, "reversal" with OKN stimulus or (a) periodicity to the oscillation.
- May decrease with induced convergence, increased fusion, extraocular muscle surgery, contact lenses, and sedation.

2. Fusion maldevelopment nystagmus syndrome

Fusion maldevelopment nystagmus syndrome (FMNS) is the new name for the old term—latent/*latent manifest nystagmus* as described in CEMAS.

Characteristic features CEMAS criteria for FMNS are summarized below:
- Infantile onset
- High frequency, low-amplitude pendular nystagmus (dual-jerk waveform), jerk in direction of fixing eye
- Intensity decreases with age.
- Ocular motor recordings show two types of slow phases linear and decelerating.
- Nystagmus is not present, when both eyes are open. It appears when one eye is covered. It is a jerk nystagmus with rapid phase towards the uncovered eye.
- While testing visual acuity in such patients, one eye should be fogged (by adding plus lenses in front) rather than occluding to minimize induction of latent nystagmus.
- May be associated with congenital esotropia and dissociated vertical deviation (DVD).
- Becomes manifest under monocular viewing conditions, i.e. in the presence of decreased vision in one eye as in anisometropic amblyopia, strabismic amblyopia, etc.

Symbolic recording of a case of FMNS is shown in Fig. 14.5.

Common associated findings
Conjugate, horizontal, uniplanar; usually no associated sensory system deficits (e.g. albinism, achromatopsia), may change with exaggerated convergence ("blockage"), head posture

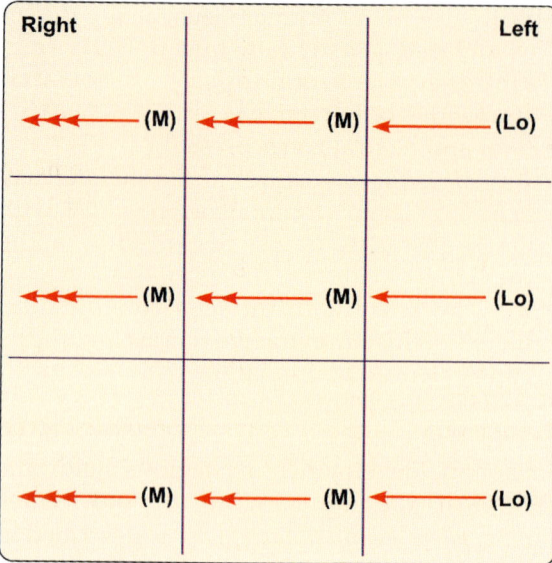

Right — **Left**

Fig. 14.5 Symbolic recording of a case of fusion maldevelopment nystagmus syndrome (FMNS) depicting right beating horizontal jerk nystagmus of medium amplitude and moderate frequency. Intensity of the nystagmus increases in the right gaze and decreases in left gaze.

associated with fixing eye in adduction, no head shaking, may exhibit "reversal" with OKN stimulus, no (a) periodicity to the oscillation. Dissociated strabismus may be present. Decreases with increased fusion (binocular function).

3. Spasmus nutans syndrome

Spasmus nutans syndrome (SNS), old name spasmus nutans (SN) is the 3rd most common nystagmus seen in infancy.

Characteristic features CEMAS criteria for SNS are as below:

• Infantile onset
• Variable conjugacy, small-frequency, low-amplitude oscillation
• Abnormal head posture and head oscillation, improves (disappears) during childhood
• Normal MRI/CT scan of visual pathways
• Ocular motility recordings—high-frequency (>10 Hz), asymmetric, variable conjugacy, pendular oscillations
• Usually spontaneously remits clinically in 2 to 8 years, remains present with eye movement recordings

Common associated findings are: Dysconjugate, asymmetric, multiplanar, family history of strabismus, may be greater in one (abducting) eye, constant, head posture/oscillation (horizontal or vertical), usually no associated sensory system deficits may have associated strabismus and amblyopia, may increase with convergence, head bobbing, head posture may be compensatory; normal fundus exam; decreases with increased fusion (binocular function).

B. ACQUIRED NYSTAGMUS

I. Nystagmus associated with diseases of the visual system

Pathogenesis

As mentioned in pathogenesis, fixation disorders can lead to nystagmus. The smooth visual fixation mechanism stops the eyes from drifting away from a stationary object of regard. This fixation mechanism depends upon the motion detection (magnocellular) portion of the visual system which is inherently slow, with a response time of about 100 milliseconds that encumbers all visually mediated eye movements, including fixation, smooth pursuit, and optokinetic responses.[4] If the response time is delayed further by disease of the visual system, then the attempts by the brain to correct eye drifts leads to ocular oscillations.

Vision is also needed for recalibrating and optimizing all types of eye movements. These functions depend on visual projections to the cerebellum. Thus, signals go from secondary visual areas concerned with motion-vision project via the pontine nuclei and middle cerebellar peduncle to the cerebellum. For calibration of the ocular motor system, visual signals are compared with eye movement commands. At present, it is not certain how or where this function is performed. A group of cells in the paramedian tracts (PMT) in the lower pons have been suggested as a probable centre.

Diseases affecting any part of the visual system, from retina to cortical visual areas, or interrupting visual projections to pons and cerebellum, may be associated with nystagmus.

to un-inhibited, prolonged vestibular impulses which leads to nystagmus.

Clinical features

- Spontaneous horizontal nystagmus, present in central gaze.
- Reverses direction approximately every 90–120 seconds. The changing direction of the waveforms is caused by an actively shifting null zone.
- Acquired PAN has the same characteristics in light or in darkness.
- Smooth pursuit and optokinetic nystagmus are usually impaired.

Jerk see-saw and hemi see-saw nystagmus

Causes

Jerk see-saw nystagmus (hemi see-saw nystagmus) occurs in patients with lesions in the region of the interstitial nucleus of Cajal (INC). The associated ocular tilt reaction is due to an imbalance of central otolithic projections from vestibular nuclei to the INC.

Clinical features

- One-half-cycle consists of elevation and intorsion of one eye and synchronous depression and extorsion of the other eye. In the next half-cycle, the vertical and torsional movements reverse (Fig. 14.9).
- The waveform may be pendular or jerk. Some authorities label the pendular form as see saw and jerk form as hemi see-saw.
- See-saw nystagmus may be congenital, or Acquired.
- Patients often have a contralateral ocular tilt reaction.

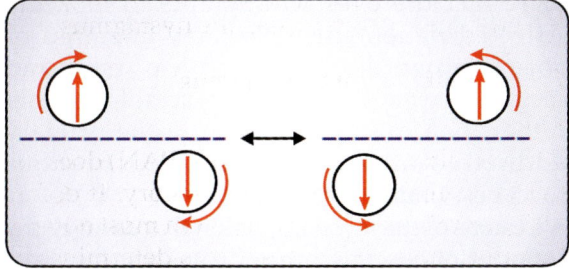

Fig. 14.9 *Symbolic recording of a case of see-saw nystagmus (for explaination see text).*

- With a right sided lesion, the reaction consists of a left head tilt, a skew deviation with a right hypertropia, tonic intorsion of the right eye and extorsion of the left eye, and misperception that earth-vertical is tilted to the left.

III. Nystagmus due to abnormalities of the mechanism for holding eccentric gaze

Gaze-evoked nystagmus

Nystagmus that is induced by turning the eye to an eccentric position in the orbit is called gaze-evoked nystagmus. It is the most common form of nystagmus encountered in clinical practice. Gaze-evoked nystagmus is a general term that includes both physiologic and pathologic nystagmus. When the nystagmus is physiologic, the term end-point nystagmus should be used. When the nystagmus is associated with a paresis of gaze, e.g. ocular motor nerve palsies or weakness of the extraocular muscles, the term gaze-paretic nystagmus is appropriate.

- Gaze-evoked nystagmus usually occurs on lateral (Fig. 14.10) or upward gaze, seldom on looking down.
- Waveform is dependent on effect of fixation.
- If fixation is impaired, the slow phases consist of exponentially decaying waveform.

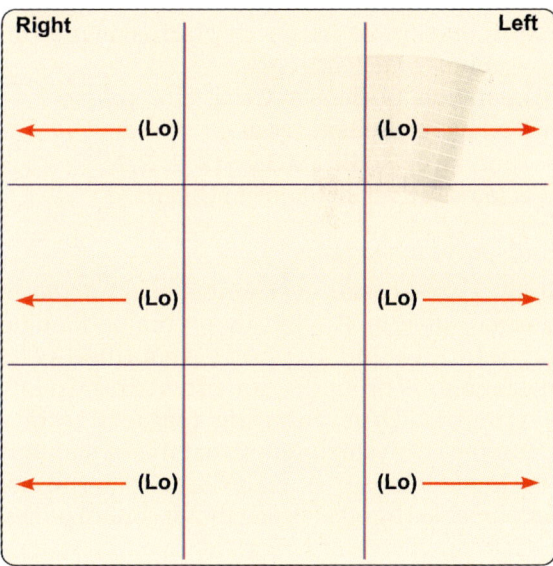

Fig. 14.10 *Symbolic recording of a case of bilateral gaze-evoked nystagmus. Note horizontal jerk nystagmus of small amplitude and low-frequency with fast phase in the direction of gaze.*

• If visual fixation is possible, however, the slow phase has a linear profile.

To hold gaze at an eccentric position, the elastic force of the fascia and ligaments has to be overcome. This is achieved by a tonic contraction of the extraocular muscles. The neural signal involved in this contraction has been termed as 'step', that is generated by the gaze-holding network, also called the neural integrator. This network includes the vestibulo-cerebellum, the medial vestibular nucleus and adjacent nucleus prepositus hypoglossy in the medulla, and the interstitial nucleus of Cajal (INC) in the midbrain.

Etiology. Gaze-evoked nystagmus is caused by a deficient step, so that the eyes cannot be maintained at an eccentric orbital position and are pulled back toward central position by the elastic forces of the orbital fascia. Corrective quick phases then move the eyes back towards the desired position in the orbit.

Additionally, lesions that produce gaze-evoked nystagmus also impair visual fixation and smooth pursuit.

Causes of gaze-evoked nystagmus include:
• Medications, including alcohol, anticonvulsants and sedatives.
• Structural lesions that damage the gaze-holding neural network.
• Nucleus prepositus hypoglossi/medial vestibular nucleus region
• Interstitial nucleus of Cajal
• Rarely, cerebellar lesions.
• Familial episodic ataxia type 2 (EA-2), which also has attack of ataxia and vertigo.

End-point nystagmus

It is a gaze-evoked nystagmus encountered in normal subjects. It typically occurs on looking far laterally and is poorly sustained. The nystagmus is primarily horizontal. It is usually symmetric. Differentiating features from a pathological nystagmus are that this nystagmus has lower intensity (i.e. slower drift) and is not accompanied by other ocular motor abnormalities.

Dissociated nystagmus (ataxic nystagmus)

It is a special type of pathologic gaze-evoked nystagmus, most commonly associated with an internuclear ophthalmoplegia (INO). Dissociated nystagmus includes a series of saccades followed by postsaccadic drift that occurs, when the patient attempts to look laterally away from the side of the lesion. Since the saccades initiate the oscillations, this is not a true nystagmus. It represents an attempt by the brain to adaptively correct hypometric saccades due to the weak medial rectus muscle, which because of Hering's law of equal innervation leads increase in the innervation to the normal, abducting eye, thereby resulting in overshooting saccades and postsaccadic drift of the normal eye if the patient attempts to fixate with the diseased eye. Thus, whenever a patient habitually prefers to fixate with a paretic eye, the normal eye, will show a dissociated nystagmus while looking in the direction of action of the paretic muscle, regardless of the pathogenesis of the weakness.

Other causes of dissociated nystagmus are:
• Previous extraocular muscle surgery
• Myasthenia gravis
• Miller Fisher syndrome

Bruns' nystagmus

Tumours in the cerebellopontine angle, produce a low-frequency, large-amplitude nystagmus, when the patient looks toward the side of the lesion, and a high-frequency, small-amplitude nystagmus, when the patient looks toward the side opposite the lesion. The nystagmus that occurs on gaze towards the side of the lesion is gaze-evoked nystagmus caused by defective gaze holding, whereas the nystagmus that occurs during gaze towards the side opposite the lesion is caused by vestibular imbalance. This is called Bruns' nystagmus (Fig. 14.11).

Convergence-retraction nystagmus

It is characterized by quick phases that converge or retract the eyes on attempts to look up. Affected patients usually have impaired or absent upward gaze for both pursuit and saccadic eye movements. It is a saccadic disorder rather than nystagmus because the primary adductive movements are asynchronous saccades. Causes include:
• Lesions of the mesencephalon that damage the posterior commissure, e.g. pineal tumours.
• Chiari malformation
• Epileptic seizures

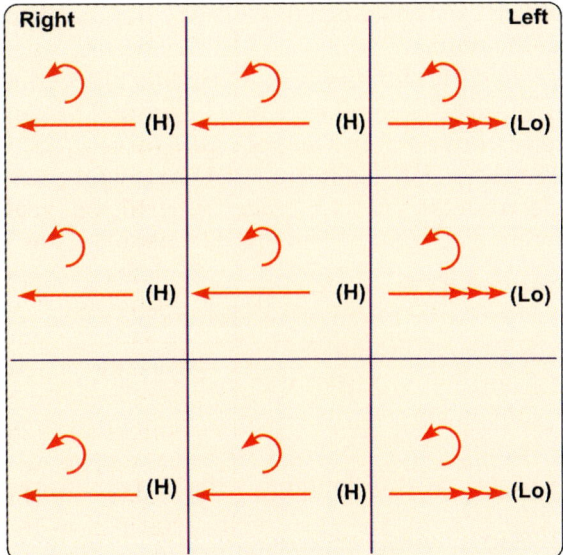

Fig. 14.11 *Symbolic recording of a case of Bruns' nystagmus depicting a high frequency, small amplitude, right-beating horizontal and rotary waveform.*

Centripetal and rebound nystagmus

If a patient with gaze-evoked nystagmus attempts to look eccentrically for a sustained period, the nystagmus begins to decrease in amplitude and may even reverse direction, this is called centripetal nystagmus. If the eyes are then returned to the central position, a short-lived nystagmus with slow drifts in the direction of the prior eccentric gaze occurs. This is called rebound nystagmus. Both centripetal and rebound nystagmus reflect an attempt by brainstem or cerebellar mechanisms to correct for the drift of gaze-evoked nystagmus. Rebound nystagmus occurs in patients with:

- Cerebellar disease
- In normal subjects with typical gaze-evoked nystagmus
- Lateral medullary infarction
- Tumour confined to the flocculus.

CLINICAL EVALUATION AND ELECTRO-PHYSIOLOGICAL RECORDING AND NEUROIMAGING

A. CLINICAL EVALUATION

It is often possible to diagnose the cause of nystagmus through careful history and systematic examination of the patient.

History

History should include:

- Duration of nystagmus
- Whether it interferes with vision and causes oscillopsia
- Accompanying neurological symptoms
- Whether nystagmus and other visual symptoms are worse with viewing far or near objects, or with patient motion, or with different gaze angles.
- If abnormal head posture is present, whether or not these features are evident on old photographs.

Examination of a patient with nystagmus

Comprehensive examination of the visual system
- *Visual acuity* assessment with and without posture, for both near and distance and both binocularly and uniocularly. Binocular acuity should be recorded before occlusion. Methods of measuring monocular vision while avoiding total occlusion include fogging the other eye with plus spheres, polarizing lenses, central field occlusion and the red-green duochrome slide test.
- *Anterior and posture segment examination* to rule out cause of low vision. Especially look for
- *Measurement of head posture.* In most patients with infantile nystagmus, the head position corresponds roughly to the null zone. However, an anomalous head posture may be present in patients with INS for reasons other than nystagmus, e.g. uncorrected astigmatism, incomitant squint, muscular torticollis. Nevertheless, presence of AHP in a patient with INS has better visual prognosis than no AHP. All the components of head posture, i.e. face turn, chin elevation or depression and head tilt should be noted. Face turn can be measured using the Goniometer (Fig. 14.12) or by simply using a scale and a protactor.

Systematic examination of each functional class of eye movements (vestibular, optokinetic, smooth-pursuit, saccades, vergence) and their effect on nystagmus.

Examination of nystagmus in a systematic manner. It is essential to have a mental checklist during clinical examination. **ABCDEF** is a suggested pneumonic for systematic examination of nystagmus where:

A is amplitude

B is basic shape or waveform

C is conjugacy

D is direction

E is effect of gaze position and fixation, e.g.

- The stability of fixation (with the eyes close to primary position) viewing near and far targets, and at eccentric gaze angles.
- In patients with head turn or tilt, the eye should be observed in various directions of gaze, when the head is in that position as well as when the head is held straight.
- During fixation, occlude each eye in turn to check for latent nystagmus.
- The effect of removal of fixation (with Frenzelor high-plus spherical lenses).

F is frequency.

Note. Details of the features of nystagmus and method of their clinical documentation has been described earlier (*see* pages 376–379).

B. ELECTROPHYSIOLOGICAL RECORDING OF EYE MOVEMENTS

Electrophysiological recording of ocular motility has provided a new basis for eye movement abnormality classification, etiology and treatment. Only salient features of some of the techniques available for ocular motility recordings are mentioned here.

1. Electro-oculography

Electro-oculography (EOG) is based on the measurement of resting potential of the eye which exists between the cornea (+ve) and back of the retina (–ve).

Technique of recording is shown in Fig. 14.13A and B. Electrodes are placed over the orbital margin near the medial and lateral canthi serve as *active electrodes* (E1–E4 in Fig. 14.13A). A forehead electrode serves as a *ground electrode* or indifferent electrodes (E5 in Fig. 14.13A).

Salient features.

- Horizontal range of measurement of 1 to 40° with a resolution of 1°.
- Useful for horizontal and some vertical movements.
- A bitnoisy–1°.
- Best clinical all rounder with good electrodes.

2. Electronystagmography

Electronystagmography (ENG) is an adaption of electro-oculography (EOG). For ENG like EOG (Fig. 14.13), a ground electrode is attached to the forehead and three recording electrodes are placed one each to the side, above and below each eye which measure the eye movement.

Tests performed with ENG include:

- *Oculomotor tests.* ENG is used to record nystagmus during oculomotor tests such as saccades, pursuit and gaze testing and optokinetics. Abnormal oculomotor test results may indicate either systemic or central pathology as opposed to peripheral (vestibular) pathology.
- *Positional testing* is performed to see the effect of head or body movements on the eye movements.
- *Caloric test* is performed to assess the vestibular system.

3. Binocular infrared reflectance oculography (BIRO)

- Useful for horizontal and some vertical movements.
- Has a restricted range.
- Noise–0.1°

4. Electromagnetic scleral search coil method

- Useful for horizontal, vertical and torsional movements.
- Good resolution and frequency response.

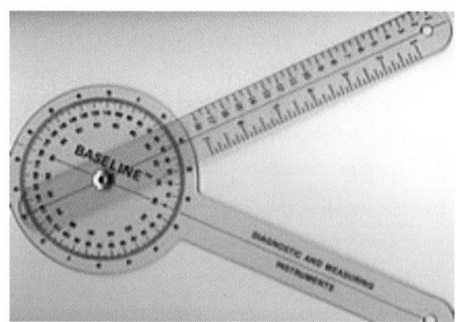

Fig. 14.12 *Goniometer: An orthopaedic instrument which can be used to measure face turn.*

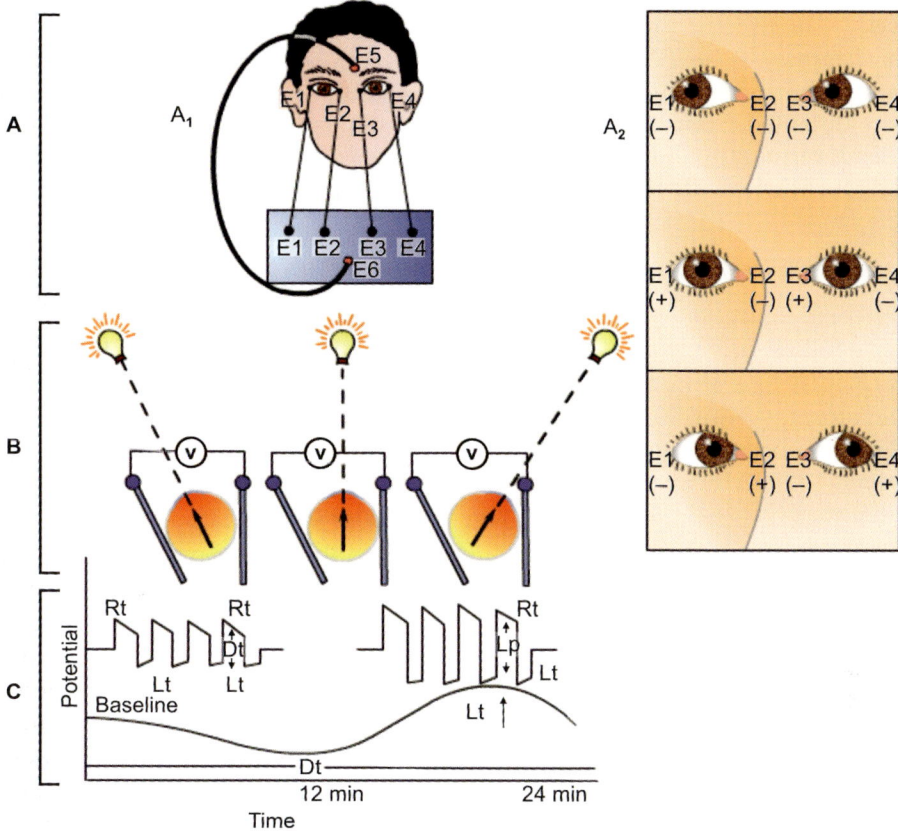

Fig. 14.13 *Technique of recording electro-oculogram: A, Position of electrodes; B, Ocular movements during recording; C, Record of EOG.*

- Requires mind bending mathematical analysis.
- Eye has to be anaesthetized and a thick silicone lens is needed.
- Expensive.

5. Videonystagmography

Videonystagmography (VNG) is a sophisticated technique in which nystagmus is recorded with the help of the infrared video camera which is incorporated in the specially designed infrared camrea goggles (worm by the patient during the recording technique (Fig. 14.14). A very sensitive head movement sensors are also incorported in it.

Tests performed with VNG. Similar to ENG, there are three parts of VNG testing:
- Ocular and optokinetic testing
- Positional nystagmus testing and
- Caloric testing

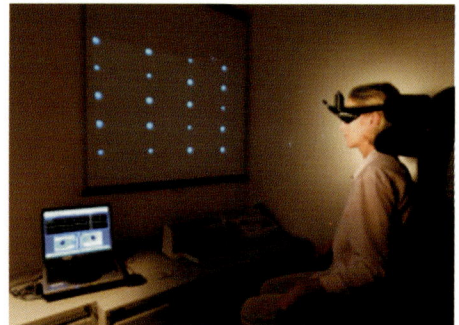

Fig. 14.14 *Technique of videonystagmography with infrared goggles worn by the patient.*

Advantages of VNG over ENG
- *Less combursome* and less time consuming as electrodes are not required.
- *Direct observation* of video images of eye movements available.
- *Simultaneous comparision* of waveform can be performed.

- *Computerised record* allows storage, processing and analysis.
- *Provides more information than ENG.* In addition to information about amplitude, frequency and intensity obtained from ENG; the VNG also provides information about slow phase velocity and foveation window with the help of intrinsic software.

Clinical uses of eye movement recording

Important clinical uses of eye movement recording are as follows:

- *Identifies congenital type of nystagmus* on the basis of waveform. About 40–60% cases of nystagmus have associated squint. About 35% of these patients have FMNS. The best method to differentiate INS form FMNS is eye movement recordings.
- *Allows classification* of acquired nystagmus with greater certainty.
- *VNG helps to evaluate the evolution of nystagmus.* Many INS waveforms begin as pendular nystagmus. Growth and development of the visual sensory system evoke evolution of waveforms during early infancy from pendular to jerk type nystagmus by development of corrective fast phases as well as breaking saccades in slow phases producing the so called 'mature' waveforms associated with better vision.
- *Measures slowness of saccades* which can be diagnostic, e.g. internuclear ophthalmoplegia.
- *Allows observation of motility* in darkness (vestibular nystagmus).
- *Allows temporal resolution* of very fast eye movements such as flutter, opsoclonus, convergence nystagmus, dysmetria which are difficult to evaluate with the naked eye.
- *Trains one to interpret what is' seen'.*
- *Helps in objective assessment of visual functions* of a patient with nystagmus by calculating foveation time, foveation eye position, and eye velocity criteria.
- *Tells about the potential for visual improvement* with treatment.
- *Useful in objective documentation* of response to treatment.
- *Helps in null point evaluation.*

C. NEUROIMAGING

Neuroimaging is indicated to find out associated CNS abnormalities especially in patients with acquired nystagmus, periodic alternating nystagmus, see saw nystagmus, spasmus nutans syndrome and infantile nystagmus syndrome with pallor disc and poor vision.

Hertle's criteria for neurological workup in patients with nystagmus are as follow:

I. *History of*:
- Onset of nystagmus after 6–9 months of age.
- History of prematurity or LBW or developmental delay.
- Abnormal pregnancy/delivery.
- Exposure to toxins/drugs.

II. *Ocular features*:
- Photophobia, delayed visual behaviour.
- Structural abnormalities like foveal or optic nerve dysplasia.
- Nystagmus pattern vertical, asymmetric, dysconjugate or associated with other ocular motor disorders (decrease pursuit, abnormal saccades, paretic gaze).

III. *General features*:
- Patient having manifest hard, soft, focal or diffuse neurologic signs.
- Localising signs of acquired nystagmus.

D. OTHER TESTS

OCT is indicated in retinal dystrophies, degenerations, foveal hypoplasia, schisis cavity, retinal thinning, choroidal thinning.

Auto fluorescence can be used for diagnosing accumulation of lipofuschin in macular dystrophies.

ERG is useful in sensory nystagmus associated with conditions like achromatopsia, CSNB, LCA and other atypical retinal dystrophies.

■ TREATMENT OF NYSTAGMUS

Aims of treatment

- To improve *visual acuity* by stabilizing the eyes
- To shift the *null zone*, if any, in the primary position, i.e. to reduce abnormal head posture.
- To correct the associated *strabismus*
- To decrease any *oscillopsia* wherever possible.

Treatment modalities

Treatment modalities for nystagmus include:
- Optical,
- Medical, and
- Surgical.

I. OPTICAL TREATMENT

1. Correction of refractive error may sometimes significantly decrease nystagmus, especially in patients with bilateral aphakia. Although refraction is difficult in the presence of nystagmus but every effort should be made to correct any significant refractive error. Retinoscopy may be performed in null zone, whenever it is present. Further, contact lenses are more useful than the spectacles (especially in high myopes), since these move with the movement of eye and so the visual axes always coincide with their optical axes. In addition to optical advantage, at actile feedback from the contact lenses have also been reported to decrease the nystagmus.

Clear or tinted contact lenses can be prescribed.
- *Accommodation may be deficient in patients with congenital nystagmus.* Dynamic retinoscopy should be performed before dilation. If accommodation is deficient, a bifocal correction should be provided.

2. Treatment of amblyopia. Amblyopia if present, should be treated with standard treatment. Penalization with plus lenses or atropinization is preferred over occlusion by some workers.

3. Stimulating accommodative convergence by over correcting minus lenses may improve visual acuity at distance fixation by dampening the nystagmus.

Patients chosen to have this treatment must show evidence of good accommodative facility.

4. Partial field occlusion. An unusual method of decreasing the intensity of congenital nystagmus, based on partial field occlusion was suggested by Sasso. "Porthole" glasses that had a clear 10 degree central field but an occluded periphery were prescribed. For some patients having torticollis and nystagmus, occlusion of some parts of peripheral field alleviated anomalous head posture. However, the data was inadequate for evaluating this concept thoroughly.

5. Prismotherapy in nystagmus may be useful as follows:

  i. *Base-out prisms* may stimulate fusional convergence (especially in patients with congenital motor nystagmus) and thus improve the visual acuity by dampening the nystagmus.

    This results in improvement of visual acuity both for distance and near. The prism power is usually split between the two eyes. Both ground in and membrane style prisms may be used. This option is best reserved for patients with good vision, normal fusion and modest nystagmus.

  ii. *Prisms with base opposite to preferred* direction of gaze may be helpful in correcting the head posture. Prisms minimize a head turn by reorienting the visual axis towards primary gaze. Often the preferred eye is held in adduction. Equal power prisms are placed before each eye and oriented in the same direction so that the apex is in the direction of preferred gaze, and the base in the direction of head turn. For example, in a patient with head turn to the left, the null zone is in dextroversion and a prism base-in before the right eye and base-out before the left eye will be helpful in correcting the abnormal headposture (Fig. 14.15).

Similarly, the appropriate prisms can also be used to correct the vertical and oblique head turns. Because of optical disadvantages, the long-term use of prisms incorrecting the head posture is discouraged. However, on the basis of patient's response to prismo therapy, the results of surgery for head turn can be predicted.

6. Galilean arrangement of contact lenses and glasses (optical device by Rushton and Cox) can be used to stabilize the retinal images in

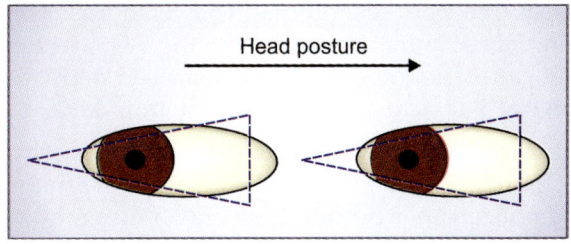

Fig. 14.15 *Use of prism to correct head posture (for explanation see text).*

patients with acquired nystagmus and oscillopsia. This device reduces the magnitude of image movement by limiting image slip along the retina. As a result the visual acuity may improve through an increase in the foveation time. There occurs a decrease in oscillopsia also because of the reduced image motion. This device consists of a high minus contact lens combined with a high plus spectacle lens. Rigid contact lenses of –58D or –28D are paired with spectacle lenses of +32D or +20D irrespectively. Stabilization of retinal image up to 90% is possible using this system. The prismatic effect of the large plus lens plays key role in stabilization of retinal image. This lens images all objects at centre of rotation of the eye, irrespective of exact direction of the visual axis. Thus if eyeball rotates, light rays from the object will remain focussed at the same central point within the eye. The minus contact lens refocuses the image on retina. As the contact lens moves with the eyes, there should be no prismatic effect from the high power plus lens. This has the added benefit of magnifying central 30° field. However the peripheral field is not stabilised, leading to ring scotoma.

II. MEDICAL TREATMENT

1. *Cyclopentolate* used as 1% eyedrops twice a day has been reported to reduce the amplitude, velocity and frequency of latent nystagmus in about 60% of patients.

2. *Botulinum toxin* injected into the retrobulbar space (dose: 10–25 U in 0.1–1 ml) every 3–4 months has been reported to dampen nystagmus and improve visual acuity in patients with acquired nystagmus and oscillopsia.

3. *Baclofen* has been observed to suppress the acquired periodic alternating nystagmus. The initial recommended dose is 5 mg TDS, which in case of no response can be increased stepwise every 3 days to a maximum of 80 mg/day.

4. *Clonazepam* may be useful in patients with downbeat nystagmus and see-saw nystagmus. Clonazepam is used in dose of (0.5–1 mg/bd).

5. *Carbamazepine* is useful in superior oblique myokymia.

6. *Propranolol* is reported to be effective for opsoclonus.

7. *Brinzolamide* (1%) eye drops used thrice a day is noted to improve foveation by 50%, with broadening of the null zone. Its effect may be equivalent to systemic acetazolamide or eye muscle surgery but intermediate between those of soft contact lenses or convergence. 80% Patients on the brinzolamide eyedrops may experience improvement in the best corrected vision corresponding to one line on the Snellen chart. Visible reduction in nystagmus takes place in 27% and reduced AHP in 22% patients and nearly 30% would experience no change.

The effect comes within one week and lasts as long as the drops are continued. There may be additive effect of the drops when used after the tenotomy and reattachment procedure. Topical brinzolamide may be contraindicated in congenital or acquired pathologies of corneal endothelium.

8. *Gabapentine* (300 mg/qid) and ***memantine*** (10 mg/qid) are reported to be useful in patients with upbeat nystagmus, acquired pendular nystagmus and alternating periodic nystagmus. These drugs can also be tried in patients with congenital nystagmus.

III. SURGICAL TREATMENT

INDICATIONS

- To eleminate abnormal head posture by shifting the null point to primary position.
- To decrease the intensity of nystagmus in patients having no abnormal head posture.
- Both of the above.
- *To improve visual acuity* (usually by 1–3 logmar lines), contrast sensitivity and reaction time (improves by 0.3 seconds) by improving foveation.
- *To correct strabismus and to restor binocular fusion and stereopsis*, where ever possible.

Important points to be considered while planning surgery for nystagmus are as follows:

1. *Surgical intervention is useful in patients* with congenital motor nystagmus and nystagmus blockage syndrome.

2. *Surgery should be performed*, only if the abnormal head posture causes a significant

cosmetic disturbance and/or visual difficulties, i.e. when head turn-or tilts more than 15°.

3. *Surgery should always be performed* after the age of 5–6 years; since spontaneous improvement in abnormal head posture can occur in some cases up to this age. Moreover, by this age, it is possible to have more reliable examination demonstrating head posture and ocular alignment. For children with strabismus, earlier intervention may provide the best opportunity for bifoveal fixation to develop. With an acquired nystagmus and torticollis, it is prudent to wait at least a year to be certain that the abnormal eye movements are consistent and the head turn is stable.

GENERAL PRINCIPLES OF SURGERY

- *Null point needs to be shifted in primary position.* For this, the eyes should always be moved in the same direction as the abnormal head posture.
- Face turn will be corrected only if the surgery is done on the fixating eye.
- In the presence of strabismus and an abnormal head posture due to nystagmus, the head position can be corrected only by operating on the fixing eye.
- Strabismus can be corrected by operating on the fixating eye or nonfixating eye.
- Surgery for face turn is performed first followed by surgery for the strabismus.
- *Surgical therapy should be based* on the greatest amount of abnormal head position that is measured at distance.

(A) SURGICAL TECHNIQUES FOR ABNORMAL HEAD POSTURE

Patients with nystagmus who have null point (other than the primary position) assume an abnormal head posture (AHP) to dampen the nystagmus. A significant AHP needs to be corrected.

Kestenbaum and Anderson were the first to report on the surgical techniques for the treatment of abnormal head posture in congenital nystagmus.

- *Kestenbaum procedure* originally comprised of recession-resection of all the four horizontal recti

- *Anderson procedure* comprised of only recessions, e.g., for right face turn recession of right MR and left LR muscle.
- *Modified Kestenbaum-Anderson procedures* have been suggested by various workers thereafter.

Different modified surgical techniques are now recommended for the face turn without trabismus, for face turn with strabismus and for nystagmus blockage syndrome.

I. Surgical techniques for face turn

1. Surgical techniques for face turn without strabismus

Modified Kestenbaum-Anderson procedure. It consists of *bilateral recess-resect* operations.

Up to 30° of face turn (e.g. in a patient with head turn to the left) the modified Kestenbaum-Anderson procedure, as described by PARK, is effective. It comprise lesser amount of recessions and also lesser amount of surgery on MR muscles as compared to LR muscles. He suggested the '5, 6, 7, 8' guidelines for a bilateral equal surgery as below (Fig. 14.16):

- Right lateral rectus (RLR) recession 7 mm
- Right medial rectus (RMR) resection 6 mm
- Left medial rectus (LMR) recession 5 mm
- Left lateral rectus (LRL) resection 8 mm

Modified Kestenbaum-Anderson procedure, as described by PARK, is also called *'classic maximum'* (Table 14.1)

Up to 45° of face turn a 40% augmentation in the above surgery is recommended (Table 14.1).

Up to 60° of face turn a 60% augmentation in Park's figures are suggested Table 14.1.

2. Surgical techniques for face turn with associated strabismus

a. Face turn with esotropia

i. *Face turn ipsilateral to the fixing eye* can be corrected by recess-resect procedure on the

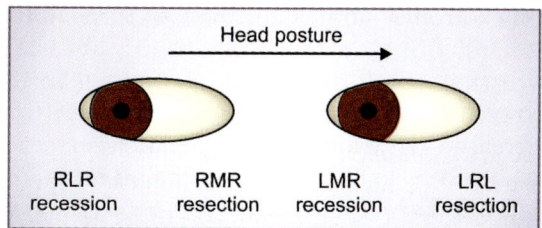

Fig. 14.16 *Diagrammatic depiction of position of eyes in a patient with left face turn and the suggested Kestenbaum procedure to correct it.*

Table 14.1 *Modified Kestenbaum-Anderson procedures for nystagmus in a patient with left face turn*

Type of surgery	Dosage extraocular muscle surgery		
	Classic maximum	40% augmentation	60% augmentation
RMR resection	6	8.4	9.6
RLR recession	7	9.8	11.2
LMR recession	5	7	8
LLR resection	8	11.2	12.8

horizontal recti of the fixing adducted eye. For example, in a patient with left esotropia having right face turn and fixating with right adducting eye, MR recession and LR resection of the right eye should be performed. This procedure will correct face turn as well as an esotropia up to 30PD. The residual esotropia, if any, can be corrected later by surgery on the other eye.

ii. *Face turn ipsilateral to the deviating esotropic eye,* should be first tackled with recess-resect procedure on the opposite fixing eye. This procedures will correct the face turn but will increase the esotropia in the deviating eye, which can be later corrected surgically. For example, in a patient with right face turn and right esotropia, surgery for the face turn should be first done on the left fixing eye (MR resection and LR recession) to move it in the direction of face turn. The resulting increased right esotropia can be later corrected surgically by right MR recession and LR resection.

b. Face turn with exotropia

i. *Face turn ipsilateral to the fixing eye* can be corrected by recess-resect procedure on the horizontal recti of the fixing adducted eye. This procedure will correct the face turn but will increase the exotropia in the deviating nonfixing eye, which can be later corrected surgically. For example, in a patient with right face turn and left exotropia, surgery for the face turn should be first done on the right fixing eye (MR recession and LR resection) to move it in the direction of right face turn. The resulting increased left exotropia can be later corrected surgically by left MR resection and LR recession.

ii. *Face turn ipsilateral to the deviating exotropic eye,* should be first tackled with recess-resect procedure on the fixing eye. This procedure, in addition to correcting face turn,

will also correct/reduce the associated exotropia. For example, in a patient with right exotropia having right face turn and fixating with left eye, surgery for the face turn should be done on the left eye (MR resection and LR recession) to move it in the direction of right face turn. This procedure will correct right face turn as well as the right exotropia. The residual exotropia, if any, can be later corrected surgically by right MR resection and LR recession.

II. Surgical techniques in patients having head tip (chin elevation or depression) associated with childhood nystagmus

Headtip occurs in patients having a null zone with eyes in depression or elevation. The basic principle for surgically correcting the headtip is like that for correcting face turns, i.e. the eyes should be moved in the direction of abnormal head posture. Symmetrical surgery on all the four recti (vertical Kestenbaum) may be useful.

Vertical Kestenbaum. Recommended procedures by Park are as follows:

1. For headtip of more than 25°

- *For chin elevation.* Bilateral 4 mm resection of the superior recti combined with bilateral 4 mm recession of the inferior recti.
- *For chin depression.* Bilateral 4 mm resection of the inferior recti combined with bilateral 4 mm recession of the superior recti.

2. For headtip of less than 25°

The operation is limited to bilateral 4 mm recession of the depressors or elevators without resection of their antagonists.

However, recently most workers recommend that the amount of surgery to be performed should be at least 5–6 mm to obtain satisfactory results.

III. Surgical techniques in patients having head-tilt associated with childhood nystagmus

Some patients with childhood nystagmus (CN) have a combination of both horizontal and rotatory components with latter being the major component. Patients which have a significant headtilt have a torsional null position, and shifting the null position by torsional Kestenbaum is suggested in such cases.

The basic principle to correct head tilt (not related to paralysis of any cyclovertical muscle) is to rotate the eyes in the direction of the headtilt, which can be accomplished by any of the following surgical techniques of torsional Kestenbaum:

1. Surgery on two oblique muscles

In this technique, for example, in a patient with head tilt towards right shoulder, the eyes can be surgically rotated to the right by:

- *Weakening of right superior oblique muscle* (either by a tenotomy or a recession of the anterior fibres), and
- *Weakening of the left inferior oblique* with a recession or some other weakening procedure.

2. Surgery on four oblique muscles

On the basis of Kestenbaum's principle, some workers have proposed symmetrical surgery on all the four oblique muscles (*torsional Kestenbaum*). For instance, in a patient with *head tilt towards the right shoulder*, the following surgery has been recommended:

Right eye is excycloducted by recessing the anterior and retropositioning the posterior aspect of the superior oblique tendon and advancing the anterior and anteropositioning the posterior aspect of the inferior oblique tendon.

Left eye is incycloducted by advancing the anterior portion and anteropositioning the posterior edge of the superior oblique tendon and by recessing the anterior portion and retro-placing the posterior position of the inferior oblique insertion.

3. Vertical transposition of the horizontal rectus muscles

Decker has reported vertical transposition of the horizontal rectus muscles, e.g. to cause excycloduction of the right eye as follows:

- Right medial rectus—transposed downwards.
- Right lateral rectus—transposed upwards.

4. Surgical slanting of the insertion of all four rectus muscles

Spielmann has recommended this surgery, for example, in a patient with head tilt towards right the right eye is excycloducted by recession of the:

- Temporal part of the superior rectus
- Nasal part of the inferior rectus
- Inferior part of the lateral rectus, and
- Superior part of the medial rectus.

Note. A special care is required to preserve the blood supply of the anterior segment of the eyeball in this operation.

5. Horizontal transpositioning of the vertical rectus muscles

von Noorden et al have recommended this surgery (as a preference over the other surgeries), for example, in a patient with head tilt towards right as follows:

Right eye should be excyclotorted by transposing the right superior rectus nasally and the right inferior rectus temporally.

Left eye should be incyclotorted by transposing the left superior rectus temporally and left inferior rectus nasally.

They have recommended that transposition of each muscle should be by one full muscle width without changing their distance from the limbus.

(B) SURGICAL TECHNIQUES FOR NYSTAGMUS BLOCKAGE (DAMPENING) SYNDROME

1. **Recession of the MR and resection of LR** of the converging eye has been recommended by Adelstein and Cuppers with good results.

2. **Bilateral medial rectus recession** sometimes combined with posterior fixation sutures has been reported to be a more effective and thus a better choice than the recess-resect procedure.

(C) SURGICAL TECHNIQUES FOR DECREASING NYSTAGMUS INTENSITY

1. **Producing an artificial divergence** (prismatically and surgically) have been reported to be of some use.

Surgical procedure consists of bilateral medial rectus recession.

Aim of the surgery is to induce a latent divergent ocular position which the patient will then overcome by exerting fusional convergence, thereby damping the nystagmus.

For the success of procedure, the patients must have adequate fusional reserves to overcome the induced deviation, so, preoperative testing with prisms is mandatory.

Indications include patient with INS and convergence dampening with near vision > distance vision.

Benifits of the surgery include:
- Dampening of nystagmus occurs by 70–80%.
- Improvement in vision in magnificant.

2. Maximal recession of all the four horizontal rectus muscles has been recommended for decreasing the nystagmus intensity. For undisturbing the balance of forces, it has been recommended that a 10 mm of bilateral MR recession and 12 mm of bilateral LR recession is the best procedure. However, before contemplating such a surgery, it should be made amply clear to the patient that this operation will only decrease its intensity and note liminate the nystagmus.

Note. Large 4-muscle recessions or muscle extirpations are not preferred presently.

3. Tenotomy and reattachment. All the four horizontal recti are detached and resutured at the same insertion.

Indications. Nystagmus with no null, primary position null or alternating null (periodic or aperiodic).

Benefits of surgery include 25% reduced intensity of nystagmus, broadening of null zone, improvement in vision by 1 to 3 logMar units in about 50% of patients and 40% increase in NAFX in 90% of patients.

4. Augmented Anderson procedure. It comprises:
- MR recession: 9 mm, and
- LR recession: 12 to 13 mm.

Indications. Patients with INS and face turn <25°.

Benefits of surgery include:
- Dampening of nystagmus by 90%.
- Improvement in vision in magnification.

NYSTAGMUS-LIKE OCULAR MOTOR OSCILLATIONS

Nystagmus-like oscillations can be described as below:
- Inappropriate saccades
- Voluntary saccadic oscillation 'nystagmus'
- Roving eye movements

INAPPROPRIATE SACCADES

Involuntary inappropriate saccades include:

Saccadic intrusions

These are basically transient breaks in fixation. These may occurs as:
- *Square wave jerks.* These are small amplitude conjugate saccades (<5°) which moves the eye away from fixation and back again (Fig. 14.17A).
- *Square wave pulses* also known as *macrosquare wave jerk* have a large ampitude (>5°) and a shorter intersaccadic latency (100–150 ms) (Fig. 14.17 B). They are usually and indication of neurological malfunction.

Saccadic oscillation

These movments oscillate across fixation and usually have amplitude large than 5°. Saccadic oscillations are of following types:
- *Macro-saccadic oscillations.* They have a similar intersaccadic latency to square wave jerk (Fig. 14.17C). They can reliably distinguished from ocular flutter only by eye movement recording.
- *Ocular flutter* occurs due to interruption of cerebellar connection to brainstem. It is characterized by horizontal oscillation and inability to fixate after change of gaze. Ocular flutter represent back to back horizontal scaddes without any interscaddic latency (Fig. 14.17D)
- *Opsoclonus* refers to combined horizontal, vertical and/or torsional oscillations associated with myoclonic movement of face, arms and legs. It is seen in patient with encephalitis. Opsoclonus has a similar waveform to ocular flutter but is multidirection and associated with ossilopsia.
- *Superior oblique myokymia* is characterized by monocular, rapid, intermittent, torsional

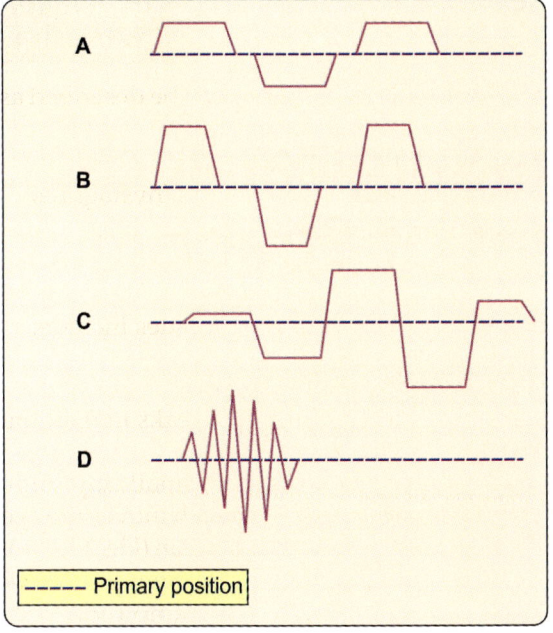

----- Primary position

Fig. 14.17 *Inappropriate saccades:* A, *Square wave jerk;* B, *Macro-square wave jerks;* C, *Macro-saccadic oscillations;* and D, *Ocular flutter.*

vertical movements (which are best seen on slit-lamp examination).

• *Ocular bobbing* refers to rapid downward deviation of the eyes with slow updrift. It occurs due to pontine dysfunctions.

VOLUNTARY SACCADIC OSCILLATIONS 'NYSTAGMUS'

Voluntary saccadic oscillations 'nystagmus' refers to the voluntary, poorly sustained conjugate oscillation of the eyes consisting of rapidly alternating small-amplitude saccades.

Characteristic features. The oscillations are conjugate, usually horizontal and symmetrical, and consist of back-to-back saccades. The oscillations can be sustained only for a matter of seconds; convergence is usually associated with either the initiation or the maintenance of the oscillation. The amplitude of the movement is small and the frequency high. There may be a familial basis for the ability to initiate voluntary 'nystagmus' or it may be learned. Voluntary 'nystagmus' can be readily differentiated from acquired nystagmus and does not require further investigation.

ROVING EYE MOVEMENTS

Roving eye movements refers to conjugate large amplitude low-frequency horizontal pendular-like movements. The movements are apparent soon after birth and are generally associated with severe anterior visual pathway disease such as Leber's congenital amaurosis and severe forms of bilateral optic nerve hypoplasia. With time the amplitude becomes smaller and a congenital nystagmus waveform may become superimposed on the roving pattern or may replace it.

BIBLIOGRAPHY

1. Boyle NJ, Dawson EL, Lee JP, Benefits of Retroequatorial Four Horizontal Muscle Recession Surgery in Congenital Idiopathic Nystagmus in Adults, JAAPOS, 2006;10:404–8.
2. Dell'Osso LF, Tenotomy and congenital nystagmus: a failure to answer the wrong question, Vision Res, 2004;44:3091–4.
3. Erbagci I, Gungor K, Bekir NA, Effectiveness of retroequatorial recession surgery in congenital nystagmus, Strabismus, 2004;12:35–40.
4. Flynn JT, Dell'Osso LF, The effects of congenital nystagmus surgery, Ophthalmology, 1979;86:1414–27.
5. Hertle RW, Dell'Osso LF, Benefits of retroequatorial four horizontal muscle recession surgery in congenital idiopathic nystagmus in adults, JPAAOS, 2007;11:313.
6. Schiavi C, Scorolli L, Campos EC, Surgical management of anomalous head posture due to supranuclear gaze palsies and acquired nystagmus. In: Spiritus M (ed.), Transactions of the 23rd Meeting of the European Strabismological Association, Nancy, 1996;229–32.
7. Sternberg-Raab A, Anderson–Kestenbaum operation for asymmetrical gaze nystagmus, Br J Ophthalmol, 1963;47: 339–45.
8. Wang Z, Dell'Osso LF, Jacobs JB, et al., Effects of tenotomy on patients with infantile nystagmus syndrome, JAAPOS, 2006;10: 552–60.
9. Wang ZI, Dell'Osso LF, Tomsak RL, Jacobs JB, Combining recessions (nystagmus and strabismus) with tenotomy improved visual function and decreased oscillopsia and diplopia in acquired downbeat nystagmus and in horizontal infantile nystagmus syndrome, JAAPOS, 2007;11:135–41.

Chapter

15

Principles of Non-Surgical and Surgical Management of Strabismus

NON-SURGICAL MANAGEMENT

Goals of Treatment of Strabismus

Goals of treatment of strabismus are:

1. To restore good visual acuity in each eye.
2. To achieve satisfactory cosmetic appearance.
3. To restore, if possible, normal single binocular vision.

To achieve these goals, treatment of squint varies for its different clinico-aetiological varieties and has been described along with the each clinical entity. However, the principles, indications and the techniques of different treatment modalities available for the squint have been described here in general. The commonly practised treatment modalities include:

- Optical treatment,
- Pharmacologic treatment,
- Orthoptics, and
- Surgical treatment.

Non-surgical treatment is essential in all most all strabismus cases and in many cases may be sufficient to successfully treat the strabismus without surgery.

A. OPTICAL TREATMENT

I. CORRECTION OF REFRACTIVE ERROR

Spectacles for correction of refractive error should be prescribed in every case. These will improve the visual acuity and provide sharp retinal image that in young children is essential as a stimulus for the use of eyes and to achieve fusion. Refractive correction also provides a proper balance between accommodation and convergence and thus at times may correct the squint partially or completely (as in accommodative esotropia). Some important points regarding refractive correction in patients with strabismus are as follows:

General principles for prescribing glasses.

1. In general, *full cycloplegic correction* should be prescribed (without making any tonus allowance for the cycloplegic used), especially in young children from infancy to preschool age, neglecting the effect of glasses on the patient's vision.
2. In school going children, the refractive correction prescribed should be such that would provide an optimal distant vision.
3. An *overcorrection of +1.0DS to +3.0DS* of the non-amblyopic eye has been advocated by some workers as penalization treatment.

Role of glasses in esotropia

1. *Refractive accommodative esotropia.* Full cycloplegic correction should be made to correct the esotropia.
2. *Non-refractive accommodative esotropia* with high AC/A ratio need to be treated with bifocal glasses giving full hyperopic correction in the distance segment and an add of +1.00 D to +3.5 D in the near segment. The minimum add required is tested in steps of 0.5D till the convergence excess for near is controlled.
3. *Esotropic patients having associated myopic* should be prescribed minimum myopic lenses that give best corrected visual acuity.
4. *Esotropic patients having associated myopia and high AC/A ratio* also require bifocals.
5. *Residual esotropia* of small amount (<15PD) should be prescribed the maximum hypermetropic correction. If this is insufficient, additional plus lenses may be tried to ascertain, if binocular single vision can be achieved.
6. *Consecutive esotropia* of small amount (<15PD), persisting after 3 weeks of surgery for intermittent exotropia can be treated by prescribing full hyperopic correction. Bifocals can be prescribed, when esotropia is for near only.

Role of glasses in exotropia

1. *Undercorrection of hypermetropic error* is recommended to reduce the degree of consecutive exotropia. However, this should not be at the cost of asthenopic symptoms.
2. *Use of over-minus glasses* has been suggested by Jampolsky for controlling the intermittent exotropia by stimulating accommodation and convergence in under 5 ear children.
3. *Inverse bifocal with a minus add for near* has been suggested for convergence insufficiency type of exotropia.

II. PRISMOTHERAPY

Prismotherapy for strabismus has become popular after the introduction of Fresnel press-on prisms.

Advantages of Fresnel press-on membrane prisms include: Light weight, cosmetically acceptable, easy to apply on the back of patient's glasses, availability in powers from 0.5D to 30D.

Indications

The indications for prismotherapy in strabismus are as follows:

I. *Role of prisms to assess the effect of surgery* (Diagnostic Prism)

1. *Prism adaptation test (PAT).* This test has been advocated by some workers to be performed before the surgical treatment is performed in patients with esotropia; while others do not agree on its utility. In PAT, base-out prisms are given to the patient, so that esotropia is slightly overcorrected, i.e. to the point of slight exotropia. The results of the PAT are interpreted as below:

Favourable response or good fusional prognostic sign is labelled, when a patient accepts the prism and demonstrates fusion, when allowed to wear prisms for several days before surgery. Such patients are likely to respond well to slight surgical overcorrection of esotropia and develop spontaneous restoration of normal retinal correspondence.

Unfavourable response or poor fusional prognostic sign is considered, if a patient overconverges in response to slight overcorrection with the prisms in PAT and, thus returns with a marked esotropia in spite of its neutralization with prism. This overconvergence can occur within minutes or hours or days or weeks after the prisms are worn. A further increase in convergence is reported after addition of prisms and, the patient is said to *eat up the prism.*

The overconvergence in response to PAT has been assumed to occur, most likely, in the presence of sensory abnormal retinal correspondence (ARC) and thus represents a peripheral motor fusional convergence. Such patients are likely to respond in a way similar to conventional surgical treatment as well and thus will have a recurrence of esotropia. However, in clinical practice, it has been observed that in many cases, ARC disappears following surgical alignment without over-correction. Because of this controversy, PAT has not become much popular and so most of the strabismologists no more practice prismotherapy for sensorial anomalies.

2. *To know the response of associated vertical deviation to surgical treatment for the horizontal deviation.* It has been reported that in some patients, associated vertical deviation also disappears following prismotherapy for the associated horizontal strabismus. It is assumed that in such cases surgical treatment for the horizontal strabismus alone will be sufficient to correct the associated vertical deviation as well. However, like PAT results of this test are also based on the assumption that the response to surgical intervention will be similar to the response to prismotherapy. While in clinical practice, it may not be cent percent true.

3. *To plan the amount of vertical muscle surgery* required in congenital or long-standing vertical muscle palsies.

II. *Role of prisms in managing dilopia and abnormal head posture* (relieving prisms)

Prism may be employed in the early management till scenario for surgical treatment is clear.

1. *Paralytic strabismus.* During recovery phase of paralytic squint, prisms are quite useful in preventing contracture of the antagonist muscle, e.g. as in:

• Superior oblique palsy, and
• Sixth nerve palsy.

2. *As a temporary measure in acquired ocular restrictive defects* such as blow-out fractures and thyroid ophthalmopathy, prisms may be employed in the early management till scenario for surgical treatment is clear.

III. *Maintenance of binocular single vision by neutralizing the deviation*

1. *Vertical deviations.* Prismotherapy is quite useful in patients with small (less than 12D) comitant vertical deviations. However, larger degrees of vertical deviations associated with greater degrees of incomitance almost always require surgery.

2. *Horizontal deviations* in which therapeutic use of prisms for relief of diplopia may be quite successful are:

• *Late onset deviations in visually mature patients* such as those associated with muscle paresis and divergence insufficiency.
• *Primary intermittent exotropia.* Some workers have recommended prismotherapy for the treatment of primary intermittent exotropia, where surgical treatment is not yet warranted. However, other workers have reported that *part time occlusion therapy* is perhaps more effective and useful in such cases rather than the prismotherapy.

3. *Surgically overcorrected exotropia.* It is generally agreed that a slight overcorrection (consecutive esotropia) for 1 to 3 weeks postoperatively is desirable in patients with intermittent exotropia. Fusional divergence usually develops spontaneously to allow the eyes to straighten. If a stable esotropia persists over one month postoperatively, it needs to be corrected by base-out prisms. For a larger overcorrection requiring resurgery, the base-out prisms may be prescribed to prevent diplopia until surgical treatment can be undertaken.

4. *Surgically undercorrected exotropia.* It has been reported that in undercorrected exotropia, the use of overcorrecting base-in prisms (10D greater than the deviation) in immediate postoperative period may be successful in establishing a good fusional result. Hardesty has described the convergence response to such prism therapy. However, it has also been reported that prisms used in this manner, probably will not be effective, if given later than three months postoperatively.

5. *Surgically undercorrected esotropia.* In many cases of esotropia with ARC in its peripheral convergence response, a small residual esotropia with monofixation will be present postoperatively. Prismotherapy in such a deviation is not indicated, since it will not convert such cases to bifoveal fixation.

6. *Surgically overcorrected convergence insufficiency* may spontaneously lead to postoperative diplopia. During this period, prismotherapy may be useful in alleviating the diplopia.

IV. *Management of convergence insufficiency*

Convergence insufficiency of hypoaccommodative type and convergence paralysis are also relieved symptomatically by base-in prisms.

V. *Management of heterophorias*

Patients with marked asthenopic symptoms, particularly those with vertical phorias respond well to prismotherapy.

VI. *Role of prisms in nystagmus* (see page 393)

Guidelines for prescribing prisms

In principle, the patient should be given the lowest powered prism which makes him/her comfortable. The guideline generally applied is to correct two-thirds of the deviation, but the variation found in different conditions and among patients with the same condition make this rule of little value. Useful guidelines are:

- *Patients with acquired vertical muscle palsies* usually require a prism equal or nearly equal to the angle of deviation.
- *Patient with congenital or long-standing palsies* and most patients with dysthyroid eye disease involving vertical eye movement, may require as little as half the amount measured. Patients with long-standing vertical strabismus caused by retinal detachment surgery also behave in a similar way.
- *Prism correction. Patients with esodeviations,* especially those which increase in the distance (divergence weakness type), are harder to control and, therefore, require a larger prism in relation to the angle of deviation than do those with exodeviations.

- *Patients with paralytic strabismus who have been deprived of binocular single vision* for many months may not be able to fuse the images immediately prisms are introduced. Although it may not be possible to demonstrate! fusion in the clinic, it is worthwhile fitting trial prisms for a period to see whether binocular single vision can be obtained with more time.
- *Patients with very incomitant deviations* are thought to be unsuitable for prism therapy because the area of binocular single vision achieved will be too small; however, even a very small field of binocular fixation is welcomed by some patients, while others find the intermittent diplopia too distracting. It is often worth a short period of trial prisms in these cases.

Methods of using prisms

Prisms can be used by following methods:
- As Fresnel prism
- In spectacle frames
- As clip-on prism

- *Fresnel prisms* are the method of choice for temporary use. Up to 30" can be applied to either eye but high-powered prisms may not be tolerated because of their adverse effect on visual acuity; usually up to 20" can be worn comfortably, at least by children.
- *In spectacle frames.* If the patient has a high refractive error, the spectacle lenses can be decentred to give the desired effect, provided that the prism strength is not too great. Patients with lower refractive errors and those who are emmetropic can be prescribed additional prisms. These methods are used, when permanent or long-term use of prisms is envisaged.
- *Clip-on prisms:* These are generally used, only when the patient cannot tolerate Fresnel prisms. The strength is limited to 10–12 Δ in front of each eye because of the weight involved. These are no longer commercially available.

■ B. PHARMACOLOGIC TREATMENT

I. Miotics (also see pages 193, 227 and 230)

Mechanism of action. Though pharmacologic actions of the miotics (parasympathomimetics) include miosis and spasm of accommodation, their utility in strabismus is through their effect on accommodation.

Miotics commonly used in strabismus management include long-acting cholinesterase inhibitors such as DFP (0.025% ointment and 0.1% solution), echothiopate (0.03%, 0.06%, 0.125% and 0.25% solution), and demecarium bromide (0.125% and 0.25% solution).

Indications for use of miotics include:
i. *Diagnostic trial* to differentiate between accommodative (refractive and non-refractive) and non-accommodative esotropia.
ii. *Therapy of accommodative esotropia* especially non-refractive type (*see* page 229).
iii. *Postoperative miotic therapy* may be useful in patients with residual esotropia as well as in consecutive esotropia (after surgery for an intermittent exotropia).
iv. *Amblyopia.* Use of miotics in the amblyopic eye and atropine in the sound eye has been advocated as penalization treatment for amblyopia (*see* page 193).

2. Atropine

Common uses of atropine in the management of strabismus are as follows:
i. *Cycloplegic refraction.* Atropine is most useful for cycloplegic refraction especially in children with strabismus.
ii. *Therapy of accommodative esotropia.* A few workers have recommended atropine in combination with overcorrection of hypermetropic refractive error for treatment of accommodative esotropia.
iii. *Amblyopia.* Use of atropine in sound eye with or without a miotic in the amblyopic eye has been recommended as penalization treatment for amblyopia.

3. Botulinum toxin

Mechanism of action. Botulinum toxin, when injected into an extraocular muscle blocks release of acetylcholine and thus causes chemical denervation and thus paralysis of the muscle for several weeks. As a result, the antagonist muscle becomes comparatively strong and thus neutralizes the deviation.

Indications. Botulinum toxin may be useful in the short-term treatment of: Infantile esotropia, paralytic strabismus especially acute 6th nerve palsy, surgical overcorrections, Graves' ophthalmopathy and nystagmus.

Dosage. Botulinum toxin is injected into the muscle to be weakened under electromyographic (EMG) control after local or general anaesthesia. When general anaesthesia is used, ketamine hydrochloride rather than barbiturates or halothane is used to preserve the EMG signal. Vertical and horizontal deviations less than 20D are treated initially with 1.25 to 2.5 units and horizontal deviations greater than 20D with 2.5 to 5 units initially in volumes of 0.05–0.15 ml. The saline reconstituted lyophylized powder must not be shaken otherwise the protein will denaturate. Reinjections may be titrated down depending on the effect achieved from the original injection.

Complications reported following injection of botulinum toxin are as follows:
i. *Diplopia* due to transient overcorrection is very common, but resolves in a few weeks.
ii. *Blepharoptosis* has been reported to occur in 25% children and 16% of adults after horizontal muscle injection, due to spillage in the orbit, which resolved within a few months.
iii. *Vertical deviations* after horizontal muscle injection have been reported to occur in 17% cases, which persisted only in 20% cases.
iv. *Perforation* of the globe and retrobulbar or subconjunctival *haemorrhage* are the other very rare complications noted.

4. Other drugs

i. *Chlordiazepoxide hydrochloride* has been reported to decrease the deviation and/or improve the fusional amplitude in patients with esodeviations.
ii. *Phenytoin (dilantin)* has been reported to reduce the near point of accommodation and AC/A ratio and thus affect accommodative and partially accommodative esotropia.
iii. *Levadopa/carbidopa combination* has been used as an adjunct to occlusion therapy in amblyopia, with no clear role. Some workers have reported its role in early initiation of the

effect of occlusion in cases of moderate to severe amblyopia.

iv. *Citicholine (CDP choline)* has also been reported to have a role in amblyopic patients. It is an essential intermediate for phosphatidyl choline synthesis. It increases cerebral blood flow and also shows neural restorative effect via its action on dopaminergic pathway for central nervous system.

C. ORTHOPTICS

Literally, the word orthoptics means 'straight eyes'. However, with regard to therapy orthoptics refers to teaching an individual to obtain the best possible use of both eyes together in the form of a comfortable binocular single vision. Practically orthoptics training is used to treat convergence insufficiency, to combat suppression, amblyopia and abnormal retinal correspondence and to improve fusional amplitudes and stereopsis.

Goals of orthoptic treatment

The ultimate goals of orthoptic treatment are:

1. Visual acuity levels in each eye should be best possible.
2. Eyes should be straight—with or without surgical help.
3. Binocular single vision.
4. Fusion with good amplitudes and reserves.
5. Reduction of refractive glasses (when involved).

Pre-requisites for a successful orthoptic treatment

1. *At the patient level.* Since orthoptics is mainly a training process chiefly concerned with helping to establish a new sensory pathway that will effect the accurate usage of the two eyes since this takes place at the cortical level, therefore, vital pre-requisites at the patient level are:

- Reasonable intelligence,
- Physical and psychological maturity,
- Good attention span and,
- Confidence and co-operation.
- Able to attend regularly.

Keeping in view the above points, the age of patient is very important. It is impossible to treat orthoptically 2–3 years old. They are too young to understand and their attention span may only be 1 or 2 minutes. There are some exceptional 4 years old who understand instructions well but whose attention span may be too short to make treatment worthwhile. The age of 5 years is usually the youngest treatable age. The average age to begin treatment is 6 years.

2. *At the parents' level.* Since parents play the key role in their child's treatment, they must:

- Realize that the reeducation process takes a long time,
- Have good understanding of the purpose of the treatment, methods and procedures used,
- Have good rapport between child and orthoptist.

3. *At the orthoptist level.* Since orthoptist is the main person concerned with the treatment, he/she should:

- Have a friendly but firm attitude towards the child,
- Have a good rapport and understanding with the treating ophthalmologist, and
- Win the confidence of child and parents.

4. *At the ophthalmologist level.* Since it is the ophthalmologist who refers the child for the orthoptic treatment, therefore, he should:

- Ensure that the other modes of treatment required, i.e. refraction and prescription of glasses, prisms, miotics, etc. have been taken care of
- Ensure that symptoms must be attributable to the deviation and not to other causes.
- Must exclued pathological causes for strabismus
- Have frequent conferences with the orthoptist about the patient's treatment, and
- Take decision about the surgical treatment whenever required.

Indications of orthoptics

1. *Diagnostic indications.* A complete orthoptic work-up is required in each and every patient suspected of having a neuromuscular anomaly of the eye.

2. *Therapeutic indications.* Orthoptic exercises and training may be required in patients with phorias and tropias, both pre- and postoperatively. The scope of orthoptic treatment includes:

- Elimination of convergence insufficiency
- Fusion training, to increase fusion amplitude
- Antisuppression exercises
- Treatment of anomalous retinal correspondence
- Treatment of amblyopia
- Control of deviation

Order of orthoptic treatment

The natural course of events, when a heterophoria slowly becomes a heterotropia and is left untreated, in order of occurrence include:

- Deterioration of amplitudes
- Occurrence of diplopia
- Development of suppression and development of amblyopia (in a monocular deviation).

However, the orthoptic treatment in a patient with heterotropia proceeds in the opposite direction as follows:

- Amblyopia is treated first, to be followed by
- Antisuppression therapy,
- Diplopia training, and
- Amplitude improvement.

Delivery of orthoptic treatment

The details of the orthoptic treatment required for various neuromuscular anomalies of the eye have been described along with the concerned anomaly. However, for a quick review, they are listed below.

1. *Treatment of convergence insufficiency.* Orthoptic treatment of convergence insufficiency is quite effective (for details, *see* page 157). It includes the following:

- Pencil convergence exercises
- Physiological diplopia exercises
- Training for increasing fusional convergence with base-out prisms or on synoptophore.

2. *Exercises for increasing fusional amplitudes.* Both convergence and divergence fusional amplitudes can be increased by fusion training using:

- Prisms or
- Major amblyoscope
  (for details, *see* pages 213 and 214)

Indications

- To compensate a latent strabismus
- To improve control of an intermittent strabismus
- As a pre- and postoperative measure in constant strabismus

3. *Orthoptic treatment of suppression* includes the following:

- Diplopia exercises
- Vergence control in heterophoria and surgical alignment of eyes in large tropias.
- Differential stimulation
- Macular massage
- Occlusion therapy
  (for details, *see* page 190)

SURGICAL MANAGEMENT

Extraocular muscle surgery is only a part of the therapeutic management of a strabismic patient. Of course, the squint surgery is aimed to produce and maintain a condition in which the visual axes of the two eyes are directed, without conscious effort to the object of fixation whatever its position. However, in some cases, this may require more than one operation and in others it may even not be possible at all. All these facts should be made amply clear to the patient and/or the parents.

INDICATIONS FOR SQUINT SURGERY

1. *To correct squint cosmetically as well as functionally.* This is possible in cases in which the visual acuity of the two eyes is equal or has been made nearly equal by appropriate occlusion treatment (so that alternation occurs easily) and in which binocular function has been improved (where possible) by appropriate orthoptic treatment, if indicated.

2. *To correct the squint only cosmetically.* This is indicated in old children and adults who have untreatable deep amblyopia, persistent abnormal retinal correspondence and absence of power of fusion. Patients having sensory squint secondary to organic disorders (e.g. optic atrophy, central chorioretinitis) are also corrected cosmetically only.

3. *To relieve marked asthenopic* symptoms squint surgery may be indicated, in some cases. These include patients with phorias and intermittent tropias which could not be treated by an active orthoptic treatment.

4. *To correct abnormal head posture* which may be assumed by some patients to relieve diplopia (e.g. in superior oblique or lateral rectus weakness) or to improve vision (e.g. with nystagmus and an eccentric null point).

5. *To relieve mechanical restriction or to improve appearance* surgery may be required sometimes in patients with hypertrophied conjunctiva or Tenon's capsule from prior muscle surgery.

OPTIMAL TIME FOR SQUINT SURGERY

Optimal time for squint surgery varies depending upon the type of squint, age of the patient and presence of various sensory adaptations as below.

1. CONCOMITANT SQUINT

Although it is difficult to be dogmatic as to precisely when to operate upon a case of concomitant squint, especially in a child, the following suggestions have been made by experienced strabismologists:

i. *Children too young for orthoptic treatment,* i.e. those below 4–5 years should be considered for operation as follows:

- If a *constant squint* is present after wearing of glasses (where indicated) for a month and the squint is an alternating one or that an early alternation has been established by appropriate occlusion, i.e. vision is almost equal in the two eyes; the child should be operated as early as possible. Such a recommendation has been made on the basis of the observation that in young children, if the visual axes are put within a few degrees of parallelism by means of operative treatment, and good binocular vision may develop per se, provided that the child already posseses some rudimentary development of his normal binocular reflexes.
- In *intermittent squint* with or without glasses, the surgery should be delayed and child should be observed and refracted every six months. Orthoptic treatment should be started

as early as possible. In many cases with intermittent squint the need for operation may be dispensed altogether with glasses and/or orthoptic treatment. However, before abandoning the idea of surgery, it must be ascertained that squint has completely disappeared and not that there has occurred mere reduction in the angle of deviation (which may be satisfactory from the cosmetic point of view but of no functional value).

ii. *In children old enough for orthoptic treatment* (i.e. those above 4–5 years), following considerations should be made:

- Before the surgery is performed for a constant squint, best possible efforts with optical and orthoptic treatment should be made to treat the associated (if any) sensory adaptation (such as suppression, amblyopia and abnormal retinal correspondence). The efforts should be aimed at developing good binocular vision with fusion amplitudes.
- In the presence of an abnormal retinal correspondence, now most surgeons recommend early surgery; since both cosmetic and functional results may be obtained in many cases (i.e. ARC disappears spontaneously after surgery).
- In the absence of a true fusion, the case may have to be assessed purely for the cosmetic effect. However, it has been reported that parallelism of the visual axes produced by an early surgery, may sometimes result in development of binocular fusion.

iii. *In older children (above 12 years of age) and adult* patients who have deep intractable amblyopia (functional or organic) the time of surgery may be decided according to personal requirements for cosmetic purposes only, since there is hardly any scope for a functional cure.

2. PARALYTIC SQUINT

The most important principle is to establish over a significant period of time that the condition is stable and that no spontaneous improvement is likely to occur. Therefore, a hastily surgical treatment may result in an over-correction of the deviation in some cases. On the other hand in some cases the condition may continue to deteriorate so that ill-time surgical interference will prove to be inadequate. However, in most cases if the condition remains static for a period of 3–6 months, the surgical treatment may be considered.

Expectations from the treating ophthalmologists regarding optimal time to operate

It is expected that the operating ophthalmologist should be ready with the following spade work and home task when he decides that it is the optimal time to operate:

- He should have accomplished all the preoperative measures which are necessary and helpful to achieve the basic three goals of squint management.
- He should have a plan as to what surgery will be performed and why.
- By this time, he must educate the parents and/or patients as to the goals, his plan of attack, the risks involved in surgery, the risks involved in not operating, and the possibility that more than one operation may be necessary.
- He should have plans for what to do postoperatively:
  - If the patient is fusing,
  - If the patient is overcorrected, and
  - If the patient is undercorrected.

TYPES OF SURGICAL TECHNIQUES FOR SQUINT CORRECTION

A. MUSCLE WEAKENING PROCEDURES

1. *Recession* of an extraocular muscle is the most commonly performed weakening procedure. This procedure weakens the muscle action by changing its arc of contact with the globe.

2. *Marginal myotomy* is infrequently indicated. This procedure weakens the muscle by reducing the number of contractile fibres and not by changing the arc of contact. Therefore, it is effective in further weakening on already maximally recessed muscle. This procedure is also indicated where recession cannot be performed as in patients with very thin sclera and in those having buckle implants.

3. *Myectomy* also weakens the muscle by reducing the contractile fibres and is seldom performed nowadays except by some surgeons especially for inferior oblique muscle.

4. *Free tenotomy* or disinsertion of the rectus muscles may be performed in desparate cases. Oblique muscle tenotomy is practised by many surgeons to weaken this muscle.

5. *Posterior fixation suture* also known as Faden operation or retropexy of an extraocular muscle is a weakening procedure that does not affect the deviation in primary position but weakens the muscle action in patients who are already orthotropic. However, it reduces the deviation in esotropic patients, when performed on medial rectus. Faden operation is performed under following circumstances:

- To correct the dissociated vertical deviation.
- Patients having incomitant strabismus with orthotropia in primary position.
- To treat upshoot and downshoot of the adducted eye in patients with Duane's retraction syndrome type I.
- Esotropia with a variable angle.
- Persistent esotropia after maximal recession and resection surgery.
- To dampen the nystagmus.

It has been reported by von Noorden that the Faden operation is most effective, when performed on the medial rectus, less effective on vertical rectus muscles and least effective on the lateral rectus muscle.

6. *Recession of conjunctiva and Tenon's capsule* may also help in augmenting the weakening effect of a rectus muscle especially in patients with large deviations of long standing where the elasticity of conjunctiva and Tenon's capsule is impaired and where scars have been formed from previous surgery.

7. *Muscle lengthening by insertion of a silicone expander or non-absorbable suture material* has been recommended as a more controlled weakening procedure for superior oblique muscle.

B. MUSCLE STRENGTHENING PROCEDURES

1. *Resection* is the most commonly performed muscle strengthening procedure. This procedure strengthens the muscle by shortening its length.

One should avoid excessive resection of a muscle, since this may restrict the eye movements in the opposite direction.

2. *Advancement* of the muscle insertion towards limbus is usually not preferred as the primary procedure alone. However, it may be combined with the resection procedure or may be used as secondary procedure in already resected muscle to further strengthen it or in cases with overcorrection due to recession of a muscle.

3. *Tucking* of an extraocular muscle also enhances its action. This procedure is not being preferred for rectus muscles. However, a superior oblique tucking is performed frequently to strengthen this muscle. This procedure, when performed on the superior oblique muscle, is quite effective in improving the depression of the adducted eye and in counteracting the excyclotropia.

C. PROCEDURES THAT CHANGE DIRECTION OF MUSCLE ACTION

1. *Vertical transpositioning of the horizontal recti* is recommended in patients with A- or V-pattern without associated oblique muscle dysfunction.

2. *Horizontal transpositioning of the vertical recti* has also been recommended by some surgeons for correction of A-V pattern.

3. *Slanting of the rectus muscle insertion* has also been recommended by some surgeons for correction of A-V-patterns. However, at present, it is not a preferred technique.

4. *Transplantation of muscles in paralytic squint* (*see* page 439).

D. PERIOSTEAL FIXATION OF THE GLOBE MEDIAL

1. *Medial periosteal fixation of globe* is recomendation in patients with third nerve palsy

2. *Lateral periosteal fixation of lateral rectus* after disinsertion is also recomended in patients with third nerve palsy.

CHOICE OF OPERATION AND AMOUNT OF SURGERY

Choice of operation and amount of extraocular muscle surgery to be performed depend upon multiple factors, i.e. type and angle of squint,

age at the time of onset of squint, duration of squint, age at the time of operation, visual status, convergence and accommodation status. Therefore, degree of squint correction versus amount of extraocular muscle manipulation required cannot be mathematically determined. A discussion on this aspect of squint management can be considered under following heads:

- General considerations for planning squint surgery
- Guidelines for planning squint surgery
- Rough estimates for amount of squint surgery

GENERAL CONSIDERATIONS FOR PLANNING SQUINT SURGERY

As we know, it is not possible to provide a readymade menu for correcting each patient with strabismus, rather the plan of surgery has to be tailor made for the individual patient. The clinical factors other than the measurement of deviation in primary position which need to be considered in the planning are as follows:

1. *Amblyopia.* As discussed under the 'optimal time for surgery', the surgery should be delayed till the vision has been made equal or nearly so by appropriate means such as glasses and amblyopia therapy, when needed. However, if the visual acuity cannot be made equal, the surgery should preferably be performed on the eye with poor vision.

2. *Vertical incomitancy.* Presence of A- or V-pattern should be taken into consideration while planning surgery for the horizontal strabismus. The surgical treatment may include an additional surgery on the oblique muscle or vertical transpositioning of the horizontal recti.

3. *Horizontal incomitancy.* In the presence of a mechanical restriction or paretic limitation of the eye movements, the deviation in left gaze and right gaze may differ significantly from the deviation in primary gaze. Surgeon should aim at making the alignment more nearly comitant after surgery.

For example, in a patient with 30° exotropia in primary position, 20° in right gaze and 40° in left gaze, the surgery may be modified as below:

- If bilateral lateral rectus recession is planned, a more recession on left than the right side may be performed to have greater reduction of the exotropia in left gaze.

- If a resect-recess procedure is planned to get a greater reduction in exotropia in left gaze, a greater recession of the left lateral rectus and less resection of the left medial rectus than the standard amounts of surgery should be performed.

In other words, testing of versions is very important in deciding the appropriate surgical technique as follows:

- *In esotropia associated with excessive adduction and normal abduction,* a maximal recession of the medial rectus and a nominal resection of the lateral rectus should be performed.
- *In esotropia associated with normal adduction and a deficient abduction,* a maximal resection of the lateral rectus and a nominal recession of the medial rectus should be performed.
- *In exotropia associated with excessive abduction and normal adduction* a maximal recession of the lateral rectus and a nominal resection of the medial rectus should be performed.
- *In exotropia associated with normal abduction and deficient adduction,* a maximal resection of the medial rectus and a nominal recession of the lateral rectus should be preferred.
- *When the strabismus is associated with a normal abduction and adduction,* one should prefer the strengthening (resection) rather than the weakening (recession) procedure.
- *When the strabismus is associated with an excessive movement in one direction and deficient on the other,* one should prefer to do maximal weakening of the muscle in the excessive movement and maximal strengthening of the muscle with deficient movement.

All the above recommendations have been made by the workers with an aim to normalize the excursions of the eyes along with correction of deviation.

4. Lateral incomitancy. One must consider the measurements in lateral gaze while planning surgery in a patient with intermittent exotropia. It has been observed that standard amounts of surgery may result in overcorrection in patients having lateral incomitancy (e.g. in a patient with exotropia of 30° in primary positioin and of 20° in right as well as left gaze). It has been recommended that amount of recession of each lateral rectus should be reduced by 1 mm in such patients.

5. *Previous surgery.* The details of the previous surgery performed (wherever possible), its results and effects (any mechanical restriction, etc.) should be duly taken into consideration while planning a repeat surgery as follows:

- Though planning for an under- or over-corrected squint should be made as for a fresh case of squint, it is preferable to operate on muscles that have not had prior surgery.
- In the presence of a mechanical restriction from excessive resection/scarring or weakness from excessive recession, reoperation on the involved muscle may provide better results.
- In multiple surgeries, one must ensure that at least one rectus muscle remains unoperated in each eye.

6. *Distance and near measurements and AC/A ratio* should also be taken into consideration while planning surgery for horizontal deviations. Duane classified horizontal deviations on the basis of distance/near measurements as follows:

Esodeviations
- *Basic esotropia*—distance deviation equals near deviation. Some surgeons prefer a monocular recession of the MR and resection of LR in such cases. While others prefer bilateral symmetrical recession of medial recti.
- *Convergence excess type esotropia*—near deviation greater than distance. Bilateral medial rectus recession is preferred by some surgeons over monocular recess-resect procedure.
- *Divergence insufficiency type esotropia*—distance deviation greater than near. Bilateral lateral rectus resection is preferred by some surgeons over uniocular recess-resect procedure.

Exodeviations
- *Basic exotropia*—distance and near deviation is equal. Some surgeons prefer a monocular recession of the LR and resection of MR in such cases. While others prefer bilateral symmetrical recession of lateral recti.
- *Convergence insufficiency type exotropia*—near devition is greater than distance. This condition rarely requires surgery. Some success has been reported with bilateral MR resections.

- *Divergence excess type exotropia*—distance deviation greater than near deviation, normal AC/A ratio, no increase in near deviation on occlusion. Bilateral lateral rectus recession is preferred by many surgeons over uniocular recess-resect procedure.
- *Pseudo or simulated divergence exces type of exotropia.* In this condition, distance deviation measures greater than near deviation on routine examination. But after occlusion test, near deviation increases to equal the distance deviation. Uniocular recess-resect procedure is preferred by most surgeons.

7. *Special considerations for cyclovertical strabismus.* While considering surgery for the vertical strabismus, one must make the note of deviation in right gaze and left gaze and also in upgaze and downgaze of the same eye. And in general, surgery should be performed on those muscles whose field of action is in the same field as the greatest vertical deviation.

8. *Forced duction test (FDT)* should always be performed before planning the surgery. In small children, FDT should be performed under general anaesthesia just before surgery, and if a mechanical restriction is detected, the original surgical plan may have to be changed accordingly. However, it should be kept in mind that when succinylcholine has been used, a sustained contraction of the extraocular muscles may occur for a period of about 20 minutes. Therefore, it is better to use a non-depolarizing muscle relaxant in squint surgery, since it will not alter the FDT.

GUIDELINES FOR PLANNING SQUINT SURGERY

General guidelines based on the experience of various squint surgeons which can help in planning the squint surgery are as follows:

1. *Surgeon factor.* Every surgeon gets a different amount of correction vis-a-vis another surgeon for the same amount of surgery. Therefore, it is advisable that each surgeon must standardise one's approximate effectiveness of a particular procedure based on review of his/her experience.

2. *Degree of squint.* The same amount of muscle surgery will give greater correction for larger deviations vis-a-vis smaller deviations.

3. *Age of the patient and duration of squint.* A more extensive surgery may be required in older children and adults having squint of long duration as compared to small children for the same amount of deviation, since in the former, secondary anatomical changes take place in muscles and fascia.

4. *Recession versus resection.* In general, weakening of a muscle by recession produces more correction per millimetre of surgery vis-a-vis strengthening of a muscle by resection. Therefore, relatively larger amounts of resection are required to produce an effect comparable to that achieved by recession of the antagonist.

5. *Intractable amblyopia.* In the presence of an intractable amblyopia, it is not possible to predict the results of surgery. This point should be made amply clear to the patient and/or parents.

6. *Medial versus lateral rectus surgery.* In general, a recession of the medial rectus muscle is more effective than the same amount of recession performed on a lateral rectus muscle.

7. *Horizontal versus vertical rectus muscles.* Recession of the vertical rectus muscles is much more effective than the recession performed on the horizontal rectus muscles.

8. *Combined recession-resection operation* provides more correction than the added results of each procedure, when performed alone. Further, this procedure is more effective in stabilizing the surgical results vis-a-vis single procedure, since the resection procedure reduces the amount of contracture that normally occurs in recessed antagonist.

ROUGH ESTIMATES OF AMOUNT OF SQUINT SURGERY

As mentioned earlier, it is not possible to provide a surgical dose-response curve or tables for correcting strabismus. Nevertheless, the conclusions drawn by experienced surgeons may serve as rough estimates for the beginners. However, once again it is stressed that surgeons should standardize their own approach by retrospectively and continuously reviewing their own results and adjusting the amount of surgery for attaining the best possible results. For standardizing their surgery, it is mandatory that surgeons should use the ocular motility measurements and judgement made by themselves. The rough estimates of surgical-

Table 15.1 *Rough estimate of amount of extraocular muscle surgery for esotropia*

Deviation in prism dioptres	Monocular surgery in mm		Binocular surgery in mm	
	Recession of +	Resection of	Bilateral or	Bilateral or
	MR	LR	MR recession	LR resection
15	3.0	4	3.0	4.0
20	3.5	5	3.5	5.0
25	4.0	5	4.0	5.5
30	4.5	6	4.5	6.0
35	5.0	7	5.0	6.5
40	5.5	7	5.5	7.0
50	6.0	8	6.0	8.0
60	6.5	9	6.5	9.0
70	7.0	10	7.0	10.0

Table 15.2 *Rough estimate of amount of extraocular muscle surgery for exotropia*

Deviation in prism dioptres	Monocular surgery in mm		Binocular surgery in mm	
	Recession of +	Resection of	Bilateral or	Bilateral
	MR	LR	MR recession	LR resection
15	4.0	3.0	4.0	3.0
20	5.0	4.0	5.0	3.5
25	6.0	4.5	5.5	4.5
30	7.0	5.0	6.0	5.5
35	7.5	5.0	6.5	6.0
40	8.0	6.0	7.0	6.5
50	9.0	7.0	8.0	7.5
60	10.0	8.0	9.5	8.0
70	10.0	10.0	8 mm bilateral LR recession + 8 mm MR resection of one eye	
80			8 mm bilateral LR recession + 8 mm bilateral MR resection	

dosage have been described along with the different types of strabismus. However, for a ready reference, they are again summarized in Tables 15.1 and 15.2.

ANAESTHESIA FOR SQUINT SURGERY

Three types of anaesthesia commonly used in strabismus surgery are:

- Topical anaesthesia
- Local anaesthesia
- General anaesthesia

TOPICAL ANAESTHESIA

Use and indications. It has been recommended that use of topical anaesthesia produces adequate analgesia without affecting the motor supply of extraocular muscles and thus allowing the readjustment of muscle position during surgery to affect cosmetic or functional results. It is specially useful where unpredicted results are anticipated.

Technique. Topical anaesthesia can be achieved by instillation of either 4% cocaine, 0.5% proparacaine or 0.5% tetracaine drops, four times every 4 minutes, before the conjunctival incision is made. It is important to note that after the conjunctiva is opened, further anaesthetic drops should not be instilled, since paralysis of extraocular muscles will occur and thus the main advantage of topical anaesthesia will be lost.

Prerequisites. Topical anaesthesia can be used in co-operative adults only. In addition, a very fine handling is required during surgery under topical anaesthesia. Excessive pulling and manipulation produces pain; so topical anaesthesia is effective for simple recession procedures, and not for resection procedures or for recession procedures involving restricted muscles where exposure is difficult. Further, it is recommended that no barbiturates or high doses of analgesics be given preoperatively, since these will affect the angle of deviation during surgery and thus the mere purpose of topical anaesthesia will be defeated. It should be ensured that a suitable target and cover device should be available in the operation theatre to check the alignment during the procedure.

Disadvantages. Topical anaesthesia is not effective in controlling the pain produced by pulling on or against a muscle and thus not suitable in all cases. Further, it can be used only in very co-operative adults and is thus not much popular.

LOCAL ANAESTHESIA

Local anaesthesia is commonly used for squint surgery in older co-operative children and adults. It allows a very comfortable and smooth surgery by producing lid and ocular anaesthesia and akinesia.

Techniques. Local anaesthesia can be achieved either by—(1) a combination of surface anaesthesia, facial nerve block and retrobulbar block or (2) a combination of surface anaesthesia and peribulbar block.

Surface and topical anaesthesia is achieved as described above.

Facial block. For intraocular surgery, it is necessary to block the facial nerve which supplies the orbicularis oculi muscle, so that patient cannot squeeze the eyelids.

Orbicularis akinesia can be achieved by blocking the facial nerve at its terminal branches (Van Lint block), superior branches (Atkinson block) or proximal trunk (O'Brien or Nadbath block).

1. *Blocking the peripheral branches of facial nerve (Van Lint's block):* This technique blocks the terminal branches of the facial nerve, producing localised akinesia of the orbicularis oculi muscle without associated facial paralysis.

In this technique, 2.5 ml of anaesthetic solution is injected in deeper tissues just above the eyebrow and just below the inferior orbital margin, through a point about 2 cm behind the lateral orbital margin, level with outer canthus (Fig. 15.1).

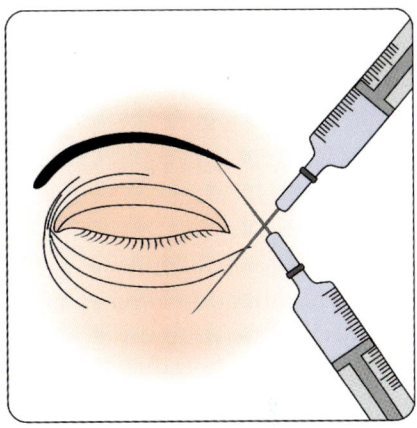

Fig. 15.1 *Technique of van Lint's facial block.*

2. *Facial nerve trunk block* at the neck of mandible (O'Brien's block). In it, facial nerve is blocked near the condyloid process. The condyle is located 1 cm anterior to the tragus. It is easily palpated, if the patient is asked to open and close the mouth with the operator's index finger located across the neck of the mandible. At this point, the needle is inserted until contact is made with the periosteum and then 4–6 ml of local anaesthetic is injected while the needle is withdrawn (Fig. 15.2).

This technique is associated with pain at the injection site and unwanted facial paralysis.

3. *Nadbath block:* In this technique, the facial nerve is blocked as it leaves the skull through the stylomastoid foramen. This block is also painful.

4. *Atkinson's block:* In it, superior branches of the facial nerve are blocked by injecting anaesthetic solution at the inferior margin of the zygomatic bone.

Retrobulbar block. It was introduced by Herman Knapp in 1884. It is administered by injecting 2 ml of anaesthetic solution (2%

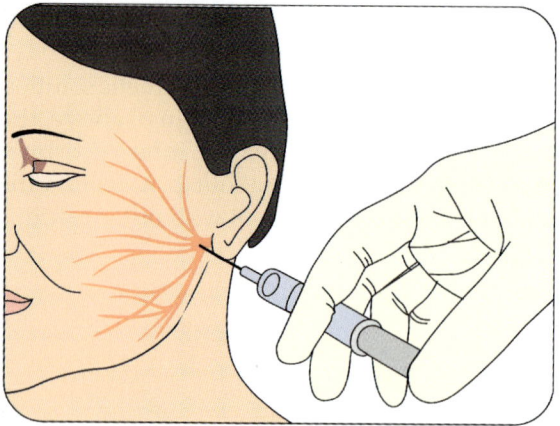

Fig. 15.2 *Distribution of facial nerve and technique of O'Brien's block.*

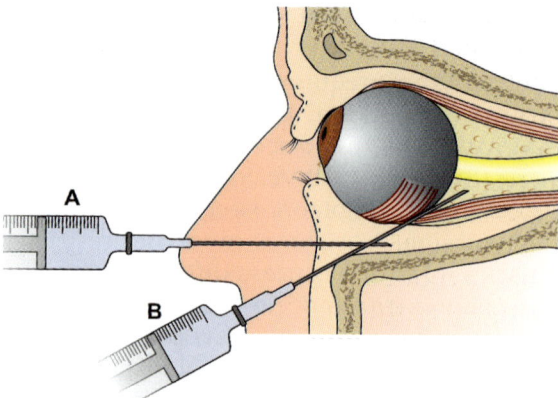

Fig. 15.4 *Position of needle for peribulbar block in the peripheral orbital space (A) and for retrobulbar block in the muscle cone (B).*

xylocaine with added hyaluronidase 5 IU/ml and with or without adrenaline one in one lac) into the muscle cone behind the eyeball. It is usual to give the injection through the inferior fornix or the skin of outer part of lower lid, with the eye in primary gaze (Fig. 15.3B). The needle is first directed straight backwards then slightly upwards and inwards towards the apex of the orbit, up to a depth of 2.5 to 3 cm (Fig. 15.4B).

Retrobular block anaesthetises the ciliary nerves, ciliary ganglion and third and sixth cranial nerves thus producing globe akinesia, anaesthesia and analgesia. The superior oblique muscle is not usually paralysed as the fourth cranial nerve is outside the muscle cone.

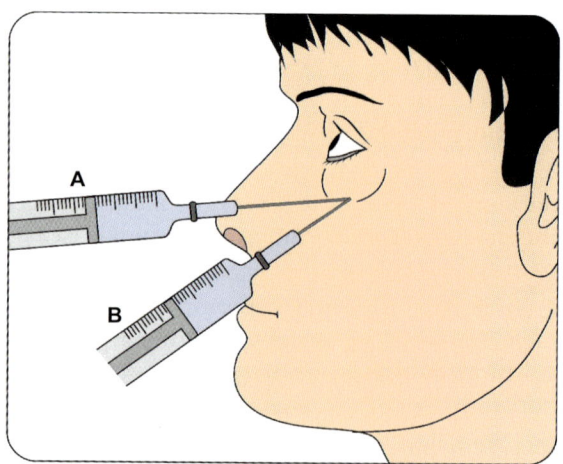

Fig. 15.3 *Position of needle on the lower eyelid skin for peribulbar block (A) and retrobulbar block (B).*

Complications encountered with it include retrobulbar haemorrhage, globe perforation, optic nerve injury, and extraocular muscle palsies.

Peribulbar block. This technique described in 1986 by Davis and Mandel has almost replaced the time tested combination of retrobulbar and facial blocks, because of its fewer complications and by obviating the need for a separate facial block.

Primarily, the technique involves the injection of 6–7 ml of local anaesthetic solution in the peripheral space of the orbit (Fig. 15.4A), from where it diffuses into the muscle cone and lids, leading to globe and orbicularis akinesia and anaesthesia. Classically, the peribulbar block is administered by two injections; first through the upper lid (at the junction of medial one-third and lateral two-thirds) and second through the lower lid (at the junction of lateral one-third and medial two-thirds) (Fig. 15.3A). After injection orbital compression for 10–15 minutes is applied with digital massage, superpinky or any other method.

The anaesthetic solution used for peribulbar anaesthesia consists of a mixture of 2% lignocaine, and 0.5–0.75% bupivacaine (in a ratio of 2:1) with hyaluronidase 5 IU/ml and adrenaline one in one lac.

GENERAL ANAESTHESIA

Indications. General anaesthesia is indicated for squint surgery in infants, small children and also in anxious, uncooperative and mentally retarded adults and those patients willing for surgery only under general anaesthesia.

Special consideration during general anaesthesia for squint surgery

- It is recommended that if the child with esotropia is on miotic therapy (phospholine iodide or other cholinestrase agents), it should be discontinued at least 6 weeks prior to surgery so that the blood cholinestrase levels can be returned to normal before surgery. If this has not been possible, the anaesthesiologist should be warned that the use of succinylcholine is contraindicated.
- Since succinylcholine causes sustained contraction of extraocular muscles for about 20 minutes, so it will alter the forced duction test (FDT). Therefore, it is better to use a non-depolarising muscle relaxant in squint surgery, since it will not alter the FDT.

Advantages of general anaesthesia. The main advantage of general anaesthesia is that it produces complete analgesia and akinesia and does not require patient's cooperation during the surgical procedure. Needless to say that while performing surgery under general anaesthesia, the ophthalmologist is most comfortable and is relieved of serious responsibilities.

Disadvantage of general anaesthesia in squint surgery. (1) In general there is increased risk, i.e. not present in topical and local anaesthesia. (2) General anaesthesia is more costly and requires services of an experienced anaesthesiologist. (3) Incidence of oculocardiac reflex (bradycardia), oculodepressor reflex (hypotension) and oculorespiratory reflex (apnoea) is higher under general anaesthesia. Therefore, it is recommended that a retrobulbar anaesthesia should be given (to block the afferent pathway of these reflexes), even when the squint surgery is being done under general anaesthesia. (4) Under general anaesthesia, it is not possible to relate eye position with the preoperative deviation and postoperative results. This preposition is to be particularly kept in mind in esotropia, since the eye under general anaesthesia may look less esotropic or even exotropic. This situation may intimidate an inexperienced surgeon, who may perform less surgery, resulting in under-correction; and thus another surgery may be required.

COMMON OPERATIVE STEPS IN SQUINT SURGERY

Fixation of the globe

For fixation and rotation of the globe in different directions, 6-0 or 5-0 Mersilene or silk suture on spatulated needle is passed through the conjunctiva and episcleral tissue *near the limbus* at following positions:

- For horizontal rectus muscle surgery—at 12 and 6 o' clock positions (Fig. 15.5A).
- For vertical rectus muscle surgery—at 9 and 3 o'clock positions.
- For inferior oblique muscle surgery—at about 4½ o'clock in left eye and at about 7½ o'clock in right eye (i.e. near the limbus in inferotemporal quadrant).

After applying the traction sutures the eyeball is rotated away from the muscle on which surgery is being performed, e.g. laterally for surgery on the medial rectus (Fig. 15.5A).

Conjunctival incision and exposure of the muscle

The conjunctival approaches recommended for exposure of the rectus muscles are: (1) Limbal incision approach, (2) transconjunctival or Swan approach, and (3) cul-de-sac or fornix approach.

The technique, advantages and disadvantages of each approach are described here in brief.

Limbal incision or von Noorden's approach

Technique

1. At the limbus, conjunctiva and Tenon's capsule are fused together. This conjoined tissue is grasped close to the limbus with forceps and a small radial incision perpendicular to the limbus is made with the help of scissors (Fig. 15.5B).

2. The dissection is then carried concentric with the limbus by spreading the blades of a blunt-tipped Westcott spring-action scissors beneath the conjoined layer; which is then severed.

3. Generally, perpendicular incision of about 4–5 mm long are made at both ends of the limbal

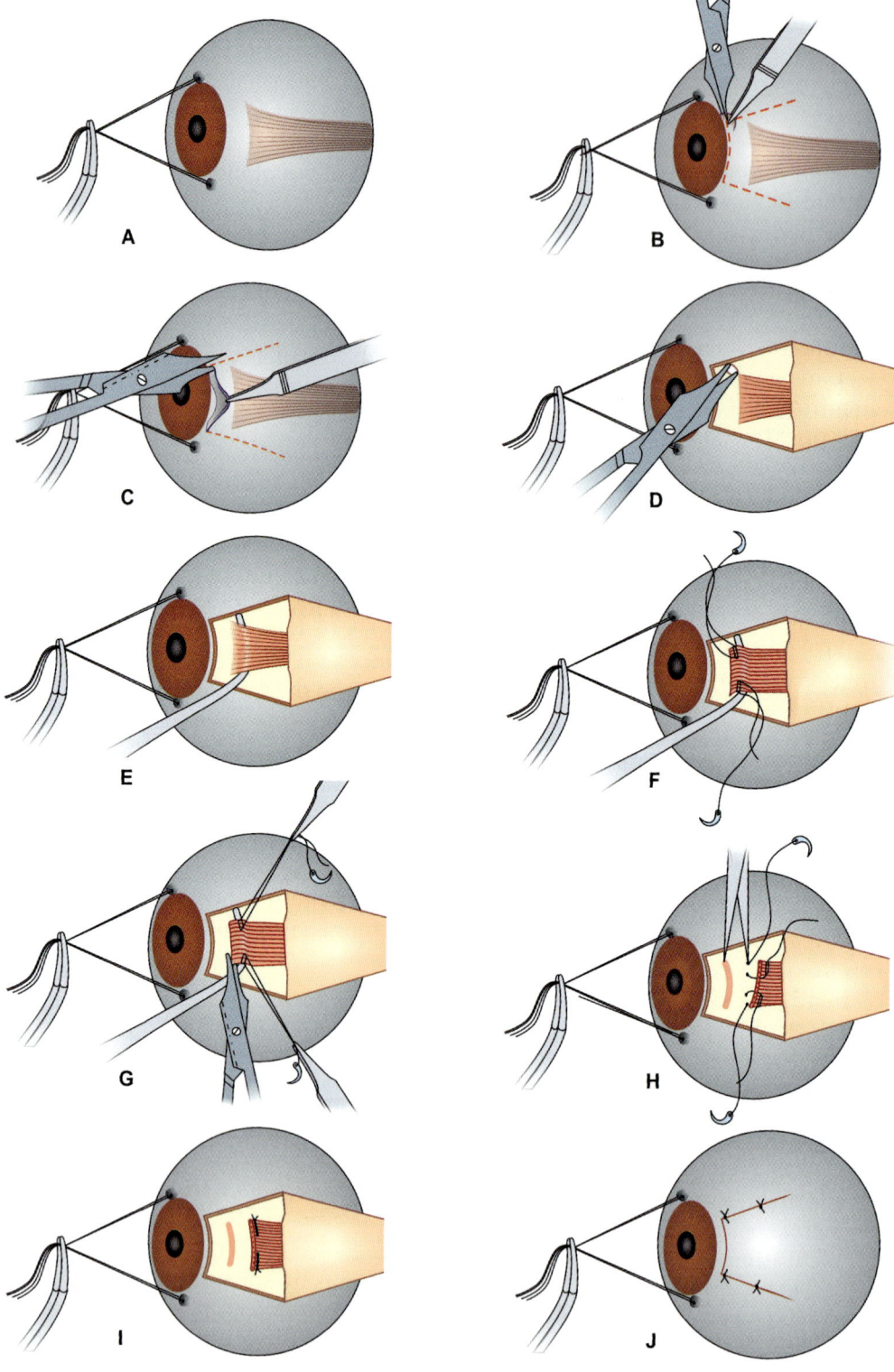

Fig. 15.5 *Surgical technique of medial rectus recession (for explanation, see text).*

incision to facilitate exposure (Fig. 15.5C). However, some surgeons prefer only one perpendicular incision.

4. The limbal incision provides a direct access to the Tenon's space. To separate the anterior Tenon's capsule and intermuscular septum from the sclera, the blades of a curved Steven's tenotomy scissors are inserted into the upper and lower quadrants and the blades are spread gently only once (Fig. 15.5E).

5. A muscle hook is then inserted below the muscle near its insertion and the muscle is engaged by rotating the hook 180° (Fig. 15.5E).

6. The muscle is made prominent by applying traction with the hook and lifting away the conjunctival flap (Fig. 15.5H).

7. For a good exposure, the borders of the muscle are then freed by sharp dissection of the facial connections and the conjunctival surface of the muscle in the anterior part is freed after severing the check ligaments.

8. The muscle surgery is then performed as per requirement (Fig. 15.5F to I) and after completion of the procedure, the wound is closed by applying sutures through the edges of the conjunctival flap and the limbal tissue near the incision. Additional sutures are applied to close the radial incision as per requirement (Fig. 15.5J).

Advantages of limbal incision

- It provides a direct access to the Tenon's space and thus a very little dissection of Tenon's capsule is required to reach the muscle insertion; this cuts down the bleeding and scarring.
- With this incision, the normal anatomic relations of Tenon's capsule and conjunctiva are least disturbed and that it allows a fine closure.
- This technique is easy and quick and allows optimal cosmetic and functional results.
- It is essential for a bare sclera closure (i.e. for conjunctival recession).
- It is the most comfortable approach for adjustable muscle surgery.

Note. Because of the above advantages, the limbal incision has become technique of choice for conjuctival recession, adjustable suture surgery, repeat surgery and muscle transpositions.

Disadvantages

The disadvantages are a reasonably frequent occurrence of dellen and retraction of the conjunctival flap postoperatively but these are minimal.

Over the muscle incision (Swan approach)

Technique

In this approach, an incision in both, the conjunctiva and Tenon's capsule is made over the muscle. For the medial rectus, the incision is placed 1–2 mm anterior to the plica semilunaris and for the lateral rectus, the incision is made midway between the limbus and the lateral fornix. The sub-Tenon's space is freed by spreading the scissors points. The muscle is engaged by the muscle hook and is freed from facial connections by sharp dissection.

Advantages

The only advantage of this approach is that limbal area is not disturbed and so there are no chances of formation of cosmetically unsatis-factory ridge at the limbus and thus no problem of dellen formation.

Disadvantages

This incision has been reported to produce fibrosis over the muscle resulting sometimes in a cosmetically unacceptable conjunctival scar and also making the resurgery (when required) more difficult. So, most of the squint surgeons are not preferring this approach.

Cul-de-sac (fornix) incision (Park's approach)

Technique

1. In this approach, a combined conjunctival and Tenon's capsule incision is made in the bulbar conjunctiva just near the cul-de-sac (1–2 mm to the limbal side of cul-de-sac). This incision is parallel to the fornix, approximately 8 mm in length and depending upon the muscle to be operated at following sites:

- For *surgery on medial rectus,* assistant is asked to grasp the limbus in the inferior nasal quadrant and rotate the eyeball upward and outward; and an incision is made in the infero-nasal quadrant which terminates just temporal to the semilunar fold.

- For *surgery on the lateral rectus,* the assistant should hold the limbus in the inferotemporal quadrant and rotate the eyeball up and in, and the incision made in the inferotemporal quadrant should extend temporally from an imaginary line dropped into the cul-de-sac that divides the lateral and middle third of the cornea.

- For *inferior rectus surgery,* incision is made in the inferior cul-de-sac with its centre at 6 o'clock position.

- For *superior rectus surgery,* incision is made in the superior cul-de-sac with its centre at 12 o'clock position.

- For surgery on *inferior oblique muscle,* incision is made in the inferotemporal quadrant (inferior cul-de-sac).

- For surgery on the *superior oblique muscle,* an incision is made in superior cul-de-sac, situated just temporal to the superior rectus muscle.

2. The Tenon's capsule and intermuscular septa are cut down to bare sclera.

3. The muscle concerned is hooked from the bare sclera exposed, freed from the various fascial connections and the muscle surgery is performed as per requirement.

4. In the end of surgery, the conjunctiva is reposited back into the fonix by a gentle massage. Usually, no suture is required to close unless an exposed, gaping wound is visible between the palpebral fissure.

Advantages

1. Often no sutures are required for closure.

2. There are no visible conjunctival or Tenon's scars.

3. This approach is useful not only for horizontal rectus surgery but also for procedures on the vertical recti and obliques.

Disadvantages

1. Technique is bit difficult as compared to the limbal approach.

2. The exposure is depended upon the technique of assistance.

Closure of the conjunctival incision

Following the completion of extraocular muscle surgery, the conjunctival wound should be closed by any of the following techniques depending upon the type of incision given:

1. *Closure of limbal incision* is accomplished by interrupted sutures (Fig. 15.5J).

2. *Closure of over the muscle conjunctival* incision can be carried out either with running sutures or with the interrupted sutures.

3. *Swan closure technique* comprises suturing of Tenon's capsule and conjunctiva independently in two layers. Usually Tenon's capsule is closed with vertical placed 6-0 Vicryl sutures and conjunctiva is closed with horizontally placed 6-0 silk sutures.

4. *Horizontal closure following a vertical incision* by interrupted or running suture is preferred by a few surgeons.

5. *Bare sclera closure technique* is indicated in cases in which previous surgery or injury has led to severe fibrosis of the conjunctiva and episcleral tissues, producing a mechanical limitation of motion. Making of the limbal incision is mandatory, when bare sclera closure technique is planned. In this technique, the conjunctiva is attached directly to the sclera by interrupted sutures, leaving a bare scleral area between the conjunctival margin and the limbus. The area heals by the gradual proliferation of conjunctival epithelium.

Note. It is important to emphasize that the conjunctiva and its closure play an important role in the surgical results. It is mandatory that, following the closure of the conjunctiva, forced ductions be carried out to make sure that the conjunctival closure does not provide any mechanical limitation.

■ RECESSION OF RECTUS MUSCLES

RECESSION OF MEDIAL RECTUS

After the muscle has been exposed by any of the above described techniques (most surgeons are preferring von Noorden's limbal approach), the salient points of the technique of medial rectus recession are as follows:

1. **Exposure of the muscle** (Fig. 15.5A to E). It is especially important on the medial rectus to free

the check ligament, since failure to do so may result in retraction of the caruncle post-operatively. It is also important to ensure whether the muscle is completely engaged or not. It is done by passing a second muscle hook repeatedly under the insertion from above or from below.

2. *Passing of sutures through muscle* (Fig. 15.5F). After the muscle has been meticulously separated, the position of the insertion is noted and two single armed sutures (6-0 Vicryl with spatulated needle) are placed and locked (by whip suture technique) at both margins of the muscle close to the insertion. After the locking stiches, the suture ends are tagged with bulldog clamps for identification.

3. *Cutting the muscle* (Fig. 15.5G). Traction to the muscle hook and sutures is applied and the muscle is cut free of the insertion from the sclera using curved Stevens tenotomy-scissors. Bleeding from the cut insertion site is controlled by applying pressure or using wet field cautery.

4. *Securing of muscle at the new insertion site on the sclera* (Fig. 15.5H). Eyeball is stabilized by grasping the stump of the insertion remaining on the sclera with a forceps and the new insertion (depending upon the predetermined amount of recession) is measured and marked with the help of a caliper. The needles are then passed through the sclera parallel to the limbus at the previously marked distance. It is important to note that needle should be visible at all times while passing through the scleral lamellae, so as to avoid perforation. The muscle is then secured to sclera by tying the sutures (Fig. 15.5I). It is important that the knots be tied securely and to the sclera directly, rather than on top of the muscle. Preferably the muscle should be spread out to its normal width. Following the completion of the reattachment of the muscle, the amount of recession actually carried out should again be measured with the help of caliper.

5. *Closure of the conjunctival incision* should be done depending upon the type of incision used (*see* page 416, Fig. 15.5J).

Limits of medial rectus recession
- *Maximal limits.* Most of the previous reports and conservative surgeons recommend that with a normally acting lateral rectus muscle,

the medial rectus muscle should not be recessed more than 5.5 mm. In the presence of a paralytic lateral rectus, the medial rectus can be recessed up to 6.5 mm. However, recent reports suggest that MR can be recessed up to 7–8 mm without producing significant limitation of adduction postoperatively.
- *Minimal limits.* It has been recommended that minimal limit for MR recession is 3 mm, because recession of MR less than 3 mm has hardly any effect.

RECESSION OF LATERAL RECTUS
- The technique of recession of lateral rectus is essentially the same as that of medial rectus recession.
- It is important to remember that owing to close proximity of the inferior oblique insertion to the inferior border of lateral rectus muscle, the former is commonly hooked and sometimes even along with the latter dissected and inserted. Therefore, an extra care is required to prevent this complication. It is recommended that preferably lateral rectus should be engaged/hooked from the superior border side.

Limits of lateral rectus recession
- *Maximal limits.* Under normal circumstances, lateral rectus should not be recessed more than 8–10 mm. However, in patients with a large degree exotropia in blind eye, the amount of LR recession may be more, but in such cases usually there is slight limitation of abduction postoperatively.
- *Minimal limits.* Minimal amount of lateral rectus recession recommended is 5 mm, since LR recession less than this has little effect per se.

RECESSION OF SUPERIOR RECTUS
- The technique of recession of superior rectus is essentially the same as that described for medial rectus.
- It is important to remember that accidently superior oblique tendon may be hooked while engaging the superior rectus muscle. Care should be taken to avoid it.

RECESSION OF INFERIOR RECTUS
- Essentially, the technique is similar to recession of any other rectus muscle.

However, one should dissect carefully the intermuscular septum and all fascial connections between the inferior rectus muscle and Lockwood's ligament as far posteriorly as possible.

- While dissecting the fascial connections of inferior rectus muscle, one should take care to avoid injury to the nerve to inferior oblique muscle, which enters this muscle just as it passes the lateral border of the inferior rectus muscle, 12 mm posterior to the inferior rectus insertion.

HANG-BACK TECHNIQUE OF RECTUS MUSCLE RECESSION

Hang-back (HB) technique of rectus muscle recession is a type of non-adjustable suspension recession (SR) technique. It is reported to be equally effective and comparatively safer than the conventional recession technique. It is performed for up to 7 mm of recessions.

Surgical steps

1. *Initial steps up to isolation* of the muscle are similar to conventional recession (*see* page 351 and Fig. 15.5A to E).

2. *Passing of suture through the muscle.* A double armed 6-0 Vicryl suture is passed through the muscle 1.0 to 1.5 mm from the insertion. Locked bites are taken at each end of the muscle (Fig. 15.6A).

3. *Disinsertion* of the muscle is then carried out with the help of tenotomy scissors.

4. *Placing of sutures on the sclera for hang-back recession* as described by Potter and Nelson are as follows:

- The suture needles are passed through angled, 5 mm scleral tunnels that are 6 mm apart from each other and begin where the posterior side of the insertion merges with flat scleral fibres and emerge anterior to the insertion as close to each other as possible (Fig. 15.6.B).
- The sutures are then pulled forward until the cut end of the muscle rests firmly against the posterior aspect of the insertion (Fig. 15.6C).
- The calipers are opened equal to the amount of recession and aligned perpendicular to the suture arms. In this position, then the sutures are clamped with a locking needle holder placed just inside the proximal caliper tip

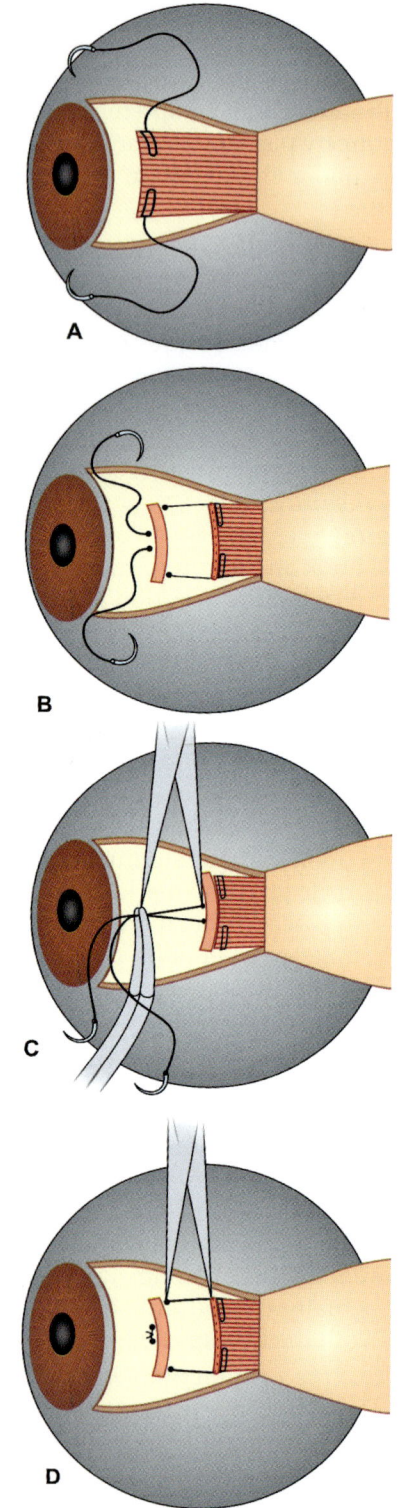

Fig. 15.6 *Hang-back technique of rectus muscle recession (for explanation, see text).*

(Fig. 15.6C). The surgeon must observe metal-to-metal (caliper tip to needle holder tip) contact during this step to pervent asymmetric suture lengths and unequal recession of the ends of the muscle. Four overhand knots are tied and trimmed while the needle holder clamps the sutures firmly.

- The needle holder is then removed and the muscle retracts until the knot rests against the insertion (Fig. 15.6D). The eye is rotated in the opposite direction with the toothed forceps to facilitate the posterior movement of the muscle.
- Finally, the caliper is placed from the insertion to the anterior end edge of the muscle to verify its position (Fig. 15.6D).

5. *Conjunctival closure* is carried out with 6-0 Vicryl sutures as usual (Fig. 15.5J).

HEMIHANG-BACK TECHNIQUE OF RECTUS MUSCLE RECESSION

Hemihang-back (HHB) technique of rectus muscle recession is a type of non-adjustable suspension recession (SR) in which the muscle is reattached and suspended from the sclera posterior to the original insertion. It is performed for more than 7 mm of recession.

Surgical technique

1. *Initial steps up to disinsertion* of the muscle are similar to hang-back technique.
2. *Placing of sutures on the sclera in hemihang-back technique* (Potter and Nelson).

- The calipers are first set on one-half of the total proposed amount of recession (e.g. for 10 mm recession, initial caliper setting should be 5 mm). As in a conventional recession, the calipers are used to mark the entrance points for the scleral tunnels posterior to the insertion. The entry points are marked 6 mm apart (Fig. 15.7A).
- The sutures needles are then passed from the entry point through angled, 3 mm scleral tunnels that emerge next to one another (Fig. 15.7A).
- Further steps to produce another 5 mm of suspension recession are similar to hang-back technique (Fig. 15.7B).
- In the end, the calipers are reset for total amount of recession (10 mm or above) and the total recession from the original insertion is varified (Fig. 15.7C).

3. *Conjunctival closure* is performed as usual.

Advantages of hang-back and hemihang-back techniques

1. The risk of scleral perforation is reduced in both procedures because the surgeon works from a comparatively more anterior site than would be selected in a conventional recession.

2. Advantage of HHB is that it minimizes awkward needle placement in the sclera.

3. These techniques avoid excessive manipulation of the eye which may lead to decreased postoperative inflammation and more effective muscle weakening.

4. Post-equatorial exposure which risks injury to the vortex veins is not required in these techniques.

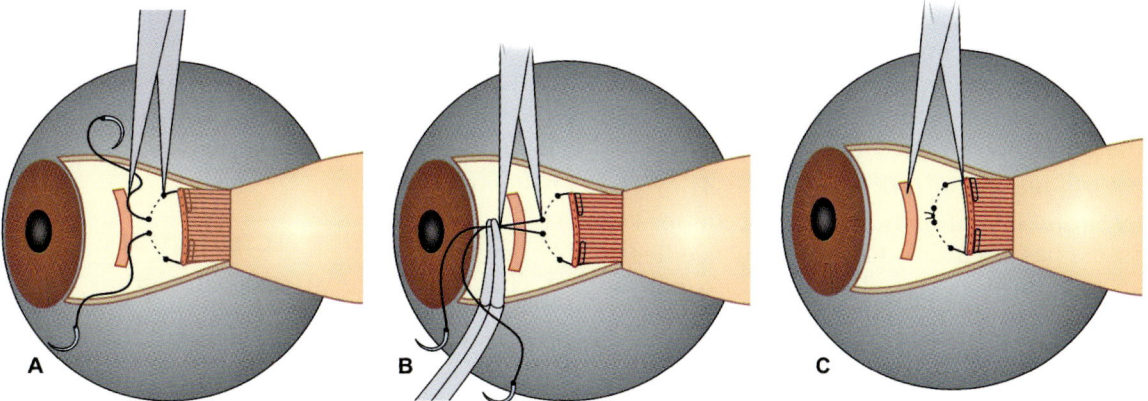

Fig. 15.7 *Hemihang-back technique of rectus muscle recession (for explanation, see text).*

5. Chances of postoperative, induced cyclo-vertical deviations, are less with suspension recession techniques.

RESECTION OF RECTUS MUSCLES

RESECTION OF MEDIAL RECTUS

Steps of the resection of the medial rectus muscle are as follows:

1. *Conjunctival incision* is similar to recession technique (*see* page 415).

2. *Exposure of muscle.* Basic technique is same as described for recession procedure (*see* page 350).

   However, while exposing the muscle for resection, the muscle should be freed only up to requirement for resection, keeping the fascial attachments intact as much as possible (c.f. recession).

3. *Passing of sutures through the muscle.* After the muscle has been meticulously separated, it is slightly stretched using two muscle hooks–one just under the insertion and another about 10 mm away from it. The amount of muscle to be resected is measured and marked with the caliper (Fig. 15.8A). Two double armed 6-0 Vicryl sutures are passed at the marked site and are locked using the whip suture technique (Fig. 15.8B). A Jamson resection clamp or any fine hemostat is applied just anterior to the suture (Fig. 15.8C).

4. *Cutting of the muscle.* The muscle hook near the insertion is stretched and the muscle is disinserted using Westcott or Stevens tenotomy scissors (Fig. 15.8D). Then the muscle tissue anterior to the clamp/hemostat is excised with the help of tenotomy scissors (Fig. 15.8E) (some surgeons do not apply any clamp and cut the muscle tissue 1 mm anterior to the sutures after crushing with a hemostat).

5. *Securing of muscle to the insertion site (technique-I).* After the requisite amount of muscle has been resected, the four needles of the two double-armed sutures are passed through the superficial scleral lamellae just below the original insertion stump in a vertical fashion; one needle of each suture being placed close to the centre of the insertion site and the other through the corresponding end

(Fig. 15.8F). After pulling the cut muscle end up to the old insertion, each suture is tied with a tripple knot (Fig. 15.8G).

Alternative technique of securing the muscle (technique-II). Some surgeons, after marking the resection site, apply the muscle clamp just anterior to it (Fig. 15.9A) and then disinsert the muscle (Fig. 15.9B and C) followed by placing 2-double-armed sutures through the insertion site (Fig. 15.9D). The sutures are then carried through the muscle which is lifted by clamp (Fig. 15.9D). The assistant then pulls the muscle with the clamp towards the old insertion site and the surgeon ties each suture with a tripple knot (Fig. 15.9E). The muscle is then crushed just anterior to the sutures with the help of a haemostat (Fig. 15.9F) and then cut using tenotomy scissors (Fig. 15.9G).

6. *Spring-back balance test of Jampolsky* should preferably be carried out after the completion of resection to prevent overcorrection. To perform this test, eyeball is grasped at the limbus with two fixation forceps (similar to forced duction test) and is rocked back and forth several times in the desired plane and then quickly released noting the velocity of spring back and final position of the eyeball. Following observations may be made:

• If, for example, medial rectus has been over corrected, the eye ball will come to rest in a position of adduction. Under such circumstances, the surgeon should recess the just resected muscle to avoid overcorrection.

• If the position of the eyeball after the spring-back balance test suggests the need for additional strengthening, then the resected muscle should be advanced 2 mm towards the limbus.

7. *Closure of the conjunctiva* is performed as usual (Fig. 15.5J).

RESECTION OF OTHER RECTUS MUSCLES

• The technique of resecting other rectus muscles is essentially the same as described for the medial rectus.

• Special points to be taken care for during each rectus muscle are same as described for the recession technique.

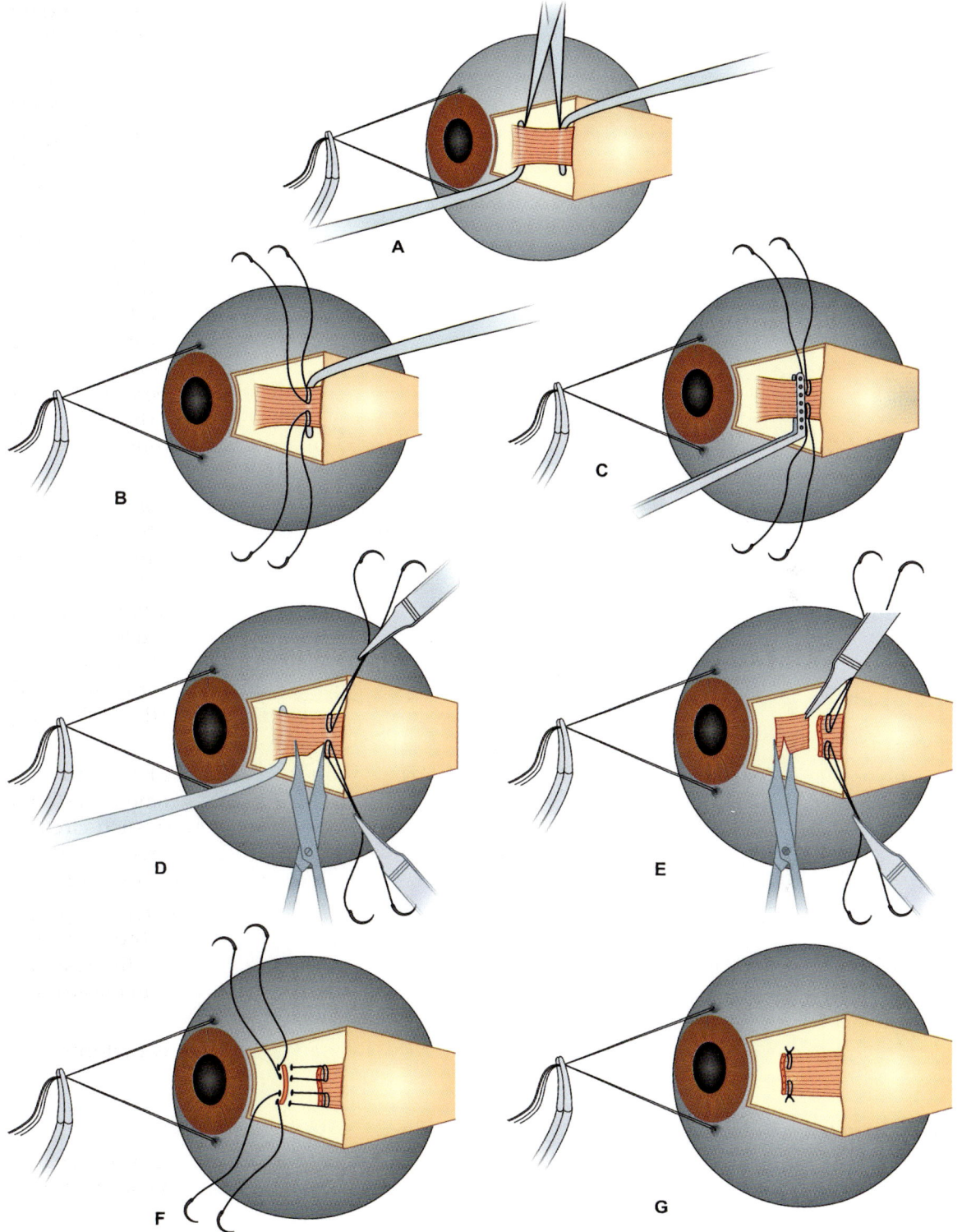

Fig. 15.8 *Surgical technique I of medial rectus resection (for explanation, see text).*

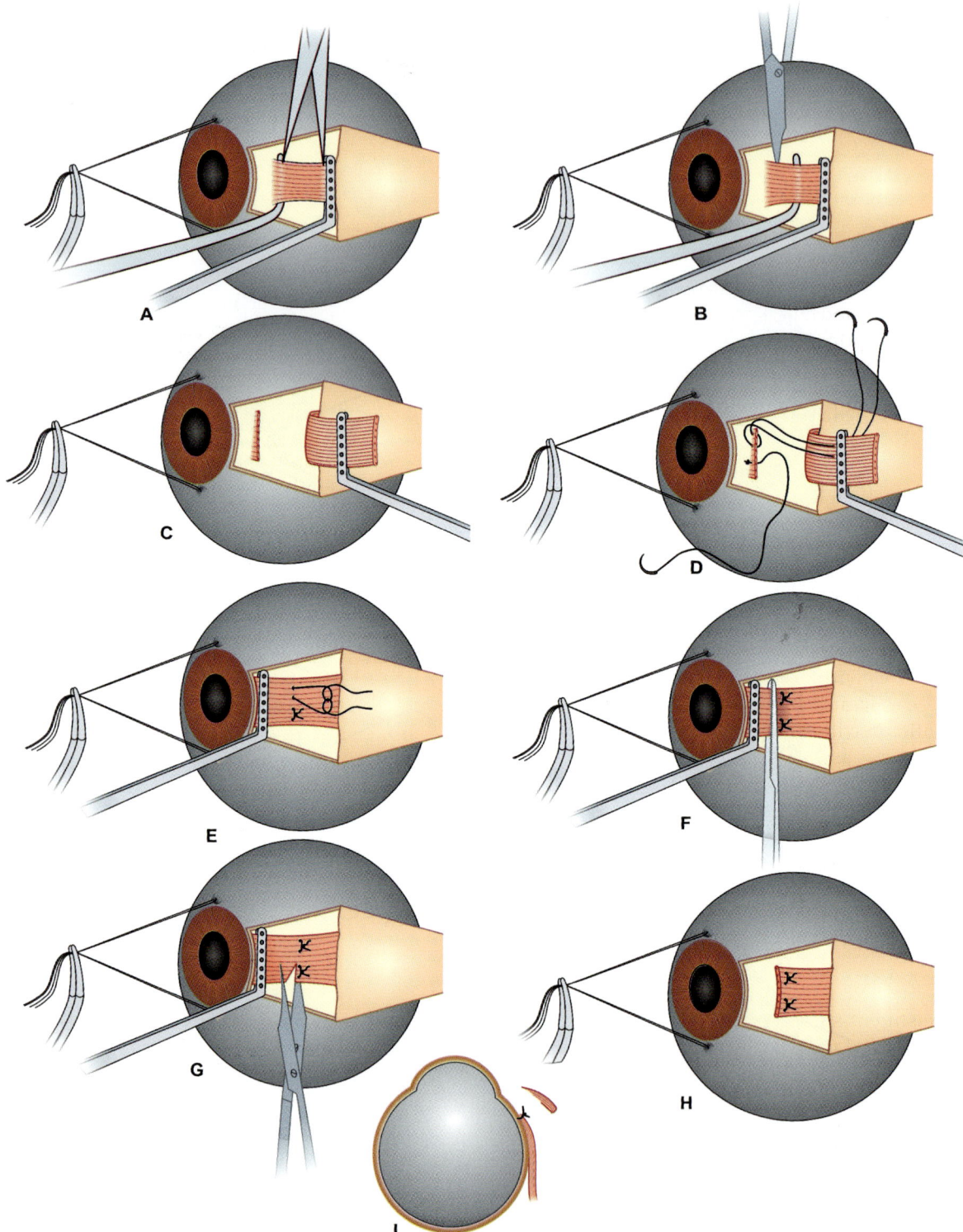

Fig. 15.9 *Surgical technique II of medial rectus resection (for explanation, see text).*

Limits of rectus muscle resection in mm

	Maximal	Minimal
Medial rectus	8–10	4
Lateral rectus	12–14	4–5
Superior rectus	5–6	2–3
Inferior Rectus	5–6	2–3

ADJUSTABLE SUTURES IN RECTUS MUSCLE SURGERY

Keeping in view the unpredictable results of strabismus surgery, the adjustable suture technique which permits alteration in the results in the immediate postoperative period, is becoming popular.

Indications

Should adjustable suture surgery be performed in every case of strabismus is controversial; no convincing data are available to show that long-term results with this technique are superior to conventional methods. However, adjustable surgery is useful in conditions where the results of strabismus surgery are comparatively less predictable, as below:
- Patients with long-standing deviation.
- Acquired strabismus with fusional potential.
- Patients with paralytic squint requiring large recession and resection.
- Patients with restrictive strabismus in which accurate assessment of muscle function is difficult.
- Re-operation.
- Strabismus due to long-standing aphakia with good visual acuity, bothered by diplopia.
- All cases of strabismus where diplopia is the prime problem and thus needs precise postoperative results.

Prerequisites

Adjustment suture surgery needs an alert and attentive patient who will co-operate for measurement of the deviation in required position. In general, adjustable suture surgery can be undertaken in adults and children above 11–12 years of age who will be able to co-operate for the procedure.

Technique

Various adjustable strabismus surgery techniques include, 'pull over (stay) sutures', 'topical anaesthesia' or 'awake strabismus surgery', post-operative adjustable (two stage) surgery and 'operation/reoperation technique'. Out of these, 'postoperative adjustable (two-stage) suture technique' is most popular. Therefore, only this technique will be discussed here.

Steps of postoperative adjustable suture technique with recession

1. *Initial surgical steps* up to meticulous exposure of the muscle are same as in usual recession procedure (*see* page 415).
2. *Passing of suture in the muscle.* A double-armed 6-0 Vicryl suture is passed and tied through the centre of tendon and then passed and locked through its upper and lower edges, near the insertion (Fig. 15.10A).
3. *Cutting of the muscle.* The muscle is severed near its insertion with tenotomy scissors.
4. *Placing of sutures in the sclera.* In this technique, instead of placing sutures in the sclera at a measured distance away from the original insertion (as done in usual recession), the sutures are passed directly through the insertional stump. To facilitate postoperative suture adjustment, the scleral tunnel created by the suture is widened by moving the sutures back and forth several times. The muscle is allowed to recede a desired amount of recession, measured by caliper (Fig. 15.10B), and the sutures are tied first with a single knot, and then with a bow knot (Fig.15.10C). The end of the suture that will open the knot is cut long for later identification.
5. *Closure of conjunctiva.* The knot is kept exposed by suturing the conjunctival flap on either side of the insertion stump using bare sclera technique of closure (Fig. 15.10C).
6. *Placing of traction suture.* Lastly, a traction suture (5-0 Mersilk) may be inserted through the superficial sclera between the limbus and the old tendon insertion. This will act as a 'globe-control handle' and facilitate exposure by rotating the globe during suture adjustment. It is important to note that at the end of the surgery, pad and bandage is done without using ophthalmic ointment, since it can make muscle suture manipulation more difficult.
7. *Postoperative adjustment.* One has to wait for the adjustment of suture till the anaesthetic effect

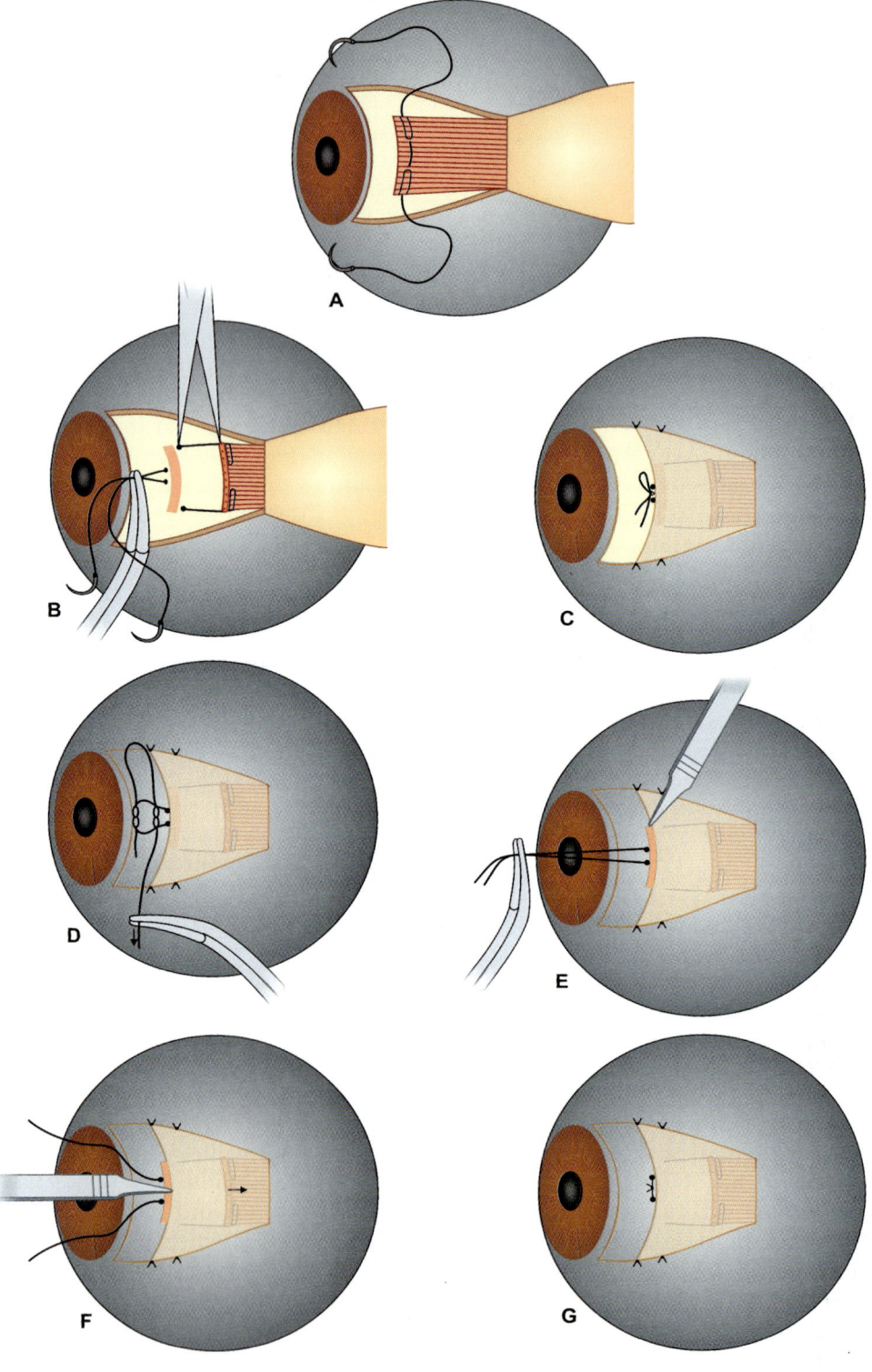

Fig. 15.10 *Surgical steps of recession using two-stage postoperative adjustable sutures technique.*

has worn off. This is variable in the individual cases. Most surgeons prefer to do it on the second day. The procedure is done while the patient sits on a chair with back rest as follows:

- *Assessment of deviation.* On second day, after removal of the patch, the amount of deviation is assessed by prism cover test. In cases of refractive error, this is done with optical correction. In case of diplopia, Maddox rod is used appropriately. Two or three measurements should be taken with 20–30 minutes interval before adjustments.

- *Topical anaesthesia and separation of lids.* Once the deviation is stabilized, topical anaesthetic drops are instilled twice or thrice into the conjunctival sac. The lids are separated by using a speculum. The bow knot is loosened, by using a needle holder and tying forceps and is adjusted accordingly (Fig. 15.10D).

- *Suture adjustment.* In case of overcorrection, the muscle is pulled forward by the sutures while the globe is fixed with help of a forceps applied at the insertion stump (Fig. 15.10E). In case of undercorrection, the muscle is pushed backward. To do this, globe is pulled with the help of traction suture or a forceps applied at the insertion stump in the opposite direction, e.g. temporally in case of medial rectus recession (Fig. 15.10F) and the patient is asked to look in the direction of field of action of the recessed muscle. This manoeuvre allows the muscle to slide further posteriorly. Practically, it is easy to pull the muscle forward rather than pushing it backward. For this reason, most of the surgeons prefer to do 1 or 2 mm more recession than the required amount. After the adjustment is completed the sutures are permanently tied with a tripple knot (Fig. 15.10G).

Steps for postoperative suture adjustment with resection

1. *Initial steps* up to exposure of the muscle are same as for usual surgery.

2. *Placing of sutures in the muscle.* While using adjustable sutures for resection, the sutures are placed approximately 3 mm posterior to the desired amount of resection. For example, if the muscle to be resected is 5 mm, the sutures are placed 8 mm from the insertion in a manner similar to that for recession.

3. *Resection of muscle.* 8 mm of the muscle segment is then resected as done for usual resection.

4. *Placing of sutures in the sclera.* The two needles of the double-armed suture are then passed under the original insertion stump similar to adjustable suture recession. The bow knot is then tied after allowing the muscle finally to rest 3 mm from the original insertion, thus effectively resulting in a 5 mm resection.

5. *Rest all other steps up to final adjustment* are similar to the adjustable suture surgery for recession.

Disadvantages of adjustable suture surgery

1. Increases the total operation time during primary surgery.
2. Requires an additional procedure.
3. A vaso vagal attack can occur while pulling on the muscle.
4. During adjustment, suture can break causing a slipped muscle.

Contraindications of adjustable suture surgery

1. Children and uncooperative adult patients.
2. Variable angle of deviation like in intermittent exotropia, where the patient tries to control the deviation.
3. Surgery involving angulation or displacement of the muscle.
4. Surgery on oblique muscles.

MARGINAL MYOTOMY

Marginal myotomy refers to weakening of a muscle by giving an incision partly through the muscle margin.

Indications

The operation is most often used, when further weakening of a maximally recessed muscle is desired. For example, a marginal myotomy of one of the recessed muscle can be done, if a patient has been undercorrected following bilateral lateral rectus recession for exotropia or bilateral medial rectus recession for esotropia.

Technique

1. *Initial steps up to exposure of the muscle* are similar to usual recession.

2. *Marginal myotomy.* After the muscle has been exposed meticulously, it is held under tension with two large hooks. Haemostasis is obtained by briefly crushing the tissue to be cut with mosquito haemostats. The inferior haemostat is applied 3–4 mm behind the insertion and the superior haemostat is applied 3–4 mm posterior to this (Fig. 15.11A). Marginal myotomy is then performed with the help of tenotomy scissors, cutting about 70% of the width of the muscle in the crushed area (Fig. 15.11B). It is important to note that posterior incision should always be made before the anterior one to prevent distortion of the muscle. Otherwise the distortion of the muscle will make it difficult to gauge the length of second incision. Figure 15.11C depicts the muscle lengthening after completion of myotomy.

3. *Closure of the conjunctiva* is done as usual for muscle surgery (Fig. 15.5J).

◼ FADEN OPERATION

Faden operation also known as *posterior fixation suture* or retroequatorial myopexy is a weakening procedure for the rectus muscles that weakens the muscle only in its field of action by decreasing the mechanical advantage of the muscle acting on the globe.

Indications

This operation was first described by Cuppers in Germany. The term Faden in German means a suture or a sling. Indications of Faden operation are as follows:

1. *Dissociated vertical deviation.* Suture is placed in the superior rectus with or without recession to treat vertical deviations.

2. *Nystagmus blockage syndrome.* Suture is placed on the medial rectus with its recession to treat the esotropia present in primary position.

3. *Incomitant strabismus.* In patients who are orthotropic in primary position but have diplopia in peripheral position of gaze sutures are placed on the appropriate muscle for the desired weakening effect.

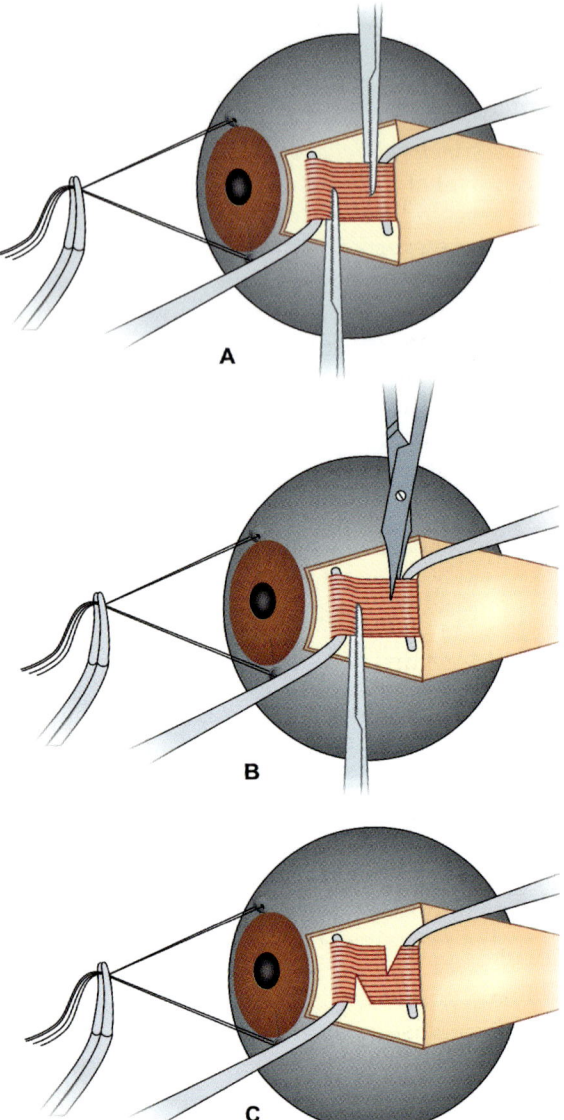

A

B

C

Fig. 15.11 *Surgical technique of marginal myotomy.*

4. *Vertical strabismus present only in down gaze.* Sutures are placed on the inferior rectus of the hypotropic eye.

5. *Duane's retraction syndrome type I.* The procedure is used to treat upshoot and downshoot of the adducted eye.

6. *Laterally incomitant exotropias* may also be managed by the Faden operation.

7. *Non-accommodative type of convergences excess esotropias* are also reported to be corrected by this procedure.

8. *Near esotropias with high AC/A ratio* which is poorly controlled with hyperopic correction, bifocals and miotics may be successfully treated with bimedial recession combined with Faden operation.

Surgical technique

1. *Initial steps* up to exposure of the muscle are similar to those described for a usual recession procedure.

2. *Rotation of the globe.* Application of posterior fixation suture requires an excessive rotation of the globe in opposite direction. This can be accomplished by applying additional traction suture at the insertion site (Fig. 15.12A).

3. *Placing of posterior sutures.* Faden operation is performed with or without recession of the muscle as per indication. When combined with recession, first the muscle is disinserted from the original insertion. The posterior fixation sutures (5–0 Mersiline non-absorbable) are placed through the superficial scleral lamellae 12–15 mm behind the original insertion (Fig. 15.12A). Then the recession procedure is completed as usual and the posterior fixation sutures are passed through the muscle and tied (Fig. 15.12B).

4. *Conjunctival closure* is done in the usual fashion (Fig. 15.5J).

Mechanics of the operation

When a posterior fixation suture is placed, the effective insertion of the muscle is shifted posteriorly. This decreases the muscle power in its field of action without affecting the position of the eyes in primary position. The weakening of the muscle power in this procedure can be understood as an artificial paresis resulting from: (1) reduction of arc of contact (Fig. 15.12C), (2) shortening of the active length of the muscle (Fig. 15.12C), (3) the power of the rectus muscle to rotate the eyeball depends upon the leverage existing between the centre of rotation, C and the line of pull of the muscle at tangential point T (Fig. 15.12D), after Faden suture the moment arm M of the lever system is decreased and more muscle force (3+) is now required to rotate the globe by the same amount (Fig. 15.12E), (4) probably some muscular damage and decrease effectiveness of the muscle contraction

and, (5) a mechanical restriction from reverse leash effect.

After this operation, the weakened (sutured) muscle will require more innervation for a particular movement. According to Hering's law of equal innervation, the increased innervation will also go to its yoke muscle. Thus indirectly this operation also strengthens the yoke muscle in the field of action (Fig. 15.12F and G).

For an appropriate effect von Noorden has recommended the distance of posterior fixation for different muscles as below:

Muscle	Distance of posterior insertion	Idieal distances
Medial rectus	12–15 mm	14 mm
Lateral rectus	13–16 mm	16 mm
Superior rectus	11–16 mm	14 mm
Inferior rectus	11–12 mm	12 mm

Advantages of Faden operation

1. There is decreased likelihood of over-adduction, especially in cases of non-accommo-dative convergence excess.
2. The upshoots and downshoots associated with extreme adduction seen in Duane's retraction syndrome are lessened.
3. Postoperative forced duction following this procedure is free.
4. Last but not the least, it also saves the ciliary blood vessels from damage associated with recession/resection.

Problems associated with Faden operation

1. The procedure needs a vigorous traction of the eyeball to facilitate suture application. Even after this, it is difficult to apply sutures.
2. Vortex vein may be injured.
3. Chances of globe perforation are more.
4. Results are variable. A weakening effect of 0 to 10 prism dioptre in the field of action of muscle is reported. Thus, either under correction or over correction may occur.

INFERIOR OBLIQUE WEAKENING PROCEDURES

Indications

1. *Primary inferior oblique overaction.* Bilateral inferior oblique weakening is indicated for bilateral overaction, even if asymmetrical.

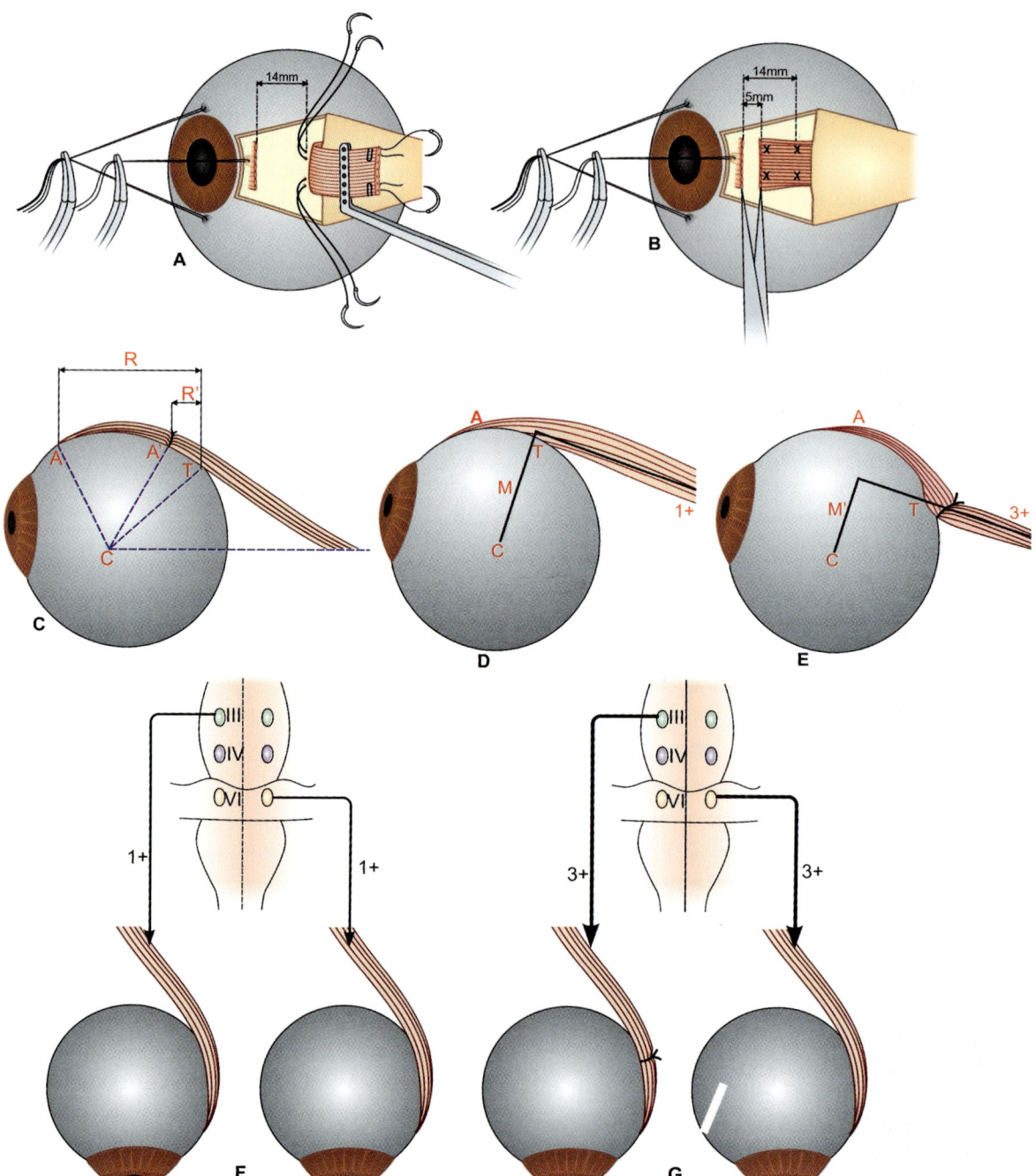

Fig. 15.12 *Surgical technique of Faden operation with recession of a rectus muscle. (A and B) and mechanics of this procedure (C to G). (C) Normal arc of contact* (R) *and reduced arc of contact* (R') *after Faden operation. (D) Normal length of moment arm* (M) *of the rectus muscle lever system; (E) Reduced length of moment arm* (M') *after Faden operation; (F) The innervation required* (1+) *to adduct the fixating nonparetic right eye is insufficient to abduct the left eye of a patient with left lateral rectus palsy; (G) A posterior fixation of the right medial rectus increases the innervational requirment* (3+) *to adduct this eye. According to Hering's law of equal innervation, this increase innervation will also flow to the yoke muscle in the fellow eye and thus will improve the abduction of the left paretic eye.* [C: Centre of rotation; A: Normal anatomical insertion; A: Anatomical insertion after Faden operation; T: Tangential point (physiological insertion); R: Normal arc of contact; R': Reduced arc of contact after Faden operation; M: Normal length of moment arm; M': Reduced length of moment arm after Faden operation].

2. *Secondary overaction of inferior oblique following superior oblique palsy.* Unilateral inferior oblique weakening is indicated.

3. *Double elevator palsy.* Inferior oblique muscle weakening is indicated in the contralateral eye.

4. *Upshoots in Duane's retraction syndrome* can be controlled by the inferior oblique muscle weakening.

Weakening procedures

1. *Disinsertion,* i.e. cutting the muscle from the globe near its insertion.

2. *Myectomy* involves the excision of a segment of muscle belly.

3. *Extirpation* refers to almost complete removal of the muscle.

4. *Recession* involves disinsertion followed by reattachment at the planned site.

5. *Recession with anterior transposition* involves disinsertion and reattachment near the lateral end of the inferior rectus insertion.

The most commonly used procedures are myectomy and recession. Some surgeons prefer disinsertion and others recession with anterior transposition. Each technique has its own inherent advantages and disadvantages. And each surgeon has his own reasons to prefer a particular technique.

DISINSERTION

Surgical technique

Disinsertion alone is carried out through the conjunctival incision placed at the inferior border of the lateral rectus (Fig. 15.13A and B). After conjunctival incision, the lateral rectus is hooked first, then a second hook is passed to engage the inferior oblique muscle near its insertion (Fig. 15.13C). With traction between the two hooks, good exposure is obtained and the muscle is severed from the globe with tenotomy scissors (Fig. 15.13C). The hook is repassed so as to make sure that all fibres of the inferior oblique have been successfully disinserted from the sclera. It is also helpful to make sure that the inferior oblique retracts into the inferior orbital area and that it does not reattach to the point from which it was severed.

Advantages

1. Procedure is very simple and easy.
2. There is no danger of placing sutures over the macular area (of recession).
3. Bleeding is minimum (of myectomy).

Disadvantages

Incidence of recurrence of overaction is very high.

INFERIOR OBLIQUE RECESSION

Surgical technique

1. *Rotation of globe.* Lids are separated with universal eye speculum. A 5-0 Mersiline suture is placed through the fused conjunctiva and Tenon's capsule near the limbus in the infero-temporal quadrant and globe is elevated and adducted by applying traction on this suture (Fig. 15.13A).

2. *Conjunctival incision.* Either cul-de-sac incision (Fig. 15.13A) or limbal incision is made in the inferotemporal quadrant.

3. *Exposure of muscle.* With meticulous dissection of the fascial connections, lateral rectus and inferior rectus muscles are identified and hooked away by the assistant. Anterior border of the fleshly inferior oblique can then be directly visualized (Fig. 15.13B). A muscle hook is then passed between the sclera and inferior oblique to engage the muscle. Inferior oblique is dissected free of the intermuscular septum and the fascia which joins it with the lateral rectus (Fig. 15.13C).

4. *Disinsertion of the muscle* (Fig. 15.13D). After the muscle insertion is exposed meticulously, it is disinserted by tenotomy scissors and the detached muscle is held by assistant with serrated forceps.

5. *Reinsertion of the muscle.* Two 6-0 Vicryl sutures are passed at its detached end and locked by the whip suture technique (Fig. 15.13E). For reinsertion of the muscle to various points on the sclera depending the degree of weakness required, following techniques are in vogue:

i. *Park's technique.* Park recommended that for a 10 mm recession of the inferior oblique, the medial needle should be passed through the sclera at a point 2 mm lateral and 3 mm

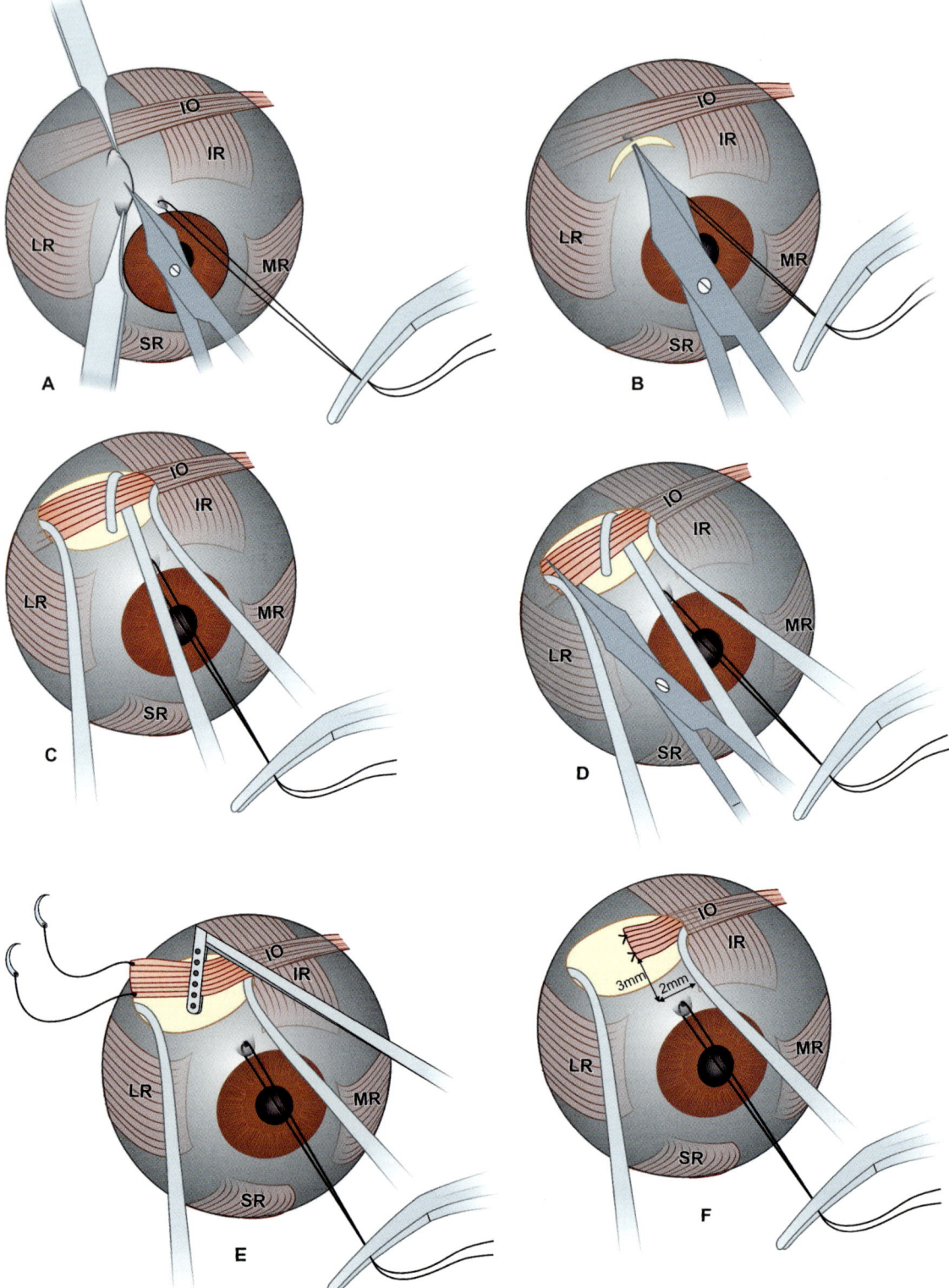

Fig. 15.13 *Surgical technique of inferior oblique disinsertion and recession (for expalnation, see text).*

posterior to the lateral aspect of insertion of the inferior rectus muscle. The lateral needle of the suture is placed more laterally according to width of inferior oblique and about 1 mm more inferiorly and the suture are tied securely (Fig. 15.13F).

It has been reported that 10 mm Park's recession is more effective in weakening vertical functions of the muscle than 10 mm Fink's recession (described below).

ii. *Fink's technique.* The classical Fink's technique utilizes the lower end of lateral rectus muscle as the landmark. For an 8 mm recession, the muscle is inserted at a point 6 mm posterior and 6 mm down to the inferior edge of the lateral rectus muscle. A point 2 mm up or 2 mm down the above point gives a recession of 6 mm and 10 mm, respectively.

iii. *Elliot and Nankin's technique.* This technique provides anterior positioning of the inferior oblique along with its recession. In this technique, whole muscle is fixed just temporal to the inferior rectus muscle insertion.

6. **Closure of the conjunctiva** is done in the end.

Advantages

Presently, recession with or without anterior positioning of the inferior oblique muscle is preferred over disinsertion and myectomy because of the following advantages:

- Recession can be graduated to produce predictable results.
- It can be always be revisited and the surgery can be undone, underdone and overdone.

Disadvantages

Recession of inferior oblique is technically difficult than the disinsertion and myectomy.

INFERIOR OBLIQUE MYECTOMY

Surgical technique

1. *Initial steps* up to exposure of the muscle are similar to those for the recession (Fig. 15.14A to C).

2. *Myectomy.* After meticulous exposures the inferior oblique muscle is clamped with two haemostats applied approximately 8 mm apart

(Fig. 15.14A) and the muscle segment in between the haemostats is excised with tenotomy scissors (Fig. 15.14B and C). It is important to observe that all of the muscle fibres have been isolated and cut. The stumps are cauterized to prevent:

- Postoperative haemorrhage,
- Reattachment of the muscle to the sclera, or
- Reattachment of the two stumps to each other.

3. *Conjunctival closure* is done as usual.

Advantages

- Technically easier to perform.
- Results are as good as recession.

Disadvantages

- Effect cannot be graduated.
- Myectomy is a destructive procedure and once done cannot be controlled.
- Results may be unpredictable depending on where the residual muscle stump reattaches.

■ SUPERIOR OBLIQUE WEAKENING PROCEDURES

Indications

1. **Unilateral weakening** of the superior oblique is not commonly performed except as part of the treatment of:

- Brown's syndrome, and
- Isolated inferior oblique muscle weakness.

2. **Bilateral weakening** of superior oblique is often performed with or without horizontal muscle surgery for A-pattern deviations. This surgery is expected to cause an eso-shift of up to 30–40 prism dioptres in downgaze, little change in primary position and almost no effect in upgaze.

Weakening Procedures

1. Tenotomy, i.e. cutting of the tendon
2. Split lengthening of tendon
3. Recession
4. Silicon expander
5. Translational recession of Prieto-Diaz
6. Posterior tenotomy of superior oblique (PTSO)

SUPERIOR OBLIQUE TENOTOMY

Superior oblique tenotomy can be performed by either nasal approach or a temporal approach.

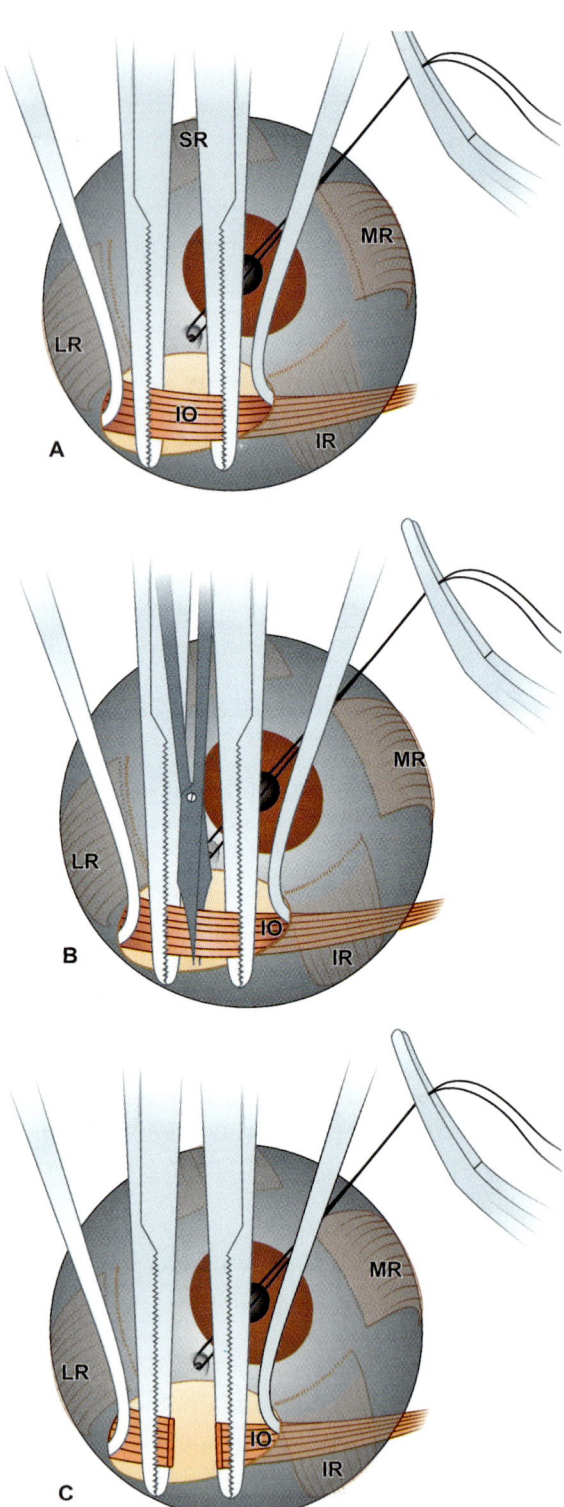

A

B

C

Fig. 15.14 *Surgical technique of inferior oblique myectomy.*

Recently, most surgeons are preferring temporal approach.

Surgical technique for temporal approach of superior oblique tenotomy

1. *Fixation of globe.* Lids are separated with universal eye speculum and a 5-0 Mersiline suture is passed through the conjunctiva and episcleral tissue near the limbus at approximately 11 o'clock position (right eye) or 1 o'clock position (left eye). The eyeball is rotated downward and inward by applying traction on these sutures (Fig. 15.15A).

2. *Conjunctival incision.* An 8 mm cul-de-sac incision is made in the superotemporal quadrant starting just temporal to superior rectus insertion.

3. *Exposure of the superior oblique tendon* is carried out taking following steps meticulously:

- After undermining the conjunctiva, the intermuscular septum (between superior rectus and lateral rectus) is buttonholed and sclera is exposed.
- *Superior rectus muscle is isolated,* and engaged in the muscle hook.
- Assistant further depresses and adducts the eyeball by pulling on the superior rectus muscle insertion with the help of muscle hook. As this is done, the insertion of the superior oblique is pulled down towards the incision.
- At this juncture, the conjunctival incision is stretched temporally and also posteriorly with the help of two separate muscle hooks or lid retractors (Fig. 15.15B).
- Thin and filmy glistening fibres of superior oblique tendon are identified below the superior rectus muscle after retracting it medially with Desmarre's retractor. Then the superior oblique tendon is engaged by a sweeping action of the muscle hook. After the superior oblique tendon is engaged, it takes substance and appears thick.

4. *Tenotomy.* After the superior oblique tendon is isolated on the muscle hook, a complete transection of it is done with the help of tenotomy scissors (Fig. 15.15C). It is recommeded that in bilateral tenotomy, the transection site on each tendon should be at same distance from these insertion point to get symmetric

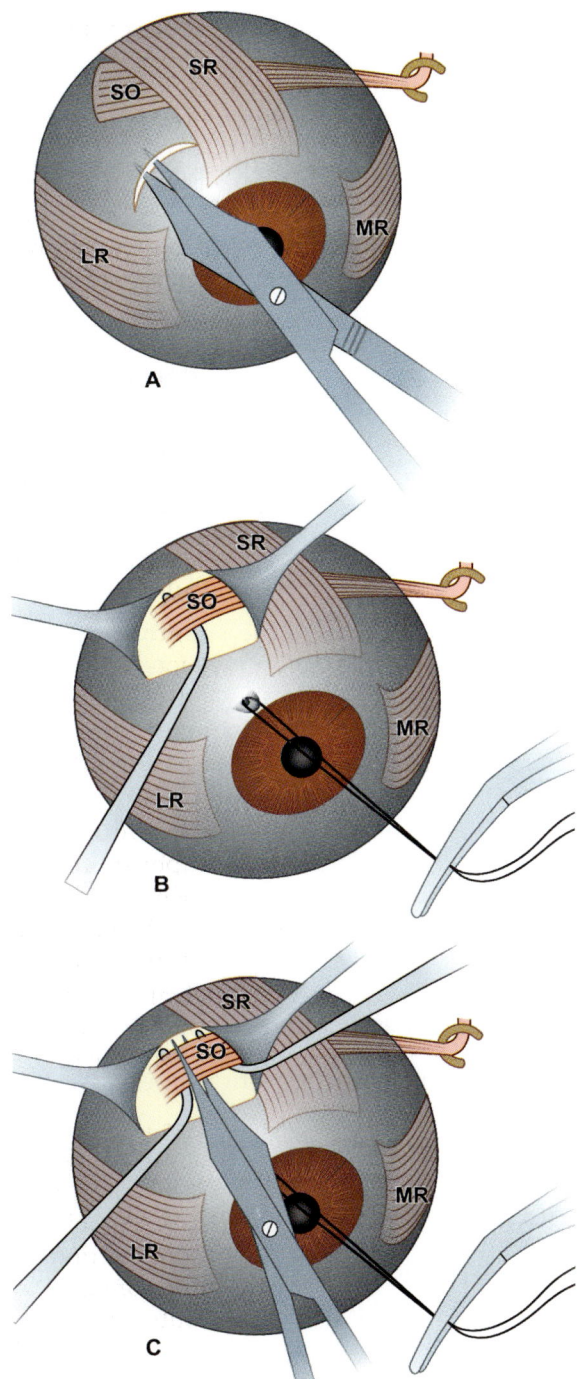

Fig. 15.15 *Surgical technique of temporal approach for superior oblique tenotomy.*

results. Such a measurement is possible with the temporal approach but not with the nasal approach.

Surgical technique for nasal approach of superior oblique tenotomy

1. *Conjunctival incision.* The cul-de-sac incision is made through the conjunctiva and Tenon's capsule in the superonasal quadrant between the medial and superior rectus muscles, about 4–5 mm behind the limbus. The wound is gently spread with the help of tenotomy scissors (Fig. 15.16A).

2. *Exposure of the tendon.* First of all the superior rectus muscle is identified and engaged with a muscle hook. The eyeball is rotated downward and outward by applying traction on this muscle hook. The upper edge of the wound is retracted with a Desmarre's retractor and the glistening white band of the superior oblique tendon is identified (Fig. 15.16B).

3. *Tenotomy.* The superior oblique tendon is engaged with a muscle hook and pulled forward and is dissected meticulously from the surrounding tissues. After the tendon is isolated clearly, it is cut with the help of scissors (Fig. 15.16C).

4. *Conjunctiva is closed* as usual.

Superior oblique tenotomy, temporal versus nasal appraoch

1. *Nasal approach* for performing superior oblique tenotomy without striping the intermuscular septum is considered better for treating Brown's syndrome. Since by this technique, the superior oblique is weakened but some action is retained because of undisturbed attachment of the intermuscular septum to the tendon. It is reported that this retained action of superior oblique avoids the postoperative complication of torsional diplopia.

2. *Temporal approach* is preferred in all other indications, especially when bilateral tenotomy is to be performed, because of the following advantages:

• Exact measurement of the site of transaction of the tendon can be obtained. This allows bilateral symmetric results.

• Complications like blepharoptosis and superior rectus weakness known with nasal approach are almost eliminated by temporal approach.

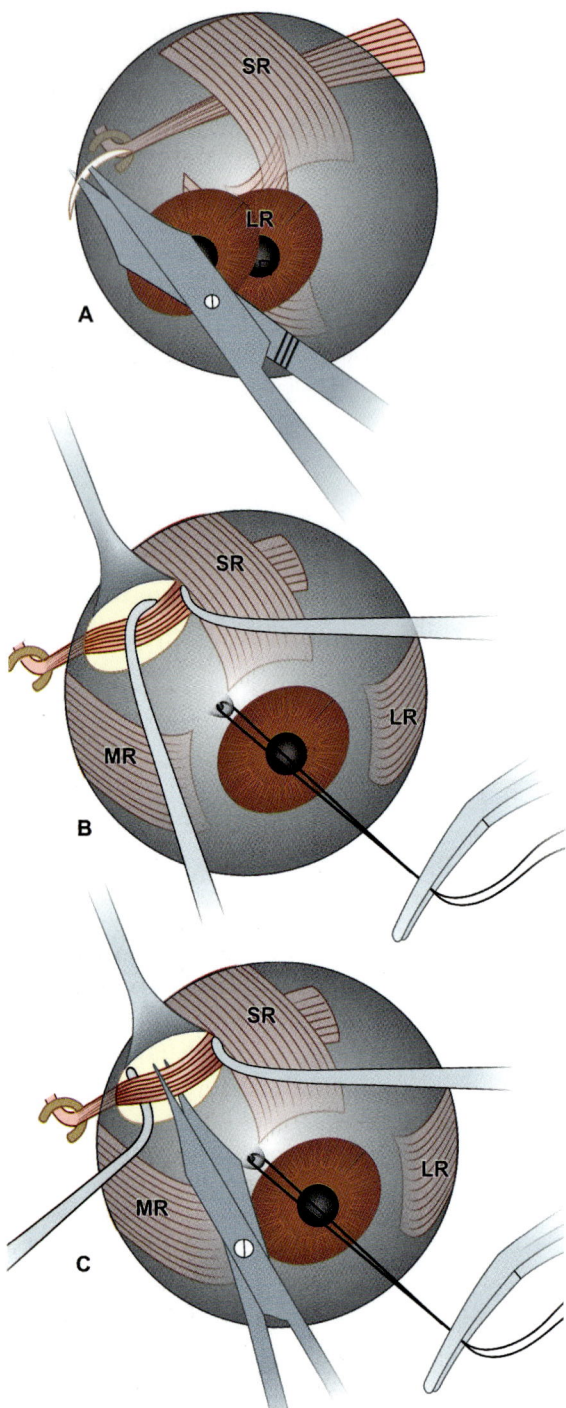

Fig. 15.16 *Surgical technique of nasal approach for superior oblique tenotomy.*

- Occurrence of transient Brown's syndrome has been reported following nasal but not with temporal approach.

- Temporal approach is technically easier than the nasal approach. However, injury to the superior temporal vortex vein is obviously a potential hazard of the temporal approach.

TECHNIQUES OF OTHER WEAKENING PROCEDURES FOR SUPERIOR OBLIQUE

1. In general, *temporal approach* is preferred over the nasal approach for superior oblique weakening procedures.

2. *Initial steps* up to the exposure of the tendon are similar to those described for superior oblique tenotomy.

3. *Final steps* for different weakening procedures are as follows:

   i. *In recession,* the superior oblique tendon is reinserted near the nasal border of superior rectus muscle, about 4 mm posterior to its insertion.

   ii. *In anteropositioning,* the superior oblique tendon is further anteriorized as compared to recession.

   iii. *In translational recession,* the anterior point of superior oblique reinsertion is 4 mm nasal from the superior rectus and 12 mm posterior from the limbus. The advantage of the translation recession is that it prevents the limitation of depression in abduction which occurs with recession or anteropositioning.

   iv. *In superior oblique expander* technique some surgeons insert 2 or 2.5 mm silicon tube (or retinal band no. 240) in between the cut ends of the superior oblique tendon 3 mm nasal to the nasal border of superior rectus muscle.

   v. *Posterior tenotomy of superior oblique (PTSO).* This operation is based on the observation that posterior fibres of superior oblique account for its vertical action. So tenotomy of the posterior fibres of the superior oblique is performed for a selective weakening of its depressor action.

SUPERIOR OBLIQUE STRENGTHENING PROCEDURES

SUPERIOR OBLIQUE TUCK

Indications

1. *In superior oblique paresis,* the tucking procedure helps in enhancing effect.

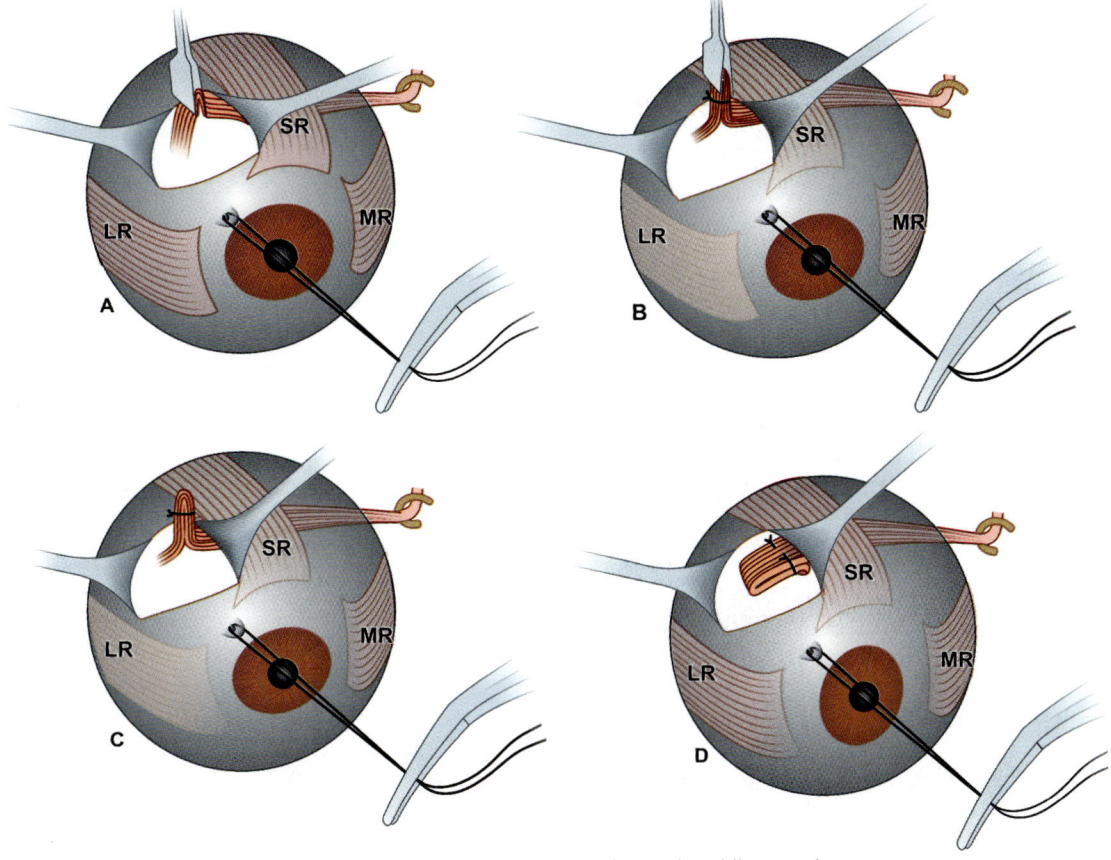

Fig. 15.17 *Surgical technique of superior oblique tuck.*

2. *In DVD,* superior oblique tucking with or without inferior oblique weakening has been advocated.

Surgical technique

1. *Initial steps* up to exposure of the superior oblique tendon are similar to those described for temporal approach for superior oblique tenotomy (*see* page 483 and Fig. 15.15A and B).

2. *Tucking procedure.* After isolating, the tendon is transferred from the muscle hook to a Burch tendon tucker or its von Noorden modification (Fig. 15.17A). The tendon is then lifted upward and pulled taut by turning the screw of the handle of the tendon tucker (Fig. 15.17B). After a sufficient (12–14 mm) tuck has been created on the tucker, two 5-0 Mersiline sutures are placed near the base of tuck (Fig. 15.17C). The sutures are secured and the tucker removed. Previously most of the surgeons used to secure the tip of the tuck to the sclera in the direction

of the original plane of the tendon by an additional suture. However, an inadvertent anterior pull on the tendon during this manoeuver may decrease the vertical effect of the operation and cause pseudo-Brown's syndrome. Therefore, many surgeons prefer not to fasten the tucked portion to the sclera (Fig. 15.17D).

3. *Forced duction test* is performed in the end to determine the degree of restriction when elevating the adducted eye. The tuck is considered adequate when mild elastic restriction is felt. If a severe restriction is encountered, the tucking should be undone followed by a lesser amount of tucking.

4. *Conjunctival closure* is done with one or two 7-0 Vicryl sutures.

Note. A transient postoperative limitation of elevation of adducted eye (psuedo-Brown's syndrome) is a common phenomenon after superior oblique tucking. Rarely a permanent Brown's syndrome may also occur.

HARADA-ITO PROCEDURE

The Harada-Ito procedure is a selective strengthening procedure for anterior fibres of the superior oblique muscle. This procedure essentially consists of anterior and lateral displacement of the anterior fibres of the muscle resulting in an advancement of its insertion around the equator by several millimetres. This operation is based on the idea that the anterior fibres of the tendon are selectively concerned with the torsional action of the superior oblique muscle and that strengthening of these fibres will enhance the incyclotropic effect thereby correcting the excyclotropia.

Indications
This procedure has been reported to be useful in patients with bilateral or unilateral superior oblique palsy for correcting an excyclotropia of 10° or more but without significant primary position vertical deviation.

Surgical technique
1. *Initial steps* up to exposure of the superior oblique tendon are same as described for superior oblique tenotomy (Fig. 15.15A and B).

2. *Anterior and lateral displacement of the anterior fibres of superior oblique tendon* is carried out, after meticulous isolation of the tendon, by any of the following techniques:

   i. *Conventional Harada-Ito technique.* A 5-0 Mersiline (non-absorbable) suture single-armed is passed through the anterior half of the tendon fibres and secured firmly with a tripple knot (Fig. 15.18A). The needle is then passed through the sclera at a point located 3 mm temporal and anterior to the insertion (Fig. 15.18B). At this juncture, secure tying of the suture over its scleral fixation will pull the anterior fibres of the tendon anteriorly and laterally.

   ii. *Fells modification over Harada-Ito technique.* A visual estimate of half the width of superior oblique tendon is made and its insertion is split parallel to its tendinous fibres. A single 6-0 Vicryl suture is placed at the edge of the

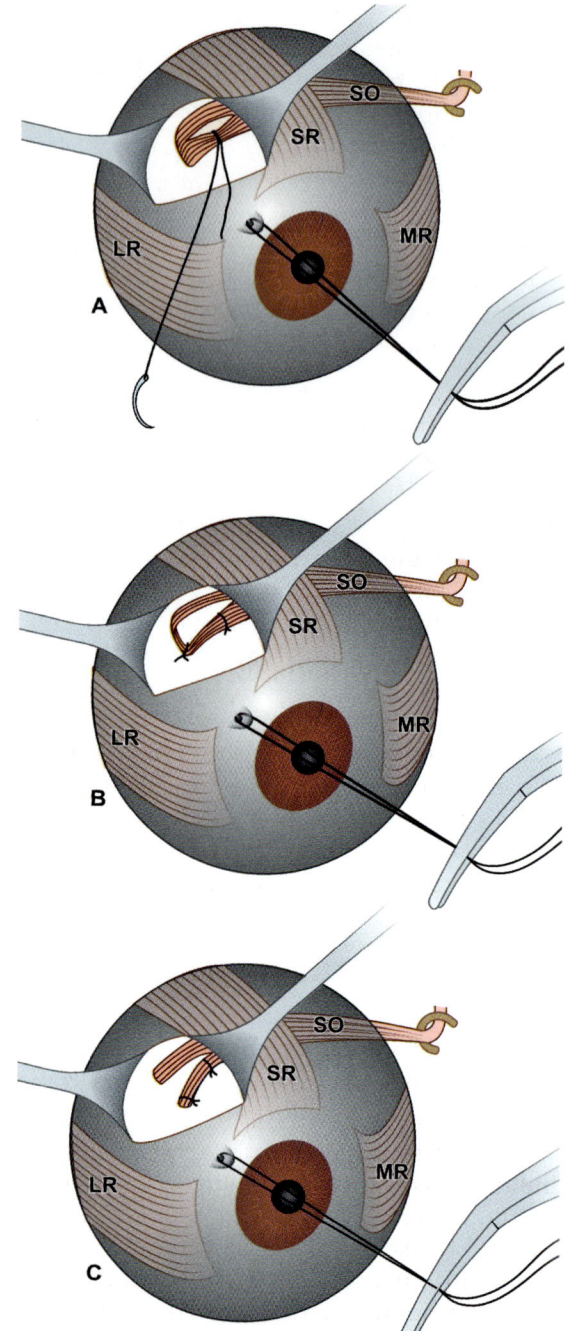

Fig. 15.18 *Surgical technique of Harada-Ito procedure (for explanation, see text).*

anterior half of the insertion. The anterior half of the tendon is then disinserted and reattached to the sclera at a point where the continuation of the lines of insertion of the superior and lateral recti meet. A second single-armed 6-0 Vicryl suture is used to secure the posterior point of the splitted and anteriorly transported anterior half of the tendon approximately 6 mm directly behind this point (Fig. 15.18C).

iii. *Harada-Ito procedure with adjustable suturing technique.* Some surgeons have suggested the use of adjustable sutures after splitting the tendon as in Fells' modification. However, not much advantages are associated with this modification.

3. *Conjunctival closure* is performed with one or two of 7-0 Vicryl sutures.

MUSCLE TRANSPOSITION PROCEDURES

Muscle transposition procedures essentially involve moving the extraocular muscles out of their original planes of action. Such procedures are generally reserved for treatment of paralytic strabismus. The usual situations in which these procedures are used include paralysis of cranial nerves III and VI as well as double elevator palsy. The muscle transposition procedures are also useful in A- and V-patterns, cyclo-deviations and small vertical and horizontal deviations. A few commonly performed muscle transposition procedures are described here.

MUSCLE TRANSPOSITION PROCEDURES IN TREATMENT OF A- AND V-PATTERNS

1. Vertical transposition of the horizontal rectus muscles and horizontal transposition of the vertical rectus muscles has been recommended for correcting A- and V-patterns.

2. Surgical technique of these procedures is similar to recession and resection procedures for rectus muscles except that muscles are reinserted by shifting the insertion between half or one full muscle width as per requirement. Important point to be noted is that even after shifting, the muscle should be reinserted parallel to the limbus.

MUSCLE TRANSPOSITION PROCEDURES FOR TREATMENT OF CYCLODEVIATIONS

1. Horizontal transposition of vertical rectus muscles and vertical transposition of horizontal rectus muscles has been recommended for:

- Correction of cyclotropia, and
- Correction of compensatory head tilt to one shoulder in patients with a nystagmus having null zone in tertiary gaze position.

2. The direction in which the vertical and horizontal rectus muscles be transposed to cause incycloduction or excycloduction of each eye is as follows:

- To cause incyclodeviation, the superior rectus should be shifted temporally and inferior rectus nasally (Fig. 15.19).
- To produce excyclodeviation, superior rectus should be shifted nasally and inferior rectus temporally.
- To produce incyclodeviation, the medial rectus should be shifted upward and lateral rectus downward (Fig.15.20).
- To cause excyclodeviation the medial rectus should be shifted downward and lateral rectus upwards.

3. Surgical technique of these procedures is similar to recession and resection procedure for these muscles, except that muscles are reinserted by shifting the insertion by one-half or one full muscle thickness, as per requirement. Even the shifted reinsertion should be parallel to limbus.

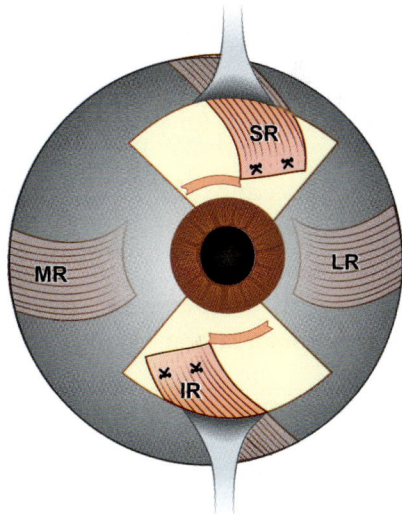

Fig. 15.19 *Temporal transposition of superior rectus tendon and nasal transposition of inferior rectus tendon to produce incyclodeviation.*

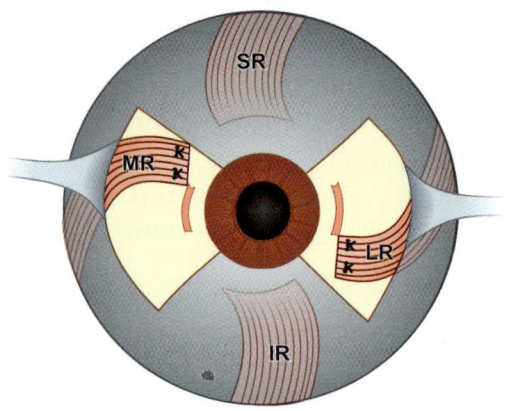

Fig. 15.20 *Upward transposition of medial rectus and downward transposition of lateral rectus to produce incyclodeviation.*

MUSCLE TRANSPOSITION PROCEDURES FOR PARALYTIC SQUINT

- It has been reported that the muscle transposition procedures are useful in paralytic squint by their mechanical effect and not by any innervational adjustment.

- The muscle transpositions are useful in paralytic squint, only if there is no restriction to passive movements of the eyeball in the paretic field of gaze. Therefore, if forced duction test reveals any restriction, it should be removed first by a maximal recession of the contracted antagonist of the paretic muscle with or without conjunctival recession depending upon the need.

- The commonly performed muscle transposition procedures for paralytic squint are as follows:
  - Knapp's procedure
  - Hummelsheim procedure
  - Jensen's procedure
  - Transposition of superior oblique tendon
  - Transposition of lateral rectus muscle

Knapp's procedure

Indication

Knapp procedure consists of transposition of the insertion of medial and lateral recti to that of superior rectus (in patients with double elevator palsy) or inferior rectus (in patients with double depressor paralysis).

Surgical technique

1. *Conjunctival incision* consists of a superior or inferior limbal peritomy of approximately 210° depending upon the indication.

2. *Exposure of the muscles.* The medial and lateral recti and either superior or inferior rectus, are exposed as described in recession for rectus muscles.

3. *Disinsertion of horizontal recti.* After meticulous isolation, as in recession procedure, 6-0 Vicryl sutures are passed near the insertion of medial and lateral recti and the muscles are disinserted from the globe.

4. *Transposition of the horizontal recti.* A Desmarre's retractor is used to hold the conjunctiva out of the surgical field and the medial and lateral recti are reattached to the globe at each corner of the insertion of either superior rectus (in patients with double elevator palsy (Fig. 15.21) or inferior rectus (in patients with double depressor palsy).

5. *Conjunctival closure* is done in the end of surgery.

Jensen's procedure

Indication

Jensen's procedure is indicated in patients with complete paralysis of lateral rectus muscle. It consists of transposition of half thickness muscle of superior and inferior recti to the lateral rectus at the level of equator.

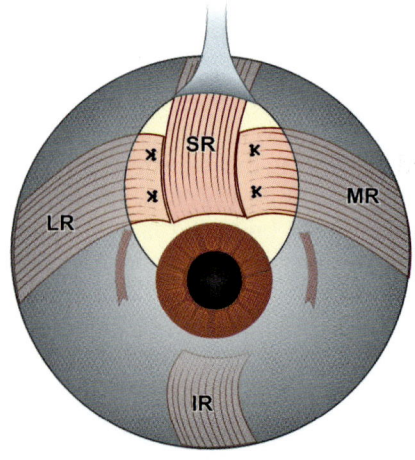

Fig. 15.21 *Knapp's procedure for double elevator palsy.*

Surgical technique

1. *Conjunctival incision* consists of 180° peritomy performed at the temporal half of the limbus.
2. *Exposure of the muscles.* The lateral, superior and inferior recti are meticulously exposed beyond the equator as in recession procedure.
3. *Transposition of the muscles.* The tendons of superior, lateral and inferior rectus muscles are isolated and split posteriorly for approximately 8 mm with the help of a muscle hook. Then the temporal halves of the superior and inferior recti are joined with the corresponding superior and inferior halves of the lateral rectus over the equator using 5-0 Mersiline suture (Fig. 15.22). It is important to note that at least one branch of the anterior ciliary vessel should remain in the nasal segment of each of the vertical recti that are not incorporated in the muscle union. Further, one must ensure that sutures are tied loosely enough to prevent strangulation and necrosis of the muscle.
4. *Recession of the medial rectus.* It is imperative that Jensen's procedure should always be combined with a maximal recession of the ipsilateral medial rectus muscle with or without conjunctival recession to obtain successful results. The recession is performed as usual. To prevent anterior segment ischaemia, especially in older individuals, the recession of medial rectus and conjunctiva should be performed at least 4 to 5 months prior to the actual Jensen's procedure.
5. *Conjunctival closure* is done as usual.

Hummelsheim procedure

Indication

This procedure is indicated in complete 6th nerve palsy in which any contracture of the medial rectus has been eliminated by a previous or simultaneous medial rectus recession.

Surgical technique

Hummelsheim procedure basically consists of total transplant of the superior and inferior rectus muscles to the insertion of the lateral rectus muscle (Fig. 15.23). The surgery is performed through a 180° temporal peritomy and the technique is essentially similar to Knapp's procedure.

Transposition of superior oblique tendon

Indication

Transposition of superior oblique tendon to the insertion of medial rectus muscle is indicated in patients with third cranial nerve palsy. This procedure is always combined with a maximal recession (10–12 mm) of the lateral rectus and resection (8–9 mm) of the medial rectus muscle.

Surgical technique

Superior oblique tendon transposition is performed by nasal approach. In this classical approach, superior oblique tendon is exposed as described for nasal approach for tenotomy (*see* page 435). A small closed mosquito haemostat is then slid along the tendon until its tip enters the pulley of the trochlea. The tendon is freed after fracturing the pulley by just opening the hemostat. The tendon is then shortened by 10–12 mm and is sutured to the sclera near the superior border of the medial rectus muscle. Results of this procedure in improving the adduction are not always encouraging.

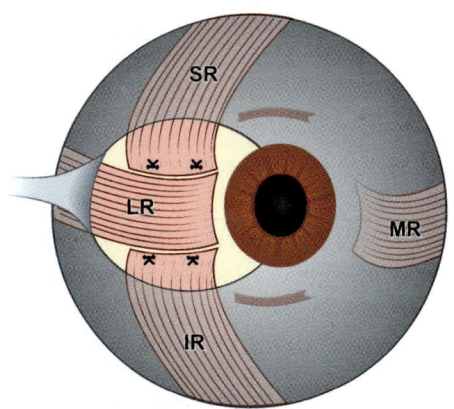

Fig. 15.23 *Surgical technique of Hummelsheim procedure for lateral rectus muscle palsy.*

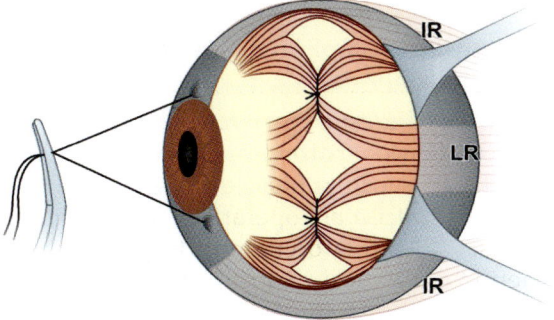

Fig. 15.22 *Jensen's procedure for lateral rectus palsy.*

Transposition of lateral rectus muscle

Some lateral rectus transposition procdures which have been recommended by some workers, for surgical management of third nerve palsy include:

- Inferior nasal transposition of lateral rectus
- Lateral rectus transposition to the nasal pole of superior rectus muscle
- Medial transposition of Y-split lateral rectus muscle

Periosteal fixation of extraocular muscles

Medial rectus orbital wall (periosteal) fixation

Medial rectus orbital wall (periosteal) fixation with the help of non-absorble 5-0 mersiline sutures through the retrocaruncular or skin approach (using DCR incision) has also been described for surgical management of third nerve palsy. However, it shows limited effectiveness.

Lateral rectus orbital (periosteal) fixation

Lateral rectus orbital (periosteal) fixation after disinserting the LR combined with 8–9 mm resection of MR has been reported to show reasonably good results in patients with third nerve palsy.

COMPLICATIONS OF EXTRAOCULAR MUSCLE SURGERY

Complications of extraocular muscle surgery are inevitable for any regularly operating strabismus surgeon. They vary in severity and frequency. Complications of extraocular muscle surgery, their prevention and management can be discussed under following headings:

- Complications of anaesthesia
- Intraoperative complications
- Postoperative complications

COMPLICATIONS OF ANAESTHESIA

Undoubtedly, general anaesthesia has become very safe in the recent days, however, it is never entirely free from danger. Even deaths due to anaesthesia to the tune of 2 per 10,000 have been reported during strabismic surgery. The potentially dangerous complications reported are as follows:

1. *Cardiac arrest.* Such a life-threatening complication may occur during operation or during recovery period. So a careful and meticulous monitoring is very important. Further, the ophthalmologist must be aware of the updated means of managing such a catastrophy and should be in a position to actively help the anaesthetist during the crisis hours. A ready tray of emergency drugs filled in syringes is mandatory in the operation theatre.

2. *Malignant hyperthermia.* It is a comparatively rare but again a life-threatening complication of anaesthesia.

Prevention. In some families susceptibility to this condition is inherent and is apparently autosomal dominant. Therefore, careful history and constant monitoring of the rectal temperature especially in predisposed patients may help in avoiding the crisis. Use of succinylcholine should be better avoided, as chances of malignant hyperthermia are comparatively more, when this drug is used.

Management. The condition is diagnosed by the occurrence of tachycardia, arrhythmia, rapidly rising temperature, acidosis and shock. The first sign of malignant hyperthermia is muscular rigidity and hyperthermia is a late sign. Once diagnosed, it should be treated energetically to prevent death by taking following measures:

- Immediately stop anaesthesia
- Provide care and surface cooling
- Correct metabolic acidosis
- Intravenous use of the drug dantrolene sodium is quite effective incontrolling malignant hyperthermia.

3. *Hepatic porphyria and suxamethonium* sensitivity are other genetic disorders which can cause serious complications during and after general anaesthesia.

4. *Oculocardiorespiratory reflexes.* The occurrence of oculocardiorespiratory reflexes is related to extraocular muscle manipulation and thus to be precise are operative complications. However, since they occur more frequently with general anaesthesia and are to be basically managed by the anaesthetist so they are discussed here. The oculocardiorespiratory

reflexes include oculocardiac reflex, oculorespiratory reflex and oculodepressor reflex.

• *Oculocardiac reflex (OCR)* refers to slowing of heart rate and/or disturbances in cardiac rhythm resulting from manipulation of extraocular muscles. It was first described by Aschner in 1908 and since then an abundant work has been done on various aspects of OCR. Its reported incidence varies from 32 to 90%.

• *Oculorespiratory reflex (ORR)*, also first described by Aschner, refers to slowing of respiration on extraocular muscle traction.

• *Oculodepressor reflex (ODR)* has recently been described by Khurana et al. to denote the significant fall in blood pressure observed during extraocular muscle traction. One might expect the cardiac output and, therefore, arterial blood pressure to fall in the presence of significant cardiac slowing due to oculocardiac reflex (OCR). However, the significant hypotension observed by the authors even after abolition of OCR by vagotomy, atropine and glycopyrronium have confirmed ODR to be distinct and independent of OCR.

• *Prevention of OCR, ORR and ODR* becomes imperative during squint surgery since the retrobulbar injection of 2% xylocaine blocks the afferent pathway of all three reflexes, its use has been recommended, even when the surgery is performed under general anaesthesia. In addition, intravenous atropine or glycopyrronium should also be used to block the efferent pathway of OCR. Further, controlled ventilation must be preferred to spontaneous breathing at least before, after and during muscle traction.

5. *Succinylcholine-induced apnoea.* Succinylcholine-induced apnoea may occur in children who are on miotics, echothiophate iodide. So it is most important to not to schedule surgery until the miotics have been discontinued for a period of at least 2–3 weeks, thus avoiding this problem. However, this problem can also occur due to primary cholinesterase deficiency which is an autosomal recessive condition reported to affect some individuals. These patients can have prolonged apnaea following succinylcholine administration in the absence of prior treatment with miotics. Making specific queries of unusual perianaesthetic problems in general, family history may sometimes be helpful in anticipating it.

INTRAOPERATIVE COMPLICATIONS

1. Haemorrhage

• *Mild surgical haemorrhage* from subconjunctival vessels is routine and is not preventable. Rarely wet field cautery may be needed to control bleeding from these vessels.

• *A moderately excessive haemorrhage* may occur, if the muscle is cut inadvertently, which is preventable if dissection is carried out meticulously. Compression for a while or wet field cautery may be needed to control it.

• *A profuse venous bleeding* indicates vortex vein rupture. It is not an uncommon complication and is caused by careless dissection or anomalous location of vortex veins. The vortex vein, i.e. most easily ruptured is the inferior temporal vortex veins. Rupture often occurs during lateral rectus and inferior oblique surgery. The best way to handle this complication is that no attempt should be made to try to clamp the vortex vein, since clamping may result in further damage. Generally speaking, there are no postoperative complications from a tear in a vortex vein during surgery.

2. Lost muscle

• Lost muscle is a serious complication of extraocular muscle surgery.

• Medial rectus is the most frequently lost muscle, because of its fewer attachments to other muscles and ligaments. For instance, inferior rectus is checked in its retraction into the orbit by Lockwood's ligament, superior rectus by its attachment to levator and lateral rectus by its association with inferior oblique muscle.

• Lost muscle can occur intraoperatively or in immediate postoperative period.

• Lost muscle occurs because of following *reasons:*

  – Inadvertant transection of the muscle.

  – Slipping of the muscle from the suture.

  – Slipping of the muscle from the resection clamp.

- *Prevention* for lost muscle includes, a gentle, meticulous and careful dissection, secure placement of sutures at preferred site and proper application of resection clamp.
- *Intraoperative muscle loss* should be managed as follows:
  - If slippage occurs during a recession procedure, flooding the area with irrigation solution may usually reveal the cut end of a tendon as a glistening white structure. If so, the muscle can be easily retrieved and resutured.
  - If the slippage occurs during resection procedure or when the above measures do not help in finding the lost muscle in recession, one should gently examine the Tenon's capsule with forceps in both hands used end over end. The tunnel in the Tenon's capsule in which the muscle course can be searched by this manoeuvre. Then one can reach back through the tunnel and grasp the muscle with forceps and pull forward. The sutures are placed and the procedure is carried out as planned.
  - If the muscle cannot be found, the best choice is to perform a maximal recession on the antagonist muscle along with a recession and Faden procedure on the yoke muscle of the lost muscle. If alignment in the primary position cannot be obtained by this, then one should perform a muscle transposition procedure. In this procedure, the adjacent halves of the two closest rectus muscles are transposed to the scleral insertion site of the lost muscle.
- *Postoperative muscle lost* occurs due to slippage of muscle not secured properly to the sclera. Possibility of a slipped muscle probably exists until the 5th or 6th postoperative day, when granulation tissue has sufficiently attached the muscle to sclera. *It is diagnosed* by following observations:
  - Patient will be unable to move the eye into the field of action of lost muscle.
  - Palpebral fissure will widen as the patient attempts to move the eye into the field of action of lost muscle.
  - Patient will either have a marked over-correction or a larger deviation than was

present before the operation, depending upon the muscle lost.

Management of postoperative slipped muscle is similar to that of intraoperative lost muscle. It is most important to note that exploration should be carried out as early as possible, since as time passes, finding the muscle becomes progressively more difficult.

3. Perforation of eyeball

Scleral perforation with or without perforation of choroid or choroid and retina, during extraocular muscle surgery may occur in one of two ways:

i. *During cutting of the muscle insertion,* sometimes scleral laceration, with or without damage to underlying tissue, may occur. This complication is most likely to occur, if the muscle is under considerable traction with the hook and the sclera is very thin especially in patients with high myopia and/or hereditary connective tissue disease. It should be managed as below:

- *Scleral perforation* should be sutured with 10–0 nylon suture. If scleral hole is large, a preserved scleral patch or a silicone patch may be applied to the area. If small and is located directly at the muscle insertion during resection procedure; the resected muscle can be sutured over the defect.
- Pupil should be dilated and the retina should be examined with the indirect ophthalmoscope.
- Prophylactic transcleral cryotherapy is recommended around the site of injury. When a retinal perforation is discovered, careful postoperative follow-up examinations with indirect ophthalmoscopy should be performed.

ii. *During placement of needles for reinsertion of the muscle,* chances of scleral and chorioretinal perforation are more than during cutting of the muscle. In fact, this complication may occur more frequently than is usually recognized or admitted. Undoubtedly, the rate of perforations has decreased since the introduction of spatula needle. It is recommended that even on slightest doubt of perforation with needle, the pupil should be dilated and a careful indirect ophthalmoscopy should be carried out. If a retinal hole is detected, it should be managed as discussed above.

Though extremely rare, but serious complications such as endophthalmitis, retinal detachment and phthisis bulbi have been reported following perforations. Therefore, a very careful watch is required for such cases.

4. *Operation on the wrong muscle*

Such a complication has also been reported occasionally under following circumstances:

- By mistake (or due to absentmindedness of the surgeon), the muscle to be resected may be recessed and vice versa.
- In excessively rotated globe, the exact position of the muscle may be shifted.
- During reoperation, the previously operated muscles may in an unusual location.
- Myectomy of the inferior rectus is a possible complication of myectomy of the inferior oblique at its origin through an inferior cul-de-sac approach.

Prevention of such a complication includes:

- Exact marking of 3, 6, 9 and 12 o'clock meridian at limbus before the conjunctival incision is made.
- To use the identifying check marks of the various muscles such as close association of the:
  - Inferior oblique with lateral rectus,
  - Superior oblique with superior rectus, and
  - Inferior oblique with inferior rectus.

5. *Inadvertent injury to the other muscles*

Inadvertent injury to the following muscles has been reported during strabismus surgery:

i. *Partial or complete disinsertion of the inferior oblique may occur during lateral rectus surgery.* This is because, it is extremely easy to hook part or all of the inferior oblique tendon, when passing a hook under the lateral rectus muscle. To prevent this complication, it is recommended that the lateral rectus be doubly hooked and that the area be carefully inspected to make sure that the inferior oblique is not incorporated and disinserted during the freeing of the inferior check ligaments and inferior intermuscular septum during a lateral rectus recession. If, however, the inferior oblique is inadvertently partially or completely disinserted, a suture may be placed in the muscle belly and sutured to the globe at its original insertion.

ii. *Partial or complete severance of superior oblique tendon and sheath* may occur while attempting to hook the superior rectus muscle. Therefore, surgeon should be very careful while engaging the superior rectus muscle. However, if this does happen, following measures should be taken:

- Inferior oblique should be recessed, so that a significant vertical deviation does not result.
- If the operation originally planned is resection of the superior rectus muscle the surgeon should decrease the amount of surgery he planned to do.
- If the operation is recession of the superior rectus, surgeon should increase the amount of recession along with weakening of the inferior oblique of the same side.

6. *Operation on the wrong eye*

Operation on the wrong eye is an embarassing complication, sometimes encountered by the surgeon. The best way to avoid this complication is examination of the patient by the surgeon himself in the morning before surgery.

- Operation on the horizontal muscles of the wrong eye may many a time correct the deviation in the affected eye; but undoubtedly the patient and/or her/this guardians and surgeon all are upset by this mistake.
- Operation on the vertical muscle of the wrong eye is always serious because the misalignment will be exaggerated. If the mistake is discovered immediately, it should be taken care of in the operation theatre there and then. However, if the mistake is discovered postoperatively, it should be managed like a new fresh case of misalignment.

POSTOPERATIVE COMPLICATIONS

1. *Postoperative infections.* Because of perfect asepsis and better quality spatulated needles, the incidence of postoperative infection have tremendously decreased. However, though quite rare, following infections are reported:

i. *Endophthalmitis* has been reported to occur following squint surgery because of following reasons:

- Introduction of an infectious organism following sclerochorioretinal perforation.
- Extension of cellulitis of extraocular muscles.

Early diagnosis and energetic management can save the useful vision.

ii. *Orbital cellulitis,* though rare but it has been reported in the literature postoperative complication of squint surgery.

iii. *Localized suture abscess* has also been reported, possibly resulting from contaminated suture material.

2. Suture reaction. Because of better quality synthetic sutures, the reactions are now very rare. However, suture reactions were common with the organic suture material. They used to occur as *acute allergic reactions* within 24 hours to 7 days of strabismus surgery and as delayed foreign body reaction after 6–8 weeks of surgery. Acute reaction is characterized by conjunctival hyperaemia, chemosis, itching and a dull red smooth mass beneath the conjunctiva at the site of muscle reattachment. It is treated by topical steroid eyedrops.

3. Conjunctival granuloma. Because of improved suture material and microsurgical techniques, the incidence of conjunctival granuloma has decreased. Conjunctival granuloma occurs as non-allergic foreign body reaction to suture material, cotton fibres, glove powder, an eyelash burried in the wound or Tenon's capsule incarcerated into the wound. Conjunctival granuloma is characterized by a localized elevated hyperaemic conjunctival mass which may sometimes be even pedunculated. Treatment consists of topical steroid eyedrops. Sometimes, even surgical excision may be required.

4. Conjunctival cyst. Conjunctival inclusion cyst may occur following inadvertent closure of the conjunctival epithelium in the wound. It appears as a subconjunctival translucent mass that develops several days to weeks after strabismus surgery. Some conjunctival cysts will resorb spontaneously. When indicated, surgical treatment consists of complete excision of the cyst.

5. Dellen. Dellen refers to a localized area of corneal thinning due to dehydration. It is more common following limbal approach.

6. Anterior segment ischaemia. It is a rare but potentially serious complication of extraocular muscle surgery which occurs due to disruption of blood supply to the anterior segment from the anterior ciliary arteries.

In anterior segment ischaemia, cornea becomes oedematous with stromal swelling and folds in Descemet's membrane. Anterior chamber shows heavy flare and cellular reaction. Lens may become cataractous.

Prevention of anterior segment ischaemia is most important since its treatment is unsatisfactory. Following measures have been recommended for its prevention:

- All four rectus muscles should never be disinserted simultaneously.
- Disinsertion of three muscles can be done safely in children, but should always be avoided in adults.
- In general, a waiting of at least 6 months in adult patients after surgery on both horizontal rectus muscles is recommended before operating on the vertical recti.
- Techniques for preservation of anterior ciliary vessels during extraocular muscle surgery which have been recommended are as follows:
  - Microdissection of the anterior ciliary vessels from the muscle under operating microscope.
  - Modified rectus tucking procedure as a strengthening procedure.
  - Muscle splitting procedures. The reliability of these procedures in preventing anterior segment ischaemia is yet to be ascertained.

Treatment of anterior segment ischaemia consists of:

- Topical steroids every 1–2 hour,
- Systemic steroids for about 0–15 days, and
- Topical atropine twice a day.

Prognosis. The anterior chamber reaction is usually controlled with the above treatment. However, iris atrophy and cataract usually occur as sequelae of the anterior segment ischaemia. Sometimes the eyeball may go into phthisis bulbi.

7. Necrotizing scleritis has been reported as an infrequent complication following strabismus surgery. Patients with systemic diseases like autoimmune vasculitis are more prone to develop this complication.

8. *Refractive error* changes mostly astigmatic have been reported following strabismus surgery. Possibly, these changes occur because of corneal curvature alterations caused by the temporary imbalance of the muscle forces.

9. *Postoperative diplopia* is a common occurrence following strabismus surgery for comitant heterotropias. It may last from a few days, a few weeks or even lifetime. Children are usually able to suppress early and so diplopia is short lasting. While in adults, it may sometimes be troublesome. Therefore, all adults opting for correction of strabismus, must be warned of this complication.

10. *Postoperative retinal detachment.* Retinal detachment has been reported as very infrequent complication following strabismus surgery. A missed scleroretinal perforation is considered the probable cause.

11. *Postoperative scarring.* Scarring of the conjunctiva and extraocular muscles can occur postoperatively and result in restriction. The affected muscles and conjunctiva may need recession. Postoperative scarring of Tenon's capsule may produce an L-deformity of the inferior oblique and a J-deformity of a rectus muscle or cicatricial advancement of a rectus muscle (*see* page 352).

12. *Adhesive syndrome* has been reported to occur following surgery on inferior oblique muscle (*see* page 352).

13. *Under- or overcorrections* are the most common postoperative complications of strabismus surgery. Their management has been discussed along with the surgical treatment of different types of heterotropia.

14. *Gaze incomitance.* Gaze incomitance may occur following in large recession large angle strabismus. Gaze palsy is also a known complication of Kestenbaum procedure especially the augmented procedure employed in patients with congenital nystagmus.

15. *Alteration in palpebral fissure*
- *Narrowing of palpebral tissue may* occur with following procedures:
  - Vertical rectus muscle resections, because of fascial attachments from the exterior surface of the muscle and adjacent lid.

  - A large recess-resect procedure on the horizontal rectus muscle, especially in a reoperation can cause slight narrowing of palpebral tissue because of slight retraction of the globe.
- *Widening of the palpebral tissue may occur with* vertical rectus muscle recessions.

16. *Psychological complications.* A multitude of psychologically rooted behavioural changes have been reported following surgery in young children and thus should be kept in mind. A few such disorders include enuresis, stuttering, night terrors etc.

POSTOPERATIVE CARE AFTER STRABISMUS SURGERY

1. *Immediate general care* includes:
- *Vital signs* should be observed for at least 24 hours after the surgery, especially when it has been performed under general anaesthesia.
- *Antiemetics* may be given, if required and diet is limited.
- *Analgesics* are rarely required following strabismus surgery, when required, usually aspirin or ibuprofen will produce comfort.

2. *Dressing.* It is useful to apply pad and bandage on the operated eye for at least 24 hours.

3. *Topical antibiotics and steroids.* Eyedrops should be instilled 3 to 4 times a day and eye ointment at night for 2 to 3 weeks following surgery.

4. *Oral antibiotics* are usually given for a period of 5–7 days. Though their role in preventing rare complications like orbital cellulitis and endophthalmitis is debatable but it definitely saves the surgeons from legal complications in case of any eventuality.

5. *Oral anti-inflammatory drug* may also be given for a period of 3 to 4 days.

6. *Warm compresses* to reduce swelling have also been recommended.

7. *Restrictions for the patient* are to avoid swimming, playing in a sand box or other possible sources of postoperative infection.

8. *Discharge from the hospital.* If every thing goes well, patient may be discharged from the hospital a day after surgery. Following tests should be done before discharging the patient:

- *Conjunctival incision* site should be examined to make sure that it is closed properly and the sutures have not broken.
- *Approximate alignment* of the eyes should be determined by cover test and Hirschberg's test.
- *Version test* should be performed to rule out the possibility of slipped muscle.
- *Presence of diplopia* should be checked and if found, the patient and or parents should be told that this is a good sign since it may be the first step towards fusion.

9. *Postoperative follow-up examinations.* At the time of discharge from hospital, patient and/or parents are instructed to dress the eyes with sterile water and to use the prescribed eyedrops and ointment.

Most patients are seen within one week postoperatively and then at weekly intervals for the next 2 weeks. And after that at 2 weeks intervals for the next 2 months. It must be emphasized that patients should be followed closely in the immediate postoperative period since this is a critical time, if one is attempting to achieve fusional results. It is during this period that situation is most plastic and that new characteristics of the motor and sensory systems are taking place.

During each follow-up visit, following tests should be performed:

- Visual acuity testing
- Tests for alignment of the eyes
- Ocular movements
- Diplopia, if present, is identified as to types

10. *Postoperative orthoptic treatment.* It will vary depending upon the preoperative parameters, operative results, type of squint, age of the patient and has been discussed with individual clinical entity.

OUTLINES OF STRABISMUS MANAGEMENT

■ HETEROPHORIA

Examination

1. Measurement of visual acuity.
2. Refraction and fundus examination.
3. Cover-uncover test.
4. Measurement of deviation.

- Prism and cover test
- Maddox rod test
- Maddox wing test

5. Assessment of ocular movements.
6. Measurement of amplitude of fusional convergence.
7. Measurement of accommodation.

Line of treatment

Exophoria

1. Correct refractive error.
2. Equalize visual acuity, if necessary.
3. Improve positive fusional convergence.
4. Surgery, when indicated.

Esophoria

1. Correct refractive error.
2. Equalize visual acuity, if necessary.
3. Improve negative fusional convergence.
4. Miotics, when exercises not sufficient and AC/A ratio is large.
5. Surgery, when indicated.

Hyperphoria

1. Correct refractive error
2. Equalize visual acuity, if necessary.
3. Prescribe prisms.
4. Surgery, when indicated.

Cyclophoria

1. Correct refractive error.
2. Equalize visual acuity.
3. Surgery—when torsion due to oblique muscle defect is present.

■ HETEROTROPIAS

Examination

1. Test visual acuity
2. Refraction and fundus examination
3. Cover test
4. Measurement of deviation
   - Synoptophore method
   - Prism bar cover test (PBCT)
5. Assessment of ocular movements
6. Assessment of accommodation, convergence and AC/A ratio

7. Assessment of fusional ability and amplitudes of fusion
8. Assessment of binocular co-operation and sensory anomalies.

Esotropia

Differential diagnosis

1. *Infantile esotropia*

a. *Additional history*
- Onset before the age of six months
- Fixates with either eye
- Constant ET

b. *Tests*
- Abduction—reluctant but intact
- Measurements—large ET, V-pattern
- Cross-fixates—equal vision
- Cycloplegic refraction—small refractive error
- Versions—possible IO overaction
- Cover-uncover—possible DVD

2. *Accommodative esotropia*

a. *Additional history*
- E (T), N > D
- Eye preference
- Worse than when tired, concentrating
- Typical age of onset—18 months to 3 years
- Range of onset—7 months to 10 years

b. *Tests*
- P + C, CC + SC—accommodative component
- Cycloplegic refraction
  - <4 D hyperopia, high AC/A
  - >4 D hyperopia, normal AC/A
- Fusion, CC—excellent usually
- Vision—amblyopia frequently

3. *LR palsy* (CN VI)

a. *Additional history*
- Severe head/neck trauma
- ET greater to right gaze, left gaze, or both sides
- Head position to right or left
- Horizontal, diplopia, variable worse at distance
- Sudden onset of ET/diplopia
- Present since birth, if congenital
- Associated with facial nerve palsy (Moebius or brainstem tumour)
- Associated with ear pain (Gradenigo)
- Worsens with fatigue (myasthenia gravis)

b. *Tests*
- Fusion with head position—recent onset
- Measurements—ET > right and/or left gaze
  - ET D > N slight A tendency
- Measure with OD, OS fix—primary/secondary deviation
- Versions/ductions, saccades—decreased LR function
- Diplopia testing—horizontal, incomitant young child may suppress
- Vision—possible amblyopia
- Forced ductions—negative

4. *Duane's retraction syndrome type I*

a. *Additional history*
- No trauma
- Lid fissure changes with gaze
- Abnormal head position
- Present since birth

b. *Tests*
- Versions, ductions—no abduction, lid fissure narrows during adduction
- Fusion with head position—fusion often
- Vision—may have amblyopia

5. *Consecutive esotropia*

a. *Additional history*
- Previous surgery for XT

b. *Tests*
- Fusion with ET corrected—fusion usually if X or X (T) preopative.

6. *Nystagmus compensation syndrome*

a. *Additional history*
- Any nystagmus seen during abduction
- Large ET present since birth
- Cross-fixates turning head to see

b. *Tests*
- Krimsky—over-converges with "correcting prism".
- Versions/ductions—jerk nystagmus in abduction, o.u.
- Cross-fixation—does not move fixing eye out of adducted position to mid-line.

7. *Cyclic esotropia*

a. *Additional history*
- 24, 48, or 96 hours schedule of alternation between ET one cycle and straight next cycle
- Fairly sudden onset during childhood.

b. *Tests*

- ET day
- Fusion—may have diplopia initially, then suppression/ARC
- PB + CT—large ET, comitant usually
- *Straight day*
- Fusion—excellent
- PB + CT—ortho or small exophoria
- Vision—may have amblyopia

8. *Strabismus fixus*

a. *Additional history*

Long-standing ET

b. *Tests*

- Forced ductions—positive MR tightening
- Measurements—large ET, greater in R and L gaze
- Versions/ductions—decreased abduction, fixed adduction
- Vision—must cross-fixate and turn head to see

9. *Divergence paralysis*

a. *Additional history*

- General health—N raised intracranial pressure
- Infections, parasites, and travel abroad
- Trauma possible

b. *Tests*

- Divergence amplitudes—nearly non-existent
- Versions/ductions—full, abduction okay
- Diplopia testing—uncrossed, worse at distance
- Measurements—may fuse at near
- Vision—equal

10. *Accommodative effort syndrome*

a. *Additional history*

- Near asthenopia, blurring, or diplopia

b. *Tests*

- NPA—normal
- PB + PC—E', possibly E (T)'
- Divergence amplitudes—poor
- Plus lenses for near—help relieve symptoms

11. *Pseudoesotropia*

a. *Additional history*

- Onset—usually since birth
- Incomitance

b. *Tests*

- Hirschberg/cover uncover—no deviation
- External—epicanthal folds frequently
- Angle kappa—negative
- Fusion—excellent, no suppression
- Versions/ductions—appears to have increasing
- ET to right and left gaze

Line of treatment

Refractive accommodative esotropia

1. Correct refractive error
2. Treat amblyopia, if neccessary
3. Overcome suppression
4. Improve negative fusional convergence
5. Surgery should be avoided

Non-refractive accommodative esotropia

1. Treat amblyopia, if necessary
2. Bifocals with a +3 add over cycloplegic refraction
3. Miotics, only if bifocals not accepted
4. Orthoptic treatment to over come suppression and improve negative fusional convergence

Mixed accommodative esotropia

1. Correct refractive error, bifocals, if AC/A is high
2. Treat amblyopia, if necessary
3. Orthoptic treatment to overcome suppression and improve the negative fusional convergence.
4. Surgery only for the remaining nonaccommodative part of squint.

Essential infantile esotropia

1. Correct refractive error
2. Amblyopia treatment, if necessary
3. Surgery by the age of 2 years

Essential late onset esotropia

1. Correct refractive error
2. Treat amblyopia, if necessary
3. Perform surgical correction
   - Basic esotropia—recess/resect
   - Convergence excess—bimedial recession
   - Divergence insufficiency type—bilateral lateral rectus resection.

Sensory esotropia
1. Correct refractive error
2. Cosmetic surgery, if necessary

Exotropia
Differential diagnosis

1. **Primary exotropia**

a. *Additional history*
- Intermittency
- Worse at distance or near
- Worse with fatigue, illness

b. *Tests*
- Fusion—usually excellent
  Measurements—exodeviation, usually comitant Basic, divergence excess type, convergence insufficiency type
- Vision—equal
- Convergence amplitudes—poor fusional convergence amps

2. **Infantile exotropia**

a. *Additional history*
- Present since birth
- Eye preference

b. *Tests*
- Vision—decreased in non-preferred eye
- Health of eyes—no specific disease of eye
- Measurements—usually large; comitant XT

3. **MR palsy/CN III palsy**

a. *Additional history*
- Present since birth, if congenital
- Severe trauma
- General health—possible headaches, myasthenia gravis
- Other signs—ipsilateral ptosis, mydriasis, cycloplegia, hypodeviation, contralateral body paralysis (Benedikt's syndrome)

b. *Tests*
- Versions/ductions—decreased adduction
- Measurements—incomitant exodeviation, greater in adduction
- Measure with OD, OS fix—primary and secondary deviation
- Vision—possible amblyopia, cycloplegia
- Head position—present, if to attain fusion

4. **Duane's retraction syndrome type II**

a. *Additional history*
- No trauma
- Lid fissure changes with gaze
- Abnormal head position
- Present since birth

b. *Tests*
- Versions/ductions—decreased adduction with lid narrowing, abduction okay
- Head position—done to achieve fusion
- Fusion with head—often present position
- Vision—may be amblyopic

5. **Sensory exotropia (due to blind eye)**

a. *Additional history*
- Age of blindness in one eye (if over 7, likely to go exo)
  Constant non-alternating XT

b. *Tests*
- Vision—blind eye
- Krimsky measurements—fairly comitant XT

6. **Consecutive exotropia**

a. *Additional history*
- Previous surgery for ET

b. *Tests*
- Measurements—XT
  Fusion—diplopia or suppression/ARC

7. **Craniofacial anomalies**

a. *Additional history*
- Alpert syndrome
- Crouzon syndrome

b. *Tests*
- Measurements —large XT, bilateral SO palsies often
- Versions/ductions—IO, overaction, SO under-action
- External—bilateral exophthalmos (Crouzon)
- Refraction—astigmatism (Alpert), progressive hyperopia (Crouzon)

8. **Convergence paralysis**

a. *Additional history:*
- Trauma
- General health—recent neurological condition possible

b. *Tests*
- Convergence amplitudes—nearly non-existent

- Measurements—comitant exodeviation N>D
- Versions/ductions—full
- Diplopia—crossed, worse at near
- Fusion—at distance only
- Vision—equal

9. Internuclear ophthalmoplegia (INO)

a. Additional history
- Bilateral—systemic multiple sclerosis
- Unilateral—vascular accident, inflammation, infection, or tumour in brainstem, possibly myasthenia gravis

b. Tests
- Versions/ductions—decreased adduction with jerk nystagmus in abducted eye
- Convergence amplitudes—intact convergence

10. Pseudoexotropia

a. Additional history:
- Constant

b. Tests
- Krimsky/cover-uncover test. No eye deviation
- Fusion—excellent, no suppression
- Angle kappa—positive
- Funduscopy—may have retinopathy of prematurity with temporally dragged fovea

Line of treatment

Primary intermittent exotropia

1. Correct refractive error; myopia should be fully corrected hypermetropia up to 2.0 DS need not be corrected.
2. Orthoptic treatment:
- Antisuppression exercises
- Exercises for positive relative convergence
- Occlusion therapy
3. Prismotherapy in children where surgery is to be postponed for some period.
4. Surgery is indicated, when:
- Exotropia occurs more than 50% working hours
- Deviation exceeds 20D
- There develops secondary convergence insufficiency with asthenopic symptoms.
- Suppression develops
- There occurs gradual deterioration of stereopsis.
- *Age for surgery:* Before 4 years

Primary constant exotropia

1. Surgical correction should be done as early as possible.
2. Orthoptic treatment both before and after surgery should be continued, if fusion ability can be demonstrated.

Sensory exotropia

1. Correct any refractive error
2. Amblyopia therapy may be tried in children with anisometropia or aphakia
3. Cosmetic surgery is the usual treatment.

Consecutive exotropia

1. Correct any refractive error
2. Assess state of binocular sensory cooperation
a. If normal regional correspondence and bifoveal fusion can be demonstrated:
  i. *Overcome suppressions*
  ii. *Improve fusional convergence*
  iii. *Perform surgery*
b. If bifoveal fusion cannot be demonstrated; assess cosmetic appearance.
  i. *If good, leave alone*
  ii. *If poor, perform cosmetic surgery.*

Vertical and cyclodeviations

Differential diagnosis

I. Isolated CN palsy (SO most common)

a. Additional history
- Trauma, may be mild
- Head tilt
- Combined horizontal and vertical diplopia
- Diplopia/asthenopia worse to right and left
- Myasthenia gravis

b. Tests
- Fusion with head position—usually fuses
- PB CT, 9 positions—incomitant HT
- B3ST—isolates EOM palsy
- Versions/ductions
  - SO: May show underactive SO, overactive IO, inhibitional palsy of contralateral (IPC) SR
  - IO: May show underactive IO, overactive SO, IPC IR
  - SR: May show underactive SR; overactive IR, IPC SO
  - IR: May show underactive IR, overactive SR, IPC IO

- Vertical amplitudes—may exist, if congenital/long-standing. No vertical amplitude, if recent onset
- Subjective torsion
  - May exist, if recent onset
  - No torsion, if congenital/long-standing palsy
  - SO, SR—extorsion
  - IO, IR—intorsion
- Look at old photographs—old head tilt, if congenital/long-standing

2. *DVD*
a. *Additional history*
- Associated with congenital/infantile ET
- One or both eyes seen to go up, neither eye ever goes hypodeviation
- Intermittent HT, either eye

b. *Tests*
- Cover-uncover—either eye elevates under cover without associated hypodeviation of the fellow eye
- PBCT—difficult to measure, variable
- Versions/ductions—rule out IO overaction as "cause"
- Red glass test
- Bielschowsky's phenomenon—positive

3. *Brown's syndrome*
a. *Additional history*
- Trauma to trochlear region of globe
- Sinus, orbital surgery
- Juvenile rheumatoid arthritis
- Present since birth, if congenital

b. *Tests*
- Versions/ductions—no elevation of globe in adduction. Eye elevates easily in abduction
- Forced ductions—restriction of globe up and in
- Fusion—often fuses in downgaze
- Vision—amblyopia may or may not be present
- Krimsky—hypotropia of affected eye, when up and in

4. *Blow-out fracture*
a. *Additional history*
- Blunt trauma—orbital fracture
- Diplopia/discomfort worse in upgaze often

b. *Tests*
- Ductions/versions

- Hypotropia worsens towards upgaze
- Restrictions of ductions—upgaze, may be down, right, or left gaze
- Forced ductions—restriction of globe, upgaze usually
- X-ray/CT scan—orbital fracture, floor frequently, or nasal wall
- Diplopia field—often has region of single binocular vision
- Exophthalmometry—often affected eye enophthalmic

5. *Double elevator palsy (DEP)*
a. *Additional history*
- Present since birth
- Ptosis on affected side
- Chin up head position
- No trauma

b. *Tests*
- Fusion with chin up—possible fusion
- Versions/ductions—constant hypotropia of affected eye
- Forced ductions—no restrictions of elevation unless very long-standing
- External—pseudoptosis on affected side

6. *Graves' ophthalmopathy*
a. *Additional history*

Thyroid dysfunction in past or present

b. *Tests*
- Ductions/versions—restriction of upgaze (IR), lateral gaze (MR), or any EOM
- Forced ductions—positive for restriction
- Fusion with head position—usually has fusion
- Diplopia—variable, vertical > horizontal

7. *Pseudohypertropia*
a. *Additional history*
b. *Tests*
- Cover-uncover—no deviation
- Lift lid—appearance of HT disappears
- Assess pupils—possible asymmetry
- Document with photos—no deviation by light reflex

Line of treatment

Comitant vertical deviatons

1. Treat amblyopia and suppression
2. Prescribe prism for deviations up to 10D:

– Minimum prismatic power that provides comfortable DSV should be prescribed.
– Distribute prism power equally in two eyes with base-down in front of the hypertropic and base-up infront of hypotropic eye.

3. Surgery is indicated for deviations larger than 10D.

• Vertical transplantation of horizontal rectus muscle insertion is sufficient for 10–14D vertical deviations associated with horizontal tropia.

• Recession of appropriate vertical muscle (3 to 4 mm) is required for larger deviations of 15D to 25D.

Dissociated vertical deviations

For significant cosmetic problem due to DVD, treatment is mainly surgical following operations may be performed:

1. Faden operation with superior rectus recession.
2. Large recession of the superior rectus muscle.
3. Resection of the inferior rectus muscle.
4. Recess-resect procedure on superior and inferior rectus muscles.
5. Recession of the inferior oblique with anteriorization of its insertion.

Inferior oblique overaction

In significant cases, inferior oblique weakening should be done by any of the following procedures:

1. Disinsertion
2. Myectomy
3. Extirpation
4. Recession
5. Recession with anterior transposition

Superior oblique overaction

1. Superior oblique tenotomy
2. Superior oblique lengthening

Cyclodeviation with vertical deviation

1. *Weakening of the offending inferior oblique* muscle should be done, when excyclodeviation with hyperdeviation is associated with secondary overaction of inferior oblique.
2. *Tucking of superior oblique muscle* should be done, when excyclodeviation with hyper-

deviation occurs in the field of paretic superior oblique without overaction of inferior oblique.
3. *Bilateral tucking of superior oblique* is required in patients with bilateral superior oblique palsy producing V-pattern esotropia and excyclodeviation.

Excyclodeviations with no vertical deviation

1. Harada-Ito procedure (anterolateral advancement of superior oblique tendon)
2. Nasal transposition of inferior rectus muscle in patients with congenital absence of superior oblique tendon or in those where it has already been tenotomized.
3. Temporal transpositioning of superior rectus muscle.

Incyclodeviation with no vertical deviation

Temporal transposition of inferior rectus along with nasal transposition of the superior rectus muscle.

Incomitant strabismus

A- and V-pattern horizontal tropias

1. Treatment of V-pattern esotropia

i. *For correction of horizontal deviation in primary position:*
   – *Bilateral medial rectus recession or*
   – *Medial rectus recession and lateral rectus resection*

ii. *For correction of V-pattern:*
   – *Inferior oblique muscle weakening–when overacting, otherwise*
   – *Infraplacement of medial recti or infraplacement of MR and supraplacement of LR.*

2. Treatment of A-pattern esotropia

i. When superior oblique overaction is associated—bilateral tenotomy of superior oblique muscles should be performed and either bilateral medial rectus recession or recess-resect procedure should be performed for correction of horizontal deviation in the primary gaze after making adjustment for 10–15 prism dioptres which is corrected by bilateral superior oblique tenotomy. Alternatively, horizontal rectus muscle surgery may be deferred for a later date.

ii. When superior oblique overaction is not present, the treatment of choice is either bilateral medial rectus recession with supraplacement of the insertions, or combined supraplacement of the medial rectus and infraplacement of the lateral rectus muscle with a recess-resect procedure.

3. *Treatment of V-pattern exotropia*

i. If inferior oblique muscle overaction is present, these muscles should be recessed and either a bilateral lateral rectus muscle recession or recess-resect procedure should be performed for the horizontal deviation in primary position.

ii. When inferior oblique overaction is not present, the treatment of choice is either bilateral lateral rectus muscle recession with supraplacement of the insertion or combined supraplacement of LR and infraplacement of MR with a recess-resect procedure.

4. *Treatment of A-pattern exotropia*

i. If superior oblique overaction is present, its bilateral tenotomies should be performed. And keeping in mind the effect of superior oblique tenotomies on the horizontal deviation in primary position, either bilateral lateral rectus recession or a recess-resect procedure should be planned.

ii. When superior oblique overaction is not present, the treatment of choice is either bilateral lateral rectus muscle recession with infraplacement of the insertion or combine infraplacement of the LR and supraplacement of MR with a recess-resect procedure.

5. *Treatment of Y-pattern exotropia*

i. No treatment is required, when the patient fuses in primary position and downward gaze, has a normal head posture, and does not have double vision in upward gaze.

ii. When chin elevation is present and there is associated overaction of the inferior oblique, surgical weakening of both inferior oblique muscles will close the Y-pattern.

iii. If the inferior obliques are not overacting, supraplace the lateral recti without recessing or infraplace the medial recti without recessing.

6. *Treatment of λ-pattern exotropia*

Despite fusion in primary position, patients with λ-pattern exotropia may have considerable difficulty with near work (i.e. in downgaze). No horizontal surgery is indicated, but following procedures may be performed:

i. If the superior obliques are overacting, perform bilateral superior oblique tenotomies.

ii. If the superior obliques are not overacting, supraplace the medial recti without recessing or infraplace the lateral recti without recessing.

Paralytic strabismus

- Investigate and treat the cause of paresis if found.
- Conservative managemnet for 6–8 months.
- Surgery, if indicated after 6–8 months depending upon the muscle involved.

Special restrictive ocular motility defects

Duane's retraction syndrome

Surgery is performed only if there is significant abnormal head posture and/or significant deviation in the primary position. In general surgical results are not very encouraging.

Brown's syndrome

Surgery to weaken the superior oblque should be performed only in the presence of a significant head tilt and/or a large vertical deviation.

BIBLIOGRAPHY

1. Abraham, SV: The use of an echothiophate phenylephrine formulation (echophenyline-B3) in the treatment of convergent strabismus and amblyopia with special emphasis on iris cysts. J Pediatr. Ophthalmol. 1:68, 1964.

2. Abraham, SV: The use of miotics in the treatment of convergent strabismus and anisometropia:a preliminary report. Am. J. Ophthalmol. 32:233, 1949.

3. Aust, W: The use of prisms in pre- and post-operative treatment. In Fells. P., editor: The First Congress of the International Strabismological Association. St. Louis. 1971, Mosby-Year Book. Inc., p. 255.

4. Basmadjian, G, LaSelle, P, and Dumas, J: Retinal detachment after strabismus surgery. Am J Ophthalmol. 79:305, 1975.

5. Bergman, JA: Idiopathic malignant hyperthermia. Arch. Ophthalmol. 93:232, 1975.

6. Breinin, GM, Chin, NB, and Ripps, H: A rationale for therapy of accommodative strabismus. Am J Ophthalmol. 61:1030, 1966.

7. Brown, HW: Complications in surgery of the extraocular muscles. In Fasanella, RM, editor: Management of complications in eye surgery, Philadelphia, 1957, WB Saunders Co.

8. Buckley, EG, and Flynn, JT: Superior oblique recession versus tenotomy: a comparison of surgical results. J Pediatr. Ophthalmol. Strabismus 20:112, 1983.

9. Burian, HM: Use of bifocal spectaclesin the treatment of accommodative esotropia. Br Orthopt. J 13:3, 1956.

10. Caldeira, JA: Graduated recession of the superior oblique muscle. Br J Ophthalmol. 59:553, 1975.

11. Cibis, GW: Incidence of inadvertent perforation in strabismus surgery. Ophthalmic Surg. 23:360, 1992.

12. Cole, JG, and cole HG: Recession of the conjunctiva in complicated eye muscle operations. Am J Ophthalmol. 53:618, 1962.

13. Costenbader. FD, and Kertesz, E: Relaxing procedures of the inferior oblique, a comparative study. Am J Ophthalmol. 57:276, 1964.

14. Dottan, SA Hoffman, P, and Oliver, MD: Astigmatism after strabismus surgery. Ophthalmic Surg. 19:128, 1988.

15. Elasas, FJ, and Witherspoon, CD: Anterior segment ischemia after strabismus surgery in a child. Am J Ophthalmol. 103:833, 1987.

16. Fells, P: Management of paralytic strabismus. Br J Ophthalmol. 58:255, 1974.

17. Fink, WH: Surgery of the oblique muscles of the eye. St. Louis, 1951, Mosby- year Book, Inc,., p 296.

18. Gifford, SR: Some notes on the treatment of strabismus. Br J Ophthalmol. 19:148, 1935.

19. Gldstein. JH: The role of miotics in strabismus. Surv. Ophthalmol. 13:31. 1968.

20. Gonzales, C, and Klein, B: Myectomy and anterior transposition of the inferior oblique muscle: a new surgical procedure and its results in 49 operations, Binoc. Vision 8:249, 1993.

21. Gross, SA Noorden, GK von, and Jones, DB: Necrotizing scleritis and transient myopia following strabismus surgery. Ophthalmic Surg. 24:839, 1993.

22. Guibor, G.P: Some uses of ophthalmic prisms. In Allen. JH editor: Strabismus ophthalmic symposium II. St. Louis, 1958, Mosby - Year Book, Inc, p.244.

23. Harada, M, and Ito, Y:Srgical correction of cyclotropia. Jpn.J. Ophthalmol. 8:88, 1964.

24. Helveston, EM: Muscle transposition procedures, Surv. Ophthalmol. 16:92, 1971.

25. Ing. MR: Infection following strabismus surgery. Ophthalmic Surg, 22:41, 1991.

26. Knapp, P: The surgical treatment of double-elevator paralysis, Trans. Am. Ophthalmol. Soc. 67:304, 1969.

27. Knapp, P: The surgical treatment of persistent squint. Doc. Ophthalmol. 34:221, 1973.

28. Knapp, P: The use of membrane prisms. Trans. Am. Acad. Ophthalmol. Otolaryngol. 79: 718., 1975.

29. Kramer, ME: Clinical orthoptics: diagnosis and treatment, St.Louis, 1949, Mosby - Year Book, Inc., p. 349.

30. Lyle, KT, and Bridgeman, GJO: Worth and Chavasse squint, ed, 9, London, 1959, Tindall and Cox, p. 51.

31. Milot, J, Jacob, JL, Blanc, VF, and Hardy, JF: The oculocardial reflex in strabismus surgery. Can. J Ophthalmol. 18:314, 1983.

32. Noorden, GK von: Indications of the posterior fixation operation in strabismus. Ophthalmology 85:512, 1978.

33. Noorden, GK von: Modification of the limbal appraoch to surgery of the rectus muscles. Arch. Ophthalmol. 82:349, 1969.

34. Noorden, GK von: The limbal approach to surgery of the rectus muscles. Arch. Ophthalmol. 80:94, 1968.

35. Nooden, GK von, and Milam, J: Penalization in the treatment of amblyopia: preliminary experiences. Am J Ophthalmol. 88:511, 1979.

36. Noorden, GK von, Morris, J, and Edelman, P: Efficacy of bifocals in the treatment of accommodative esotropia. Am J Ophthalmol. 85:829. 1978.

37. Parks MM: Fornix incision forhorizontal rectus muscle surgery. Am J Ophthalmol. 65:907, 1968.

38. Parks, MM: The weakening surgical procedures for eliminating overaction of the inferior oblique muscle. Am J Ophthalmol. 73:107, 1972.

39. Parks, MM, and Helveston, EM: Direct visualization of the superior oblique tendon. Arch. Ophthalmol. 84:491, 1970.

40. Plager, D.A., and Parks, MM: Recognition and repair of the "lost" rectus muscle, Ophthalmology 97:131, 1990.

41. Repka, MX, and Ray, JM: The efficacy of optical and pharmacological penalization. Ophthalmology 100: 769, 1993.

42. Schlossman, A: Prognosis, management, and results of pleoptic treatment. Int. Ophthalmol. Clin. 1:829, 1961.

43. Scott, AB: Botulinum toxin injection into extraocular muscles as an alternative to strabismus surgery. Ophthalmology 87:1044, 1980.

44. Scott, AB: Botulinum toxin injection of the eye muscles to correct strabismus. Trans. Am Ophthalmol. Soc, 79:734, 1981.

45. Scott, AB, Rosenbaum, A, and Collins, CC: Pharmocologic weakening of extraocular muscles. Invest. Ophthalmol. vis. Sci. 12: 924, 1973.

46. Sharma, P, Arya, AV, and Prakash, P: Scleral dellen in strabismus surgery. Acta Ophthalmol. 68:493, 1990.

47. Snir, M, Nissenkorn, l, Buckman, G, Cohen, S, and Ben-Sira, l: Postoperative refractive changes in children with congenital esotropia: a preliminary study. Ophthalmic Surg. 20:57, 1989.

48. Thompson, WE, and Reinecke, RD: The changes in refractive status following routine strabismus surgery. J Pediatr. Ophthalmol. Strabismus 17:372, 1980.